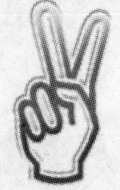

Objective

Biotechnology

for Competitive Examinations

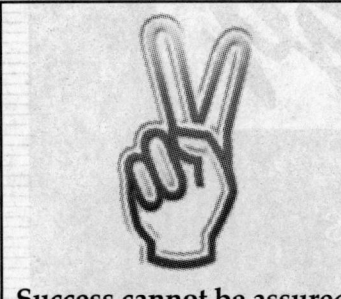

Success cannot be assured
It has to be attained

Objective
Biotechnology
for Competitive Examinations

Useful for

- ASRB, ARS-NET, ICAR-SRF, ICMR,CSIR-JRF and NET, NAARM DBT, IARI, NDRI, JNV, and all Entrance Examination for Admission to MSc and PhD Programmes
- UPSC Administrative Service (pre- and mains)
- State Public Services Commission (pre- and mains)
- Undergraduate and Postgraduate courses for all Indian Universities

RS Sengar PhD
Officer-in-Charge, Department of
Agriculture Biotechnology

Amit Kumar MSc, MPhil
College of Agriculture
Sardar Vallabhbhai Patel
University of Agriculture and Technology
Meerut

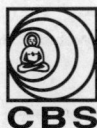

CBS Publishers & Distributors Pvt Ltd

New Delhi • Bengaluru • Chennai • Kochi • Mumbai • Pune
Hyderabad • Kolkata • Nagpur • Patna • Vijayawada

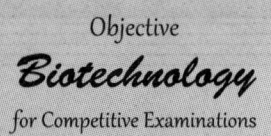

Objective
Biotechnology
for Competitive Examinations

ISBN: 978-81-239-2365-9

First Edition: 2014

Published by Satish Kumar Jain for

CBS Publishers & Distributors Pvt Ltd
4819/XI Prahlad Street, 24 Ansari Road, Daryaganj, New Delhi 110 002, India.

Ph: 23289259, 23266861, 23266867   Fax: 011-23243014   Website: www.cbspd.com
e-mail: delhi@cbspd.com; cbspubs@airtelmail.in

Corporate Office: 204 FIE, Industrial Area, Patparganj, Delhi 110 092
Ph: 4934 4934   Fax: 4934 4935   e-mail: publishing@cbspd.com; publicity@cbspd.com

Branches

- **Bengaluru:** Seema House 2975, 17th Cross, K.R. Road,
  Banasankari 2nd Stage, Bengaluru 560 070, Karnataka
  Ph: +91-80-26771678/79   Fax: +91-80-26771680   e-mail: bangalore@cbspd.com
- **Chennai:** 20, West Park Road, Shenoy Nagar, Chennai 600 030, Tamil Nadu
  Ph: +91-44-26260666, 26208620   Fax: +91-44-42032115   e-mail: chennai@cbspd.com
- **Kochi:** 36/14 Kalluvilakam, Lissie Hospital Road, Kochi 682 018, Kerala
  Ph: +91-484-4059061-65   Fax: +91-484-4059065   e-mail: kochi@cbspd.com
- **Mumbai:** 83-C, Dr E Moses Road, Worli, Mumbai-400018, Maharashtra
  Ph: +91-9833017933   e-mail: mumbai@cbspd.com
- **Pune:** Bhuruk Prestige, Sr. No. 52/12/2+1+3/2 Narhe, Haveli
  (Near Katraj-Dehu Road Bypass), Pune 411 041, Maharashtra
  Ph: +91-20-64704058, 64704059, 32392277 Fax: +91-20-24300160   e-mail: pune@cbspd.com

Representatives

- **Hyderabad** 0-9885175004
- **Nagpur** 0-9021734563
- **Kolkata** 0-9831437309, 0-9051152362
- **Patna** 0-9334159340
- **Vijayawada** 0-9000660880

Printed at India Binding House, Noida, UP

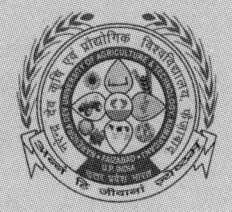

Dr RS Kureel
Vice-Chancellor
Narendra Deva University of
Agriculture and Technology
Kumarganj, Faizabad

Foreword

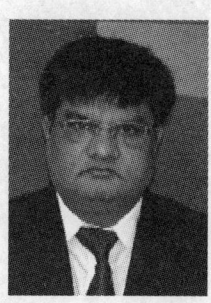

Two scientists are bringing out the first edition of its publication on question bank of biotechnology for the benefit of the faculty and students. This is a useful and innovative publication. The idea of bringing out such a publication has primarily been conceived as effective education and teaching. Set of questions with answers at a glance can solve many problems of students preparing for different competitive examinations and also for their undergraduate and postgraduate examinations. Setting the right questions in the form of cross-examination is a good method of teaching, which helps in quick learning and understanding the subject. Competitive examinations are the order of the day. All colleges conducting professional courses at postgraduate levels are admitting students based on common entrance examinations, which are of objective type.

I am happy to know that Dr RS Sengar, Associate Professor and Officer-in-Charge, and Amit Kumar, Department of Agriculture Biotechnology, Sardar Vallabhbhai Patel University of Agriculture and Technology, Meerut, and their colleagues are bringing out the book for the objective biotechnology for the help of undergraduate and postgraduate students in the field of biotechnology for developing their skills to perform better in competitive examinations. The subject matter covered in this book has been documented systematically and comprehensively. I believe that this book would be of immense use to the students of biotechnology appearing for various competitive examinations, i.e. JRF, SRF, ARS/NET, ASRB, SAUs, PCS civil services and other such competitive examinations.

The main purpose of this book is to bring together objective type questions on the subject matter to provide up-to-date information for better understanding of the readers. It would serve as a useful reference material for researchers, students and consultants. I hope this book would be of great help to all those concerned with the science or biotechnology. I do hope this book will help the faculty members to make their teaching effective and efficient. The book will also help the students to understand the subject of their studies in depth and provide them the necessary insight to prepare themselves for different competitive examinations and interviews for their career advancement.

I congratulate Dr RS Sengar and his young and energetic faculty colleagues for their sincere efforts and hard work in bringing out the first edition of objective biotechnology publication.

Dr RS Kureel
Vice-Chancellor

Preface

The book entitled *Objective Biotechnology* owes its foundation to the sincere and careful analysis of questions on biotechnology being asked in the examinations conducted by ASRB for ARS, SRF-JRF/NET, CATET/SAUs/UPSE, PCS, ICMR, CSIR-JRF and NET, NAARM, DBT, IARI, NDRI, JNU, PhD and various agricultural universities. The main objective of this book is to help the graduate and postgraduate students of agriculture/BTech (biotechnology) to quickly grasp the facts comprehensively. It is a collection and compilation work from various sources and has been endeavoured to include as much as information could be possible. It is realized that the coverage of material in this book is likely to be far from complete as the information available in biotechnology is immense. So you will find all types of questions at one place. Answers of all objective type questions are also provided which will make your life a bit easier. The question bank comprises more than 7,000 objective type questions with answers and eight model papers for practices and many of them have already been asked in the previous examinations of JRF-NET. The questions presented in this book are mostly memory-based which were asked in various examinations. These sets of questions will give the candidates an idea about the model questions and will help them to be focused. The main objective of this book is to help the readers to quickly grasp the facts comprehensively and systematically covering various branches of biotechnology. However, I should consider my efforts well rewarded only if this book serves the need of all concerned. Readers are welcomed to point out errors, if any, and send their valuable suggestions for improving the quality of the book.

We are highly thankful and obliged to Dr HS Gour, Vice-Chancellor of our Sardar Vallabhbhai Patel University of Agriculture and Technology, Meerut, for his persistent encouragement and valuable suggestions for the successful completion of the present manuscript. We have received generous help from many scientists, and senior and fellow teachers for the preparation of objective biotechnology book (Dr. Shivendra Vikram Sahi, Prof and Head, Department of Biotechnology, Ogden College of Science and Engineering, Western Kentucky University, Bowling Green Ky. 42101, USA). We will ever remain indebted to our respected teacher Prof VP Singh, Head and Dean, Department of Plant Science, MJP Rohilkhand University, Bareilly, for his invaluable and concrete suggestions in this connection.

Dr Anil Gupta, Professor and Head, Department of Molecular Biology and Biotechnology, College of Basic and Tech., Pantnagar; Prof Vinay Kumar Sharma and Gyan Singh Sikhawat, Department of Biosciences and Biotechnology, Banasthali University, Rajasthan; Prof RP Singh, Department of Biotechnology, IIT-Roorkee; Prof NS Sikhawat, Department of Biotechnology, JNV University, Jodhpur; Dr NK Singh and Dr TR Sharma, Principal Scientist, Biotechnology, National Research Center on Plant Biotechnology, New Delhi; Prof Akhilash Tyagi, Director, NIPGR, New Delhi; Rakesh Tuli, NABI, Mohali, Chandigarh; Prof BD Singh, BHU, Varanasi; Prof PK Gupta, CCS University, Meerut; Prof RL Singh, Dr RMLA University, Faizabad; Prof KN Singh and Dr RP Singh, ND University of Agriculture and Technology, Kumarganj, Faizabad; Dr Sundeep Kumar Sharma, NBPGR, New Delhi, Dr AK Sharma, Ramie Research Station (ICAR), Sorbhog, Barpeta, Assam; Reshu Chaudhary, Vivekanand Pratap Rao and Amit Kumar, Research Scholars, for their extraordinary help in shaping the *Objective Biotechnology* book. We are highly thankful to our colleagues and faculty members of College of Biotechnology and Department of Agriculture Biotechnology, SVPUA&T, Meerut, for extending valuable comments and help, directly and indirectly. It would rather be impossible to list all those who have provided encouragement and help in the preparation of this book. I am extremely thankful to all of them.

The first author will ever remain grateful to his reverend parents (Dr Sanwal Singh Sengar and Smt Kamala Sengar) who have kindly inspired him for this contribution. My wife Sarita and kids (Divyanshu and Kartikey) gave me persistent encouragement by their smiling faces to enable us to write the manuscript. As a First author I express my due gratitude to my younger brother (Dr Rajesh Singh Sengar), his better half (Smt Kalpana Sengar) and kids

(Saumay and Amranshu) for their affection, continuous help and cooperation during the preparation of the manuscript. We will not forget to keep on record the pains taken by Shri SK Jain, Managing Director, CBS Publishers & Distributors, New Delhi, for his encouragement and help in bringing out this publication in a presentable form.

I take this opportunity to express my sincere gratitude towards my mentor Late Prof HS Srivastava, who has always been a source of strength and moral support in all my endeavours especially in the field of life science. I hope this book will satisfy the needs of majority of academicians, scholars and students. Benediction of many dignitaries from ICAR Institutes, SAUs and IITs has led me to the completion of this herculean task well in time. In future I expect their same co-operation for quality improvement and wish I would serve the society at large in better way. I am indebted to everyone who is directly or indirectly involved in successful completion of this book. At the end, the potential of this question book lies in how you explore it. And right exploration is an indicator of the success of question bank. I am sure that you are the right person who will carve out the success story from this book.

RS Sengar

Contents

CSIR-UGC National Eligibility Test (NET) for Junior Research Fellowship and Lecturership

SYLLABUS FOR LIFE SCIENCES PAPER I AND PAPER II

1. *Molecules and their Interaction Relevant to Biology*

A. Structure of atoms, molecules and chemical bonds.

B. Composition, structure and function of biomolecules (carbohydrates, lipids, proteins, nucleic acids and vitamins).

C. Stablizing interactions (Van der Waals, electrostatic, hydrogen bonding, hydrophobic interaction, etc.).

D. Principles of biophysical chemistry (pH, buffer, reaction kinetics, thermodynamics, colligative properties).

E. Bioenergetics, glycolysis, oxidative phosphorylation, coupled reaction, group transfer, biological energy transducers.

F. Principles of catalysis, enzymes and enzyme kinetics, enzyme regulation, mechanism of enzyme catalysis, isozymes.

G. Conformation of proteins (Ramachandran plot, secondary, tertiary and quaternary structure; domains; motif and folds).

H. Conformation of nucleic acids (A-, B-, Z-,DNA), t-RNA, micro-RNA).

I. Stability of protein and nucleic acid structures.

J. Metabolism of carbohydrates, lipids, amino acids, nucleotides and vitamins.

2. *Cellular Organization*

A. **Membrane structure and function:** Structure of model membrane, lipid bilayer and membrane protein diffusion, osmosis, ion channels, active transport, ion pumps, mechanism of sorting and regulation of intracellular transport, electrical properties of membranes.

B. **Structural organization and function of intracellular organelles:** Cell wall, nucleus, mitochondria, Golgi bodies, lysosomes, endoplasmic reticulum, peroxisomes, plastids, vacuoles, chloroplast, structure & function of cytoskeleton and its role in motility.

C. **Organization of genes and chromosomes:** Operon, interrupted genes, gene families, structure of chromatin and chromosomes, unique and repetitive DNA, heterochromatin, euchromatin, transposons.

D. **Cell division and cell cycle:** Mitosis and meiosis, their regulation, steps in cell cycle, and control of cell cycle.

E. **Microbial Physiology:** Growth, yield and characteristics, strategies of cell division, stress response.

3. *Fundamental Process*

A. **DNA replication, repair and recombination:** Unit of replication, enzymes involved, replication origin and replication fork, fidelity of replication, extrachromosomal replicons, DNA damage and repair mechanisms.

B. **RNA synthesis and processing:** Transcription factors and machinery, formation of initiation complex, transcription activators and repressors, RNA polymerases, capping, elongation and termination, RNA processing, RNA editing, splicing, polyadenylation, structure and function of different types of RNA, RNA transport.

C. **Protein synthesis and processing:** Ribosome, formation of initiation complex, initiation factors and their regulation, elongation and elongation factors, termination, genetic code, aminoacylation of tRNA, tRNA-identity, aminoacyl tRNA synthetase, translational proof-reading, translational inhibitors, post- translational modification of proteins.

D. **Control of gene expression at transcription and translation level:** Regulation of phages, viruses, prokaryotic and eukaryotic gene expression, role of chromatin in regulating gene expression and gene silencing.

4. Cell Communication and Cell Signaling

A. **Host parasite interaction:** Recognition and entry processes of different pathogens like bacteria, viruses into animal and plant host cells, alteration of host cell behavior by pathogens, virus-induced cell transformation, pathogen-induced diseases in animals and plants, cell-cell fusion in both normal and abnormal cells.

B. **Cell signaling:** Hormones and their receptors, cell surface receptor, signaling through G-protein coupled receptors, signal transduction pathways, second messengers, regulation of signaling pathways, bacterial and plant two-component signaling systems, bacterial chemotaxis and quorum sensing.

C. **Cellular communication:** Regulation of hematopoiesis, general principles of cell communication, cell adhesion and roles of different adhesion molecules, gap junctions, extracellular matrix, integrins, neurotransmission and its regulation.

D. **Cancer:** Genetic rearrangements in progenitor cells, oncogenes, tumor suppressor genes, cancer and the cell cycle, virus-induced cancer, metastasis, interaction of cancer cells with normal

5. Developmental Biology

A. **Basic concepts of development:** Potency, commitment, specification, induction, competence, determination and differentiation; morphogenetic gradients; cell fate and cell lineages; stem cells; genomic equivalence and the cytoplasmic determinants; imprinting; mutants and transgenics in analysis of development.

B. **Gametogenesis, fertilization and early development:** Production of gametes, cell surface molecules in sperm-egg recognition in animals; embryo sac development and double fertilization in plants; zygote formation, cleavage, blastula formation, embryonic fields, gastrulation and formation of germ layers in animals; embryogenesis, establishment of symmetry in plants; seed formation and germination.

C. **Morphogenesis and organogenesis in animals:** Cell aggregation and differentiation in *Dictyostelium*; axes and pattern formation in *Drosophila*, amphibia and chick; organogenesis – vulva formation in *Caenorhabditis elegans*; eye lens induction, limb development and regeneration in vertebrates; differentiation of neurons, post embryonic development-larval formation, metamorphosis; environmental regulation of normal development; sex determination.

D. **Morphogenesis and organogenesis in plants:** Organization of shoot and root apical meristem; shoot and root development; leaf development and phyllotaxy; transition to flowering, floral meristems and floral development in *Arabidopsis* and *Antirrhinum.*

E. Programmed cell death, aging and senescence.

6. System Physiology-Plant

A. **Photosynthesis:** Light harvesting complexes; mechanisms of electron transport; photoprotective mechanisms; CO_2 fixation-C_3, C_4 and CAM pathways.

B. **Respiration and photorespiration:** Citric acid cycle; plant mitochondrial electron transport and ATP synthesis; alternate oxidase; photorespiratory pathway.

C. **Nitrogen metabolism:** Nitrate and ammonium assimilation; amino acid biosynthesis.

D. **Plant hormones:** Biosynthesis, storage, breakdown and transport; physiological effects and mechanisms of action.

E. **Sensory photobiology:** Structure, function and mechanisms of action of phytochromes, cryptochromes and phototropins; stomatal movement; photoperiodism and biological clocks.

F. **Solute transport and photoassimilate translocation:** Uptake, transport and translocation of water, ions, solutes and macromolecules from soil, through cells, across membranes, through xylem and phloem; transpiration; mechanisms of loading and unloading of photoassimilates.

G. **Secondary metabolites** - Biosynthesis of terpenes, phenols and nitrogenous compounds and their roles.

H. **Stress physiology:** Responses of plants to biotic (pathogen and insects) and abiotic (water, temperature and salt) stresses; mechanisms of resistance to biotic stress and tolerance to abiotic stress

7. System Physiology-Animal

A. **Blood and circulation:** Blood corpuscles, haemopoiesis and formed elements, plasma function, blood volume, blood volume regulation, blood groups, haemoglobin, immunity, haemostasis.

B. **Cardiovascular System:** Comparative anatomy of heart structure, myogenic heart, specialized tissue, ECG – its principle and significance, cardiac cycle, heart as a pump, blood pressure, neural and chemical regulation of all above.

C. **Respiratory system:** comparison of respiration in different species, anatomical consideration, transport of gases, exchanges of gases, waste elimination, neural and chemical regulation of respiration.

D. **Nervous system**: Neurons, action potential, gross neuroanatomy of the brain and spial cord, central and peripheral nervous system, neural control of muscle tone and posture.

E. **Excretory system**: Comparative physiology of excretion, kidney, urine formation, urine concentration, waste elimination, micturition, regulation of water balance, blood volume, blood pressure, electrolyte balance, acid-base balance.

F. **Sense Organ**: Vision, hearing and tactile response

G. **Stress and adaptation**

I. **Digestive system**: Digestion, absorption, energy balance, BMR.

J. **Endocrinology and reproduction**: Endocrine glands, basic mechanism of hormone action, hormones and diseases; reproductive processes, neuroendocrine regulation.

8. Inheritance Biology

A. **Mendelian principles**: Dominance, segregation, independent assortment, deviation from Mendelian inheritance.

B. **Concept of gene**: Allele, multiple alleles, pseudoallele, complementation tests.

C. **Extensions of Mendelian principles**: Codominance, incomplete dominance, gene interactions, pleiotropy, genomic imprinting, penetrance and expressivity, phenocopy, linkage and crossing over, sex linkage, sex limited and sex influenced characters.

D. **Gene mapping methods**: Linkage maps, tetrad analysis, mapping with molecular markers, mapping by using somatic cell hybrids, development of mapping population in plants.

E. **Extra chromosomal inheritance**: Inheritance of mitochondrial and chloroplast genes, maternal inheritance.

F. **Microbial genetics**: Methods of genetic transfers – transformation, conjugation, transduction and sex-duction, mapping genes by interrupted mating, fine structure analysis of genes.

G. **Human genetics**: Pedigree analysis, lod score for linkage testing, karyotypes, genetic disorders.

H. **Quantitative genetics**: Polygenic inheritance, heritability and its measurements, QTL mapping.

I. **Mutation**: Types, causes and detection, mutant types – lethal, conditional, biochemical, loss of function, gain of function, germinal verses somatic mutants, insertional mutagenesis.

J. **Structural and numerical alterations of chromosomes**: Deletion, duplication, inversion, translocation, ploidy and their genetic implications.

K. **Recombination**: Homologous and non-homologous recombination, including transposition, site-specific recombination.

9. Diversity of Life Forms

A. **Principles and methods of taxonomy:**Concepts of species and hierarchical taxa, biological nomenclature, classical and quantititative methods of taxonomy of plants, animals and microorganisms.

B. **Levels of structural organization**: Unicellular, colonial and multicellular forms; levels of organization of tissues, organs and systems; comparative anatomy.

C. **Outline classification of plants, animals and microorganisms:**Important criteria used for classification in each taxon; classification of plants, animals and microorganisms; evolutionary relationships among taxa.

D. **Natural history of Indian subcontinent**: Major habitat types of the subcontinent, geographic origins and migrations of species; common Indian mammals, birds; seasonality and phenology of the subcontinent.

E. **Organisms of health and agricultural importance**: Common parasites and pathogens of humans, domestic animals and crops.

10. Ecological Principles

A. **The Environment**: Physical environment; biotic environment; biotic and abiotic interactions.

B. **Habitat and niche**: Concept of habitat and niche; niche width and overlap; fundamental and realized niche; resource partitioning; character displacement.

C. **Population ecology**: Characteristics of a population; population growth curves; population regulation; life history strategies (*r* and *K* selection); concept of metapopulation – demes and dispersal, interdemic extinctions, age structured populations.

D. **Species interactions**: Types of interactions, interspecific competition, herbivory, carnivory, pollination, symbiosis.

E. **Community ecology**: Nature of communities; community structure and attributes; levels of species diversity and its measurement; edges and ecotones.

F. **Ecological succession:** Types; mechanisms; changes involved in succession; concept of climax.

G. **Ecosystem:** Structure and function; energy flow and mineral cycling (CNP); primary production and decomposition; structure and function of some Indian ecosystems: terrestrial (forest, grassland) and aquatic (fresh water, marine, eustarine).

H. **Biogeography:** Major terrestrial biomes; theory of island biogeography; biogeographical zones of India.

I. **Applied ecology:** Environmental pollution; global environmental change; biodiversity-status, monitoring and documentation; major drivers of biodiversity change; biodiversity management approaches.

J. **Conservation biology:** Principles of conservation, major approaches to management, Indian case studies on conservation/management strategy (Project Tiger, Biosphere reserves).

11. Evolution and Behaviour

A. **Emergence of evolutionary thoughts:** Lamarck; Darwin–concepts of variation, adaptation, struggle, fitness and natural selection; Mendelism; spontaneity of mutations; the evolutionary synthesis.

B. **Origin of cells and unicellular evolution:** Origin of basic biological molecules; abiotic synthesis of organic monomers and polymers; concept of Oparin and Haldane; experiment of Miller (1953); the first cell; evolution of prokaryotes; origin of eukaryotic cells; evolution of unicellular eukaryotes; anaerobic metabolism, photosynthesis and aerobic metabolism.

C. **Paleontology and evolutionary history:** The evolutionary time scale; eras, periods and epoch; major events in the evolutionary time scale; origins of unicellular and multicellular organisms; major groups of plants and animals; stages in primate evolution including Homo. D. Molecular Evolution: concepts of neutral evolution, molecular divergence and molecular clocks; molecular tools in phylogeny, classification and identification; protein and nucleotide sequence analysis; origin of new genes and proteins; gene duplication and divergence.

D. **The Mechanisms:** Population genetics – populations, gene pool, gene frequency; Hardy-Weinberg law; concepts and rate of change in gene frequency through natural selection, migration and random genetic drift; adaptive radiation and modifications; isolating mechanisms; speciation; allopatricity and sympatricity; convergent evolution; sexual selection; co-evolution.

E. **Brain, Behavior and Evolution:** Approaches and methods in study of behavior; proximate and ultimate causation; altruism and evolution-group selection, kin selection, reciprocal altruism; neural basis of learning, memory, cognition, sleep and arousal; biological clocks; development of behavior; social communication; social dominance; use of space and territoriality; mating systems, parental investment and reproductive success; parental care; aggressive behavior; habitat selection and optimality in foraging; migration, orientation and navigation; domestication and behavioral changes.

12. Applied Biology

A. Microbial fermentation and production of small and macro molecules.

B. Application of immunological principles (vaccines, diagnostics). tissue and cell culture methods for plants and animals.

C. Transgenic animals and plants, molecular approaches to diagnosis and strain identification.

D. Genomics and its application to health and agriculture, including gene therapy.

E. Bioresource and uses of biodiversity.

F. Breeding in plants and animals, including marker – assisted selection.

G. Bioremediation and phytoremediation.

H. Biosensors.

13. Methods in Biology

A. **Molecular biology and recombinant DNA methods:** Isolation and purification of RNA , DNA (genomic and plasmid) and proteins, different separation methods; analysis of RNA, DNA and proteins by one and two dimensional gel electrophoresis, isoelectric focusing gels; molecular cloning of DNA or RNA fragments in bacterial and eukaryotic systems; expression of recombinant proteins using bacterial, animal and plant vectors; isolation of specific nucleic acid sequences; generation of genomic and cDNA libraries in plasmid, phage, cosmid, BAC and YAC vectors; in vitro mutagenesis and deletion techniques, gene knock out in bacterial and eukaryotic organisms; protein sequencing methods, detection of post-translation modification of proteins; DNA sequencing methods, strategies for genome sequencing; methods for analysis of gene expression at RNA and protein level, large scale expression analysis, such as micro array based techniques; isolation, separation and analysis of carbohydrate and lipid molecules; RFLP, RAPD and AFLP techniques

B. **Histochemical and immunotechniques:** Antibody generation, detection of molecules using ELISA, RIA, western blot, immunoprecipitation, floweytometry and immunofluorescence microscopy, detection of molecules in living cells, *in situ* localization by techniques such as FISH and GISH.

C. **Biophysical methods:** Analysis of biomolecules using UV/visible, fluorescence, circular dichroism, NMR and ESR spectroscopy, structure determination using X-ray diffraction and NMR; analysis using light scattering, different types of mass spectrometry and surface plasma resonance methods.

D. **Statistical Methods:** Measures of central tendency and dispersal; probability distributions (Binomial, Poisson and normal); sampling distribution; difference between parametric and non-parametric statistics; confidence interval; errors; levels of significance; regression and correlation; t-test; analysis of variance; X^2 test; basic introduction to Muetrovariate statistics, etc.

E. **Radiolabeling techniques:** Properties of different types of radioisotopes normally used in biology, their detection and measurement; incorporation of radioisotopes in biological tissues and cells, molecular imaging of radioactive material, safety guidelines.

F. **Microscopic techniques:** Visulization of cells and subcellular components by light microscopy, resolving powers of different microscopes, microscopy of living cells, scanning and transmission microscopes, different fixation and staining techniques for EM, freeze-etch and freeze-fracture methods for EM, image processing methods in microscopy.

G. **Electrophysiological methods:** Single neuron recording, patch-clamp recording, ECG, Brain activity recording, lesion and stimulation of brain, pharmacological testing, PET, MRI, fMRI, CAT

H. **Methods in Field Biology:** Methods of estimating population density of animals and plants, ranging patterns through direct, indirect and remote observations, sampling methods in the study of behavior, habitat characterization-ground and remote sensing methods.

I. **Computational methods:** Nucleic acid and protein sequence databases; data mining methods for sequence analysis, web-based tools for sequence searches, motif analysis and presentation.

Syllabus for Agricultural Biotechnology in ICAR–NET Examination

Unit 1: Cell Structure and Function

Prokaryotic and eukaryotic cell architecture, Cell wall, plasma membrane, Structure and function of cell organelles: vacuoles, mitochondria, plastids, golgi apparatus, ER, peroxisomes, glyoxisomes. Cell division, regulation of cell cycle, Protein secretion and targeting, Cell division, growth and differentiation.

Unit 2: Biomolecules and Metabolism

Structure and function of carbohydrates, lipids, proteins and nucleic acids, Synthesis of carbohydrate, glycolysis, HMP, Citric acid cycle and metabolic regulation, Oxidative phosphorylation and substrate level phosphorylation, Vitamins, plant and animal hormones. Functional molecules, antioxidants, nutrient precursor, HSPs, anti-viral compounds.

Unit 3: Enzymology

Enzymes, structure conformation, classification, assay, isolation, purification and characterization, catariysis specificity, mechanism of action, active site, regulation of enzyme activity, multienzyme complexes, immobilized enzymes and protein engineering, immobilized enzymes and their application.

Unit 4: Molecular Genetics

Concept of gene, Prokaryotes as genetic system, Prokaryotic and eukaryotic chromosomes, methods of gene isolation and identification, Split genes, overlapping genes and pseudo genes, Organization of prokaryotic and eukaryotic genes and genomes including operan, exon, intron, enhancer promoter sequences and other regulatory elements. Mutation – spontaneous, induced and site-directed, recombination in bacteria, fungi and viruses, transformation, transduction, conjugation, transposable elements and transposition.

Unit 5: Gene Expression

Expression of genetic information, operon concept, Transcription – mechanism of transcription in prokaryotes and eukaryotes, transcription unit, regulatory sequences and enhancers, activators, repressors, co-activators, Co-repressors in prokaryotes and eukaryotes, inducible genes and promoters, Transcription factors post transcriptional modification and protein transport, DNA-protein interaction, Genetic code. Mechanism of translation and its control, post translational modifications.

Unit 6: Molecular Biology Techniques

Isolation and purification of nucleic acids. Nucleic acids hybridization: Southern, northern and western blotting hybridization. Immune response monoclonal and polyclonal antibodies and ELISA, DNA sequencing. Construction and screening of genomic and C-DNA libraries. Gel electrophoretic techniques. Polymerase chain reactor spectroscopy, rtPCR ultracentrifugation, chromatography, FISH, RIA etc.

Unit 7: Gene Cloning

Restriction enzymes and their uses. Salient features and uses of most commonly used vectors i.e. plasmids, bacteriophages, phagmids, cosmids, BACs, PACs and YACs, binary vectors, expression vectors. Gene cloning and sub-cloning strategies, chromosome walking, genetic transformation, Basis of animal cloning. Biology. Risk assessment and IPR.

Unit 8: Molecular Biology

Ribosome structure and function. Protein biosynthesis in prokaryotes and ekaryotes. Post-translational modification. Gene regulation, RNA processing and Post transcriptional modifications. Bioprospecting, biofortification, gene pryrimiding and gene fusion, nbozyme technology.

Unit 9: Plant Molecular Biology

Photoregulation and phytochrome regulation of nuclear and chloroplastic gene expression. Molecular mechanism of nitrogen fixation. Molecular biology of various stresses, *viz.* abiotic stresses like drought, salt, heavy metals and temperature; and biotic stresses like bacterial, fungal and viral diseases. Signal transduction and its molecular basis, molecular mechanism of plant hormone action mitochondrial control of fertility, structure, organization and regulation of nuclear gene concerning storage proteins and starch synthesis.

Unit 10: Tissue Culture

Basic techniques in cell culture and somatic cell genetics. Regulation of cell cycle and cell division.. Clonal propagation. Concept of cellular totipotency. Anther culture, somaclonal and gametoclonal variations. Hybrid embryo culture and embryo rescue, somatic hybridization and cybridization. Application of tissue culture in crop improvement. Secondary metabolite production. *In vitro*, mutagenesis, cryopreservation and plant tissue culture repository.

Unit 11: Plant Genetic Engineering

Isolation of genes of economic importance. Gene constructs for tissue-specific expression. Different methods of gene transfer to plants, *viz.* direct and vectormediated. Molecular analysis of transformants. Potential applications of plant genetic engineering for crop improvement, i.e. insect-pest resistance (insect, viral, fungal and bacterial disease resistance), abiotic stress resistance, herbicide resistance, storage protein quality, increasing shelf-life, oil quality, Current status of transgenics, biosafty norms and controlled field trials and release of transgenics (GMOs).

Unit 12: Molecular Markers and Genomics

DNA molecular markers: Principles, type and applications; restriction fragment length polymorphism (RFLP), amplified fragment length polymorphism (AFLP), randomly amplified polymorphic DNA sequences (RAPD), Simple sequence repeats (SSR), Single nucleotide polymorphism (SNP), Structural and functional genomics, gene mapping, genome mapping, gene tagging and comparative genomics and application of genomics.

Syllabus for ICAR's All India Entrance Examination for Admission to Pg Degree Programmes and ICAR–JRF (Pgs)

Biotechnology (Agriculture Science)

Section 1: Cell Structure and Function

Ultrastructure of prokaryotic and eukaryotic cells. Cyloskelton. Cell wall and plasma membrane. Cell organelles including vacuoles, plastids, galgi apparatus, ER, peroxisomes, glyoxisomes, etc., their organization and function. Cell division. Different stages of mitosis and meiosis.

Section 2: Biomolecules and Metabolism

Structure, characterization and functions of carbohydrates, lipids, proteins and nucleic acids, isolation and purification of enzymes, their classification, catalytic ste, mechanism of action, regulation of enzyme activity, basic enzyme kinetics, inhibition, immobilized enzymes and their application, Catabolism, syntheses of carbohydrate, glycolysis, HMP, citric acid cycle, purine and pyrimidine biosynthesis, metabolic regulation, bioenergetics, etc. Oxidative phosphorylation and substrate level phosphorylation.

Section 3: Molecular Genetics

Concept of gene mutation, recombination, transformation, transduction, conjugation and transpositon. Organisation of prokaryotic and eukaryotic genes and genomes including operon, exon intron, enhance sequences and other regulatory elements in prokaryotes and eukaryotes.

Section 4: Gene Expression

Replication, transcription and transposition of genetic material prokaryotes and eukaryots. RNA processing and posttranscriptional modifications, post-translational modification and their significance. DNA modification and repair mechanism. Function of mitochondrial and chloroplast genome.

Section 5: Biophysical

Photoregulation and phytochrome regulation of nuclear and chloroplastic gene expression. Molecular biology of light and dark reaction of photosynthesis. Molecular mechanism of nitrogen fixation, nitrate reductase, and genetics of nif genes. Molecular biology of various stresses. viz. drought, salt, heat and cold. Signal transduction.

Section 6: Molecular Biology Techniques

Isolation and hybridization of nucleic acids. Cot analysis, southern, northern and western blottings and hybridization. Construction and screening of genomic and DNA libraries. Current methods of radioactive and nonradioactive labelling of proteins and nucleic acids. DNA sequencing. Restriction fragment length polymorphism (RFLP), randomly amplified polymorphic DNA sequences (RAPD), gene mapping, genome mapping, gene tagging and targetting, polymerase chain reaction (PCR). DNA synthesis, monoclonal and polyclonal antibodies, ribozyme, antisense RNA methodology, radioimmune assay, enzymelinked immunosorbent assay (ELISA).

Section 7: Gene Cloning

Restriction enzymes. Salient features and uses of most commonly used vectors i.e., plasmids, bacteriophages, phagmids and cosmids: expression vectors. Cloning, sub-cloning strategies and transformation. Plant genetic vectors.

Section 8: Tissue Culture

Basic technizues in cell culture and somatic cell genetics. Clonal propagation. Concept of cellular totiopotency. Anther and pollen culture for haploid and double haploid production; somatoclonal and gametoclonal variations. Hybrid embryo culture, somatic hybridization and hybridization. Gemplasm conservation and exchange. Plant bioreactors and production of industrial compounds. Application of tissue culture in crop improvement.

Section 9: Plant Genetic Engineering

Isolation of genes of interest. Gene constructs for tissue specific expression. Different methods of gene transfer to plants viz. direct and vector mediated. Potential applications to crop improvement through plant genetic engineering, i.e. specific and non-specific resistance (defence) genes to disease, pest and herbicide resistance. Storage protein quality, stress resistance and post-harvest, production of secondary metabolites and alien proteins. Current status of transgenics.

Section 10: Fermentation Technology

Principles of fermentation processes, bioreactors and biosensors. Protein engineering. Single cell proteins

Syllabus for Environmental Science in UGC–NET

Unit 1 Introduction

Definition, principles and scope of Environmental Science

    Earth, Man and Environment, Ecosystems, pathways in Ecosystem

    Physic-chemical and Biological factors in the environment

    Geographical classification and zones

    Structure and composition of atmospheres, hydrosphere, lithosphere, Mass and energy transfer across the variation interfaces, material balance, First and Second law of thermodynamics, heat transfer processes. Scale of meteorology, pressure, tempreture, precipitation, humidity, radiation and wind.

    Atmospheric stability, inversions and mixing heights, windroses

Natural resources, conservation and sustainable development

Unit 2 Environmental Chemistry

FUNDAMENTALS of Environmental chemistry: Stochiometry, Gibbs' free energy, chemical potential, chemical equilibria, acid-base reaction, solubility products, solubility of gases in water, the carbonates system, unsaturated and saturated hydrocarbons, radionuclides.

    Chemical Compostion of Air: Classification of elements, chemical speciation. Particles, ions and radicles in the atmosphere. Chemical processes for formation of inorganic and organic particulate matter. Thermochemical and photochemical reaction in the atmosphere. Oxygen and ozone chemistry. Chemistry of air pollutants, photochemical smog.

    Water Chemistry: Chemistry of water, concept of DO, BOD, COD, sedimentation, coagulation, filtration and redox potential

    Soil chemistry: Inorganic and organic components of soil, Nitrogen pathways and NPK in soils, toxic chemicals in the Environment- air, water: Pesticides in water. Biochemical aspects of arsenic, cadmium, lead, mercury, carbon monoxide, O3 and PAN pesticides, insecticides, MIC, carcinogens in the air

    Principles of Analytical Methods: Titrimetry, Gravimetry, Colourimetry, Spectrophotometry, Chromatography, Gas Chromatography, Atomic absorption Spectrophotometry, GLC, HLC, Electrohoresis, X-rays fluorescence, X-ray diffraction, flame photometry

Unit 3 Ecology and Environment

Definition, principles and scope of ecology, human ecology and human settlement, evolutions, origin of life and speciation

    Ecosystems: structure and functions, abiotic and biotic components, energy flows, food chains, food web, ecological pyramids, types and diversity

    Ecological succession, population, community ecology and parasitism, prey-predator relationship common flora and fauna in India-Aquatic: phytoplankton, zooplankton and macrophytes; terrestrial Forest' Endangered and threatened species

    Biodiversity and its conservation: Definition, 'Hotspots' of biodiversity, strategies for biodiversity conservation, National parks and sanctuaries, Gene pool

    Microflora of Atmosphere: Air sampling techniques; identification of aeroallergens: air borne disease and allergies

Environmental Biotechnology: fermentation technology, vermiculture technology, biofertilizer technology

Unit 4 Environmental Geosciences

Environmental Geosciences-Fundamental concept.

The earth systems and Biosphere: Conservation of matter in various geospheres-Lithosphere hydrospheres, atmosphere and biosphere. Energy budget of the earth. Earth's thermal environment and seasons. Ecosystems flow of energy and matter. Co existence in communities-food webs. Earth's major ecosystem- terrestrial and aquatic. General relationship between landscape, biomes and climate. Climates of India , Indian Monsoon, EI Nino, droughts, tropical cyclones and western Disturbances

Earth's processes and Geological Hazards: Earth's processes: concept of residence, time and rates of natural cycles, catastrophic geological hazards. Study of floods, landslides, earthquakes, volcanism and avalanche. Predictin and perception of the hazards and adjustments to hazardous activities.

Mineral Resources and Environment: Resources and reserves, minerals and population. Oceans as new area for exploration of mineral resoureces, ocean ore and recycling of resources. Environmental impact of exploitation, precessing and smelting of minerals

Water resources and Environment: Global water balance. Ice sheets and fluctuations of sea levels Origin and compositin of sea water. Hydrological cycle. Factors influencing the surfaces water.

Types of water. Resources of oceans .Ocean pollution by toxic wastes. Human use of surface and groundwaters. Groundwater pollution

Land use planning. The land use plan. Soil sryeys in relation to land use planning. Methods of site selection and evaluation

Environmental Geochemistry: Concept of major, trace and REE. Classification of trace elements mobility of trace elements, Geochemical cycles, biogeochemials factors in environmental health. Human use, trace elements and health. Possible effects of imbalance of some trace elements. Diseases induced by human use of land

Principles of remote sensing and its application in Environmental Sciences, Application of GIS in Environmental managements.

Unit 5 Sources of Energy

Sun as source of energy: Solar radiation and its spectral characteristics; fossil fuels- Classification composition, physic-chemical characteristics and energy content of coal, petroleum and natural gas principles of generation of hydroelectric power, tidal ocean thermal energy conversion, wind, geothermal genergy, solar coliectors, photovoltaics, solar ponds; nuclear energy-fission and fusion;magnetohydrodynamic power, bioenergy-energy from biomass and biogas, anaerobic digestion, energy use pattern in different parts of the world

Environmental implication of energy use: CO_2 emissions, global warming: air and thermal pollution; radioactive waste and radioactivity from nuclear reactors; impacts of large-scale exploitation of solar, wind, hydro and ocean energy

Unit 6 Sources of Pollution

Air: natural and anthropogenic sources of pollution. Primary and secondary pollutant. Transport and diffusion of pollutants. Gas laws governing the behaviour of pollutants in the atmosphere. Methods of monitoring and control of air pollution SO_2, NOx, Co, SPM. Efects of pollutants on human beings, plants, animals, materials and on climate, Acid rain. Air quality standards

Water: Types, sources and consequences of water pollution. Physic-chemical and bacteriological sampling and analysis of water quality standards, seqage and waste water treatment and recycling. Water quality standard

Soil: Physic-chemical and bacteriological sampling as analysis of soil quality. Soil pollution control. Industrial waste effluents and heavy metals, their interactins with soil components. Soil micro-organisms and their function. Degradation of different insecticides, fungicides and weedicides in soil. Different kind of synthetic fertilizers and their interactions with different components of soil.

Noise: Sources of noise pollution, measurement of noise and indices, effect of meterological parameters on noise propagation. Noise exposure levels and standards, noise control and abatement measure.. impact of noise on human health

Mairine: Source of marine pollution and control, Criteria employed for disposal of pollutants in Radioactive and thermal pollution.

Unit 7 Environmental Impact Analysis

Introduction to environmental impact analysis

Environmental impact statement and environmental management plan

EIA guidelines 1994, notification of Government of India

Impact assessment methodologies

Generalized approach to impact analysis

Procedure for reviewing environmental impact analysis and statement

Guidelines for environmental audit

Introduction to environmental planning

Base ling information and prediction

Restoration and rehabilitation technology

Landuse policy for india

Urban planning for india

Rural planning and landuse pattern

Concept and strategies of sustainable development

Cost benefit analysis

Environmental priorities in India and sustainable development

Unit 8 Solid Wastes Managements

Sources and generation of solid wastes, their characterization, chemical composition and classification. Different methods of disposal and management of solid wastes. Recycling of wastes material. Waste minimization technologies

Hazardous wastes management and handling rules, 1989, Resource management, disaster management and risk analysis

Environment protectin-issures and problems, International and national efforts for environment protection, provision of constitution of India regarding environment (Article 48 A and 58A)

Environmental policy resolution, Legislation, Public policy strategies in pollution control, wildlife protection Act, 1972 amended 1991, Forest Conservation Act, 1980, Indian Forests Act (Revised)1982, Air (Prevention and control of pollution) Act, 1981 as amended by Amendment Act, 1987 and Rule 1982, Motor Vehicle Act, 1988, the water (prevention and control of pollution Act, 1974 as amended up to 1988 and Rules 1975. The environment (Protection) Act, 1986 and Rule 1986 scheme of labelling of environmentally friendly products, public liability Insurance Act, 1991 and Rule 1991

Unit 9 Statistical Analysis in Environmental Studies

Basic elements and tools of statistical analysis; probability, ampling, measurement and distribution of attributes; Distribution- normal, t and ÷, postion and binomial, arithmetic, geometric and harmonic means, moments, matrices, simultaneous linear equations; tests of hypothesis and significance

Introduction to environmental system analysis; approaches to development of models; linear simple and multiple regression models, validation and forecasting. Models of population growth and interactions- Lotka-Volterra model, Leslie's matrix model, point source stream pollution model, box model, Gaussian plume model

Unit 10 Environmental Education and Awareness

Environmental Education and Awareness

Environmental ethics and global imperatives

Global environmental problems-ozone depletion, global warming and climatic change

Current environmental issues in India; context: Narmada Dam, Tehri Dam, Almetti Dam, soil erosion, formation and reclamation pf Usar, alkaline and saline soil

Waste lands and their reclamation

Desertification and its control

Vehicular pollution and urban air quality

Depletion of natural resource

Biodiversity conservation and Agenda 21

Waste disposal, recycling and power generation, fly ash utilization

Water crises-conservation of water

Environmental hazards

Eutrophication and restoration of Indian Lakes

Rain water harvesting

Wet land conservation

Epidemiological issues (e.g. Goitre, Fluorosis, Arsenic).

Objective

Biotechnology

for Competitive Examinations

UNIT 1

UNIT 1

1

Cell Structure and Function

1. First successful tissue culture was that of

a. Tomato root   b. Carrot root
c. Potato stem   d. Tobacco callus

Ans. (a) Tomato root

2. Tissue-used by Steward et al (1957) to prove cellular totipotency was

a. Pith of root   b. Pith of stem
c. Phloem of root   d. Phloem of stem

Ans. (c) Phloem of root

3. White performed successful tissue culture in

a. 1939   b. 1932
c. 1929   d. 1922

Ans. (b) 1932

4. The smallest animal egg is that of

a. Ostrich   b. Human female
c. Duck   d. Hen

Ans. (b) Human female

5. Largest animal cell is that of

a. Ostrich   b. Duck
c. Human   d. Hen

Ans. (a) Ostrich

6. Human egg is larger than human sperm because it has

a. Larger nucleus   b. More membranes
c. More cytoplasm   d. All of the above

Ans. (c) More cytoplasm

7. Larger sized organisms usually have

a. Large sized cells
b. More noncellular material
c. Higher number of cells
d. More cellular excretions

Ans. (c) Higher number of cells

8. Large cells have

a. High metabolic rate
b. High respiration rate
c. Low surface: volume ratio
d. High surface: volume ratio

Ans. (c) Low surface: volume ratio

9. Metabolically activity cells have

a. Lower nucleocytoplasmic ratio
b. Higher nucleocytoplasmic ratio
c. Higher surface: volume ratio
d. Both B and C

Ans. (d) Both B and C

10. Alga *Acetabularia* is

a. Unicellular prokaryote
b. Multicellular prokaryote
c. Unicellular eukaryote
d. Multicellular eukaryote

Ans. (c) Unicellular eukaryote

11. Size of *Acetabularia* is

a. 10 cm   b. 10 mm
c. 1.0 mm   d. 0.1 mm

Ans. (a) 10 cm

12. Largest cell of the human body is

a. Voluntary muscle fibre cell
b. Nerve cell
c. Striated muscle fibre cell
d. Cardiac muscle fibre cell

Ans. (b) Nerve cell

13. Average size of human body cells is

a. 5–10 μm
b. 10–15 μm
c. 20–30 μm
d. 70–80 μm

Ans. (c) 20–30 μm

14. Large plant cells are

    a. Xylem vessel cells   b. Parenchyma cells

    c. Sieve tube cells   d. Sclerenchyma fibres

Ans. (d) Sclerenchyma fibres

15. Jute fibres have a length of

    a. 30–40 mm   b. 300–400 mm

    c. 30–90 cm   d. 3–9 m

Ans. (c) 30–90 cm

16. Human egg has a volume larger than human sperm by time

    a. 100,000   b. 10,000

    c. 1000   d. 100

Ans. (a) 100,000

17. Efficient large sized cells should be

    a. Elongated

    b. Branched

    c. With membrane extensions

    d. Any of the above

Ans. (d) Any of the above

18. The term protoplasm was coined by

    a. Corti   b. Dujardin

    c. Purkinje   d. Dutrochet

Ans. (c) Purkinje

19. Purkinje coined the term protoplasm in

    a. 1739   b. 1839

    c. 1779   d. 1879

Ans. (b) 1839

20. A cilium beats

    a. Asymmetrically by sweeping action

    b. Symmetrically by sweeping action

    c. Symmetrically by undulatory action

    d. Asymmetrically by undulatory action

Ans. (a) Asymmetrically by sweeping action

21. Cell theory was put forward by

    a. Schleiden and Schwann   b. Sutton and Boveri

    c. Watson and Crick   d. Darwin and Wallace

Ans. (a) Schleiden and Schwann

22. The term cell was coined by or the cell was first seen by

    a. Robert hooke   b. Leeuwenhoek

    c. Schleiden and Schwann   d. Altmann and Kolliker

Ans. (a) Robert hooke

23. Figures of cork cells observed by Robert Hooke were published in

    a. Genera plantarum   b. Species plantarum

    c. Origin of species   d. Micrographia

Ans. (d) Micrographia

24. The cells discovered in thin sections of cork by Robert hooke were actually

    a. Cell walls   b. Cellulose

    c. Protoplasm   d. Nuclei

Ans. (a) Cell walls

25. Nucleus was discovered by

    a. Robert brown   b. Leeuwenhoek

    c. Robert hooke   d. Schleiden and Schwann

Ans. (a) Robert brown

26. Smaller cell is

    a. Less active metabolically

    b. With smaller nucleus

    c. With larger nucleus

    d. More active metabolically

Ans. (d) More active metabolically

27. Credit for establishing nucleus as biological entity goes to

    a. Leeuwen hoek   b. Schwann

    c. Koch   d. Robert brown

Ans. (d) Robert brown

28. Names of Schleiden and Schwann are associated with

    a. Protoplasm as the physical basis of life

    b. Cell theory

    c. Theory of cell lineage

    d. Nucleus functions as control centre of cell

Ans. (b) Cell theory

29. Which is correct about cell theory in view of current status of our knowledge about cell structure

    a. It needs modification due to discovery of subcellular structures like chloroplasts and mitochondria

    b. Modified cell theory means that all living beings are composed of cells capable of reproducing

    c. Cell theory does not hold good because all living beings (e.g, viruse) do not have cellular organization

    d. Cell theory means that all living objects consist of cells whether or not capable of reproducing

Ans. (c) Cell theory does not hold good because all living beings (e.g. viruse) do not have cellular organization

30. Minimum cell size seen under light microscope is

a. 1 μm b. 0.1 μm
c. 0.25 μm d. 0.5 μm

Ans. (c) 0.25 μm

31. An exception to cell theory is

a. Mycoplasma b. Virus
c. Protistans d. Algae

Ans. (b) Virus

32. Cellular totipotency means

a. Synthesis of new cells
b. Formation of new species
c. Formation of new plants
d. Capability of a plant cell to form complete plant

Ans. (d) Capability of a plant cell to form complete plant

33. Who proposed cell lineage/cell always arises from pre-existing cell?

a. Lamarck b. Virchow
c. Schwann d. Darwin

Ans. (b) Virchow

34. The suffix s in ribosome unit indicates

a. Sedimentation coefficient
b. Solubility
c. Surface area
d. Size

Ans. (a) Sedimentation coefficient

35. Letter S in the structural unit of ribosome denotes

a. Concentration unit b. Svedberg unit
c. Polymerization unit d. Stability unit

Ans. (b) Svedberg unit

36. Who proposed that cell is a unit of life and that a tissue is made of cells?

a. Schleiden b. Schwann
c. Dutrochet d. Steward

Ans. (b) Schwann

37. Longest cells in human body are

a. Nerve cells b. Bone cells
c. Leg muscle cells d. Heart muscle cells

Ans. (a) Nerve cells

38. A plant cell has potential to develop into full plant. The property is called

a. Tissue culture
b. Pleuripotency

c. Totipotency
d. Gene cloning

Ans. (c) Totipotency

39. Protoplasm forms percentage of total weight of the body

a. 45% b. 70%
c. 95% d. 15%

Ans. (c) 95%

40. According to cell theory

a. Cells are fundamental structural units of organisms
b. Cells reproduce
c. Cells are living
d. Cells have nuclei

Ans. (a) Cells are fundamental structural units of organisms

41. Protoplasm is

a. Emulsion
b. Complex colloidal solution
c. Molecular solution
d. Suspension

Ans. (b) Complex colloidal solution

42. The term sarcode was used for living substance of cell by

a. Hooke b. Dujardin
c. Purkinje d. Brown

Ans. (b) Dujardin

43. Protoplasm is

a. Nonliving matter
b. Bearer of hereditary characters
c. Living matter without function
d. Physical basis of life

Ans. (d) Physical basis of life

44. The ability of a cell to form the whole organism is

a. Regeneration b. Cloning
c. Totipotency d. Development

Ans. (c) Totipotency

45. Schleiden and Schwann proposed cell theory in

a. 1836–37 b. 1838–39
c. 1901–02 d. 1938–39

Ans. (b) 1838–39

46. An individual has a number of different types of cells was first stated by

a. Dujardin
b. Robert brown

c. Dutrochet

d. Schleiden and schwann

Ans. (c) Dutrochet

47. Callus is

a. Material used in healing in phloem

b. Secondary tissue developed by woody plants

c. An undifferentiated mass of cells

d. All of the above

Ans. (c) An undifferentiated mass of cells

48. Which one is enucleated

a. Squamous epithelial cells

b. Mature leucocyte of man

c. Mature erythrocyte of frog

d. Mature erythrocyte of man

Ans. (d) Mature erythrocyte of man

49. One of the following is anucleate

a. Sieve tube

b. Companion cell

c. Medullary ray

d. All of the above

Ans. (a) Sieve tube

50. A cell can form many phenotypes. The property is called

a. Pleuripotency

b. Totipotency

c. Parasexuality

d. Parthenogenesis

Ans. (a) Pleuripotency

51. A flagellum beats

a. Independently, undulatory and asymmetrically

b. Independently, undulatory and symmetrically

c. Coordinated, pendular and symmetric

d. Coordinated, pendular and asymmetric

Ans. (b) Independently, undulatory and symmetrically

52. The coordinated beating of cilia is

a. Undulatory

b. Metachronous

c. Metachronous and isochronous

d. Both a and b

Ans. (c) Metachronous and isochronous

53. A typical vacuole possesses

a. Nucleoplasm

b. Cytoplasm

c. Hydroplasm

d. Both b and c

Ans. (c) Hydroplasm

54. Hydroplasm of vacuole possesses

a. Water

b. Minerals

c. Water and mineral

d. Air

Ans. (c) Water and mineral

55. A vacuole without a regular covering membrane is

a. Contractile vacuole

b. Food vacuole

c. Sap vacuole

d. Gas vacuole

Ans. (d) Gas vacuole

56. Which one possesses only a protein membrane

a. Feeding canals of contractile vacuole

b. Vesicles of a gas vacuole

c. Contractile vacuole

d. Gas vacuole

Ans. (b) Vesicles of a gas vacuole

57. Gas vacuoles occur in

a. Prokaryotes

b. Protistans

c. Both a and b

d. Fishes

Ans. (a) Prokaryotes

58. Gas vacuole takes part in

a. Storage of metabolic gases

b. Protection from intense radiations

c. Buoyancy regulation

d. All the above

Ans. (d) All the above

59. Food vacuole is formed from

a. Absorbed and digested food

b. Phagosome + Lysosome

c. Feeding canals + Lysosome

d. Feeding canals + Phagosome

Ans. (b) Phagosome + Lysosome

60. Vacuoles are

a. Cytoplasmic organelles

b. Noncytoplasmic organelles

c. Noncytoplasmic sacs

d. Cytoplasmic sacs

Ans. (c) Noncytoplasmic sacs

61. Contractile vacuoles take part in

a. Storage of wastes

b. Osmoregulation

c. Excretion

d. Both b and c

Ans. (d) Both b and c

62. **Filling of contractile vacuole and its swelling is called**

    a. Diastole   b. Diapauses
    c. Systole   d. Both a and b

Ans. (a) Diastole

63. **Bursting of contractile vacuole to throw its contents is**

    a. Ephagy   b. Systole
    c. Diapause   d. Dehydration

Ans. (b) Systole

64. **Number of sap vacuoles present in an animal cell is**

    a. One and large   b. Many and large
    c. Many and small   d. None of the above

Ans. (c) Many and small

65. **Young plant cells possess sap vacuoles**

    a. One, large and central
    b. Many, large and dispersed
    c. Many, small and dispersed
    d. None of the above

Ans. (c) Many, small and dispersed

66. **A single large central vacuole occurs in**

    a. Mature animal cells
    b. Mature plant cells
    c. Developing animal cells
    d. Developing plants cells

Ans. (b) Mature plant cells

67. **Liquid content of a vacuole is called**

    a. Cell sap   b. Matrix
    c. Nucleoid   d. Core

Ans. (a) Cell sap

68. **Protoplasm present inside the nucleus is called**

    a. Hyaloplasm   b. Nucleoplasm
    c. Nuclear matrix   d. Hydroplasm

Ans. (b) Nucleoplasm

69. **Nucleus was discovered by Robert Brown in**

    a. Orchid root cells   b. Bean root cells
    c. Maize stem cells   d. Wheat stem cells

Ans. (a) Orchid root cells

70. **A well organized nucleus is present in**

    a. Bacteria   b. Prokaryotes
    c. Blue green algae   d. Eukaryotes

Ans. (d) Eukaryotes

71. **A plant (cell) having more than two nuclei is known as**

    a. Syncytial   b. Coenocyte
    c. Polynucleate   d. Plasmodium

Ans. (b) Coenocyte

72. **An animal cell with numerous nuclei is called**

    a. Coenocyte   b. Syncytial
    c. Plasmodium   d. Both a and b

Ans. (b) Syncytial

73. **Nuclear envelope is composed of**

    a. Single membrane
    b. Two membranes
    c. Proteinaceous strand
    d. Both a and c

Ans. (b) Two membranes

74. **A biological membrane containing true pores is**

    a. Nuclear envelope
    b. Plasma membrane
    c. Vitelline membrane
    d. Plastid envelope

Ans. (a) Nuclear envelope

75. **Karyotheca is derived from**

    a. Envelop remains   b. ER
    c. Golgi apparatus   d. Both a and b

Ans. (d) Both a and b

76. **Perinuclear space has a width of**

    a. 100–150 Å   b. 100–300 Å
    c. 400–700 Å   d. 100–150 nm

Ans. (b) 100–300 Å

77. **Diameter of the nuclear pores is**

    a. 50–150 Å   b. 100–200 Å
    c. 300–500 Å   d. 300–1000 Å

Ans. (d) 300–1000 Å

78. **Nucleoplasm is also called**

    a. Nuclear sap   b. Karyolymph
    c. Both a and b   d. Nuclear matrix

Ans. (c) Both a and b

79. **Nucleus controls cytoplasmic functioning by sending out**

    a. Cholesterol   b. Protein
    c. RNAs   d. DNA copies

Ans. (c) RNAs

80. In nondividing cell, most of DNA is located in

    a. Mitochondria   b. Chloroplasts

    c. Chromosomes   d. Chromatin

Ans. (d) Chromatin

81. Chromatin material which remains condensed during interphase is called

    a. Heterochromatin   b. Euchromatin

    c. Chromonemata   d. Megachromatin

Ans. (a) Heterochromatin

82. Heterochromatin is genetically and metabolically

    a. Very active

    b. Inert

    c. Very active genetically

    d. Inert metabolically

Ans. (d) Inert metabolically

83. Nucleolus is a

    a. Distinct membrane bound organelle

    b. Part of chromosome

    c. Ribonucleoprotein entity

    d. DNA component

Ans. (c) Ribonucleoprotein entity

84. Nucleolus was discovered by

    a. Robert brown   b. Leeuwenhoek

    c. Robert hooke   d. Fontana

Ans. (d) Fontana

85. Size of nucleolus is large where

    a. Protein synthesis is active

    b. Protein synthesis is small

    c. No protein synthesis occurs

    d. Lipid metabolism is rapid

Ans. (a) Protein synthesis is active

86. Nucleolus contains

    a. Genetic instructions

    b. Ribosome assembly line

    c. Protein synthesis machinery

    d. Enzymes for polysaccharide formation

Ans. (b) Ribosome assembly line

87. Organelle having a significant role in mitosis is

    a. Lysosomes

    b. Mitochondria

    c. Golgi bodies

    d. Nucleolus

Ans. (d) Mitochondria

88. Granules of nucleolus are precursors of

    a. Chromosomes   b. Ribosomes

    c. RNA   d. All the above

Ans. (b) Ribosomes

89. Nucleolus is formed from

    a. Nucleus

    b. Nuclear sap

    c. Sat chromosome

    d. Giant chromosome

Ans. (c) Sat chromosome

90. Temporary inactivation of one chromosome of a pair is

    a. Facultative heterochromatin

    b. Constitutive heterochromatin

    c. Inactivated chromatin

    d. None of the above

Ans. (a) Facultative heterochromatin

91. Barr body is

    a. Nucleolus

    b. Facultative heterochromatin

    c. Constitutive heterochromatin

    d. Euchromatin

Ans. (b) Facultative heterochromatin

92. Components of nucleus are

    a. Karyotheca, nucleolus, chromatin, nucleoplasm and nuclear matrix

    b. Nuclear envelope, nucleolus, chromatin and nucleoplasm

    c. Nuclear envelop, nucleoplasm asn chromatin

    d. All the above

Ans. (a) Karyotheca, nucleolus, chromatin, nucleoplasm and nuclear matrix

93. Nuclear matrix is

    a. Heterochromatin complex

    b. Crystallo-colloidal complex

    c. Fibrous complex

    d. Nucleoplasm

Ans. (c) Fibrous complex

94. Nuclear matrix is formed of

    a. Histones

    b. Neutral proteins

    c. Acid proteins

    d. Nucleosomes

Ans. (c) Acid proteins

95. Dense fibrous complex lying adjacent to inner membrane of nuclear envelope is

a. Chromatin　　　　b. Fibrous lamina

c. Nuclear lamina　　d. Both b and c

Ans. (d) Both b and c

96. Structural element of chromatin is

a. Histone

b. Acid protein and DNA

c. Nucleosomes

d. Nuclear matrix

Ans. (d) Nuclear matrix

97. Largest organelle of the cell is

a. Nucleus　　　　　b. Chloroplast

c. Mitochondrion　　d. Vacuole

Ans. (a) Nucleus

98. The term chromatin was coined by

a. Heitz　　　　　　b. Flemming

c. Fontana　　　　　d. Bowman

Ans. (b) Flemming

99. The term nucleoplasm was given by

a. Strasburger　　　b. Flemming

c. Harris and James　d. Bowman

Ans. (a) Strasburger

100. Nucleolus contains

a. No membrane covering

b. Amorphous matrix and granular zone

c. Fibrillar zone and chromatin

d. All the above

Ans. (d) All the above

101. Living beings are made up of cells. This was first stated by

a. Lamarck

b. Von Helmont

c. Schleiden and schwann

d. Hugo de Vries

Ans. (a) Lamarck

102. In tissue culture embryoids are formed from pollen grains due to

a. Test tube culture

b. Double fertilization

c. Cellular totipotency

d. Organogenesis

Ans. (c) Cellular totipotency

103. Cellular totipotency is demonstrated by

a. Only gymnosperm cells

b. All plant cells

c. All eukaryotic cells

d. Only bacterial cells

Ans. (b) All plant cells

104. Fertilization of an egg with sperm was discovered by

a. Hertwig　　　　　b. Flemming

c. Waldeyer　　　　 d. Malpighi

Ans. (a) Hertwig

105. The volume of which the following is given in right sequence

a. Ostrich egg > Hen egg > Human egg > Smallest virus

b. Human egg > Ostrich > Smallest bacteria

c. Bacteria > Virus > Human sperm

d. Virus > Bacteria > Human sperm > Human egg

Ans. (a) Ostrich egg > Hen egg > Human egg > Smallest virus

106. Basic unit of life is

a. Cell　　　　　　　b. Tissue

c. Organ　　　　　　d. Organ system

Ans. (a) Cell

107. Cell is a unit of

a. Structure　　　　　b. Function

c. Mass of protoplasm　d. All of the above

Ans. (d) All of the above

108. Study of the cell structure under microscope is

a. Cytology　　　　　b. Cell biology

c. Cytochemistry　　　d. Microanatomy

Ans. (a) Cytology

109. Study of cells in all aspects is

a. Cytotaxonomy　　　b. Cytology

c. Cell biology　　　　d. Cytochemistry

Ans. (c) Cell biology

110. Cells were observed prior to Robert Hooke by

a. Aristole　　　　　　b. Malpighi

c. Bauhin　　　　　　d. Eicher

Ans. (b) Malpighi

111. Who initiated cell concept

a. Robert Hooke　　　b. Leeuwenhoek

c. Grew　　　　　　　d. Schleiden and Schwann

Ans. (c) Grew

112. Cell was discovered by

a. Swanson
b. Leeuwenhoek
c. Robert Hooke
d. Robert Brown

Ans. (c) Robert Hooke

113. The cell was discovered in

a. 18th century
b. 19th century
c. First half of 17th century
d. Second half of 17th century

Ans. (d) Second half of 17th century

114. Cell, as basic unit of plants, was discovered by

a. Robert Brown
b. Robert Hooke
c. Virchow
d. Schleiden

Ans. (d) Schleiden

115. Cell theory state that

a. All cells are living
b. All cells have nucleus
c. Cells are fundamental structural units of living organisms
d. Cell reproduce by mitosis and meiosis

Ans. (c) Cells are fundamental structural units of living organisms

116. Robert Brown is known for his discovery of

a. Chloroplasts
b. Respirometer
c. Nucleus
d. Mitochondria

Ans. (c) Nucleus

117. Who applied cell theory to plants

a. Schwann
b. Schleiden
c. Swanson
d. Jenssen

Ans. (b) Schleiden

118. The living substance of cell was named sarcode by

a. Corti
b. Dujardin
c. Lamarck
d. Dutrochet

Ans. (b) Dujardin

119. The modern cell theory is called

a. Protoplasmic theory
b. Cell Principle
c. Cell Doctrine
d. Both B and C

Ans. (d) Both B and C

120. Which ones do not have cellular structure

a. PPLO
b. Rickettsia
c. Viruses
d. Archaebacteria

Ans. (c) Viruses

121. Robert Hooke discovered cell in

a. 1665
b. 1725
c. 1545
d. 1595

Ans. (a) 1665

122. 'Micrographia' was written by

a. Grew
b. Hooke
c. Brown
d. Lamarck

Ans. (b) Hooke

123. Cell theory was first modified by

a. Schleiden
b. Brown
c. Schwann
d. Grew

Ans. (c) Schwann

124. Omnis cellula e cellula is generalization given by

a. Lamarck
b. Dutrochet
c. Leeuwenhoek
d. Virchow

Ans. (d) Virchow

125. Cells of Robert Hooke were actually

a. Cell walls
b. Protoplasts
c. Wall-less cells
d. Walled cells

Ans. (a) Cell walls

126. Cell principle is not applicable to

a. Bacteria
b. Viruses
c. Algae
d. Fungi

Ans. (b) Viruses

127. Distinction of individual cells is absent in coenocytic organism

a. Ulothrix
b. Volvox
c. Escherichia
d. Rhizopus

Ans. (d) Rhizopus

128. Who believed in the individuality of cells?

a. Leeuwenhoek
b. Lamarck
c. Dutrochet
d. Malpighi

Ans. (c) Dutrochet

129. Who saw the living matter for the first time?

a. Leeuwenhoek
b. Hooke
c. Grew
d. Corti

Ans. (d) Corti

130. A nucleus is absent in the mature

a. Sieve tube cells
b. Mammalian erythrocytes

c. Monocytes

d. Both A and B

Ans. (d) Both A and B

131. A tissue having more nonliving material than the living matter is

a. Epithelial tissue

b. Parenchyma

c. Connective tissue

d. Nervous system

Ans. (c) Connective tissue

132. Who proposed protoplasmic theory as opposed to cell theory?

a. Virchow

b. Schultze

c. Sachs

d. Strasburger

Ans. (b) Schultze

133. The theory proposing that body of an organism consists of incompletely divided cells is

a. Organismal theory

b. Protoplasmic theory

c. Cell theory

d. Theory of cell lineage

Ans. (a) Organismal theory

134. Organismal theory was proposed by

a. Van Mohl

b. Sachs

c. Virchow

d. Haberlandt

Ans. (b) Sachs

135. Cells are autonomous because

a. They synthesise components of living protoplasm from nonliving materials

b. They are able to grow and divide

c. Each cell has its own life span

d. All of the above

Ans. (d) All of the above

136. "Each cell leads a double life" was first proposed by

a. Schleiden

b. Grew

c. Von Mohl

d. Malpighi

Ans. (a) Schleiden

137. Ageing is slow or absent in

a. Plants

b. Parrot

c. Hydra

d. Unicells

Ans. (d) Unicells

138. Which are less efficient?

a. Multicellular animals

b. Multicellular plants

c. Colonial organisms

d. Unicellular organisms

Ans. (d) Unicellular organisms

139. A multicellular organism possesses

a. Differentiated cells

b. Undifferentiated cells

c. Dedifferentiated cells

d. All of the above

Ans. (d) All of the above

140. Number of types of cells found in human body is

a. 20

b. 30

c. 200

d. 300

Ans. (c) 200

141. Cells which lose their nucleus during differentiation are

a. Nerve cells

b. Muscle cells

c. Erythrocytes

d. Leucocytes

Ans. (c) Erythrocytes

142. A nucleated differentiated cell that has lost the power to dedifferentiate is

a. Nerve cell

b. Kidney cell

c. Liver cell

d. All of the above

Ans. (a) Nerve cell

143. First successful culture was obtained by

a. Haberlandt

b. White

c. Skoog and Miller

d. Steward et al

Ans. (b) White

144. Callus was grown successfully for the first time by

a. White

b. Gautheret

c. Nabecourt

d. All of the above

Ans. (d) All of the above

145. Morphogenesis in tissue culture was discovered by

a. G autheret

b. Skoog and Miller

c. Muir et al

d. Steward et al

Ans. (b) Skoog and Miller

146. Who proposed for the first time that cells are totipotent?

a. White

b. Haberlandt

c. Steward

d. Halperrin and Wetherell

Ans. (b) Haberlandt

147. Steward et al performed experiment to prove cellular totipotency of

   a. Tomato   b. Carrot

   c. Tobacco   d. Potato

Ans. (b) Carrot

148. Explants is

   a. Propagule

   b. Callus used for subculturing

   c. Part of plant used in tissue culture

   d. Part of tissue culture used for planting

Ans. (c) Part of plant used in tissue culture

149. What was done by Steward et al in order to separate individual cells of Carrot root?

   a. Shaking in liquid medium

   b. Homogenization

   c. Pressure sieving

   d. Microsurgery

Ans. (a) Shaking in liquid medium

150. Single cells in Steward's culture formed

   a. Cellular clumps

   b. Embryoids

   c. Plantlets

   d. All of the above

Ans. (d) Embryoids

151. Embryoids are

   a. Somatic embryo-like structures

   b. Small embryos through fertilization in culture

   c. Early embryo stages used for propagation in tissue culture

   d. All of the above

Ans. (a) Somatic embryo-like structures

152. In animals, cellular totipotency has been restricted only to

   a. Germinal cells

   b. Epithelial cells

   c. Zygote

   d. Zygote and early blastosomes

Ans. (d) Zygote and early blastosomes

153. Animal cloning is carried out by

   a. Artificial fertilization of ovum

   b. Direct growth of ovum

   c. Ovum with somatic nucleus

   d. All of the above

Ans. (c) Ovum with somatic nucleus

154. The first successful animal cloning, Dolly, was accomplished by

   a. Fisher and Velton

   b. Wilmut and Campbell

   c. Morgan

   d. Bernstein

Ans. (b) Wilmut and Campbell

155. Cells capable of division are

   a. Stem cells

   b. Meristematic cells

   c. Undifferentiated cells

   d. All of the above

Ans. (d) All of the above

156. Differentiated cells are

   a. Premiotic specialized

   b. Post-miotic specialized

   c. Premeiotic specialized

   d. Post-meiotic specialized

Ans. (b) Post-miotic specialized

157. RBCs are

   a. Differentiated cells

   b. Undifferentiated cells

   c. Dedifferentiated cells

   d. Dead cells

Ans. (a) Differentiated cells

158. During differentiation, RBCs lose

   a. Aerobic respiration   b. DNA replication

   c. RNA synthesis   d. All of the above

Ans. (d) All of the above

159. Dedifferentiated cells are formed in the region of

   a. Injury   b. Regeneration

   c. Secondary growth   d. All of the above

Ans. (d) All of the above

160. Functionally important dead cells are

   a. Cork cells   b. Tracheary elements

   c. Both A and B   d. Endothelial cells

Ans. (c) Both A and B

161. Rapidly dividing unorganized mass of cells in tissue culture is

   a. Callose   b. Callus

   c. Embryoid   d. Plantlet

Ans. (b) Callus

162. Mitosis allows the eukaryotic cells to
   a. Expose DNA for protein synthesis
   b. Grow in size
   c. Multiply
   d. Become specialized

Ans. (c) Multiply

163. In prophase and metaphase a chromosome contains two
   a. Chromatids
   b. Chrommomeres
   c. Centromeres
   d. Centrioles

Ans. (a) Chromatids

164. The centromere does not divide till the end of metaphase. This is important because centromere
   a. Is connected with nuclear envelop
   b. Produces spindle fibres
   c. Contains genes that control prophase and metaphase
   d. Holds the replicated DNAs together

Ans. (d) Holds the replicated DNAs together

165. Microtubules appearing around centriole pair in the beginning of prophase in animal cells form
   a. Spindle
   b. Aster
   c. Spindle pole
   d. Chromosome fibres

Ans. (b) Aster

166. The stage at which cytokinesis begins in plant cell is
   a. Anaphase
   b. Telophase
   c. G_0 phase
   d. Interphase

Ans. (a) Anaphase

167. The stage at which cleavage or cytokinesis begins in animal cells is
   a. Anaphase
   b. Telophase
   c. G_0 phase
   d. Interphase

Ans. (d) Interphase

168. A circle of vesicles appears at the equator of spindle towards the end of anaphase. It will form
   a. Cleavage furrow
   b. Phragmoplast
   c. Cell plate
   d. Middle lamella

Ans. (c) Cell plate

169. The correct sequence of different phases of mitosis is
   a. Anaphase → Metaphase → Prophase → Telophase → Interphase
   b. Interphase → Telophase → Metaphase → Anaphase → Prophase
   c. Metaphase → Anaphase → Telophase → Prophase
   d. Interphase → Prophase → Metaphase → Anaphase → Telophase

Ans. (d) Interphase → Prophase → Metaphase → Anaphase → Telophase

170. Which one of the organelles is responsible for the formation of aster in cell division?
   a. Ribosome
   b. Centrosome
   c. Lysosome
   d. Chromosome

Ans. (b) Centrosome

171. Region of chromosome where force is exerted during chromatid separation is
   a. Telomere
   b. Centromere
   c. Chromomere
   d. Chromonemata

Ans. (b) Centromere

172. Separation of chromosome daughters takes place at
   a. Telophase
   b. Metaphase
   c. Anaphase
   d. Prophase

Ans. (c) Anaphase

173. Mitosis is usually studied in smears or sections of
   a. Root tips
   b. Stem tips
   c. Floral buds
   d. All the above

Ans. (a) Root tips

174. Mitosis takes place in
   a. All types of cells except those involved in gamete formation
   b. Gonads
   c. Axillary buds situated near the apical bud
   d. Cells of mature leaf

Ans. (a) All types of cells except those involved in gamete formation

175. Distribution of chromosomes in dividing cells occurs during
   a. Telophase
   b. Prophase
   c. Metaphase
   d. Anaphase

Ans. (d) Anaphase

176. Plant and animal cell division differ in
   a. Cell plate
   b. Prophase
   c. Telophase
   d. Metaphase

Ans. (a) Cell plate

177. Cytoplasmic structures involved in cell division are

a. Mitochondria
b. Ribosomes
c. Lysosomes
d. Centrioles

Ans. (d) Centrioles

178. Which one occurs once in life cycle?

a. Replication of DNA
b. Replication of chromosomes
c. Meiosis
d. Mitosis

Ans. (c) Meiosis

179. Bouquet stage occurs during

a. Leptotene
b. Zygotene
c. Pachytene
d. Diplotene

Ans. (a) Leptotene

180. Synapsis of homologous chromosomes chromosomes was first observed by

a. Winiwater
b. Montgomery
c. Johanssen
d. Zickler

Ans. (b) Montgomery

181. Syneptinemal complex is found associated with

a. Paired meiotic chromosomes
b. Lampbrush chromosomes
c. Polytene chromosomes
d. Mitotic chromosomes

Ans. (a) Paired meiotic chromosomes

182. In meiosis, chromosome replication occurs during

a. Interphase
b. Interkinesis
c. Prophase I
d. Prophase II

Ans. (a) Interphase

183. The transition between meiosis I and meiosis II is

a. Interphase
b. Interkinesis
c. Telophase I
d. Prophase II

Ans. (b) Interkinesis

184. Chromosomes similar in size, shape, genes and gene sequences are

a. Sister chromatids
b. Chromomeres
c. Homologous chromosomes
d. Parental chromosomes

Ans. (c) Homologous chromosomes

185. Function of meiosis I is to separate

a. Homologous chromosomes
b. Sister chromatids
c. Cross-overs
d. Parental chromosomes

Ans. (a) Homologous chromosomes

186. Crossing over occurs in meiosis during

a. Prophase I
b. Prophase II
c. Interphase
d. Interkinesis

Ans. (a) Prophase I

187. Pairing of homologous chromosomes is

a. Chiasma formation
b. Synapsis
c. Disjunction
d. Crossing over

Ans. (b) Synapsis

188. Separation of homologous chromosomes is called

a. Dispersion
b. Bivalent formation
c. Disjunction
d. Crossing over

Ans. (c) Disjunction

189. Homologous chromosomes separate during

a. Prophase I
b. Prophase II
c. Metaphase I
d. Anaphase I

Ans. (d) Anaphase I

190. Name the stage in meiosis when there are two cells each with sister chromatids aligned at the equator of the spindle

a. Prophase
b. Metaphase II
c. Metaphase I
d. Anaphase II

Ans. (b) Metaphase II

191. The points of crossing over in meiosis appear as

a. Synaptinemal complexes
b. Protein axes
c. Chiasmata
d. Diakinesis

Ans. (c) Chiasmata

192. Number of bivalents are 8 in prophase I. what is the number of chromosomes during anaphase II?

a. 8
b. 4
c. 16
d. 32

Ans. (a) 8

193. Chromosomes normally occur as homologous pairs in

a. Egg　　　　　　b. Sperm

c. Gamete　　　　d. Zygote

Ans. (d) Zygote

194. Genome is

a. Genes of haploid of chromosomes

b. Genes of diploid of chromosomes

c. A single chromosome

d. None of the above

Ans. (a) Genes of haploid of chromosomes

195. Synapsis means

a. Pairing of any two chromosomes

b. Homologous chromosomes start separating

c. Pairing of homologous chromosomes

d. None of the above

Ans. (c) Pairing of homologous chromosomes

196. Chiasmata are formed during

a. Zygotene　　　b. Pachytene

c. Diplotene　　　d. Leptotene

Ans. (c) Diplotene

197. Meiosis is studied in smears of

a. Developing anthers　　b. Testes

c. Both a and b　　　　　d. Axillary buds

Ans. (c) Both a and b

198. Chromosome syndesis or bivalent formation occurs in

a. Leptotene　　　b. Zygotene

c. Pachytene　　　d. Diplotene

Ans. (b) Zygotene

199. Meiosis occurs in

a. Haploid cells

b. Mostly haploid cells but occasionally diploid cells

c. Diploid cells

d. Mostly diploid cells but occasionally haploid cells

Ans. (c) Diploid cells

200. Oogenesis is an example of

a. Mitosis

b. Meiosis

c. Specialization of cell

d. DNA replication

Ans. (b) Meiosis

201. Disjunction is

a. Chromosome separation during mitosis

b. Chromosome separation during prophase I

c. Chromosome separation in anaphase I

d. Chromosome separation during metaphase I

Ans. (c) Chromosome separation in anaphase I

202. At which stage of meiosis I, the homologous chromosomes separate but are held by chiasmata

a. Diakinesis　　　b. Diplotene

c. Pachytene　　　d. Zygotene

Ans. (b) Diplotene

203. Swellings present over the chromosomes are

a. Centromeres　　b. Centrosome

c. Puffs　　　　　d. Chromomeres

Ans. (d) Chromomeres

204. Number of cells daily replaced in human body is

a. 1×10^9　　　b. 5×10^9

c. 1×10^{10}　　d. 5×10^{10}

Ans. (b) 5×10^9

205. The term eumitosis is used for

a. Mitosis is higher in plants

b. Mitosis in animals

c. Mitosis where spindle is extranuclear

d. Mitosis with intranuclear spindle

Ans. (c) Mitosis where spindle is extranuclear

206. Premitosis is

a. Amitosis

b. G_1

c. G_2

d. Intranuclear mitosis

Ans. (d) G_1

207. In leptotene, the chromosomes are

a. Attached to nuclear by one end

b. Attached to nuclear by both ends directly

c. Attached to nuclear by both ends through attachment plate

d. Both b and c

Ans. (c) Attached to nuclear by both ends through attachment plate

208. Cell division was first studied by

a. Leeuwenhoek　　b. Virchow

c. Prevost and Dumas　　d. Flemming

Ans. (c) Prevost and Dumas

209. Who found that new cells develop from pre-existing cells?

    a. Remak   b. Virchow

    c. Prevost and Dumas   d. Strasburger

Ans. (a) Remak

210. Cell lineage theory was proposed by

    a. Strasburger   b. Virchow

    c. Winiwater   d. Van Beneden

Ans. (b) Virchow

211. Nucleus develops from a pre-existing nucleus. The finding was made by

    a. Farmer and Moore   b. Winiwater

    c. Sutton   d. Strasburger

Ans. (d) Strasburger

212. A mitogen of plant origin is

    a. Colchicine

    b. Epidermal growth factor

    c. Cytokinin

    d. Lymphokine

Ans. (c) Cytokinin

213. A mitogen of animal origin is

    a. Cyanide

    b. Azide

    c. Chalone

    d. Platelet derived growth factor

Ans. (d) Platelet derived growth factor

214. Which one is not a mitogen?

    a. Epidermal growth factor

    b. Platelet derived growth factor

    c. Lymphokine

    d. None of the above

Ans. (d) None of the above

215. Colchicine is

    a. Mitotic poison   b. Prophase poison

    c. Cytokinesis poison   d. None of the above

Ans. (a) Mitotic poison

216. Colchicine prevents

    a. Interphase

    b. Completion of metaphase

    c. Condensation of chromosomes

    d. Replication of chromosomes

Ans. (b) Completion of metaphase

217. Autumn Crocus is source of

    a. Azides   b. Chalones

    c. Colchicine   d. Cytokinin

Ans. (c) Colchicine

218. Which one induces cell division?

    a. Critical decrease in surface volume ratio

    b. Critical decrease in nucleocytoplasmic or kernplasma ratio

    c. Both a and b

    d. Decrease in cell size

Ans. (c) Both a and b

219. The term mitosis was introduced by

    a. Watson and Crick   b. Beadle and Tatum

    c. Farmer and Moore   d. Flemming

Ans. (d) Flemming

220. The term meiosis was introduced by

    a. Watson and Crick

    b. Beadle and Tatum

    c. Farmer and Moore

    d. Strasburger

Ans. (c) Farmer and Moore

221. Abnormal unlimited and uncontrolled cell division results in

    a. Pleurisy   b. Cancer

    c. Tumour   d. Asphyxia

Ans. (b) Cancer

222. Cells having large nucleus in proportion to cytoplasm are

    a. Dead   b. Dividing

    c. Active   d. None of the above

Ans. (b) Dividing

223. Colchicines results in doubling of chromosome number because of

    a. Nonformation of spindle

    b. Double replication of chromosomes

    c. Nonpairing of chromosomes

    d. Splitting of chromosomes

Ans. (a) Nonformation of spindle

224. Generation time represents period of

    a. Cell cycle   b. Interphase

    c. M-phase   d. S-phase

Ans. (a) Cell cycle

225. Which one is the longest phase of cell cycle?

a. Prophase
b. Telophase
c. G_1-phase
d. G_2-phase

Ans. (c) G_1-phase

226. Invisible stage of M-phase is

a. G_1-phase
b. S-phase
c. G_2-phase
d. G_0-phase

Ans. (b) S-phase

227. Histones are synthesized in

a. Prophase
b. G_1-phase
c. S-phase
d. Metaphase

Ans. (c) S-phase

228. Intermitosis is

a. Stage between meiosis I and meiosis II
b. Stage between two mitotic divisions
c. Interphase
d. Both b and c

Ans. (d) Both b and c

229. Which one is stored in G_1-phase?

a. ATP
b. Tubulin
c. Histone
d. All the above

Ans. (a) ATP

230. Centriole replication occurs in

a. Early prophase
b. G_1-phase
c. S-phase
d. G_0-phase

Ans. (c) S-phase

231. Post-mitotic phase is

a. G_0-phase
b. G_1-phase
c. S-phase
d. G_2-phase

Ans. (b) G_1-phase

232. Cell cycle was discovered by

a. Farmer and Moore
b. Prevost and Dumas
c. Howard and Pele
d. Remak

Ans. (c) Howard and Pele

233. Decision of G_0-phase occurs

a. Towards the end of G_1-phase
b. Towards middle of G_1-phase
c. At the end of telophase
d. Towards end of cytokinesis

Ans. (b) Towards middle of G_1-phase

234. Which specific protein is formed in G_2-phase?

a. Histone
b. DNA-polymerase
c. Scaffold proteins
d. Tubulin

Ans. (d) Tubulin

235. The stage at which DNA/chromosome replication occurs is

a. Prophase
b. Interphase
c. Metaphase
d. Previous telophase

Ans. (b) Interphase

236. Each cell grows during the cell cycle in

a. Interphase
b. Prophase
c. Metaphase
d. Anaphase

Ans. (a) Interphase

237. The cell size doubles in a stage of cell cycle called

a. M
b. G_2
c. S
d. G_1

Ans. (d) G_1

238. The decision for cell division is taken

a. Before the start of prophase
b. G_1-phase
c. S-phase
d. G_2-phase

Ans. (b) G_1-phase

239. Chromatin fibres are observed only in the

a. Prophase
b. Metaphase
c. Telophase
d. Interphase

Ans. (d) Interphase

240. Chromosome replication occurs during

a. Metaphase
b. S-phase
c. Anaphase
d. G_2-phase

Ans. (b) S-phase

241. It is very difficult to stop cell division when the cell has entered

a. G_1-phase
b. G_2-phase
c. S-phase
d. Prophase

Ans. (c) S-phase

242. At the time of fission, meganucleus of *Paramecium* undergoes

a. Dispersion
b. Mitosis
c. Amitosis
d. Budding

Ans. (c) Amitosis

243. Amitosis occurs during cell division in

a. Foetal membranes   b. Endosperm
c. Cartilage cells   d. All the above

Ans. (d) All the above

244. The division in which chromosomes do not differentiate is

a. Amitosis   b. Free nuclear division
c. Intracellular division   d. All the above

Ans. (a) Amitosis

245. Amitosis was discovered by Remak in

a. 1841   b. 1855
c. 1880   d. 1905

Ans. (b) 1855

246. Dividing animal cells become nearly rounded in

a. Interphase   b. Early prophase
c. Late prophase   d. Metaphase

Ans. (b) Early prophase

247. When do viscosity and refractivity of cytoplasm increase?

a. G_1-phase   b. S-phase
c. Prophase   d. Metaphase

Ans. (c) Prophase

248. Congression occurs during

a. Early prophase   b. Late prophase
c. Early metaphase   d. Late metaphase

Ans. (c) Early metaphase

249. In mitotic metaphase the limbs of the chromosomes occur

a. On the equator
b. In different directions
c. In divaricate condition
d. All the above

Ans. (b) In different directions

250. Phase of shortest duration is

a. Prophase   b. Metaphase
c. Anaphase   d. S-phase

Ans. (c) Anaphase

251. In animal cytokinesis, cleavage occurs with the help of

a. Microtubules   b. Spindle fibres
c. Microfibrils   d. Microfilaments

Ans. (d) Microfilaments

252. A mid body is formed during

a. Animal cytokinesis   b. Plant cytokinesis
c. Metaphase   d. Both a and b

Ans. (a) Animal cytokinesis

253. After mitosis, the number of chromosomes in the daughter cell shall be

a. One fourth of parent cell
b. One half of parent cell
c. Twice of the parent cell
d. Same as the parent cell

Ans. (d) Same as the parent cell

254. The term nucleolus was coined by

a. Bowman   b. Fontana
c. Hanstein   d. Strasburger

Ans. (a) Bowman

255. Constitutive heterochromatin is

a. Condensed chromatin
b. Present in all cells
c. Made of repetitive bases
d. All the above

Ans. (d) All the above

256. Nonliving cell inclusions are called

a. Ergastic substances
b. Deuteroplasmic substances
c. Paraplasmic substances
d. All the above

Ans. (d) All the above

257. Idioblast is

a. Plant cell different from others
b. Plant cell having cell inclusions
c. Both a and b
d. Animal cell different from others

Ans. (c) Both a and b

258. Chromomeres were discovered by

a. Strasburger   b. Van Beneden
c. Pfitzner   d. Winiwater

Ans. (c) Pfitzner

259. The modern concept of chromosome structure was put forward by

a. Du Praw   b. Laemli
c. Ris   d. Kornbery

Ans. (b) Laemli

260. NOR is

a. Nucleotide organizing replicase
b. Nucleotide occluding region
c. Number of replicons
d. Nucleolar organizing region

Ans. (d) Nucleolar organizing region

261. NOR occurs in the region of

a. Secondary constriction
b. Primary constriction
c. Telomere
d. Centromere

Ans. (a) Secondary constriction

262. The term chromosome was introduced by

a. Strasburger
b. Benda
c. Waldeyer
d. Hofmeister

Ans. (c) Waldeyer

263. Chromosomes having slightly unequal arms is called

a. Metacentric
b. Submetacentric
c. Telocentric
d. Acrocentric

Ans. (b) Submetacentric

264. If the centromere is terminal, the chromosome is

a. Metacentric
b. Submetacentric
c. Telocentric
d. Acrocentric

Ans. (c) Telocentric

265. In salivary gland chromosomes/polytene chromosomes, pairing is

a. Absent
b. Occasional
c. Formed between nonhomologous chromosomes
d. Formed between homologous chromosomes

Ans. (d) Formed between homologous chromosomes

266. Polytene chromosomes was first observed by

a. Stevens and Wilson
b. Heitz and Bauer
c. Balbiani
d. Khorana

Ans. (c) Balbiani

267. Chromosomes were first seen by

a. Hofmeister
b. Waldeyer
c. Walter S. Sutton
d. Crick and Watson

Ans. (a) Hofmeister

268. Chromosomes having equal or almost equal arms are called

a. Metacentric
b. Acrocentric
c. Polycentric
d. Acentric

Ans. (a) Metacentric

269. Chromosomes which remain condensed during interphase are called

a. Heterochromosomes
b. Euchromosomes
c. Mega chromosomes
d. Polytene chromosomes

Ans. (a) Heterochromosomes

270. Diagrammatic representation of the chromosomes of an organism arranged according to their size is known as

a. Genome
b. Karyotype
c. Idiogram
d. None of the above

Ans. (c) Idiogram

271. Eukaryotic chromosomes are composed of

a. DNA + Protein
b. DNA + RNA
c. RNA + Protein
d. Only DNA

Ans. (a) DNA + Protein

272. Chromosomes other than sex chromosomes are called

a. Allosomes
b. Autosomes
c. Microsomes
d. All the above

Ans. (b) Autosomes

273. Lampbrush chromosomes are also called diplotene chromosomes because they

a. Show chiasmata
b. Resemble diplotene chromosomes
c. Are in permanent diplotene stage
d. All the above

Ans. (d) All the above

274. During staining, chromosomes get stained with

a. Eosine
b. Borax carmine
c. Acetocarmine
d. Safranin

Ans. (c) Acetocarmine

275. Polytene chromosomes are noticed in

a. Man
b. Pisum sativum
c. Mice
d. Drosophila

Ans. (d) Drosophila

276. The hereditary vehicle is

a. Chromosome   b. Centromere

c. Nucleus   d. Nucleolus

Ans. (a) Chromosome

277. Balbiani rings are

a. Uncoiling of chromonemata

b. Coiling of chromonemata

c. Enlargements of centromere

d. None of the above

Ans. (a) Uncoiling of chromonemata

278. Polytene chromosome in *Drosophila* is

a. 10 times larger than somatic chromosome

b. 50 times larger than somatic chromosome

c. 10 to 50 times larger than somatic chromosome

d. About 500 times larger than somatic chromosome

Ans. (d) About 500 times larger than somatic chromosome

279. Satellite means

a. Terminal part of the chromosome beyond secondary constriction

b. Terminal part of the chromosome beyond primary constriction

c. Terminal part of the chromosome beyond tertiary constriction

d. None of the above

Ans. (a) Terminal part of the chromosome beyond secondary constriction

280. Length of chromosomes is directly proportional to

a. Size of the cell   b. Size of nucleus

c. Number of genes   d. All the above

Ans. (c) Number of genes

281. A constriction on the chromosome is

a. Centromere   b. Centrosome

c. Centriole   d. Chromomere

Ans. (a) Centromere

282. Chromosome banding was discovered by

a. Casperson et al   b. Muller

c. Berg et al   d. Christian de Duve

Ans. (a) Casperson et al

283. Banding techniques used in case of plant chromosomes are

a. G and R   b. C and G

c. C and N   d. Q and G

Ans. (c) C and N

284. The technique used to locate specific DNA sequences over the chromosome is

a. Flow cytometry

b. Banding technique

c. Fluorescence *in situ* hybridization

d. Electrophoresis

Ans. (c) Fluorescence *in situ* hybridization

285. Flow cytometry prepares

a. Chromosome histogram

b. Idiogram

c. Karyotype

d. All the above

Ans. (a) Chromosome histogram

286. Mc FISH is used in

a. Locating a specific DNA sequence over a chromosome

b. Locating two or more DNA sequences on the same chromosome

c. Location deletion

d. Finding duplicated segments

Ans. (b) Locating two or more DNA sequences on the same chromosome

287. Asymmetric karyotype is the one in which

a. There are more metacentric chromosomes

b. A few metacentric chromosomes

c. Differences between smallest and largest chromosome is large

d. Both b and c

Ans. (d) Both b and c

288. The term cell membrane was coined by

a. Nageli and Cramer   b. Flemming

c. Sachs   d. Plowe

Ans. (a) Nageli and Cramer

289. The term plasmalemma was coined by

a. Robertson

b. Plowe

c. Strasburger

d. Overton

Ans. (b) Plowe

290. Cell membrane is visible under

a. Electron microscope

b. Optical microscope

c. Both optical and electron microscope

d. Oil immersion lens

Ans. (a) Electron microscope

291. Average thickness of plasmalemma is

a. 0.25 nm   b. 2.5 nm

c. 0.75 nm   d. 7.5 nm

Ans. (d) 7.5 nm

292. Cell membrane is

a. Unilaminar

b. Bilaminar

c. Trilaminar

d. Quadrilaminar

Ans. (c) Trilaminar

293. Tripartite nature of plasmalemma was discovered by

a. Davson   b. Robertson

c. Danieli   d. Both a and b

Ans. (b) Robertson

294. Who proposed the first lamellar model of biomembranes

a. Danielli and Davson

b. Robertson

c. Helleir and Hoffmann

d. Singer and Nicolson

Ans. (a) Danielli and Davson

295. The concept of unit membrane was propounded by

a. Overton   b. Gorter and Grendel

c. Davson   d. Robertson

Ans. (d) Robertson

296. What is the latest and most acceptable model of cell membranes

a. Lamellar model

b. Fluid mosaic model

c. Micellar model

d. Unit membrane concept

Ans. (b) Fluid mosaic model

297. Cell membrane is composed of

a. Phospholipid   b. Nucleoprotein

c. Polysaccharides   d. Lipoprotein

Ans. (d) Lipoprotein

298. A biomembrane is made of

a. Proteins, lipids and carbohydrates

b. Proteins, lipids and RNA

c. Proteins, lipids and DNA

d. Proteins, lipids and hormones

Ans. (a) Proteins, lipids and carbohydrates

299. Biomembranes are similar to "protein icebergs in sea of lipids" was saying of

a. Singer and Nicolson

b. Danielli and Davson

c. Gorter and Grendel

d. Helleir and Hoffmann

Ans. (a) Singer and Nicolson

300. A cell membrane has

a. Middle electron dense layer

b. Middle electron transparent layer

c. Outer electron transparent layer

d. Inner electron transparent layer

Ans. (b) Middle electron transparent layer

301. Which one forms the continuous part of cell membrane

a. Proteins   b. Carbohydrates

c. Lipids   d. All the above

Ans. (c) Lipids

302. Most abundant lipid of cell membrane is

a. Cholesterol   b. Phospholipid

c. Glycolipid   d. Cerebroside

Ans. (b) Phospholipid

303. Integral proteins of plasmalemma occur

a. On the outer surface

b. On the inner surface

c. On both the surfaces

d. In the phospholipid matrix

Ans. (d) In the phospholipid matrix

304. Hydrophilic chemical of cell wall is

a. Pectin   b. Suberin

c. Fat   d. Lignin

Ans. (a) Pectin

305. Structural element of cell wall is

a. Matrix

b. Microfibrils

c. Microtubules

d. Arabinogalactans

Ans. (b) Microfibrils

306. Cellulose microfibrils get bound to pectins of matrix through

a. Hemicelluloses   b. Lignin

c. Peptidoglycan   d. Glycoprotein

Ans. (a) Hemicelluloses

307. Different layers of cell wall are

a. Middle lamella and primary wall
b. Primary wall and secondary wall
c. Middle lamella, primary wall and secondary wall
d. Wall layer exclude middle lamella

Ans. (c) Middle lamella, primary wall and secondary wall

308. Which is the outermost structure of cell wall

a. Primary wall
b. Secondary wall
c. Tertiary wall
d. Middle lamella, if present

Ans. (d) Middle lamella, if present

309. The first wall layer of cell is

a. Tertiary wall, if present
b. Secondary wall
c. Primary wall
d. Middle lamella, if present

Ans. (c) Primary wall

310. The innermost layer of cell wall is

a. Tertiary wall, if present
b. Secondary wall
c. Primary wall
d. Middle lamella, if present

Ans. (a) Tertiary wall, if present

311. Which is component of cell wall is normally in contact with plasmalemma

a. Primary wall
b. Secondary wall
c. Plasmodesmata
d. Middle lamella

Ans. (b) Secondary wall

312. Primary wall grows by

a. Accretion
b. Introgression
c. Intussusception
d. All the above

Ans. (c) Intussusception

313. Secondary wall grows in thickness by

a. Intercalation
b. Introgression
c. Accretion
d. Epiboly

Ans. (c) Accretion

314. Secondary wall is commonly formed of

a. Single layer
b. Many layers
c. Two layers
d. Three layers

Ans. (d) Three layers

315. Load bearing parts of the plant cells is

a. Middle lamella
b. Secondary wall
c. Primary wall
d. Tertiary wall

Ans. (b) Secondary wall

316. Primary wall has a thickness of

a. 0.1–3.0 µm
b. 0.01–0.03 µm
c. 0.1–0.5 µm
d. 0.5–1.5 µm

Ans. (a) 0.1–3.0 µm

317. Primary wall is generally elastic due to absence of

a. Lignin
b. Suberin
c. Cutin
d. Silica

Ans. (a) Lignin

318. Plant cells are distinguishable from animal cell in containing

a. Mitochondria
b. Ribosomes
c. ER
d. Cell wall

Ans. (d) Cell wall

319. The structural material of fungal cell wall is

a. Pectin
b. Cellulose
c. Peptidoglycan
d. Chitin

Ans. (d) Chitin

320. Ripe fruits soften due to

a. Degeneration of cell walls
b. Partial solubilisation of pectic compounds
c. Metabolism of tannins
d. Exosmosis

Ans. (b) Partial solubilisation of pectic compounds

321. Hardness of woody tissue is due to

a. Silica
b. Lignin
c. Cellulose
d. Suberin

Ans. (b) Lignin

322. Impermeability of cork is related to

a. Silica
b. Lignin
c. Cellulose
d. Suberin

Ans. (d) Suberin

323. Cutin occurs in

a. Phloem tissue
b. Xylem tissue
c. Endodermis
d. Epidermis

Ans. (d) Epidermis

324. In primary wall, cellulose microfibrils are

a. Small, loose and wavy
b. Long, loose and wavy
c. Small, compact and straight
d. Long, compact and straight

Ans. (a) Small, loose and wavy

325. Cellulose content is high in

a. Primary wall
b. Secondary wall
c. Tertiary wall
d. Middle lamella

Ans. (b) Secondary wall

326. Tertiary wall is known from

a. Compression wood of dicots
b. Tension wood of gymnosperms
c. Cotton fibres
d. All hard woods

Ans. (b) Tension wood of gymnosperms

327. Plasmodesmata were discovered by

a. Hanstein
b. Kolliker
c. Strasburger
d. Granier

Ans. (c) Strasburger

328. Part of endoplasmic reticulum present in a plasmodesma is called

a. Desmotubule
b. Cisterna
c. Vesicle
d. Myeloid body

Ans. (a) Desmotubule

329. Uncutinised and non-suberised cell wall is

a. Semipermeable
b. Permeable
c. Impermeable
d. Selectively permeable

Ans. (b) Permeable

330. Adjacent tracheids and vessels can transfer sap through thin areas in their walls called

a. Plasmodesmata
b. Gap junctions
c. Tight junctions
d. Pits

Ans. (d) Pits

331. Pits are

a. Depressions in primary walls
b. Depressions in secondary walls
c. Both a and b
d. Plasmodesmal connections

Ans. (b) Depressions in secondary walls

332. A complete pit is

a. Depression in secondary wall
b. Pit chamber and primary wall
c. Pit chambers of two adjacent cells and pit membrane
d. Pit chamber, primary wall and middle lamella

Ans. (c) Pit chambers of two adjacent cells and pit membrane

333. Pit membrane consists of

a. Primary wall
b. Middle lamella
c. Middle lamella + primary wall
d. Primary wall + middle lamella + primary wall

Ans. (d) Primary wall + middle lamella + primary wall

334. A pit present in the wall of cell lying adjacent to an intracellular space is

a. Complete pit
b. Blind pit
c. A pit without its partner
d. Both b and c

Ans. (d) Both b and c

335. A disc-shaped thickening present on the pit membrane is

a. Torus
b. Callus
c. Tylosis
d. Stoma

Ans. (a) Torus

336. Apoplast is

a. Cytoplasm and plasmalemma
b. Protoplast and plasmodesmata
c. Cell walls
d. Nonliving continuum made of free or outer spaces of cells

Ans. (d) Nonliving continuum made of free or outer spaces of cells

337. Cell coat consists of

a. Glycocalyx
b. Cellulose
c. Cellulose + Hemicellulose + Pectin
d. Protein

Ans. (a) Glycocalyx

338. Glycocalyx is

a. Glycoproteins and glycolipids
b. Oligosaccharide part of glycolipids and glycoproteins

c. lipid and protein parts of glycolipids and glycoproteins
d. mucopolysaccharides attached to cell wall

Ans. (b) Oligosaccharide part of glycolipids and glycoproteins

339. Separated cells of two sponge species are mixed up. They will

a. Remain separate
b. Aggregate tissue-wise
c. Aggregate and fuse to form hybrids
d. Aggregate species wise and reconstruct the sponges

Ans. (d) Remain separate

340. Separated cells of two vertebrates are mixed up. They will

a. Aggregate species-wise
b. Aggregate tissue-wise
c. Aggregate species-wise and then tissue-wise
d. Aggregate species-wise and then reconstruct the animals

Ans. (b) Aggregate tissue-wise

341. Glycocalyx is responsible for

a. Antigens like those of blood groups ABO
b. Immune reactions and histocompatibility
c. Hormone receptors
d. All the above

Ans. (d) All the above

342. The term protoplasm was coined by

a. Huxley   b. Purkinje
c. Dujardin   d. Schultze

Ans. (b) Purkinje

343. A unit of protoplasm having a nucleus and covered by plasmalemma is called

a. Ectoplast   b. Cell
c. Cytoplast   d. All the above

Ans. (b) Cell

344. Protoplasm is

a. Alveolar   b. Granular
c. Fibrillar   d. Crystallo-colloidal

Ans. (d) Crystallo-colloidal

345. Who proposed cryastallo-coloidal nature of protoplasm

a. Kolliker   b. Fromann
c. Velton   d. Hanstein

Ans. (a) Kolliker

346. Protoplast is

a. Granular protoplasm
b. Whole protoplasm of an organism
c. Unit of protoplasm contained in a cell
d. All the above

Ans. (c) Unit of protoplasm contained in a cell

347. The term protoplast was coined by

a. Strasburger   b. Hanstein
c. Butschli   d. Fischer

Ans. b

348. Who differentiated prokaryotic and eukaryotic cells

a. Huxley   b. Linnaeous
c. Whittaker   d. Dougherty

Ans. (d) Dougherty

349. Mesokaryotic condition was distinguished by

a. Whittaker   b. Dodge
c. Copeland   d. Haeckel

Ans. (b) Dodge

350. An akaryotic cell is

a. Single nucleated   b. Prokaryotic
c. Denucleated   d. Both b and c

Ans. (d) Both b and c

351. Protoplast excluding nucleus is called

a. Cytoplasm   b. Endoplasm
c. Ectoplasm   d. Protoplasm

Ans. (a) Cytoplasm

352. Cell structure between plasmalemma and karyotheca is

a. Vacuole   b. Nucleoplasm
c. Endoplasm   d. Cytoplasm

Ans. (d) Cytoplasm

353. Which one is an extracytoplasmic cell organelle

a. Vacuole   b. ER
c. Nucleus   d. Golgi apparatus

Ans. (c) Nucleus

354. In a membrane phospholipids, there are

a. One polar head and two nonpolar tails
b. Two polar head and one nonpolar tails
c. One nonpolar head and two polar tails
d. Two nonpolar head and one polar tails

Ans. (a) One polar head and two nonpolar tails

355. Extrinsic proteins of cell membrane are

a. Present superficially and are easily separable

b. Present superficially and are not separable

c. Attached to intrinsic proteins but are easily separable

d. Attached to intrinsic but are not easily separable

Ans. (c) Attached to intrinsic proteins but are easily separable

356. Main function of plasma membrane is to

a. Control cell movements

b. Control cell activities

c. Maintain cell shape and size

d. Regulate exchange of materials

Ans. (d) Regulate exchange of materials

357. Plasmalemma is

a. Permeable

b. Selectively permeable

c. Nonpermeable

d. Semipermeable

Ans. (b) Selectively permeable

358. The process of taking in liquid material by infolding of membrane is known as

a. Phagocytosis   b. Osmosis

c. Active transport   d. Pinocytosis

Ans. (d) Pinocytosis

359. Taking in of food particles or foreign bodies through cell membrane is

a. Phagocytosis   b. Pinocytosis

c. Osmosis   d. Active transport

Ans. (a) Phagocytosis

360. Pinocytosis was studied for the first time by

a. Metchnikoff   b. Lewis

c. Plowe   d. Nageli

Ans. (b) Lewis

361. A prokaryotic cell is characterized by

a. Cellulose cell wall

b. Single envelope system

c. Double envelope system

d. Presence of histones

Ans. (b) Single envelope system

362. Bacteria do not possess

a. DNA   b. RNA

c. Nucleus   d. Lipids

Ans. (c) Nucleus

363. Bacteria with tuft of flagella at one end is

a. Monotrichous   b. Lophotrichous

c. Peritrichous   d. Atrichous

Ans. (b) Lophotrichous

364. Vibrio cholera is

a. Monotrichous   b. Amphitrichous

c. Lophotrichous   d. Peritrichous

Ans. (a) Monotrichous

365. A bacterium is stained with Gram stain. It retains purple stain even after washing with acetone. The bacterium is

a. Gram (+)   b. Gram (–)

c. Gram neutral   d. Eosinophil

Ans. (a) Gram (+)

366. Which one is Gram (+)

a. Pseudomonas   b. Escherichia

c. Pneumococcus   d. Cyanobacteria

Ans. (c) Pneumococcus

367. A Gram (–) prokaryotic is

a. Mycoplasma   b. Rickettsia

c. Chlamydia   d. All the above

Ans. (d) All the above

368. Cell envelope is

a. Glycocalyx

b. Mucilage sheath

c. Mucilage sheath and cell wall

d. Mucilage cheath, cell wall and plasmalemma

Ans. (d) Mucilage cheath, cell wall and plasmalemma

369. Teichoic acid is present in

a. Mycobacterium   b. Haemophilus

c. Gram (+) bacteria   d. Gram (–) bacteria

Ans. (c) Gram (+) bacteria

370. Mycotic acid occurs in the wall of

a. Eubacteria   b. Actinomycetes

c. Archaebacteria   d. Blue green algae

Ans. (b) Actinomycetes

371. Periplasmic space occurs in between

a. Outer wall and inner wall

b. Outer wall membrane and inner membrane

c. Wall and plasmalemma

d. Plasmalemma and cytoplasma

Ans. (c) Wall and plasmalemma

372. Wall is

a. Single layered and wavy in Gram (–) bacteria
b. Two layered and smooth in Gram (+) bacteria
c. Two layered and wavy in Gram (+) bacteria
d. Two layered and wavy in Gram (–) bacteria

Ans. (d) Two layered and wavy in Gram (–) bacteria

373. In Gram (–) bacteria, peptidoglycan is

a. 70 – 80% and present in outer wall layer
b. 10 – 20% and present in inner wall layer
c. 10 – 20% and present in outer wall layer
d. 70 – 80% and found in inner wall layer

Ans. (b) 10 – 20% and present in inner wall layer

374. Bacterial wall contains

a. Cellulose
b. Peptidoglycan
c. Murein
d. Both B and C

Ans. (d) Both B and C

375. Murein peptidoglycan of bacterial wall is formed of

a. Glucose and peptide
b. Acetyl glucosamine and peptide
c. Acetyl muramic acid and acetyl glucosamine
d. Acetyl glucosamine and acetyl muramic acid cross linked with small peptides.

Ans. (d) Acetyl glucosamine and acetyl muramic acid cross linked with small peptides.

376. Antibiotic penicillin and cyclosporine kill bacteria by

a. Hydrolyzing pepidoglycans
b. Preventing cross-linking of acetyl glucosamine and acetyl muramic acid
c. Hydrolyzing plasmalemma
d. Preventing ATP synthesis

Ans. (b) Preventing cross-linking of acetyl glucosamine and acetyl muramic acid

377. Porins occur in

a. Outer wall of Gram (–) bacteria
b. Inner wall of Gram (–) bacteria
c. Wall of Gram (+) bacteria
d. Wall of all types of bacteria

Ans. (a) Outer wall of Gram (–) bacteria

378. Plasmalemma of bacteria contains

a. Cholesterol
b. Hopanoids
c. Cerebrosides
d. All the above

Ans. (b) Hopanoids

379. Chondriod is

a. A small mitochondrion found in prokaryotes
b. Anaerobic bacterium
c. A respiratory mesosome
d. A spiral aggregate of ribosomes

Ans. (c) A respiratory mesosome

380. Components of 70 S ribosome are

a. 50 S and 30 S
b. 50 S and 20 S
c. 40 S and 40 S
d. 40 S and 30 S

Ans. (a) 50 S and 30 S

381. Chromoplasm occurs in

a. Bacteria
b. Actinomyces
c. Cyanobacteria
d. Mycoplasma

Ans. (c) Cyanobacteria

382. Chlorosomes occur in

a. Purple bacteria
b. Cyanobacteria
c. Green bacteria
d. All the above

Ans. (c) Green bacteria

383. Chlorosomes are peculiar in having

a. Bacteriochlorophyll
b. Bacteriophaeophytin
c. Carotenoids
d. Non-unit protein membrane

Ans. (d) Non-unit protein membrane

384. Chromoneme is the term used for

a. Plasmid
b. Nucleoid
c. Genophore
d. Both B and C

Ans. (d) Both B and C

385. Prokaryotic DNA is naked because it is not

a. Covered by nuclear envelope
b. Associated with histone
c. Organized into nucleus
d. All the above

Ans. (b) Associated with histone

386. A plasmid which gets associated with nucleoid is called

a. Episome
b. Cryptic plasmid
c. Proplasmid
d. Temperate

Ans. (a) Episome

387. A bacterial cell inclusion which does not have its own covering membrane is

    a. Gas vesicle   b. Gas vacuole
    c. Sulphur granule   d. PHB granules

Ans. (b) Gas vacuole

388. Which one are called metachromatic granules?

    a. Volutin granules
    b. Magnetite granules
    c. Sulphur and iron granules
    d. All the above

Ans. (d) All the above

389. Magnetic granules occur in

    a. Aquaspirillium   b. Spirulina
    c. Cladothrix   d. Thiobacillus

Ans. (a) Aquaspirillium

390. Which one is a proteinaceous food reserve

    a. α-granules   b. β-granules
    c. Cyanophycin   d. PHB granules

Ans. (c) Cyanophycin

391. Bacterial flagella are

    a. Unistranded solid   b. Unistranded hollow
    c. Multistranded solid   d. Multistranded hollow

Ans. (b) Unistranded hollow

392. Which one takes part in bacterial conjugation

    a. Flagellum   b. Pilus
    c. Fimbria   d. Plasmodesma

Ans. (b) Pilus

393. Number of basal body rings present in Gram (–) bacteria is

    a. One   b. Two
    c. Three   d. Four

Ans. (d) Four

394. Number of network present in a plant cell wall is

    a. Three   b. Two
    c. One   d. Four

Ans. (a) Three

395. Besides cellulose microfibrils, the other two cell wall networks are

    a. Protein and hemicelluloses
    b. Hemicelluloses and protein
    c. Pectin and glycoprotein
    d. Pectin and hemicelluloses

Ans. (c) Pectin and glycoprotein

396. Mitochondria and plastids multiply through

    a. Binary fission
    b. Multiple fission
    c. Budding
    d. All the above

Ans. (a) Binary fission

397. A nonliving structure of cell is

    a. Cell wall
    b. Plasma membrane
    c. Cytoplasm
    d. Nucleus

Ans. (a) Cell wall

398. The chemical present in the cell wall is

    a. Pectin   b. Lignin
    c. Cellulose   d. All the above

Ans. (d) All the above

399. All plant cells possess

    a. Middle lamella   b. Primary wall
    c. Lysosomes   d. Centriole

Ans. (b) Primary wall

400. Middle lamella occurs

    a. Inner to primary wall
    b. Inner to secondary wall
    c. Outer to secondary wall
    d. Outer to primary wall

Ans. (d) Outer to primary wall

401. Middle lamella contains

    a. Cellulose   b. Pectate
    c. Lignin   d. Cutin

Ans. (b) Pectate

402. Matrix of cell wall is made of

    a. Pectin   b. Hemicelluloses
    c. Glycoprotein   d. Cellulose

Ans. (a) Pectin

403. Chemical absent from matrix of cell wall is

    a. Lipid   b. Water
    c. Glycoprotein   d. Cellulose

Ans. (d) Cellulose

404. The term cytoplasm was coined by

    a. Sachs   b. Strasburger
    c. Hanstein   d. Flemming

Ans. (b) Strasburger

405. Jelly-like semifluid complex of cytoplasm is called

a. Endoplast   b. Cytosol
c. Cytoplasmic matrix   d. Both b and c

Ans. (d) Both b and c

406. Plasmagel or gel part of cytosol in contact with plasmalemma is

a. Ectoplast   b. Hyaloplasm
c. Hyalosome   d. Both a and b

Ans. (a) Ectoplast

407. Plasmasol or sol part of cytosol is known as

a. Hyalosome   b. Hyaloplasm
c. Endoplast   d. Both b and c

Ans. (d) Both b and c

408. Which part of protoplast show streaming or cyclosis

a. Ectoplast   b. Endoplast
c. Endoplasmic matrix   d. Nucleoplasm

Ans. (b) Endoplast

409. Cytoplasmic streaming or cyclosis is absent in

a. Plant cells   b. Animal cells
c. Protozoan protists   d. Prokaryotes

Ans. (d) Prokaryotes

410. Cyclosis was first studied by

a. Robert brown   b. Dalton and Felix
c. Amici   d. Sachs

Ans. (c) Amici

411. Amici (1818) studied cyclosis for the first time in

a. Hydrilla   b. Amoeba
c. Chara   d. Acetabularia

Ans. (c) Chara

412. Cyclosis is caused by activity of

a. Microtubules   b. Microfilaments
c. Intermediate filaments   d. All the above

Ans. (b) Microfilaments

413. Circulation type of protoplasmic streaming is studied in

a. Stamina hair cell of Tradescantia
b. Hydrilla leaf cells
c. Vallisneria leaf cells
d. Both b and c

Ans. (a) Stamina hair cell of Tradescantia

414. In circulation streaming protoplasm moves in

a. One direction
b. Two opposite directions around a vacuole
c. Different directions around different vacuoles
d. Both a and b

Ans. (c) Different directions around different vacuoles

415. In rotation type of cyclosis, the cytoplasmic matrix flows in

a. One direction
b. Two opposite directions
c. Different directions
d. Side-ways

Ans. (a) One direction

416. The term organoid is used for

a. III defend organ   b. A distinct tissue
c. Idioblast   d. Cell organelle

Ans. (d) Cell organelle

417. A membrane-lined system of channels present throughout the cytoplasm is

a. Endoplasmic reticulum
b. Golgi apparatus
c. Microtubules
d. Both b and c

Ans. (a) Endoplasmic reticulum

418. Percentage of cell membranes contained in ER is

a. 10–20 %   b. 20–30%
c. 30–60%   d. 60–75%

Ans. (c) 30–60%

419. ER is absent in

a. Animal cells   b. Prokaryotes
c. Plant cells   d. Protista and fungi

Ans. (b) Prokaryotes

420. Eukaryotic cells devoid of ER are

a. Liver cells   b. Kidney cells
c. Mature leucocytes   d. Mature erythrocytes

Ans. (d) Mature erythrocytes

421. An intracellular structure believed to be formed by inpushing of plasmalemma is

a. Endoplasmic reticulum
b. Nuclear envelope
c. Mitochondrion
d. Chloroplasts

Ans. (a) Endoplasmic reticulum

422. Eukaryotic cells which contain very little of ER are

a. Early embryonic cells   b. Ova

c. Resting cells   d. All the above

Ans. (d) All the above

423. ER is made of

a. Cisternae   b. Tubules

c. Vesicles   d. All the above

Ans. (d) All the above

424. Spermatocytes possess ER in the form of

a. A few vesicles

b. A few tubules

c. Abundant tubules and vesicles

d. Cisternae, tubules and vesicles

Ans. (a) A few vesicles

425. Sacroplasmic reticulum is endoplasmic reticulum of

a. Adipose cells   b. Muscle cells

c. Nerve cells   d. Leucocytes

Ans. (b) Leucocytes

426. In nerve cells, ER forms

a. Myeloid bodies   b. Neurotubules

c. Nissl granules   d. Neurofilaments

Ans. (d) Neurofilaments

427. Myeloid bodies are granular structures formed of ER in

a. Retinal cells   b. Adipose cells

c. Plasma cells   d. Reticulocytes

Ans. (a) Retinal cells

428. In adipose cells, ER is represented by

a. Cisternae and tubules

b. A few tubules

c. Cisternae and vesicles

d. A few vesicles

Ans. (b) A few tubules

429. ER was discovered by

a. Palade   b. Porter et al

c. Thompson   d. Both b and c

Ans. (d) Both b and c

430. The term endoplasmic reticulum was coined by

a. Thompson   b. Palade

c. Porter   d. Garnier

Ans. (c) Porter

431. The term ergastoplasm was given to basophilic membranous structures by

a. Palade   b. Garnier

c. Schimper   d. Fleming

Ans. (b) Garnier

432. ER was discovered from

a. Liver cells   b. Kidney cells

c. Muscle cells   d. Nerve cells

Ans. (a) Liver cells

433. Membrane thickness of ER is

a. 75 Å   b. 90 Å

c. 50–60 Å   d. 30–40 Å

Ans. (c) 50–60 Å

434. ER without association with ribosomes is called

a. Transitional ER   b. SER

c. Agranal ER   d. Both b and c

Ans. (d) Both b and c

435. Rough endoplasmic reticulum is the one that contains

a. Abundant tubules

b. Association with ribosomes

c. Fenestrations

d. Both b and c

Ans. (b) Association with ribosomes

436. RER is

a. Neutrophilic   b. Acidophilic

c. Basophilic   d. Neutrogenic

Ans. (c) Basophilic

437. What is more abundant in SER

a. Cisternae and vesicles

b. Cisternae and tubules

c. Tubules and vesicles

d. Cisternae

Ans. (c) Tubules and vesicles

438. What is more abundant in RER

a. Cisternae   b. Vesicles

c. Tubules   d. Both a and b

Ans. (a) Cisternae

439. P_{450} and P_{448} occurs over

a. SER   b. RER

c. Annulate ER   d. Transitional ER

Ans. (a) SER

440. SER takes part in synthesis of

    a. Lipids and steroids   b. Vitamins

    c. Carbohydrates   d. All the above

Ans. (d) All the above

441. RER is specialized for synthesis of

    a. Local proteins

    b. Local proenzymes

    c. Proteins and proenzymes for transport

    d. Hormones

Ans. (c) Proteins and proenzymes for transport

442. Pollutants and carcinogens are detoxified by

    a. P_{450} and P_{448} b. SER in liver

    c. RER in liver   d. Both a and b

Ans. (d) Both a and b

443. Ribophorins are required for

    a. Synthesis of ribosomes in nucleolus

    b. Attachment of ribosomes over RER

    c. Attachment of ribosome subunits

    d. Attachment of mRNA to ribosomes for protein synthesis

Ans. (b) Attachment of ribosomes over RER

444. Which of the following provides mechanical support to cell

    a. Ribosomes

    b. Golgi bodies

    c. Lysosomes

    d. Endoplasmic reticulum

Ans. (d) Endoplasmic reticulum

445. Endoplasmic reticulum occurs in the form

    a. Vesicles

    b. Cisternae

    c. Tubules

    d. All the above

Ans. (d) All the above

446. Cells specialized in secretion of proteinaceous substances possess

    a. Bound ribosomes   b. Free ribosomes

    c. Abundant amino acids   d. Abundant mRNA

Ans. (a) Bound ribosomes

447. Besides proteins, ribosomes contain

    a. DNA   b. RNA

    c. Both DNA and RNA   d. Lipids

Ans. (b) RNA

448. Sedimentation unit of ribosome is

    a. μ (micron)   b. μm (milimicron)

    c. Å (Angstrom)   d. S (Svedberg)

Ans. (d) S (Svedberg)

449. Cytoribosomes of eukaryotes are different from those of bacterial cells in having

    a. Smaller size (70 S type)

    b. Larger size (80 S type)

    c. Differential chemical structure

    d. All the above

Ans. (b) Larger size (80 S type)

450. A ribosome is composed of

    a. A single unit   b. Two subunits

    c. Three subunits   d. Four subunits

Ans. (b) Two subunits

451. Ribosome develop from

    a. Nucleus   b. Nucleolus

    c. Endoplasmic reticulum d. Mitochondria

Ans. (b) Nucleolus

452. Polysome is a chain of

    a. Oxysomes   b. Sphareosomes

    c. Ribosomes   d. Dicytosomes

Ans. (c) Ribosomes

453. Enzyme peptidyl transferase occurs in

    a. Large subunit of ribosome

    b. Smaller subunit of ribosome

    c. Endoplasmic reticulum

    d. Lysosomes

Ans. (a) Large subunit of ribosome

454. Hydrolases identified from different lysosomes are

    a. 30   b. 35

    c. 50   d. 70

Ans. (c) 50

455. An enzyme often present in lysosomes and having antiseptic property is

    a. Lysozyme   b. Plasminogen activator

    c. Lipofucin   d. Both b and c

Ans. (a) Lysozyme

456. Secondary lysosome are

    a. Digestive vacuoles   b. Autophagic vacuoles

    c. Residual vacuoles   d. All the above

Ans. (d) All the above

457. Lysosomes containing inactive enzymes are called

a. Primary lysosomes
b. Secondary lysosomes
c. Autophagosomes
d. Residual bodies

Ans. (a) Primary lysosomes

458. Lysosomes alongwith food content is known as

a. Primary lysosomes   b. Secondary lysosomes
c. Microbodies   d. Residual bodies

Ans. (b) Secondary lysosomes

459. Autophagic vacuoles digest

a. Cell organelles
b. Solid particles of phagosomes
c. Fluid droplets of pinosomes
d. All the above

Ans. (a) Cell organelles

460. Residual vacuoles throw their undigested materials by

a. Pinocytosis   b. Phagocytosis
c. Ephagy   d. Diffusion

Ans. (c) Ephagy

461. Lipofuscin granules present in nerve cells are actually

a. Primary lysosomes
b. Digestive vacuoles
c. Residual bodies
d. Newly digested lipids

Ans. (c) Residual bodies

462. Cartilage matrix is digested during its osteogenesis through

a. Intracellular autophagic activity
b. Extracellular lysosomal activity
c. Intracellular heterophagic activity
d. Both b and c

Ans. (b) Extracellular lysosomal activity

463. Disease caused by hyperactivity of lysosomes is

a. Arthritis   b. Gout
c. Lung fibrosis   d. All the above

Ans. (d) All the above

464. A disease caused by reduced ephagic activity of residual bodies is

a. Hepatitis   b. Polynephritis
c. Hypertension   d. Both a and b

Ans. (d) Both a and b

465. Which one is lysosomal activity

a. Reabsorption of tadpole tail
b. Mobilization of stored substances
c. Removal of obstructions
d. All the above

Ans. (d) All the above

466. When are lysosomes extra-active

a. Seed maturation   b. Seed germination
c. Flowering   d. Fruiting

Ans. (b) Seed germination

467. Cell organelles getting stained with redox dye Janus Green is

a. Lysosome   b. Mitochondrion
c. Ribosome   d. Golgi apparatus

Ans. (b) Mitochondrion

468. An early name of mitochondrion was

a. Fila   b. Sacrosome
c. Bioplast   d. All the above

Ans. (d) All the above

469. Mitochondria were discovered by

a. Michaelis   b. Benda
c. Kolliker   d. Krebs

Ans. (c) Kolliker

470. The scientist who related mitochondria to aerobic respiration is

a. Kinsbury   b. Michaelis
c. Seekevitz   d. Fernandes-Moran

Ans. (a) Kinsbury

471. A eukaryotic aerobic cell that does not possess mitochondria is

a. Liver cell   b. Kidney cell
c. Erythrocyte   d. Leucocyte

Ans. (c) Erythrocyte

472. Single mitochondria is found in

a. Microasterias   b. Chlorella
c. Micromonas   d. All the above

Ans. (d) All the above

473. Number of mitochondria present in a sperm is

a. 4–6   b. 12–14
c. 20–24   d. 40–50

Ans. (c) 20–24

474. Number of mitochondria found in a kidney cell is

    a. 100–150   b. 300–400

    c. 500–600   d. 1000–1200

Ans. (b) 300–400

475. A liver cell contains mitochondria

    a. 500–600   b. 1000–1200

    c. 1500–2000   d. 2000–4000

Ans. (a) 500–600

476. Giant Amoeba (*Chaos chaos*) has mitochondria

    a. 5000–10000   b. 50,000

    c. 80,000   d. 100,000

Ans. (b) 50,000

477. Number of mitochondria found in flight muscle cell can be

    a. 500,000   b. 200,000

    c. 100,000   d. 50,000-100,000

Ans. (b) 200,000

478. In animal cell, a mitochondrion is

    a. Largest organelle

    b. Second largest organelle

    c. Third largest organelle

    d. None of the above

Ans. (b) Second largest organelle

479. Outer mitochondrial membrane resembles bacterial membrane and outer chloroplast membrane having

    a. Selective permeability   b. Single ion channels

    c. Porin   d. All the above

Ans. (c) Porin

480. Cristae were discovered by

    a. Palade   b. Fernandes-Moran

    c. Nass and Afzelius   d. Luck and Rich

Ans. (a) Palade

481. Power houses of the cell are

    a. ATP   b. Lysosomes

    c. Mitochondria   d. Chloroplasts

Ans. (c) Mitochondria

482. Number of oxisomes present in a mitochondrion is believed to be

    a. 10^3–10^4 b. 10^4–10^5

    c. 10^5–10^6 d. 10^6–10^7

Ans. (b) 10^4–10^5

483. In the inner mitochondrial membrane, proton channel is constituted by

    a. F_0 b. F_1

    c. NADH (H^+)   d. Cytochrome oxidase

Ans. (a) F_0

484. Mitochondrial matrix contains

    a. Enzymes   b. DNA and RNA

    c. Ribosomes   d. All the above

Ans. (d) All the above

485. Small particles attached to inner mitochondrial membrane are

    a. Ergosomes   b. Cristae

    c. Elementary particles   d. Quantasomes

Ans. (c) Elementary particles

486. Mitochondria are concerned with

    a. Oxidative phosphorylation

    b. Intermediate metabolism

    c. Krebs cycle

    d. All the above

Ans. (d) All the above

487. In prokaryotes oxidative phosphorylation is carried out by

    a. Chondriome   b. Plasma membrane

    c. Lomasome   d. Chromatophore

Ans. (b) Plasma membrane

488. Mitochondria are semi-autonomous due to

    a. Presence and functional naked DNA

    b. Presence of ribosomes

    c. Ability to divide

    d. All the above

Ans. (d) All the above

489. Pigment free plastids are

    a. Chloroplasts   b. Chromoplasts

    c. Lysosomes   d. Leucoplasts

Ans. (d) Leucoplasts

490. The term plastids was given by

    a. Schimper   b. Haeckel

    c. Hanstein   d. Strasburger

Ans. (b) Haeckel

491. All types of plastids are formed from

    a. Protoplastids   b. Leucoplasts

    c. Amyloplasts   d. Aleuroplasts

Ans. (a) Protoplastids

492. Protoplastids are found in
   a. Root cells   b. Storage cells
   c. Meristematic cells   d. Cortical cells

Ans. (c) Meristematic cells

493. The plastid which can form all other types of plastids is
   a. Leucoplast   b. Amyloplast
   c. Chloroplast   d. Chromoplast

Ans. (a) Leucoplast

494. Chromoplasts are formed from chloroplasts during
   a. Ripening of tomato   b. Ripening of chilli
   c. Development of carrot   d. Both a and b

Ans. (d) Both a and b

495. Chromoplasts are formed from leucoplasts in
   a. Rose petals   b. Carrot
   c. Dahlia florets   d. All the above

Ans. (b) Carrot

496. The plastids with irregular shape are
   a. Leucoplasts   b. Chloroplasts
   c. Chromoplasts   d. Amyloplasts

Ans. (c) Chromoplasts

497. Irregular shape of chromoplasts is due to
   a. Genetic differences
   b. Crystallization of carotenoids
   c. Formation of lipids
   d. Destruction of lamellae

Ans. (b) Crystallization of carotenoids

498. Leucoplasts are present in
   a. Green cells
   b. Pigmented cells other than green
   c. Nonpigmented cells
   d. Both a and b

Ans. (c) Nonpigmented cells

499. Organelle covered by double membrane is
   a. Nucleus   b. Mitochondrion
   c. Plastid   d. All the above

Ans. (d) All the above

500. Plastids with 3 or 4 membrane covering are found in
   a. Gymnosperms
   b. Pteridophytes
   c. Euglenoids and Brown Algae
   d. Bryophytes

Ans. (c) Euglenoids and Brown Algae

501. Plastids contain
   a. Double membrane covering
   b. DNA, RNA and ribosomes
   c. Lamellae
   d. All the above

Ans. (d) All the above

502. Starch is stored in
   a. Chromoplasts   b. Amyloplasts
   c. Chloroplasts   d. Both b and c

Ans. (d) Amyloplasts and Chloroplasts (d) Both b and c

503. Plastids storing proteins are called
   a. Elaioplasts   b. Oleosomes
   c. Aleuroplasts   d. Phaeoplasts

Ans. (c) Aleuroplasts

504. Organelle ribosomes occur in
   a. Bacteria
   b. Blue-Green algae
   c. Plastids and mitochondria
   d. Nucleus

Ans. (c) Plastids and mitochondria

505. Organelle ribosomes resembles
   a. Organelle ribosomes of prokaryotes
   b. Cytoribosomes of prokaryotes
   c. Cytoribosomes of eukaryotes
   d. All the above

Ans. (b) Cytoribosomes of prokaryotes

506. Ribosomes was first observed by
   a. Claude   b. Palade
   c. George   d. De Duve

Ans. (a) Claude

507. Palade granules are
   a. Glycoprotein particles   b. Pigment granules
   c. Excretory vesicles   d. Ribosomes

Ans. (d) Ribosomes

508. Ribosomes were discovered by
   a. Robinson and Brown   b. Thompson
   c. Perner   d. Schimper

Ans. (a) Robinson and Brown

509. Organelle and prokaryotic ribosomes are generally

    a. 80 S   b. 100 S

    c. 70 S   d. 45 S

Ans. (c) 70 S

510. Eukaryotes possess ribosomes

    a. 60 S   b. 70 S

    c. 80 S   d. Bothe b and c

Ans. (d) Bothe b and c

511. An organelle devoid of membrane covering is

    a. Lysosome   b. Peroxisome

    c. Ribosome   d. Sap vacuole

Ans. (c) Ribosome

512. Element required for bringing about union of ribosome subunit is

    a. Ca^{2+} b. Mg^{2+}

    c. Fe^{2+} d. Cu^+

Ans. (b) Mg^{2+}

513. Size of 80S, ribosome is

    a. 150–200 Å × 135–150 Å

    b. 200–290 Å × 170–210 Å

    c. 250–300 Å × 180–220 Å

    d. 300–340 Å × 200–240 Å

Ans. (d) 300–340 Å × 200–240 Å

514. Dalton weight of 70S ribosome is

    a. 2.7–3.0 million   b. 3.1–3.5 million

    c. 3.6–4.0 million   d. 4.0–4.5 million

Ans. (a) 2.7–3.0 million

515. rRNA: protein ratio of 80 S ribosome is

    a. 40–44 : 56–60

    b. 45–50 : 50–55

    c. 50–55 : 45–50

    d. 60–65 : 35–40

Ans. (a) 40–44 : 56–60

516. rRNA present in 40 S subunit of ribosome is

    a. 5 S   b. 5.8 S

    c. 28 S   d. All the above

Ans. (d) All the above

517. rRNA present in 60 S subunit of ribosome is

    a. 5 S   b. 5.8 s

    c. 28 s   d. All the above

Ans. (d) All the above

518. rRNA present in 50 S subunit of ribosome is

    a. 23 S   b. 5 S

    c. Both a and b   d. 23 S, 5.8 S and 5 S

Ans. (c) Both a and b

519. Number of proteins associated with 60 S ribosome subunit is

    a. 40   b. 34

    c. 30   d. 21

Ans. (a) 40

520. Chloramphenicol prevents protein synthesis over

    a. Prokaryotic ribosomes   b. Organelle ribosomes

    c. Both a and b   d. 80 S ribosomes

Ans. (c) Both a and b

521. Most abundant organelles of the cell are

    a. Mitochondria   b. Plastids

    c. Ribosomes   d. Microbodies

Ans. (c) Ribosomes

522. Golgi apparatus was first seen by

    a. George   b. Golgi

    c. Cajal   d. Robinson and Brown

Ans. (a) George

523. Who studied Golgi apparatus for the first time

    a. Golgi   b. George

    c. Cajal   d. Koltzoff

Ans. (a) Golgi

524. Golgi was able to differentiate Golgi apparatus through

    a. Phase contrast microscopy

    b. Metallic impregnation technique

    c. Electron microscopy

    d. Special redox dye

Ans. (b) Metallic impregnation technique

525. Golgi studied Golgi apparatus in

    a. Nerve cells of dog and fish

    b. Goblet cells of dog's stomach

    c. Nerve cells of barn owl and cat

    d. Goblet cells of barn owl and cat

Ans. (c) Nerve cells of barn owl and cat

526. Metallic stain used by Golgi was

    a. Lead acetate

    b. Osmium chloride and silver salts

c. Phosphotungstate

d. Palladium

Ans. (b) Osmium chloride and silver salts

527. Golgi apparatus was first seen under electron microscope by

a. Novikoff

b. Dalton and Felix

c. Rhodin

d. De Robertis and Franchi

Ans. (b) Dalton and Felix

528. A cell organelle with a definite polarity is

a. Ribosome   b. Mitochondrion

c. Golgi apparatus   d. Chloroplast

Ans. (c) Golgi apparatus

529. Golgi apparatus is made of

a. Cisternae   b. Tubules and vesicles

c. Golgian vacuoles d. All the above

Ans. (d) All the above

530. On which side of golgi apparatus are the membranes thin

a. Concave distal side

b. Concave proximal side

c. Convex distal side

d. Convex proximal side

Ans. (d) Convex proximal side

531. Golgian vacuoles develop from

a. Tubules

b. Convex proximal cisterna

c. Concave distal cisterna

d. Transition vesicles

Ans. (c) Concave distal cisterna

532. Golgi apparatus receives biochemicals with the help of transition vesicles formed by

a. ER

b. Plasmalemma

c. Lysosomes

d. Nuclear blebs

Ans. (a) ER

533. Number of cisternae present in Golgi apparatus of an animal cell is

a. 4–8   b. 8–13

c. 13–20   d. 20–30

Ans. (a) 4–8

534. Space between adjacent cisternae of Golgi apparatus is

a. 15 Å   b. 30 Å

c. 80–100 Å   d. 100–300 Å

Ans. (d) 100–300 Å

535. Inter-cisternal space is occupied by

a. Cytosol   b. Cementing materials

c. Fibrils   d. All the above

Ans. (d) All the above

536. Which one is the function of Golgi apparatus

a. Cell plate formation

b. Matrix formation of connective tissue

c. Secretion of tears

d. All the above

Ans. (d) All the above

537. Golgi apparatus is concerned with

a. Excretion   b. Secretion

c. ATP synthesis   d. RNA synthesis

Ans. (a) Excretion

538. Golgi complex is not found in

a. Nerve cells   b. RBCs

c. Germ cells   d. All the above

Ans. (b) RBCs

539. Golgi apparatus is found in

a. Cryptogams only   b. Phanerogams only

c. Prokaryotic cells d. Eukaryotic cells

Ans. (d) Eukaryotic cells

540. Cell organelle specialized in forming acrosome part of sperm is

a. Mitochondrion   b. Centriole

c. Peroxisome   d. Golgi apparatus

Ans. (d) Golgi apparatus

541. Amongst plants, Golgi apparatus is absent in

a. Sieve tube cells

b. Sperms of bryophytes

c. Sperms of pteridophytes

d. All the above

Ans. (d) All the above

542. Membrane flow occurs in

a. Golgi apparatus   b. ER

c. Karyotheca   d. Contractile vacuoles

Ans. (a) Golgi apparatus

543. Isolated units of Golgi apparatus found in plant cells are called

a. Golgisomes   b. Dictyosomes
c. Lipochondria   d. Cisternae

Ans. (b) Dictyosomes

544. Dictyosomes are unicisternal in

a. Fungi   b. Protistans
c. Algae   d. Bryophytes

Ans. (a) Fungi

545. Which cell organelle is involved in formation of saliva, tears and sweat

a. RER
b. SER
c. Golgi apparatus
d. Both b and c

Ans. (c) Golgi apparatus

546. Golgi apparatus takes part in synthesis of

a. Carbohydrates   b. Glycoproteins
c. Hormones   d. All the above

Ans. (d) All the above

547. Lysosomes were first seen and named by

a. De Duve   b. Palade
c. Novikoff   d. Robertson

Ans. (c) Novikoff

548. Lysosomes originated from

a. Plasmalemma   b. Golgi apparatus
c. Bothe a and b   d. RER

Ans. (b) Golgi apparatus

549. Main function of lysosomes is

a. Secretion
b. Respiration
c. Extracellular digestion
d. Intracellular digestion

Ans. (d) Intracellular digestion

550. Lysosomes are

a. All alike   b. Of three types
c. Of four types   d. Of two types

Ans. (c) Of four types

551. De Duve discovered lysosomes from

a. Orchid root cells   b. Rat liver cells
c. Rat kidney cells   d. Leaf cells

Ans. (b) Rat liver cells

552. Lysosomes are absent in animal cells

a. Erythrocytes   b. Plasma cells
c. Nerve cells   d. Muscle cells

Ans. (a) Erythrocytes

553. pH of lysosome interior is

a. 10–12   b. 8–10
c. 5–7   d. 4–5

Ans. (d) 4–5

554. The three types of plastids were named by

a. Meyer   b. Schimper
c. Hanstein   d. Pyrenoids

Ans. (b) Schimper

555. Autoplasts of Meyer are

a. Leucoplasts   b. Proplastids
c. Chloroplasts   d. Both a and b

Ans. (c) Chloroplasts

556. Structural elements of chloroplasts are

a. Plastoglobuli
b. Photosynthetic pigments
c. Thylakoids
d. Quantosomes

Ans. (c) Thylakoids

557. Thylakoids of chloroplasts are also called

a. Lamellae   b. Fret membranes
c. Loculi   d. Grana

Ans. (a) Lamellae

558. In a chloroplasts. The photosynthetic pigments occur

a. In matrix
b. Grana
c. Membranes of thylakoids
d. Loculi and fret channels of thylakoids

Ans. (c) Membranes of thylakoids

559. Grana are present in

a. Mitochondria   b. Chloroplasts
c. Golgi bodies   d. Ribosomes

Ans. (b) Chloroplasts

560. Grana are

a. Protein storing plastids
b. Coloured plastids
c. Stacks og thylakoids
d. Individual thylakoids present in stroma

Ans. (c) Stacks og thylakoids

561. Number of grana present in a chloroplast is

    a. 10–20   b. 20–30

    c. 30–40   d. 40–60

Ans. (d) 40–60

562. Number of thylakoids present in a granum is

    a. 10–100   b. 5–10

    c. 100–200   d. 200–500

Ans. (a) 10–100

563. Particles of thylakoid membranes involved in ATP synthesis are called

    a. Quantosomes   b. CF_0–CF_1

    c. Photosystems   d. Pyrenoids

Ans. (b) CF_0–CF_1

564. Structure associated with chloroplast of green algae is

    a. Pyrenoid   b. Stigma

    c. Both a and b   d. Endoplasmic reticulum

Ans. (c) Both a and b

565. Plastids which provide bright colour to the flowers and fruits are

    a. Chloroplasts   b. Leucoplasts

    c. Chromoplasts   d. Proplastids

Ans. (c) Chromoplasts

566. Peroxisomes and glyoxisomes are

    a. Energy transforming organelles

    b. Membrane-less organelles

    c. Macrobodies

    d. Microbodies

Ans. (d) Microbodies

567. Which one is a microbody

    a. Sphaerosome   b. Lysosome

    c. Peroxisome   d. All the above

Ans. (c) Peroxisome

568. Organelle covered by a single membrane is

    a. Sphareosomes   b. Peroxisomes

    c. Glyoxisomes   d. All the above

Ans. (d) All the above

569. Microbody present only in plants is

    a. Sphareosomes   b. Peroxisomes

    c. Glyoxisomes   d. Both b and c

Ans. (c) Glyoxisomes

570. Microbodies resemble mitochondria in

    a. Using oxygen

    b. Producing reducing power

    c. Having catalase

    d. Formation of ATP

Ans. (a) Using oxygen

571. Microbodies differ from mitochondria in

    a. Single membrane   b. Absence of DNA

    c. Direct oxidation   d. All the above

Ans. (d) All the above

572. New spherosomes develop from

    a. Old sphaerosomes   b. ER

    c. Golgi apparatus   d. Prospherosomes

Ans. (b) ER

573. Spherosomes are involved in

    a. Utilization of alcohol

    b. Storage of fat

    c. Synthesis and storage of fat

    d. Synthesis and storage of carbohydrates

Ans. (c) Synthesis and storage of fat

574. Scientist credited with discovery of spherosome is

    a. Rhodin   b. Perner

    c. Koltzokk   d. Claude

Ans. (b) Perner

575. An organelle reported to have lysosomal activity in plants is

    a. Sphaerosome   b. Glyoxisome

    c. Peroxisome   d. All the above

Ans. (a) Sphaerosome

576. A cell organelle called uricosome is

    a. Lysosome   b. Sphaerosome

    c. Peroxisome   d. Glyoxysome

Ans. (c) Peroxisome

577. Microbodies possess

    a. Hydrolases   b. Oxidases

    c. Isomerases   d. All the above

Ans. (b) Oxidases

578. Peroxisome was discovered by

    a. De Duve   b. Rhodin

    c. De Roertis and Franchi d. Beevers

Ans. (a) De Duve

579. Cell organelle having enzyme uricase or urate oxidase is

    a. Lysosome   b. Glyoxisome

    c. Peroxisome   d. Sphaerosome

Ans. (c) Peroxisome

580. Major function of peroxisomes is oxidation of

    a. Excess purine   b. Surplus amino acids

    c. Alcohol and drugs d. All the above

Ans. (d) All the above

581. Glyoxisomes occur in

    a. Leaf cells   b. Fatty seeds

    c. Roots   d. Meristematic cells

Ans. (b) Fatty seeds

582. Glyoxisomes are useful in

    a. Converting sugars to fats

    b. Converting fats to sugars

    c. Deamination and converting amino acids to fatty acids

    d. Amination and changing fatty acids to amino acids

Ans. (b) Converting fats to sugars

583. The term cytoskeleton was given by

    a. Koltzoff   b. Rhodin

    c. Menke   d. Park

Ans. (a) Koltzoff

584. The term microtubule was coined by

    a. De Robertis and Franchi b. Mayer

    c. Palade   d. Slautterback

Ans. (d) Slautterback

585. A microtubule has a diameter of

    a. 100 Å   b. 150 Å

    c. 250 Å   d. 100 nm

Ans. (c) 250 Å

586. A microtubule is made of

    a. Protofilaments   b. Microfilaments

    c. Microfibrils   d. Elementary fibrils

Ans. (a) Protofilaments

587. Number of protofilaments in a microtubule is

    a. 10   b. 13

    c. 16   d. 18

Ans. (b) 13

588. Microtubules are formed of a protein called

    a. Tubulin   b. Actin

    c. Flagellin   d. Myosin

Ans. (a) Tubulin

589. Microtubules are present in

    a. Bacteria   b. Viruses

    c. Eukaryotic cells   d. Mycoplasma

Ans. (c) Eukaryotic cells

590. Protein tubulin occurs in microtubules as

    a. Monomers   b. Homodimers

    c. Heterodimers   d. Heteropolymers

Ans. (c) Heterodimers

591. Microtubule assembly is inhibited by

    a. GTP   b. Ca^{2+}

    c. Mg^{2+} d. Colchicine

Ans. (d) Colchicine

592. Microtubule assembly is promoted by

    a. Calmodulin   b. GTP

    c. Ca^{2+} and Mg^{2+} d. All the above

Ans. (d) All the above

593. Microfilaments were discovered by

    a. Slautterback

    b. Paleviz et al

    c. Altman

    d. Ledbetter and Porter

Ans. (b) Paleviz et al

594. Diameter of a microfilament is

    a. 5–6 nm   b. 10 nm

    c. 15 nm   d. 25 nm

Ans. (a) 5–6 nm

595. Microfilaments are required for

    a. Movement of flagella and cilia

    b. Cell polarity

    c. Sol-gel changes

    d. All the above

Ans. (c) Sol-gel changes

596. Cell polarity is determined by

    a. Intermediate filaments

    b. Microtubules

    c. Protofilaments

    d. Centrioles

Ans. (b) Microtubules

597. Cytoskeleton components that determine orientation of cellulose microfibrils are

    a. Microfilaments

    b. Microtubules

    c. Intermediate filaments

    d. Basal bodies

Ans. (b) Microtubules

598. Which one provides support to microvilli, membrane ruffling and pseudopodia

    a. Microfilaments

    b. Desmin and vimentin filaments

    c. Microtubules

    d. ER

Ans. (a) Microfilaments

599. The contractile constituent of cytoskeleton is

    a. Microtubules

    b. Intermediate filaments

    c. Microfilaments

    d. Microfibrils

Ans. (c) Microfilaments

600. The diameter of intermediate filament is

    a. 1 nm   b. 5 nm

    c. 7–8 nm   d. 10 nm

Ans. (d) 10 nm

601. Tonofibrils are

    a. Intermediate filaments

    b. Microfilaments

    c. Cross-linked microtubules

    d. Both a and b

Ans. (a) Intermediate filaments

602. In nerve fibres, intermediate filaments form

    a. Neurotubules   b. Neurofilaments

    c. Neurofibrils   d. Dendrites

Ans. (c) Neurofibrils

603. In muscle cells, intermediate filaments produce

    a. Z-line   b. M-line

    c. H-line   d. Both a and b

Ans. (d) Both a and b

604. Centrioles are found

    a. Singly   b. Pairs

    c. Triplets   d. Quadruplets

Ans. (b) Pairs

605. The centriole pair occurs in a complex called

    a. Centrosome   b. Centromere

    c. Kinetochore   d. Basal plate

Ans. (a) Centrosome

606. The two centrioles of a pair occur

    a. Parallel to each other

    b. At right angles to each other

    c. At an angle other than 90°

    d. End to end

Ans. (b) At right angles to each other

607. Each centriole has on its periphery MTOCs called

    a. Spokes

    b. Pericentriolar thickenings

    c. Massules

    d. Both a and b

Ans. (c) Massules

608. Centrosome was discovered by

    a. Boveri   b. Porter

    c. Thompson   d. Schimper

Ans. (a) Boveri

609. Cell organelle having a cartwheel constitution is

    a. Centriole and basal body b. Microtubule

    c. Microfilament   d. Basal plate

Ans. (a) Centriole and basal body

610. The pattern of organization in centrioles is

    a. 9 + 2   b. 9 + 3

    c. 9 + 0   d. 9 + 1

Ans. (c) 9 + 0

611. In ultrastructure blepharoplasts resemble

    a. Centrioles   b. Flagella

    c. Cilia   d. None of the above

Ans. (a) Centrioles

612. Subfibres of cilia and flagella are made of

    a. Tubulin   b. Elastin

    c. Myosin   d. Actin

Ans. (a) Tubulin

613. Pattern of organization of eukaryotic cilia and flagella is

    a. 9 + 0   b. 9 + 1

    c. 9 + 2   d. 9 + 3

Ans. (c) 9 + 2

614. Bacterial flagellum is made of

a. Flagellin
b. Actin
c. Elastin
d. Myosin

Ans. (a) Flagellin

615. Number of microtubules present in a centriole is

a. 20
b. 25
c. 27
d. 18

Ans. (c) 27

616. Number of microtubules found in cilium or flagellum is

a. 11
b. 13
c. 18
d. 20

Ans. (d) 20

617. Doublet fibrils of a cilium or flagellum are tilted at an angle of

a. 5°
b. 10°
c. 15°
d. 20°

Ans. (b) 10°

618. Triplet fibrils of a centriole are tilted at an angle of

a. 40°
b. 30°
c. 20°
d. 10°

Ans. (a) 40°

619. Which microtubule or subfibre of the triplet disappears while passing through basal plate

a. C
b. A
c. B
d. None of the above

Ans. (a) C

620. Number of dynein arms

a. Four attached to subfibre B
b. Two attached to subfibre B
c. Two attached to subfibre A
d. Four attached to subfibre A

Ans. (c) Two attached to subfibre A

621. Cilium or flagellum is structurally bilateral due to presence of

a. Central sheath
b. Singlet fibrils
c. Double bridge
d. Both b and c

Ans. (d) Both b and c

CHECK YOU GRASP

1. **The stage at which cytokinesis begins in plant cell is**

   a. Anaphase   b. Telophase
   c. G_0 phase   d. Interphase

2. **The stage at which cleavage or cytokinesis begins in animal cells is**

   a. Anaphase   b. Telophase
   c. G_0 phase   d. Interphase

3. **Meiosis is studied in smears of**

   a. Developing anthers
   b. Testes
   c. Both a and b
   d. Axillary buds

4. **Chromosome syndesis or bivalent formation occurs in**

   a. Leptotene   b. Zygotene
   c. Pachytene   d. Diplotene

5. **Separation of chromosome daughters takes place at**

   a. Telophase   b. Metaphase
   c. Anaphase   d. Prophase

6. **Amitosis was discovered by Remak in**

   a. 1841   b. 1855
   c. 1880   d. 1905

7. **Mitosis is usually studied in smears or sections of**

   a. Root tips
   b. Stem tips
   c. Floral buds
   d. All the above

8. **Mitosis takes place in**

   a. All types of cells except those involved in gamete formation
   b. Gonads
   c. Axillary buds situated near the apical bud
   d. Cells of mature leaf

9. **Homologous chromosomes separate during**

   a. Prophase I   b. Prophase II
   c. Metaphase I   d. Anaphase I

10. **Bouquet stage occurs during**

    a. Leptotene   b. Zygotene
    c. Pachytene   d. Diplotene

11. **Large plant cells are**

    a. Xylem vessel cells   b. Parenchyma cells
    c. Sieve tube cells   d. Sclerenchyma fibres

12. **Study of the cell structure under microscope is**

    a. Cytology   b. Cell biology
    c. Cytochemistry   d. Microanatomy

13. **Study of cells in all aspects is**

    a. Cytotaxonomy   b. Cytology
    c. Cell biology   d. Cytochemistry

14. **Schleiden and Schwann proposed cell theory in**

    a. 1836–37   b. 1838–39
    c. 1901–02   d. 1938–39

15. **Minimum cell size seen under light microscope is**

    a. 1 µm   b. 0.1 µm
    c. 0.25 µm   d. 0.5 µm

In case of less than 80% score, go through brief Review and Glance one again from chapter

Key: 1-a 2-a 3-c 4-b 5-c 6-b 7-a 8-a 9-d 10-a 11-d 12-a 13-c 14-b 15-c

2

Molecular Biology

1. **A palindrome is a sequence of nucleotides in DNA that**
   a. Has local symmetry and may serve as recognition site for various protein
   b. Is a structural gene
   c. Is part of the introns of eukaryotic genes
   d. Is highly reiterated

Ans. (a) Has local symmetry and may serve as recognition site for various protein

2. **A polypeptide having 15 amino acid residues can form any of the**
   a. 15 amino acid sequences
   b. 15^{20} amino acid sequences
   c. 20^{15} amino acid sequences
   d. None of these

Ans. (c) 20^{15} amino acid sequences

3. **A transitioin mutation**
   a. Occurs when a purine is substituted from a pyrimidine of vice-versa
   b. Result from insertion of one or two bases in to the DNA chain
   c. Always a missense mutation
   d. Results from the substitution of one purine for another or of one pyrimidine for another

Ans. (d) Results from the substitution of one purine for another or of one pyrimidine for another

4. **Acetylcholine receptor is**
   a. Cl^- channel
   b. Na^+ channel
   c. Ca^{+2} channel
   d. K^+ channel

Ans. (b) Na^+ channel

5. **ADAR is an enzyme which plays a significant role in**
   a. RNA editing in prokaryotes
   b. RNA editing in eukaryotes
   c. 5′ capping
   d. Chromatin remodelling

Ans. (b) RNA editing in eukaryotes

6. **Addition of manose-6-phosphate to a protein results in its location in**
   a. Lysosome
   b. Ribosome
   c. Golgi body
   d. Nuclei

Ans. (a) Lysosome

7. **Agar-Agar is the polymer of**
   a. Galactose
   b. Glucose
   c. Fructose
   d. Xylose

Ans. (a) Galactose

8. **Alcohol is used as disinfectant because it can destroy the surrounding bacteria by breaking**
   a. Hydrogen bonds of bacterial protein
   b. Ionic bonds of bacterial protein
   c. Hydrophobic and disulphide bonds of bacterial protein
   d. None of these

Ans. (b) Ionic bonds of bacterial protein

9. **Alfalfa is used as biofertilizer due to presence of**
   a. Sinorhizobium
   b. Rhizobium
   c. Mesorhizobium
   d. Azorhizobium

Ans. (a) Sinorhizobium

10. **All the amino acids are specified by more than one codon *except***
    a. Phenylalanine and tyrosine
    b. Tryptophan and serine
    c. Methionine and tryptophan
    d. Alanine and tyrosine

Ans. (c) Methionine and tryptophan

11. **Amino acid sequence for a protein is known, we can estimate the sequence of m-RNA coding that protein**
    a. Precisely
    b. Can't be predicted

c. Precisely to certain extent if codon frequency is known

d. Data not sufficient

Ans. (c) **Precisely to certain extent if codon frequency is known**

12. **Amino acids are translocated by intestinal epithelial cells by**

a. K+/ amino acid co-transporters

b. Na+/ amino acid co-transporters

c. H+/ amino acid co-transporters

d. Amino acid / glucose anti porters

Ans. (b) **Na+/ amino acid co-transporters**

13. **Among closely lying cells signal are communicated by**

a. Hormones

b. Gap junction

c. Neurotransmitters

d. Cell membrane protein

Ans. (b) **Gap junction**

14. **Among the following enzymes which is not involved in DNA replication process**

a. RNA polymerase   b. DNA polymerase

c. Ligase   d. Helicase

Ans. (a) **RNA polymerase**

15. **Among the following which mutagen induces formation of thymidine dimmers in DNA**

a. Nitrous oxide

b. Ethylmethyl sulphate

c. UV light

d. Ethydium bromide

Ans. (c) **UV light**

16. **An operon is inducible means**

a. The operon is for catabolic process

b. The operon is for anabolic process

c. There is another operator in the system

d. None of these

Ans. (a) **The operon is for catabolic process**

17. **V. Ramakrishnan shared noble prize for chemistry in the year 2009 for describing the detailed structure of**

a. 50s ribosomal subunit

b. 40s ribosomal subunit

c. 30s ribosomal subunit

d. None of these

Ans. (c) **30s ribosomal subunit**

18. **Bacterial DNA polymerase I can cause nick translation. This property of the enzyme is due to**

a. $3' \rightarrow 5'$exonuclease activity

b. $3' \rightarrow 5'$polymerase activity

c. $5' \rightarrow 3'$exonuclease activity

d. $5' \rightarrow 3'$ polymerase activity

Ans. (c) **$5' \rightarrow 3'$exonuclease activity**

19. **Biologically not common but sometimes playing regulatory role in gene expression, the DNA is**

a. B-form   b. Z-form

c. E-form   d. All of the above

Ans. (b) **Z-form**

20. **CAAT box and GC box are component of the promoter of**

a. Halo bacteria   b. Arabidopsis

c. mycoplasma   d. Bacteria

Ans. (b) **Arabidopsis**

21. **Ca+2 binding proteins is**

a. Tropomysosin   b. Myosin

c. Actin   d. Troponin

Ans. (d) **Troponin**

22. **Calmodulin, a calcium binding protein, is found in living organisms except**

a. Prokaryotes   b. Eukaryotes

c. Plant   d. Animals

Ans. (a) **Prokaryotes**

23. **Which of the following sequences least a averages the compounds named in order of increasing molecular weight?**

a. DNA, NAD, ADP, ATP

b. Alanine, ATP, NAD, DNA

c. Alanine, ATP, DNA, NAD

d. ATP, alanine, DNA, NAD

Ans. (b) **Alanine, ATP, NAD, DNA**

24. **c-AMP is directly involved in regulation of**

a. GTP   b. ATP

c. PFK   d. Protein kinase A

Ans. (d) **Protein kinase A**

25. **The snuffiest who first synthesized DNA in vitro was**

a. A garrod   b. J. D watson

c. A K frnberg   d. Ochoa

Ans. (c) **A K frnberg**

26. CD 4 receptors are specialized for

a. MHC I
b. MHC II
c. CDK
d. Ig G

Ans. (b) MHC II

27. The nitrogen bases in DNA are

a. AUGC
b. UTGC
c. ATGC
d. ATUC

Ans. (c) ATGC

28. RNA is absent in

a. Ribosome
b. Chromosom
c. Plasma membrane
d. Cytoplasm

Ans. (d) Cytoplasm

29. Cdk-1/cyclin A complex acts at

a. S to G2 transition
b. G1 to S transition point
c. Restriction point
d. G2 to M transition point

Ans. (a) S to G2 transition

30. Cdk-1, with cyclin B acts at

a. G1 phase
b. G2 phase
c. S phase
d. M phase

Ans. (d) M phase

31. Cdk4/cyclin D complex acts on

a. Cell cycle progression through S pahse
b. Restriction point
c. G1/S transition
d. G2/M transition

Ans. (b) Restriction point

32. β-1,4 glycosidic linkage is not found in

a. Sucrose
b. Fructose
c. Maltose
d. Lacose

Ans. (a) Sucrose

33. Who was awarded Nobel Prize for the synthesis of RNA in 1959?

a. A K frnberg
b. H. Khorna
c. S. Ochoa
d. Nirenbirg

Ans. (a) S. Ochoa

34. Cellular proteins are degraded by

a. Cyclosomes
b. Chymotripsins
c. Proteasomes
d. Lysosomes

Ans. (c) Proteasomes

35. Fuelgen reaction is a specific test for establishing the presence of

a. RNA
b. DNA
c. Sugar
d. Protein

Ans. (b) DNA

36. Change from purine to pyrimidine or pyrimidine to purine is

a. Transversion
b. Transitition
c. Deletion
d. Frame-shift

Ans. (a) Transversion

37. Codon degeneracy has evolutionary significance because

a. It reduces the number of t-RNA performing translation for 61 codon
b. It creates new reading frame and promotes formation of new polypeptides
c. It maintains wild-type eliminating lethal affects of mutation
d. None of these

Ans. (c) It maintains wild-type eliminating lethal affects of mutation

38. Colchicines treated cells are arrested in

a. Meta phase
b. G1 phase
c. S phase
d. G2 phase

Ans. (a) Meta phase

39. Cooperativity effect in proteins is the result of

a. Tertiary structure of protein
b. Quaternary structure of protein
c. Secondary structure of protein
d. All of these

Ans. (b) Quaternary structure of protein

40. COP II vesicle transport proteins froms

a. Rough ER to the golgi
b. From the cis golgi to the rough ER
c. From plasma membrane and the trans golgi to late endosomes
d. From trans golgi to the lysosome

Ans. (a) Rough ER to the golgi

41. Copy error mutation is an example of

a. Transition
b. Transversion
c. Frameshift
d. Deletion

Ans. (a) Transition

42. Copy error mutation is thought to occur due to

a. Tautomeric shift
b. Nitous oxide
c. UV rays
d. DNA methylation

Ans. (a) Tautomeric shift

43. Crossing over is not found in

a. Male drosophila
b. Maize
c. Evening primrose
d. Female drosophila

Ans. (a) Male drosophila

44. Crossing over occurs at

a. Pachytene
b. Diplotene
c. Zygotene
d. Leptotene

Ans. (a) Pachytene

45. C-value paradox is

a. Percentage of junk DNA in eukaryotes
b. Lack of correlation between genome size and complexity
c. Correct correlation between genome size and complexity
d. None of these

Ans. (b) Lack of correlation between genome size and complexity

46. C-value refers to

a. Diploid level of DNA
b. Haploid level of DNA
c. Triploidy
d. Polyploidy

Ans. (b) Haploid level of DNA

47. Cytoplasmic polyadenylation is a criticl aspect of gene expression in

a. Early embryo cell death
b. Programmed cell death
c. Aging
d. Cancer cells

Ans. (a) Early embryo cell death

48. Cytoplasmic streaming is associated with

a. Microtubules
b. Microfilaments
c. Intermediate filament
d. None of these

Ans. (b) Microfilaments

49. Cytoplasmic streaming results in to mobility of substances and organelles it involves interaction of

a. Tubulin, myosin
b. Actin, myosin
c. Tubulin kinesin
d. Actin, kinesin

Ans. (b) Actin, myosin

50. Degeneracy of the genetic code denotes the existence of

a. Multiple amino acids for a single codon
b. Codons that include one or more of the unusual bases
c. Cocoons consisting of only two bases
d. Multiple amino acids for a single amino acid

Ans. (d) Multiple amino acids for a single amino acid

51. You have isolated a motile, gram positive cell with no visible nucleus, you can assume this cell has

a. Ribosome
b. Mitochondria
c. Golgi complex
d. ER

Ans. (a) Ribosome

52. Dicentric bridges are formed in

a. Reciprocal translocation
b. Pericentric inversion
c. Paracentric inversion
d. Terminal deletion

Ans. (c) Paracentric inversion

53. X-rays induce mutagenic changes mainly by

a. Chromosomal breakage
b. Transition
c. Frame shifting
d. Transversion

Ans. (a) Chromosomal breakage

54. Disulfide bond formation in proteins takes place in

a. Smooth ER
b. Rough ER
c. Golgi complex
d. Cytosol

Ans. (b) Rough ER

55. Disulphide bond can not be formed within cytosol because

a. It's environment is highly reducing due to presence of free radicals
b. It's environment is highly reducing due to presence of glutathione
c. It lacks PDI
d. None of these

Ans. (b) It's environment is highly reducing due to presence of glutathione

56. DNA fossile are

a. Very primitive sequence of DNA
b. DNA is extracted from fossils
c. Inactive transposons in human genome
d. All of the above

Ans. (c) Inactive transposons in human genome

57. DNA gyrase is inhibited by

a. Puromycin
b. Streptomycin
c. Nalidixic acid
d. All of the above

Ans. (c) Nalidixic acid

58. Wobble hypothesis explains that

a. A single t-RNA molecule can recognize more than one codon
b. In mitochondria genetic code does not follow universal rule of genetic code
c. In some viruses and bacteria genetic code is overlapping
d. None of these

Ans. (a) A single t-RNA molecule can recognize more than one codon

59. DNA in the form of minicircles and maxicircles is found in

a. Chloroplast genome
b. Mitochondrial genome
c. Apicoplast
d. Kinetoplast

Ans. (d) Kinetoplast

60. DNA replication occurs in 5'-3' direction because

a. It enhances fidelity of the DNA
b. It is thermodynamically favourable
c. DNA is right handed
d. It reduces mismatch pairing

Ans. (b) It is thermodynamically favourable

61. Double stranded DNA break can be repaired by

a. Homologous recombination
b. Mismatch repair
c. Nucleotide excision repair
d. Direct repair

Ans. (a) Homologous recombination

62. Down's syndrome results in mental retardation in human. This condition is characterized by having

a. Monosomy for 21
b. Trisomy for chromosome X
c. Trisomy for chromosome Y
d. Trisomy for chromosome 21

Ans. (d) Trisomy for chromosome 21

63. Drug detoxification occur in

a. Rough ER
b. Smooth ER
c. Glyoxysomes
d. Peroxisomes

Ans. (b) Smooth ER

64. During cell division the transition of the cell into the S phase is controlled by?

a. CDK2
b. CDK1
c. CDK25
d. CDK4/CDK5

Ans. (a) CDK2

65. During chromatid separation microtubules attached to the

a. Telomere
b. Kinetochore
c. Centromere
d. Secondary construction

Ans. (c) Centromere

66. During DNA replication in eukaryotes RNA primers are removed by

a. RNase H
b. DNA Polymerase I
c. DNA polymerase II
d. RNA polymerase I

Ans. (a) RNase H

67. During DNA synthesis frame reading is form

a. 3'–5'
b. 5'–3'
c. Both simultaneously
d. None of these

Ans. (a) 3'-5'

68. During glycosylation of protein the oligosaccharide groups are modified by

a. Glycosidase
b. Glycosyl transferases
c. Proteases
d. None of these

Ans. (b) Glycosyl transferases

69. During meiosis centromere divides at

a. Metaphase
b. Anaphase
c. Teleophase
d. Anaphase II

Ans. (d) Anaphase II

70. During meiosis cohesion protein is broken down at

a. Anaphase I
b. Anaphase II
c. metaphase
d. interkinesis

Ans. (b) Anaphase II

71. During photoreactivation reaction DNA photolyase utilizes

a. Red light
b. Blue light
c. Far red light
d. Green light

Ans. (b) Blue light

72. During RNA processing splicing is mediated by

a. m-RNA
b. r-RNA
c. t-RNA
d. Sn RNA

Ans. (d) Sn RNA

73. During termination of protein synthesis the release factor RF3 recognizes

a. UAA
b. UAG
c. Both UAA and UAG
d. UGA and UAA

Ans. (d) UAG

74. During transcription holoenzyme RNA polymerase binds to a DNA sequence and the DNA assumes a saddle-like structure at that point. What is the sequence called?

a. AAAT box
b. CAAT box
c. TATA box
d. GGTT box

Ans. (c) TATA box

75. During transcription RNA polymerase binds to the

a. Promoter
b. Operator
c. Structural
d. Regulator

Ans. (a) Promoter

76. During translation proof reading activity is performed by

a. Ribosome
b. Aminoacyl transfer RNA synthetase
c. Translation factor
d. Peptidyl transferase

Ans. (b) Aminoacyl transfer RNA synthetase

77. Enhancers of eukaryotic gene may have a special form of DNA called

a. A-DNA
b. C-DNA
c. B-DNA
d. Z-DNA

Ans. (d) Z-DNA

78. Epinephrine plays its role in glycogenolysis by

a. Activating glycogen synthase
b. Activating phophorylase kinase
c. Inactivating adenylyl cyclase
d. None of these

Ans. (b) Activating phophorylase kinase

79. Epinephrine promotes glycogenolysis there by

a. Hydrolysizing cAMP
b. Synthesizing c-AMP
c. Inactivating G-protein
d. Inactivating Adenylyl cyclase

Ans. (b) Synthesizing c-AMP

80. Eukaryotic chromosomes are transcriptionally most active during

a. Prophase
b. Metaphase
c. Anaphase
d. Interphase

Ans. (d) Interphase

81. Eukaryotic organisms lack

a. DNA photolyase
b. DNA glycosylase
c. AP endonuclease
d. Excinucleases

Ans. (a) DNA photolyase

82. Eukaryotic transcription

a. Is independent of the presence of consensus sequences upstream from the start of transcription.
b. May involve a promoter located with in the region transcribed rather than upstream
c. Is affected by enhancer sequences only if they are adjacent to the promoter
d. None of the these

Ans. (b) May involve a promoter located with in the region transcribed rather than upstream

83. With which of the following base compositions will the Tm be highest in a double-stranded DNA molecule?

a. 30% thymine
b. 25% guanine
c. 5% thymine
d. 5% guanine

Ans. (c) 5% thymine

84. Full expression of the lac operon requires

a. Allolactose
b. Lactose
c. Lactose and c-AMP
d. Allolactose and c-AMP

Ans. (b) Lactose

85. G band corresponds to large regions of the human genome that have unusually

a. Low A + T content
b. High A + T content
c. Low G + C content
d. High G + C content

Ans. (d) High G + C content

86. Which statement is not true for DNA transcription?

a. Template strand is used as coding strand
b. Transcription is in 5'–3' direction
c. Template strand and m-RNA have complementary
d. None of these

Ans. (a) Template strand is used as coding strand

87. Genetic code is not degenerate for

a. Leucine
b. Isoleucine
c. Glycine
d. Cysteine

Ans. (c) Glycine

88. Guide RNA are involved in

a. Cutting event of m-RNA
b. RNA editing
c. End modification of hn-RNA
d. Splicing

Ans. (b) RNA editing

89. Histones are replaced by protamines in

a. Nerve cell
b. Muscle cell
c. Heart cell
d. Sperm cell

Ans. (d) Sperm cell

90. Holiday junction are formed during

a. DNA replication
b. DNA repair
c. Chromosomal aberration
d. Recombination

Ans. (d) Recombination

91. Holiday structure is used to explain

a. Site specific recombination
b. Homologous recombination
c. Gene transfer
d. Nonhomologous recombination

Ans. (b) Homologous recombination

92. Holocentric chromosomes are found in

a. Man
b. Luzula
c. Chimpanzee
d. Birds

Ans. (b) Luzula

93. Hopanoids are sterol like-molecules which are found in the plasma membrane of

a. Fungi
b. Mycoplasma
c. Archaebacteria
d. Certain bacteria and cyanobacteria

Ans. (d) Certain bacteria and cyanobacteria

94. How many kinetochores are present in a human cell?

a. 41
b. 42
c. 45
d. 46

Ans. (d) 46

95. How many linkage groups are found in human cell?

a. 21
b. 22
c. 23
d. 24

Ans. (d) 24

96. If there is 20% cytosine in DNA, what is the percentage of adenine?

a. 35%
b. 30%
c. 45%
d. 40%

Ans. (b) 30%

97. If there is mutation in cdk/cyclin, the key molecule in regulating the cell cycle, then

a. There would be uncontrolled growth
b. Cells will arrest to G_0 phase
c. The level of cdki/cyclins will enhance
d. Cell will not pass to S phase

Ans. (a) There would be uncontrolled growth

98. In an intact cell the DNA double helix is right handed because

a. The bases are asymmetric
b. It consists of D-ribose only
c. It is more stable than left handed
d. None of these

Ans. (b) It consists of D-ribose only

99. In B-DNA the distance between two base pair is

a. 0.24
b. 0.35
c. 0.34
d. 0.45

Ans. (c) 0.34

100. In cell–cycle centrioles replicate in

a. G1- phase
b. G2-phase
c. S-phase
d. M-phase

Ans. (c) S-phase

101. In cell cycle which of the following is usually not a check point?

a. G2-check point
b. G1-check point
c. S-check point
d. None of these

Ans. (c) S-check point

102. In comparison to their natural environments biologically active cell are

a. Hypotonic
b. Hypertonic
c. Isotonic
d. Vary from condition to condition

Ans. (b) Hypertonic

103. In culture, cells may reversibly be arrested in the mitotic phase by treatment with

a. Radiation   b. Gentamycin

c. Colchicines   d. Mitomycin-C

Ans. (c) Colchicines

104. In DNA the histone responsible for higher order chromatin structure is

a. H1   b. H2A

c. H2B   d. H3 AND H4

Ans. (a) H1

105. In humans t-RNA genes are transcribed by

a. RNA Polymerase I

b. RNA polymerase II

c. RNA polymerase III

d. All of the above

Ans. (c) RNA polymerase III

106. In lac operon CAP binding site is found

a. Upstream the RNA binding site

b. Downstream the RNA binding site

c. Any where the RNA binding site

d. Structural gene

Ans. (a) Upstream the RNA binding site

107. Which sequence is the best target for damage by UV radiation

a. AGGCAAA   b. AGGCAAA

c. GUAAAAU   d. CTTTTGA

Ans. (d) CTTTTGA

108. Kinetochore is a proteinaceous structure of centromere. It is important for cell division because

a. It causes spindle formation

b. Microtubules attach to kinetochore during separation of chromosome

c. It causes spindle formation

d. None of these

Ans. (b) Microtubules attach to kinetochore during separation of chromosome

109. Lactose operon is both negatively and positively regulated, this means that lactose is used

a. Along with glucose

b. After glucose has been used

c. Preferentially

d. All of these

Ans. (b) After glucose has been used

110. DNA replication under going in an E.Coli cell resulted into two circular DNAs interlocked with each other; this may be due to a defective gene encoding

a. Primase

b. DNA topoisomerase I

c. DNA topoisomerase II

d. DNA polymerase

Ans. (c) DNA topoisomerase II

111. In prokaryotes, the lagging primers are removed by...

a. 3′ to 5′ exonuclease   b. DNA ligase

c. DNA polymerase I   d. DNA polymerase III

Ans. (c) DNA polymerase I

112. The essential initiator protein at the E. Coli origin of replication is

a. DnaA   b. DnaB

c. DnaC   d. DnaE

Ans. (a) DnaA

113. Which phase would a cell enter if it was starved of mitogens before the R point?

a. G1   b. S

c. G2   d. G0

Ans. (d) G0

114. Prokaryotic plasmids can replicate in yeast cells if they contain a cloned yeast

a. ORC   b. CDK

c. ARS   d. RNA

Ans. (c) ARS

115. Which enzyme removes the RNA primer and fills in deoxyribonucleotides in prokaryotic replicons?

a. DNA polymerase III

b. DNA polymerase II

c. DNA polymerase I

d. None of these

Ans. (c) DNA polymerase I

116. The bacterial enzyme that changes positively supercoiled DNA into negatively supercoiled DNA is

a. DNA helicase

b. DNA gyrase

c. Single stranded binding protein

d. Polymerase

Ans. (b) DNA gyrase

117. **Characteristic unique in DNA is**
    a. Denaturation and renaturation
    b. Polymer complex
    c. Replication
    d. resistance to temperature change

Ans. (c) **Replication**

118. **Isotopes used for proving semiconservative replication of DNA are**
    a. N^{14} and P^{31} b. N^{14} and N^{15}
    c. N^{14} and C^{14} d. C^{14} and P^{31}

Ans. (b) N^{14} **and** N^{15}

119. **T4 DNA ligase**
    a. Requires ATP
    b. Joins double-stranded DNA fragments with an adjacent 3′-phosphate and 5′-OH
    c. Requires NADH
    d. Joins single-stranded DNA

Ans. (a) **Requires ATP**

120. **Which of the following is used in rolling circle DNA replication but not in normal cellular DNA replication?**
    a. Endonuclease
    b. Exonuclease
    c. Primase
    d. DNA ligase

Ans. (a) **Endonuclease**

121. **In eukaryotes. RNA primers are removed after replication by**
    a. DNA Pol α   b. DNA Pol δ
    c. helicase   d. FEN I

Ans. (d) **FEN I**

122. **Which of the following DNA Pol has proofreading property in animal cells**
    a. DNA Pol α
    b. DNA Pol δ
    c. DNA Pol β
    d. All

Ans. (b) **DNA Pol δ**

123. **Choose the incorrect statement**
    a. Mitochondrial DNA replicates by D-loop formation
    b. rolling circle replication is also known as σ replication
    c. DNA Pol I is made up of single polypeptide
    d. DNA Pol III has ability of nick translation

Ans. (d) **DNA Pol III has ability of nick translation**

124. **Which of the following DNA Pol in eukaryote has 5′ → 3′ exonuclease activity**
    a. DNA Pol α   b. DNA Pol β
    c. DNA Pol δ   d. None

Ans. (d) **None**

125. **Mitochondrial DNA is replicated from**
    a. A single ori site bidirectionally
    b. Two different ori sites in the same direction
    c. Two different ori sites at different times in opposite directions
    d. Many sites bidirectionally, like nuclear chromosomes

Ans. (c) **Two different ori sites at different times in opposite directions**

126. **Chloroplast DNA is replicated from**
    a. A single ori site bidirectionally
    b. Two different ori sites in the same direction
    c. Two different ori sites simultaneously and in opposite directions
    d. Many sites bidirectionally, like nuclear chromosomes

Ans. (c) **Two different ori sites simultaneously and in opposite directions**

127. **In eukaryotes, the lagging strand DNA is synthesized by DNA polymerase β**
    a. β   b. δ
    c. γ   d. ε

Ans. (d) **ε**

128. **C-bands are deeply stained chromosomal regions which represents the**
    a. Euchromatin
    b. Constitutive heterochromatin
    c. Cytosine dominant regions of chromosome
    d. Metaphase chromosome

Ans. (b) **Constitutive heterochromatin**

129. **Bar bodies are found in**
    a. Interphase of male cells
    b. Interphase of female cells
    c. Prophase of female cells
    d. Prophase of male cells

Ans. (b) **Interphase of female cells**

130. **According to operon concept, in the tryptophan operon the regulator gene forms**
    a. Inducer   b. Repressor
    c. Aporepressor   d. General inhibitor

Ans. (c) **Aporepressor**

131. Similarities between RNA polymerase and DNA Polymerase activities in prokaryotes include

a. Requirement for a template
b. Requirement for a primer
c. Synthesis of the nascent chain in 5′ to 3′ direction
d. 3′ to 5′ exonuclease editing function

Ans. (c) Synthesis of the nascent chain in 5′ to 3′ direction

132. Post-transcriptional modification of prokaryote RNA molecule includes

a. Cleavage of primary transcripts to form functional molecules of rRNA and tRNA
b. Addition of a CCA 3′terminus to all tRNA molecules
c. Methylation of bases using S-adenosylmethionine as methyl donor
d. Addition of a cap structure to the 5′ end of mRNA

Ans. (c) Methylation of bases using S-adenosylmethionine as methyl donor

133. A transesterification reaction

a. Requires no ATP
b. Breaks one bond and forms one bond
c. Involves the nucleophilic attack of an OH group on the sugar phosphate backbone
d. All of the above

Ans. (d) All of the above

134. Polycistronic messengers RNA are common in

a. Homo sapiens
b. Saccharomyces cerevisiae
c. E. coli
d. Dinosaur

Ans. (c) E. coli

135. Which one of the following does not require a primer?

a. RNA dependent DNA Polymerase
b. DNA dependent RNA Polymerase
c. DNA dependent DNA Polymerase
d. Taq DNA Polymerase

Ans. (b) RNA dependent DNA Polymerase

136. The poly A end of eukaryotic mRNAs originates from

a. Addition of a pre- synthesized poly A tail to the 3′ end of the primary transcript
b. Transcription of corresponding poly T region of the respective gene
c. Sequential addition of A residues at the 3′ end of the primary transcript
d. None

Ans. (c) Sequential addition of A residues at the 3′ end of the primary transcript

137. Regulation of polygenic transcription in prokaryotes can be at the level of

a. RNA polymerase holoenzyme recruitment to DNA
b. Enhancer binding protein induced isomerisation of the binary complex
c. Repressor and antitermination of transcription
d. All of the above

Ans. (d) All of the above

138. Catabolite activator protein acts as

a. Apo repressor   b. Co- repressor
c. Apo inducer   d. Inducer

Ans. (c) Apo inducer

139. Term 'Homeobox' was used by

a. Walter Gehring   b. Dr. Hogness
c. Goldberg   d. Lewis

Ans. (a) Walter Gehring

140. Genes whose products are constantly needed for cellular activity are called

a. Regulator genes   b. Structural genes
c. House keeping genes d. Smart genes

Ans. (c) House keeping genes

141. Bacteria utilize glucose first, even if other sugars are present, through a mechanism called

a. Operon repression   b. Enzyme repression
c. Catabolite repression d. Glucose utilization

Ans. (c) Catabolite repression

142. If there is a deletion mutation in the "operator" for lac operon, expression of lac structural gene will be

a. Permanently stop
b. Constitutively expressed
c. Not expressed
d. Resistant to catabolite expression

Ans. (b) Constitutively expressed

143. 'Zinc fingers' are important in cellular function because they are

a. Catalytic site of many metabolic enzymes
b. Structural motifs in many DNA binding proteins
c. Structures with high redox potential
d. Characteristic of palindromic strtches of unique DNA sequence

Ans. (b) Structural motifs in many DNA binding proteins

144. Lac operon is negatively regulated by repressor encoded by lacI gene. A mutation in lacI that prevents binding of lactose will result in

a. Constitutive phenotype that will be recessive

b. Uninducible phenotype that will be dominant

c. Constitutive phenotype that will be dominant

d. Uninducible phenotype that will be recessive

Ans. (c) Constitutive phenotype that will be dominant

145. Amplification of genes involves

a. Removal of histones from DNA to allow transcription of gene

b. Multiple duplications of gene via replication

c. Multiplication of extra chromosomal elements only

d. Invertebrate genomes only

Ans. (b) Multiple duplications of gene via replication

146. Full expression of lac operon requires

a. Lactose and cAMP

b. Allolactose and cAMP

c. Lactose

d. Allolactose

Ans. (b) Allolactose and cAMP

147. Which one of the following partial diploids will express β-galactosidase constitutively?

a. F' lacO^c lacZ$^+$ / lacO$^+$ lacZ$^+$

b. F' lacO$^-$ lacZ$^+$ / lacI$^+$ lacZ$^+$

c. F' lacO$^+$ lacZ$^+$ / lacI$^-$ lacZ$^+$

d. F' lacO^c lacZ$^-$ / lacO$^+$ lacZ$^+$

Ans. (b) F' lacO$^-$ lacZ$^+$ / lacI$^+$ lacZ$^+$

148. Synthesis of β-galactosidase will be constitutive in a strain with the genotype

a. I$^+$ Z$^+$ Y$^+$

b. I$^-$ Z$^+$ Y$^+$

c. I$^+$ Z$^-$ Y$^+$

d. I$^+$ Z$^+$ Y$^-$

Ans. (b) I$^-$ Z$^+$ Y$^+$

149. House keeping genes are

a. Inducible genes

b. Expressed in tumour cells

c. Expressed in all cells

d. Do not express at all

Ans. (c) Expressed in all cells

150. What is the chemical basis of gene imprinting?

a. Phosphorylation of DNA

b. Methylation of DNA

c. Oxidation of DNA

d. Glycosylation of DNA

Ans. (b) Methylation of DNA

151. The leader region (trpL) of tryptophan biosynthetic operon codes for RNA that may function as the operon's

a. Corepressor

b. Holorepressor

c. Aporepressor

d. Attenuator

Ans. (d) Attenuator

152. Chaperone proteins help in

a. Protein folding and assembly

b. Protein stability

c. Both

d. None

Ans. (c) Both

153. How many energy bonds are expended in formation of a peptide bond?

a. 2

b. 4

c. 3

d. 6

Ans. (b) 4

154. 'Kozak' is associated with

a. Transcription

b. DNA replication

c. DNA repair

d. Translation

Ans. (b) DNA replication

155. GUG codes for valine in both prokaryotes and eukaryotes but when GUG is initiation codon, this codes

a. Methionine

b. Valine

c. tryptophan

d. None

Ans. (a) Methionine

156. An antibiotic which inhibits in both prokaryotes and eukaryotes is

a. Chloromycetin

b. Puromycin

c. Actinomycin-D

d. Tetracycline

Ans. (b) Puromycin

157. At initiation the two ribosomal subunits combine with mRNA and

a. Threonine charged tRNA

b. Methionine charged tRNA

c. Serine charged tRNA

d. Proline charged tRNA

Ans. (b) Methionine charged tRNA

158. Chloramphenicol inhibits

a. Cell wall synthesis in bacteria

b. Protein synthesis on 70S ribosome

c. Protein synthesis on 80S ribosome

d. DNA replication

Ans. (b) Protein synthesis on 70S ribosome

159. An antibiotic that resembles 3′ end of a charged tRNA molecule is

a. Streptomycin   b. Penicillin

c. Tetracycline   d. Puromycin

Ans. (d) Puromycin

160. Which of the following is involved in the majority of ATP dependent cytosolic degradation of proteins in eukaryotes?

a. Cathepsins   b. Calpains

c. Lysosome   d. 26S proteosome

Ans. (d) 26S proteosome

161. Peptide bond synthesis not requires an input of energy during

a. Amino acid activation

b. Formation of 70S initiation complex of prokaryotes

c. Binding of aminoacyl-tRNA to the A site on ribosome

d. Movement of peptidyl- tRNA to the P site and associated movement of mRNA

Ans. (d) Movement of peptidyl- tRNA to the P site and associated movement of mRNA

162. What is the E site of ribosome?

a. Site where eukaryotic mRNA is processed

b. Exciting term made up by your instructor

c. Site where tRNA exits the prokaryotic ribosome

d. Site where endonuclease EcoRI restricts ribosome

Ans. (c) Site where tRNA exits the prokaryotic ribosome

163. E. coli release factor1 recognizes which codons?

a. UAA only

b. UGA

c. UAA and UGA

d. UAG and UAA

Ans. (d) UAG and UAA

164. All aminoglycoside antibiotics inhibits Protein synthesis by

a. Binding to small ribosomal subunit

b. Binding to large ribosomal subunit

c. Binding to both small and large ribosomal subunit

d. Inactivating eEF-2

Ans. (a) Binding to small ribosomal subunit

165. In the Protein synthesis, tRNA carrying initiating amino acid enters in which site of ribosome?

a. A site   b. P site

c. Anticodon   d. Recognition site

Ans. (b) P site

166. In the case of humans lysine is an essential acid because

a. It is present in all proteins

b. It is highly nutritive

c. It is not formed in body and had to be supplied the diet

d. It is required for protein synthesis

Ans. (c) It is not formed in body and had to be supplied the diet

167. To clone a gene corresponding to a protein with partial amino acid sequence. Met-Trp-Cys Trp (no. of codons for Met = 1, Cys = 2, trp = 1), no. of oligonucleotides that need to be designed to screen cDNA library is

a. 2   b. 4

c. 5   d. 8

Ans. (a) 2

168. Three of the four eukaryotic rRNAs are synthesized from a single transcription unit consisting of the rDNA. Which one of the following does not belong to this group?

a. 5.8S   b. 5S

c. 18S   d. 28S

Ans. (b) 5S

169. Synthesis of peptide bond is catalyzed by

a. A site of ribosome   b. P site of ribosome

c. 23S rRNA   d. tRNA

Ans. (c) 23S rRNA

170. How many polypeptide chains can be formed simultaneously by a given ribosome?

a. One

b. Up to 30

c. Variable, depending on the length of mRNA

d. Variable, depending both on the length or mRNA and temperature

Ans. (a) One

171. A single nucleotide pair is inserted near the 5′ end of a protein coding DNA sequence. The most likely effect will be production of

a. A protein with a single altered amino acid

b. A protein with an almost completely altered sequence

c. A greatly truncated protein

d. No protein

Ans. (b) A protein with an almost completely altered sequence

172. A recessive mutation is one which

a. Is not expressed

b. Is expressed only when in heterozygous

c. Is expressed only when in homozygous or hemizygous

d. Is eliminated by natural selection

Ans. (c) Is expressed only when in homozygous or hemizygous

173. Thmine dimer formation during replication of DNA is caused due to

a. Gamma radiation   b. UV radiation

c. X-rays   d. IR radiation

Ans. (b) UV radiation

174. The fluctuation tests done by Luria and Delbruck showed that

a. Antibiotics induce the development of resistance in bacteria

b. Growth of bacteria fluctuates based on the conc. of antibiotics in the media

c. The conc. of antibiotics fluctuates in response to the no. of bacteria in a sample

d. Phage T1 not induce mutation in wild type E. Coli

Ans. (d) Phage T1 not induce mutation in wild type E. Coli

175. Ames test is used to determine if a chemical

a. Increases rate at which bacterial cell divides

b. Decreases no. of cells in a culture

c. Induces mutations in cell's DNA

d. Decreases ability of a cell to photosynthesize

Ans. (c) Induces mutations in cell's DNA

176. Sites where mutations occur at rates higher than normal are known as

a. Suppressor sites   b. Hotspots

c. Mutator sites   d. Cistrons

Ans. (c) Mutator sites

177. In bacteria, which enzyme binds single stranded DNA, denatures double stranded DNA and matches single stranded DNA with complementary denatured DNA?

a. RecA   b. RecBCD

c. UvrABC   d. UvrD

Ans. (a) RecA

178. High energy phosphate bond of adenosine diphosphate is used in biological systems by

a. Hydrolysis of terminal phosphate to give adenosine monophosphate

b. Coupling of hydrolysis of terminal phosphate to another reaction via common intermediates

c. Transfer of terminal phosphate to glucose or similar substrates

d. Transfer of terminal phosphate of one adenosine diphosphate to another ADP to form adenosine triphosphate

Ans. (b) Coupling of hydrolysis of terminal phosphate to another reaction via common intermediates

179. If the ratio (A+G)/ (T+C) in one strand of DNA is 0.7, what is the same ratio in the complementary strand?

a. 0.7   b. 1.43

c. 0.35   d. None

Ans. (b) 1.43

180. Rate of renaturation of DNA is proportional to the

a. Square of the conc. of single strand

b. conc. of single strand

c. Square of length of single strand

d. None

Ans. (a) Square of the conc. of single strand

181. Molecular weight of mRNA that codes for a protein of molecular weight 75000 is closest to

a. 6000   b. 60000

c. 600000   d. 600

Ans. (c) 600000

182. Mammalian kinases are able to convert which of the following nucleosides to nucleotides?

a. Adenosine   b. Inosine

c. glutamine   d. Guanine

Ans. (a) Adenosine

183. End product of purine catabolism in normal humans is

a. Urea   b. Uric acid

c. Creatinine   d. Xanthine

Ans. (b) Uric acid

184. Ring structure of glucose is due to formation of hemiacetal and ring formation between

a. C_1 and C_5 b. C_1 and C_4

c. C_1 and C_3 d. C_2 and C_4

Ans. (a) C_1 and C_5

185. The scientists involved in discovery of DNA as chemical basis of heredity were

a. Hershey and Chase
b. Griffith and Avery
c. Avery, Mac Leod and Mc Carty
d. Watson and Crick

Ans. (c) Avery, Mac Leod and Mc Carty

186. One turn of DNA possesses

a. One base pair
b. Two base pairs
c. Five base pairs
d. Ten base pairs

Ans. (d) Ten base pairs

187. Number of codons in the genetic triplet code is

a. 4
b. 16
c. 32
d. 64

Ans. (d) 64

188. Initiation codons for protein synthesis are

a. UUU and GGG
b. AAU and UAA
c. AUG and GUA
d. GUG and AUG

Ans. (d) GUG and AUG

189. Termination codons for protein synthesis are

a. AUU, AUG and GUU
b. UGA, UAA and UAG
c. UAU, UAG and UUA
d. AAA, UUU and UGA

Ans. (b) UGA, UAA and UAG

190. The two antiparallel strands of DNA are

a. Equidistant and run in $5' \rightarrow 3'$ direction
b. Equidistant and run in $5' \rightarrow 3'$ and $3' \rightarrow 5'$ directions
c. Unequal and run in opposite directions
d. Unequal and diverge from each other

Ans. (b) Equidistant and run in $5' \rightarrow 3'$ and $3' \rightarrow 5'$ directions

191. The process of multiplication of DNA from DNA is known as

a. Replication
b. Duplication
c. Transcription
d. Translation

Ans. (a) Replication

192. Formation of RNA over the template of DNA is

a. Replication
b. Translation
c. Transversion
d. Transcription

Ans. (d) Transcription

193. The area of unwinding and separation of DNA strands during replication is called

a. Origin
b. Initiation point
c. Primer
d. Replication fork

Ans. (a) Origin

194. Topoisomerase is involved in

a. Producing RNA primer
b. Joining of DNA segments
c. Producing nick in DNA
d. Separation of DNA strands

Ans. (c) Producing nick in DNA

195. In DNA replication, the primer is

a. Small deoxyribonucleotide polymer
b. Small ribonucleotide polymer
c. Helix destabilising protein
d. Enzyme taking part in joining nucleotides to their complementary template bases

Ans. (b) Small ribonucleotide polymer

196. DNA strand is synthesized in the direction

a. $5' \rightarrow 3'$
b. $3' \rightarrow 5'$
c. $1' \rightarrow 4'$
d. $6' \rightarrow 1'$

Ans. (a) $5' \rightarrow 3'$

197. Okazaki segments are

a. Small segments of RNA
b. Small peptides
c. Small DNA segments
d. Small DNA segments formed over DNA template running in $3' \rightarrow 5'$ direction

Ans. (d) Small DNA segments formed over DNA template running in $3' \rightarrow 5'$ direction

198. Okazaki fragments are joined by

a. DNA polymerase III
b. DNA ligase
c. DNA polymerase II
d. DNA polymerase I

Ans. (b) DNA ligase

199. Okazaki fragments give rise to

a. Master strand
b. Sense strand
c. Lagging strand
d. Leading strand

Ans. (c) Lagging strand

200. Leading strand during DNA replication is formed

a. Continuously
b. In short segments
c. First
d. Ahead of replication

Ans. (a) Continuously

201. In proof reading during DNA replication

a. Wrong nucleotides are inserted
b. Wrong nucleotides are taken out
c. Wrong nucleotides are removes and correct ones inserted
d. Mutations are prevented

Ans. (c) Wrong nucleotides are removes and correct ones inserted

202. Nonsense codons take part in

    a. Helping protein synthesis

    b. Termination gene message for polypeptide synthesis

    c. Initiating gene message for polypeptide synthesis

    d. Synthesis of nonprotein amino acids

Ans. (b) Termination gene message for polypeptide synthesis

203. The two strand of DNA are

    a. Similar and parallel

    b. Similar but antiparallel

    c. Complementary and antiparallel

    d. Complementary and parallel

Ans. (c) Complementary and antiparallel

204. Transcription involves

    a. Protein synthesis over ribosomes

    b. Removal of worn out organelles by lysosomes

    c. Synthesis of RNA over DNA

    d. Synthesis of DNA over DNA

Ans. (c) Synthesis of RNA over DNA

205. DNA acts as a template for synthesis of

    a. DNA   b. RNA

    c. Both a and b   d. Protein

Ans. (c) Both a and b

206. Code transfer for synthesis of polypeptide involves

    a. DNA, tRNA, rRNA and mRNA

    b. mRNA, tRNA, rRNA and DNA

    c. tRNA, DNA, mRNA and rRNA

    d. DNA, mRNA, tRNA and amino acids

Ans. (d) DNA, mRNA, tRNA and amino acids

207. In polypeptide synthesis, amino acids are brought over ribosome-mRNA complex by

    a. rRNA   b. tRNA

    c. DNA   d. Nucleotides

Ans. (b) tRNA

208. tRNA attaches amino acid at its

    a. 3'-end   b. 5'-end

    c. Anticodon   d. Loop

Ans. (a) 3'-end

209. Blender experiment to prove DNA as genetic material was performed by

    a. Hershey and chase   b. Messelson and stahl

    c. Watson and crick   d. Rosalind and franklin

Ans. (a) Hershey and chase

210. The strain of *Neurospora*, which grows on minimal medium is called

    a. Autotroph   b. Prototroph

    c. Auxotroph   d. Heterotroph

Ans. (b) Prototroph

211. For their contribution in biochemical genetics the scientists who received Nobel prize in 1958 were

    a. Beadle and Tatum   b. Beadle and Lederberg

    c. Lederberg and Zinder   d. Zinder and Morgan

Ans. (a) Beadle and Tatum

212. Gentic information is carried out by long chain molecule made up of

    a. Amino acids   b. Enzymes

    c. Nucleotides   d. Histone proteins

Ans. (c) Nucleotides

213. One gene one enzyme hypothesis was proposed by

    a. Khorana and Nirenberg

    b. Beadle and Tatum

    c. Bateson and Punnet

    d. Bridges

Ans. (b) Beadle and Tatum

214. A mutant strain of *Neurospora* which fails to grow on a minimal medium unless supplemented with a nutrient is called

    a. Auxotroph   b. Autotroph

    c. Heterotroph   d. Prototroph

Ans. (a) Auxotroph

215. The terms triplet code and genetic code were coined by

    a. Watson and Crick   b. Nirenberg

    c. Gamow   d. Conrat

Ans. (c) Gamow

216. Beadle and Tatum produced mutant strain of *Neurospora* by

    a. X-rays   b. UV rays

    c. Beta rays   d. Gamma rays

Ans. (a) X-rays

217. The technique of detecting and screening the nutritional mutants in *Neurospora crassa* was developed by

    a. Mendel   b. Morgan

    c. Bateson and Punnet   d. Beadle and Tatum

Ans. (d) Beadle and Tatum

218. A gene that takes part in the synthesis of polypeptide is

a. Structural gene   b. Regulator gene
c. Operator gene   d. Promoter gene

Ans. (a) Structural gene

219. Components of an operon are

a. Operator, promoter and regulator genes
b. Regulator, promoter, operator and structural genes
c. Operator, regulator and structural genes
d. Regulator, promoter and structural genes

Ans. (b) Regulator, promoter, operator and structural genes

220. Regulated unit of genetic material is termed as

a. Operon   b. Regulator gene
c. Operator gene   d. Okazaki segment

Ans. (a) Operon

221. A codon specifies the same amino acid in *Brassica* and *Homo* because codons are

a. Nonoverlapping   b. Commaless
c. Universal   d. Nonambiguous

Ans. (c) Universal

222. In eukaryotes mRNA is synthesized with the aid of

a. RNA polymerase III   b. RNA polymerase II
c. RNA polymerase I   d. Reverse transcriptase

Ans. (b) RNA polymerase II

223. A bacterium grown over medium having radioactive ^{35}S incorporates radioactivity in

a. Carbohydrates   b. Proteins
c. DNA   d. RNA

Ans. (b) Proteins

224. GUG specifies amino acid valine. However, when functioning as initiation codon it specifies

a. Methionine   b. Valine
c. Lysine   d. Isoleucine

Ans. (a) Methionine

225. New strand formation on a DNA template can be initiated only by

a. DNA polymerase I
b. DNA polymerase III
c. RNA primer
d. DNA primer

Ans. (c) RNA primer

226. What is true about ori

a. One in all organisms
b. Several in all organisms
c. One in eukaryotes and several in prokaryotes
d. One in prokaryotes and several in eukaryotes

Ans. (d) One in prokaryotes and several in eukaryotes

227. DNA has alternate grooves

a. One major and one minor
b. Two major and one minor
c. One major and two minor
d. Two major and two minor

Ans. (a) One major and one minor

228. Number of DNA coils of a nucleosome is

a. 2 ¾   b. 2 ¼
c. 1 ¾   d. 1 ¼

Ans. (c) 1 ¾

229. Energy for activation of amino acids during protein synthesis comes from

a. ATP   b. GTP
c. CTP   d. UTP

Ans. (a) ATP

230. AUG initiation codon occurs over

a. 3′ end of mRNA   b. 5′ end of mRNA
c. Short arm of tRNA   d. Long arm of tRNA

Ans. (b) 5′ end of mRNA

231. Central dogma is not directly connected with synthesis of

a. mRNA   b. Polypeptide
c. Both a and b   d. Amino acids

Ans. (d) Amino acids

232. In *Streptococcus pneumoniae*

a. Virulent form is smooth
b. Virulent form is rough
c. Nonvirulent form is capsulated
d. All forms are rough

Ans. (a) Virulent form is smooth

233. Codon is triplet of

a. Template strand of DNA
b. Non-template strand of DNA
c. mRNA
d. tRNA

Ans. (b) Non-template strand of DNA

234. Enzyme required during DNA replication is

a. DNA polymerase   b. DNA ligase

c. Both a and b   d. Sigma factor

Ans. (c) Both a and b

235. A codon is read in

a. $3 \rightarrow 5'$ direction   b. $5 \rightarrow 3'$ direction

c. $3 \rightarrow 6'$ direction   d. $6 \rightarrow 3'$ direction

Ans. (b) $5 \rightarrow 3'$ direction

236. All nonsense codons have first base

a. Adenine   b. Cytosine

c. Uracil   d. Guanine

Ans. (c) Uracil

237. First triplet codon to be deciphered was

a. UUU   b. AAA

c. CTA   d. CCC

Ans. (a) UUU

238. Triplet pair deciphered by Khorana was

a. Serine and Threonine

b. Threonine and Histidine

c. Cysteine and Valine

d. Phenylalanine and Isoleucine

Ans. (c) Cysteine and Valine

239. The codon for anticodon 3′ UUUA - 5′ is

a. 5′ AAAU - 3′

b. 5′ UAAA - 3′

c. 3′ UAAD - 5′

d. 3′ AAAU - 5′

Ans. (a) 5′ AAAU - 3′

240. Central dogma of modern genetics is

a. RNA $\rightarrow$ RNA $\rightarrow$ DNA $\rightarrow$ Protein

b. DNA $\rightarrow$ DNA $\rightarrow$ RNA $\rightarrow$ Protein

c. DNA $\rightarrow$ RNA $\rightarrow$ Protein

d. RNA $\rightarrow$ DNA $\rightarrow$ RNA $\rightarrow$ Protein

Ans. (b) DNA $\rightarrow$ DNA $\rightarrow$ RNA $\rightarrow$ Protein

241. What is true of Watson and Crick's model of DNA. It is duplex with

a. 10 base pairs and 34 Å distance for every turn

b. 10 base pairs and 3.4 Å distance for each turn of spiral

c. 20 base pairs and 34 Å for each turn

d. None of the above

Ans. (a) 10 base pairs and 34 Å distance for every turn

242. Protein cover of virus is

a. Capsid   b. Virion

c. Viroid   d. Mucopeptide

Ans. (a) Capsid

243. A gene is

a. Three letter code in DNA

b. Equivalent to chromosome

c. Part of chromosome producing a set of enzymes (protein)

d. Part of chromosome producing only one enzymes (protein)

Ans. (d) Part of chromosome producing only one enzymes (protein)

244. tRNA recognizes ribosome by

a. TΨC loop   b. DHU loop

c. Anticodon   d. AA-site

Ans. (a) TΨC loop

245. tRNA recognizes amino acyl synthetase enzyme by

a. Anticodon   b. DHU loop

c. TΨC loop   d. AA-site

Ans. (b) DHU loop

246. Amino acid binding site of tRNA is

a. 5′ end   b. Anticodon loop

c. DHU loop   d. –CCA 3′-end

Ans. (d) –CCA 3′-end

247. Type of coiling in DNA is

a. Right handed   b. Left handed

c. Zigzag   d. Opposite

Ans. (a) Right handed

248. Hereditary characteristics are passed on from parent to the offspring mainly through

a. Enzymes

b. Genes

c. Mutants

d. Centrosomes

Ans. (b) Genes

249. The pneumococcus experiment proves that

a. RNA sometimes controls the production of DNA and proteins

b. Bacteria under go binary fission

c. DNA is the genetic material

d. Bacteria do not reproduce sexually

Ans. (c) DNA is the genetic material

250. The strongest evidence that DNA is the genetic material comes from

    a. The fact that chromosomes are made of DNA

    b. Studies on the transformation of bacterial cells

    c. The knowledge that DNA is present in the nucleus

    d. The findings that DNA is present in the cytoplasm

Ans. (b) Studies on the transformation of bacterial cells

251. When DNA is transformed from a culture of capsulated bacteria to a culture of non-capsulated bacteria converting the latter into the former type, the process is known as

    a. Transcription   b. Translocation

    c. Transduction   d. Transformation

Ans. (d) Transformation

252. A gene is made up of

    a. DNA   b. RNA

    c. Either DNA or RNA   d. Amino acids

Ans. (c) Either DNA or RNA

253. Genes are chemically

    a. Polynucleotides   b. Histones

    c. Iipoproteins   d. Hydrocarbons

Ans. (a) Polynucleotides

254. Which is entirely responsible for the transfer of hereditary traits

    a. DNA   b. RNA

    c. Chloroplast   d. Aestivation

Ans. (a) DNA

255. A link between generations is provided precisely by

    a. Chromosomes   b. Nucleic acids

    c. Nucleus   d. Cytoplasm

Ans. (b) Nucleic acids

256. The first undoubted evidence about DNA being the genetic material came from

    a. Transformation of rough-coated strain of *Diplococcus pneumonia* into smooth coated strain

    b. The establishment of DNA as the chief chemical constituent of chromosomes

    c. The establishment of DNA as a self-replicating substance

    d. Transduction of bacteria by action of bacteriophage

Ans. (a) Transformation of rough-coated strain of *Diplococcus pneumonia* into smooth coated strain

257. Duplication of DNA is called

    a. Replication   b. Transduction

    c. Transcription   d. Translation

Ans. (a) Replication

258. The usual method of DNA replication is

    a. Conservative   b. Dispersive

    c. Non-conservative   d. Semi-conservative

Ans. (d) Semi-conservative

259. A DNA molecule in which both strands have radioactive thymidine is allowed to duplicate in an environment containing non-radioactive thymidine. What will be the exact number of DNA molecules that contain some radioactive thymidine after 3 duplications?

    a. One   b. Two

    c. Four   d. Eight

Ans. (b) Two

260. A bacterium containing 100% N^{15} nitrogen bases is allowed to replicate in a medium containing N^{14} bases. After one round of duplication, the result would be

    a. All individuals would be identical to parents

    b. All individuals would be radioactive but the percentage of radioactivity in DNA would be 50%

    c. Only 50% individuals would be radioactive

    d. All individuals would be similar to parents but different among themselves

Ans. (b) All individuals would be similar to parents but different among themselves

261. A bacterium *E. coli* with completely radioactive DNA was allowed to replicate in a non-radioactive medium for two generations. What % of the bacteria should contain radioactive DNA

    a. 100%   b. 50%

    c. 25%   d. 12.5%

Ans. (b) 50%

262. Semi-conservative mode of replication of chromosome was demonstrated by (or experimental demonstration of the semi-conservative model of DNA replication was given by)

    a. Messelson and Stahl

    b. Watson and crick

    c. Stahl and Urey

    d. Bawden and Ririe

Ans. (a) Messelson and Stahl

263. If one wants to obtain precise information regarding the exact time and location of synthesis of new DNA, which of the following methods would be most effective for such a study

    a. Electron microscopy

    b. Carbon dating

    c. Isolating and extracting DNA after regular intervals and estimating DNA amount

    d. Using radioactive precursors of nucleic acids

Ans. (d) Using radioactive precursors of nucleic acids

264. The experimental system used in studies of the discovery of replication of DNA has been (or DNA replication was conducted in)

    a. *Drosophila melanogaster*

    b. *Pneumococcus*

    c. *Escherichia coli*

    d. None of these

Ans. (c) *Escherichia coli*

265. Experiments using ^{15}N (heavy nitrogen) to confirm the semi-conservative replication of DNA were carried out by

    a. Messelson and Stahl   b. Hershey and Chase

    c. Beadle and Tatum   d. Watson and Crick

Ans. (a) Messelson and Stahl

266. A DNA molecule of *Escherichia coli* is heavy (full labeled with N^{15}) and is allowed to duplicate in a medium containing N^{14}. After one generation, the two daughter strands molecules

    a. Have same density but do not resemble their parent DNA

    b. Have different densities but resemble their parent DNA

    c. Have different densities and also do not resemble the parent DNA

    d. Both the strands differ in density, but resemble their parent DNA

Ans. (a) Have same density but do not resemble their parent DNA

267. Replication of DNA takes place with the help of

    a. DNA polymerase   b. Lyase

    c. RNAase   d. DNAase

Ans. (a) DNA polymerase

268. The following is needed during DNA replication

    a. DNA polymerase and DNA ligase

    b. RNA polymerase and translocase

    c. DNA polymerase only

    d. DNA ligase only

Ans. (a) DNA polymerase and DNA ligase

269. DNA polymerase is needed for

    a. Replication of DNA   b. Synthesis of DNA

    c. Elongation of DNA   d. All the above

Ans. (a) Replication of DNA

270. DNA polymerase is required for the synthesis of

    a. DNA from DNA

    b. DNA from RNA

    c. DNA from nucleotides

    d. DNA from nucleosides

Ans. (c) DNA from nucleotides

271. The enzyme DNA polymerase can add nucleotide to the

    a. 3' carbon position

    b. 5' carbon position

    c. Both 3' and 5' carbon positions

    d. 4' carbon position

Ans. (a) 3' carbon position

272. The enzyme(s) responsible for unwinding of DNA helix during replication is/are

    a. Helicases   b. Topisomerases

    c. DNA polymerase   d. Primase

Ans. (a) Helicases

273. The enzyme topoisomerase is helpful in

    a. Unwinding of the helix

    b. Breaking of DNA strand

    c. Proof reading of replicating DNA

    d. Synthesis of primer

Ans. (b) Breaking of DNA strand

274. The expected frequency of introduction of a wrong base during DNA replication is

    a. 1:100   b. 1:1000

    c. 1:1 million   d. 1:1 billion

Ans. (d) 1:1 billion

275. Ligase enzyme is used for

    a. Denaturation of DNA

    b. Splitting of DNA into small bits

    c. Joining bits of DNA

    d. Digestion of lipids

Ans. (c) Joining bits of DNA

276. The bits of DNA segments formed are joined with each other by an enzyme

    a. Polymerase   b. Ligase

    c. Lipase   d. Kinase

Ans. (b) Ligase

277. Okazaki segments are

a. DNA segments capable of free replication

b. DNA segments formed during replication

c. Nucleotide segments formed during transcription

d. Segments of genes which undergo mutation and recombination

Ans. (b) DNA segments formed during replication

278. DNA polymerase enzyme was discovered by

a. Komberg   b. Nirenberg

c. Watson   d. Crick

Ans. (a) Komberg

279. Synthesis of DNA takes place by

a. Transduction   b. Transcription

c. Transformation   d. Replication

Ans. (d) Replication

280. Replication of DNA in eukaryotes commences from

a. One end of the chromatid extending to the other end

b. Both ends of the chromatid simultaneously

c. The centromere to either of the ends of chromatids

d. Several sites along the DNA of the chromatid simultaneously

Ans. (d) Several sites along the DNA of the chromatid simultaneously

281. The modern concept of gene is that it is

a. A segment of DNA capable of crossing over

b. A functional unit of DNA

c. A segment of DNA

d. A segment of chromosome

Ans. (b) A functional unit of DNA

282. Eukaryotes differ from prokaryotes in the mechanism of DNA replication due to

a. Different enzymes (instead of same enzyme) for synthesis of lagging and leading strands

b. Discontinuous rather than semi-discontinuous replication

c. Use of DNA primers rather than RNA primers

d. Unidirectional rather than bidirectional replication

Ans. (a) Different enzymes (instead of same enzyme) for synthesis of lagging and leading strands

283. These are special proteins which help to open up DNA double helix in front of the replication fork. These proteins are

a. DNA gyrase   b. DNA polymerase I

c. DNa ligase   d. DNA topoisomerase

Ans. (a) DNA gyrase

284. The nuclease enzyme which begins its attack from a free end of a polynucleotide is

a. Exonuclease   b. Kinase

c. Polymerase   d. Endonuclease

Ans. (a) Exonuclease

285. One gene-one polypeptide hypothesis was proposed by

a. Linus pauling   b. V. ingram

c. Yanofsky   d. Brenner

Ans. (c) Yanofsky

286. A functional unit of gene which specifies the synthesis of one polypeptide is known as

a. Recon   b. Clone

c. Codon   d. Cistron

Ans. (d) Cistron

287. The smallest gene affected by mutation is

a. Exon   b. Recon

c. Cistron   d. Muton

Ans. (d) Muton

288. The smallest unit of DNA which is capable of undergoing crossing over and recombination is called

a. Recon   b. Muton

c. Cistron   d. Intron

Ans. (a) Recon

289. The terms cistron, recon anc muton were proposed by

a. W. Ingram   b. Bateson

c. J. Lederberg   d. S. Benzer

Ans. (d) S. Benzer

290. Gene is

a. A segment of DNA

b. A segment of DNA and histone

c. A segment of DNA, RNA and Histone

d. All of the above

Ans. (a) A segment of DNA

291. The idea that genes control the production of enzyme was given by

a. E.L. Tatum

b. T.H. Morgan

c. A.E. Garrod

d. R.S. Kornberg

Ans. (c) A.E. Garrod

292. One gene one enzyme theory (hypothesis) was proposed by

a. Beadle and Tatum   b. Avery and McCarty

c. Jacob and Monad   d. Luria and Delburck

Ans. (a) Beadle and Tatum

293. Co-linearity between genes and polypeptides was established by

a. Linus Pauling   b. V. Ingram

c. Yanofsky   d. Brenner

Ans. (c) Yanofsky

294. Garrod's views on the relationship between genes and enzymes can be best stated as

a. One mutant gene-one metabolic block concept

b. One gene-one enzyme hypothesis

c. One gene-one polypeptide hypothesis

d. One cistron-one polypeptide hypothesis

Ans. (a) One mutant gene-one metabolic block concept

295. Gene controls

a. Protein synthesis but not heredity

b. Protein synthesis and heredity

c. Heredity but not protein synthesis

d. Biochemical reaction of some enzymes

Ans. (b) Protein synthesis and heredity

296. Beadle and Tatum worked on genetics of *Neurospora* which resulted in the development of a new science called

a. Genetic engineering   b. Biochemical genetics

c. Biotechnology   d. Dendrochronology

Ans. (b) Biochemical genetics

297. The chief advantage of the linear arrangement of the ascospores in *Neurospora* is that, in genetic studies, it permits

a. Easy inference of the orientation of chromatids during meiosis

b. Ready conservation of mutant phenotype

c. Accurate counting of spores

d. Easy collection of ascospores

Ans. (b) Ready conservation of mutant phenotype

298. In *Neurospora*, 8 ascospores are formed. These are 2a, 4A, 2a...it shows that

a. First generation division

b. Second generation division

c. No crossing over

d. Some meiosis occurs

Ans. (b) Second generation division

299. RNA and DNA were artificially synthesized *in vitro* by

a. Ochoa and Nirenberg

b. Ochoa and Kornberg

c. Kornberg and Nirenberg

d. Nirenberg and Khorana

Ans. (b) Ochoa and Kornberg

300. Who suggested that an intermediate RNA molecule would be needed to read the codons on messenger RNA

a. M. Nirenberg   b. H.G. Khorana

c. F. Crick   d. Kornberg

Ans. (c) F. Crick

301. The process of RNA synthesis on the DNA template is

a. Transduction   b. Translation

c. Transcription   d. Transformation

Ans. (c) Transcription

302. Transcription is synthesis of

a. Protein   b. mRNA

c. tRNA   d. rRNA

Ans. (b) mRNA

303. Transcription is the process by which

a. RNA molecule is synthesized on a DNA strand (or template)

b. Two daughter strands of DNA are synthesized

c. Amino acids are joined to form polypeptides

d. RNA molecule is synthesized within a ribosome

Ans. (a) RNA molecule is synthesized on a DNA strand (or template)

304. Genetic code determines

a. Structural pattern of an organism

b. Sequence of amino acid in protein chain

c. Variation in offsprings

d. Constancy of morphological trait

Ans. (b) Sequence of amino acid in protein chain

305. Genetic code was discovered by

a. Nirenberg and Mathei   b. Novick and Szilard

c. Kornberg   d. Willkins

Ans. (a) Nirenberg and Mathei

306. Site of protein synthesis

a. Lysosome   b. Peroxisome

c. Ribosome   d. Splisosome

Ans. (c) Ribosome

307. Dr. Hargobind Khorana has been awarded Noble Prize for research on

a. Oral contraceptives   b. Hormones

c. Genetic code   d. Immunology

Ans. (c) Genetic code

308. There are 64 codons in genetic code dictionary because

a. There are 64 type of tRNAs found in the cell

b. There are 44 meaningless and 20 codons for amino acids

c. There are 64 amino acids to be coded

d. Genetic code is triplet

Ans. (d) Genetic code is triplet

309. Genetic code was deciphered through chemical synthesis of trinucleotides by

a. Watson and Crick   b. Beadle and Tatum

c. Briggs and King   d. M.W. Nirenberg

Ans. (d) M.W. Nirenberg

310. Nirenberg synthesized a mRNA containing 34 poly-adenine (A-A-A-A-A-A......) and found a polypeptide formed of 11 polylysine. It proved that the genetic code for lysine is

a. Lone adenine   b. A-A doublet

c. A-A-A triplet   d. Many adenines

Ans. (c) A-A-A triplet

311. Khorana and his colleagues synthesized an RNA molecule with ripening sequence of UG N-bases (UGUGUGUGUGUG). It produced a tetrapeptide with altering sequence of cystien and valine. It proves that codon for cysteine and valine is

a. UGG and GUU   b. UUG and GGU

c. UGU and GUG   d. GUG and UGU

Ans. (c) UGU and GUG

312. Dr. H.G. Khorana deciphered first the triplet codon of

a. Serine and isoleucine

b. Phenylalanine and methionine

c. Threonine and histidine

d. Tyrosine and tryptophan

Ans. (a) Serine and isoleucine

313. 5′-end of the tRNA always ends in the base

a. Adenine   b. Guanine

c. Cytosine   d. Thymine

Ans. (b) Guanine

314. UGA in the yeast mitochondria codes for

a. Stop signal   b. Tryptophan

c. Glutamine   d. Aspartic acid

Ans. (d) Aspartic acid

315. The amount of which of these is least in a cell

a. mRNA

b. rRNA

c. tRNA

d. Nothing can be said definitely

Ans. (a) mRNA

316. The genetic code is

a. Universal

b. Nearly universal

c. Similar in the members of a genus

d. Different for every species

Ans. (b) Nearly universal

317. The minimum length of cistron in base pair which synthesizes a polypeptide of 50 amino acids is

a. 50 bp   b. 100 bp

c. 150 bp   d. 200 bp

Ans. (c) 150 bp

318. Considering that we have four nucleotides A, G, C, T, the number of base substitutions that can occur in the amino acid codons are

a. 549   b. 535

c. 261   d. 264

Ans. (a) 549

319. In the DNA codons are ATG ATG ATG and a cytosine base is inserted at the beginning, which of the following will result

a. A non-sense mutation   b. CA TGA TGA TG

c. CAT GAT GAT G   d. C ATG ATG ATG

Ans. (c) CAT GAT GAT G

320. Genetic code consists of

a. Adenine and guanine   b. Guanine and cytosine

c. Cytosine and uracil   d. All

Ans. (d) All

321. A single anticodon can recognize more than one codon of mRNA. This phenomenon is termed as

a. Richmond and lang effect

b. Gene flow hypothesis

c. Wobble hypothesis

d. Template hypothesis

Ans. (c) Wobble hypothesis

322. What becomes established from the Wobble hypothesis?

a. Process of peptide chain elongation
b. Economy of the number of tRNA molecules
c. Process of peptide chain initiation
d. Process of chain termination

Ans. (b) Economy of the number of tRNA molecules

323. In a codon, wobbling is generally restricted to

a. First N base
b. Second N base
c. Third N base
d. Aromatic amino acids

Ans. (c) Third N base

324. DNA is the major source of genetic information which is transmitted by transcription into RNA molecules. These RNA molecules are responsible to get this genetic information translated into proteins and thus the central dogma of molecular biology is

a. RNA → DNA → Proteins
b. DNA → RNA → Proteins
c. RNA → Proteins
d. RNA → Proteins → DNA

Ans. (b) DNA → RNA → Proteins

325. Which of the following is called amber

a. AUG
b. UAA
c. UAG
d. UGA

Ans. (c) UAG

326. Transcription is

a. Assembly of amino acids by mRNA in the form of polypeptides
b. Recognition of amino acids by RNA synthesis
c. Transfer of genetic information from DNA to mRNA
d. Recognition of base sequence on mRNA

Ans. (c) Transfer of genetic information from DNA to mRNA

327. The genetic information if carried by long chain molecules of

a. Enzymes
b. Amino acids
c. Nucleotides
d. Chromosomes

Ans. (c) Nucleotides

328. tRNA is also known is

a. Microsomal RNA
b. Messenger RNA
c. Soluble RNA
d. Ribosomal RNA

Ans. (d) Messenger RNA

329. In order to enable a chemical to serve as a genetic code, it is essential that the chemical should be

a. Able to duplicate itself
b. Able to form itself into long spiral molecules
c. A compound of pyrimidines and purines
d. Easily changed

Ans. (a) Able to duplicate itself

330. *E. coli* RNA polymerase consists of different polypeptide chains which are

a. Two in number
b. Three in number
c. Four in number
d. Five in number

Ans. (d) Five in number

331. The core enzyme constituting the *E. coli* RNA polymerase consists of following subunits

a. β, β′, σ, α
b. β, β′ α, ω
c. β, β′, σ, ω
d. β, σ, α, ω

Ans. (b) β, β′, α, ω

332. How many different types of RNA polymerases catalyse the synthesis of RNA in eukaryotes

a. Two
b. Three
c. Four
d. Five

Ans. (b) Three

333. Formation of RNA from DNA is known as

a. Translation
b. Translocation
c. Transformation
d. Transcription

Ans. (d) Transcription

334. The process by which DNA of the nucleus passes genetic information to mRNA is called

a. Transcription
b. Transportation
c. Translocation
d. Translation

Ans. (a) Transcription

335. Transcription is

a. Synthesis of DNA on RNA
b. Synthesis of RNA on DNA
c. Production of proteins on RNA
d. Replication of DNA

Ans. (b) Synthesis of RNA on DNA

336. Enzyme necessary for transcription is (or transcription of DNA is aided by)

a. DNA polymerase
b. RNA polymerase
c. Endonuclease
d. RNAase

Ans. (b) RNA polymerase

337. A DNA strand is directly involved in the synthesis of all the following *except*:

a. tRNA molecule
b. mRNA molecule
c. Another DNA strand
d. Protein synthesis

Ans. (d) Protein synthesis

338. The mRNA is formed

a. In the nucleus
b. By free ribosomes
c. From the ribosomes on endoplasmic reticulum
d. From DNA in nucleus

Ans. (d) From DNA in nucleus

339. In which of the following places, messenger RNA is found in a living cell?

a. Inside the endoplasmic reticulum
b. Inside the mitochondria
c. Inside the nucleus but outside the nucleolus
d. Inside the nucleolus

Ans. (c) Inside the nucleus but outside the nucleolus

340. Which site of a tRNA molecule hydrogen bonds to a m-RNA molecule?

a. Anticodon
b. Codon
c. 5′-end of the tRNA molecule
d. 3′-end of a tRNA molecule

Ans. (d) Anticodon

341. The formation of polyribosomes from ribosomes is done in the presence of

a. Na^+ ions
b. K^+ ions
c. Ca^{++} ions
d. Mg^{++} ions

Ans. (d) Mg^{++} ions

342. In protein synthesis, the codon used as a start signal is

a. AUG
b. UGA
c. GUA
d. UAG, UAA

Ans. (a) AUG

343. If the DNA strand has the nitrogenous base sequence ATT GCC, the mRNA will have

a. ATT GCA
b. ATC GCC
c. UGG ACC
d. UAA CGG

Ans. (d) UAA CGG

344. If the sequence of bases in DNA is ATTCGATG, then the sequence of bases in its transcript will be

a. GUAGCUUA
b. UAAGCUAC
c. CAUCGAAU
d. AUUCGAUG

Ans. (b) UAAGCUAC

345. From a DNA template with the sequence CTGATAGC, the mRNA sequence formed would be

a. GUCTUTCG
b. GACUAUCG
c. UACTATCU
d. GAUTATUG

Ans. (b) GACUAUCG

346. The function of a non-sense codon is

a. To release polypeptide chain from tRNA
b. To form an unspecified amino acid
c. To terminate the message of gene controlled protein synthesis
d. To convert a sense DNA into non-sense DNA

Ans. (c) To terminate the message of gene controlled protein synthesis

347. Termination of chain growth in protein synthesis is brought about by

a. UUG, UGC, UCA
b. UCG, GCG, ACC
c. UAA, UAG, UGA
d. UUG, UAG, UCG

Ans. (c) UAA, UAG, UGA

348. Each codon present on mRNA and anticodon present on tRNA is composed of

a. One N base only
b. A set of two N base
c. A set of three N base
d. A set of three out of U, C, A, G

Ans. (d) A set of three out of U, C, A, G

349. The process by which proteins are synthesized in a cell is called

a. Transcription
b. Translation
c. Translocation
d. Transduction

Ans. (b) Translation

350. During protein synthesis, amino acids recognize and get attached to tRNA with the help of

a. Ribosomes; Sigma and Rho factors
b. mRNA
c. Amino acyl tRNA synthetase
d. tRNA

Ans. (c) Amino acyl tRNA synthetase

351. Khorana synthesized a biologically functional tyrosine suppressor tRNA of *E. coli* in 1979 it contained

a. 77 nucleotide pairs   b. 207 nucleotide pairs
c. 312 nucleotide pairs   d. 333 nucleotide pairs

Ans. (b) 207 nucleotide pairs

352. An antibiotic which inhibits translation in eukaryotes is

a. Chloromycetin   b. Penicillin
c. Puromycin   d. Tetracycline

Ans. (c) Puromycin

353. Initiation of polypeptide chain in protein synthesis is induced by

a. Methionine   b. Glycine
c. Leucine   d. Lysine

Ans. (a) Methionine

354. Who among the following established that RNA is the genetic material

a. Lederberg   b. Griffith
c. Nirenberg and holley   d. Frankel conrat

Ans. (d) Frankel conrat

355. Which one of the following chemical characteristics is not common to all living beings

a. Similar triplet codes for amino acids
b. Energy is store by high energy-rich phosphate bonds
c. Types of protein present in the body
d. Ribosomes act as sites for protein synthesis

Ans. (c) Types of protein present in the body

356. The functional unit in the protein synthesis is

a. Peroxisome   b. Dictyosome
c. Lysosome   d. Polysome

Ans. (d) Polysome

357. In protein synthesis, polymerization of amino acids involves three steps. Which one of the following is not involved in protein synthesis

a. Elongation   b. Transcription
c. Termination   d. Initiation

Ans. (b) Transcription

358. Reverse transcriptase is

a. RNA dependent RNA polymerase
b. DNA dependent r-RNA polymerase
c. DNA dependent DNA polymerase
d. DNA dependent RNA polymerase

Ans. (d) DNA dependent RNA polymerase

359. Genes which are inactive for long periods, have the tendency to be bound to

a. Each other   b. Methyl groups
c. Actin and myosin   d. Nucleolus

Ans. (b) Methyl groups

360. The percentage of DNA in a eukaryotic cell expressed at a given time is about

a. 1%   b. 20%
c. 50%   d. 80%

Ans. (a) 1%

361. The scientist who first synthesized DNA *in vitro* was

a. A. Kornberg   b. A. Garrod
c. J.D. Watson   d. H.G. Khorana

Ans. (a) A. Kornberg

362. Artificial synthesis of DNA was done by

a. Nirenberg   b. Kornberg
c. Khorana   d. Watson and Crick

Ans. (b) Kornberg

363. Nobel prize to A. Kornberg and S. Ochoa was given for

a. Artificial synthesis of DNA and RNA
b. Theory of natural selection
c. One gene one enzyme theory
d. Mutation theory

Ans. (a) Artificial synthesis of DNA and RNA

364. In 1980, F. Sanger was awarded Nobel prize second time to be shared by Gilbert and Moseum for their work on

a. Genetic mapping of chromosomes
b. Determining amino acid sequence of insulin
c. Determining the base sequences of DNA of a virus
d. Determining the structure of DNA

Ans. (c) Determining the base sequences of DNA of a virus

365. Operon model for enzyme activity (or the concept of operon) was proposed by

a. Jacob   b. Monod
c. Boveri   d. Jacob and Monod

Ans. (d) Jacob and Monod

366. The lac operon in an example of

a. Arabonise operon   b. Inducible operon
c. Repressible operon   d. Overlapping gene

Ans. (b) Inducible operon

367. In *E. coli*, "Lac" operon is induced by

    a. β-galactosidase

    b. Lactose

    c. 'I' gene

    d. Promoter gene

Ans. (b) Lactose

368. Wild type *E. coli* cells are growing in normal medium with glucose. They are transferred to a medium containing lactose only as the sugar. Which one of the following changes take place?

    a. The lac operon is repressed

    b. All operons are induced

    c. *E. coli* cells stop dividing

    d. The lac operon is induced

Ans. (d) The lac operon is induced

369. In an *E. coli* cell, according to the operon theory an operator gene combines with

    a. Inducer gene to "switch on" structural gene transcription

    b. Regulator gene "switch off" structural gene transcription

    c. Regulator protein to "switch off" structural gene transcription

    d. Regulator protein to "switch on" structural gene transcription

Ans. (c) Regulator protein to "switch off" structural gene transcription

370. According to operon concept, the regulatory gene regulates biochemical reaction in a cell by

    a. Inhibiting transcription

    b. Inactivating enzymes

    c. Inactivating substrate

    d. Inhibiting migration of mRNA

Ans. (a) Inhibiting transcription

371. Rapid transcription of lac operon in *E. coli* requires

    a. Presence of lactose

    b. Presence of glucose

    c. Presence of glucose but absence of lactose

    d. Presence of lactose but absence of glucose

Ans. (d) Presence of lactose but absence of glucose

372. A gene which synthesizes a repressor protein is

    a. Regulator gene

    b. Promoter gene

    c. Operator gene

    d. Structural gene

Ans. (a) Regulator gene

373. In an operon, the RNA polymerase binds to

    a. Regulator   b. Promoter gene

    c. Operator gene   d. Constitutive gene

Ans. (b) Promoter gene

374. Lac operon is related to

    a. Synthesis of enzyme of lactose anabolism

    b. Synthesis of enzyme of lactose catabolism

    c. Synthesis of lac by lac insect

    d. Degradation of lac in the body of lac insect

Ans. (b) Synthesis of enzyme of lactose catabolism

375. The genes are responsible for growth and differentiation in an organism through regulation of

    a. Translocation

    b. Transformation

    c. Transduction and translation

    d. Translation and transcription

Ans. (d) Translation and transcription

376. The lac operon requires a 'helper' protein which, by binding to the promoter and by facilitating the attachment of RNA polymerase, accelerates the rate of transcription. The protein is

    a. Amino acid activating enzyme

    b. Essential metabolite

    c. Inactive repression protein

    d. Catabolite activator protein

Ans. (d) Catabolite activator protein

377. Which of the following is first recombinant DNA?

    a. DNA of one bacteria with another bacteria

    b. DNA of a virus and a bacterium

    c. DNA of bacteria and man

    d. DNA of two viruses

Ans. (b) DNA of a virus and a bacterium

378. Which of the following is employed in recombinant DNA technology?

    a. Plastids   b. Plasmids

    c. Ribosomes   d. Histones

Ans. (b) Plasmids

379. Which one of the following unit is unrelated to DNA or gene?

    a. Rishon

    b. Recon

    c. Cistron

    d. Operon

Ans. (a) Rishon

380. Genetic engineering would not have been possible if one of these were absent

a. DNA polymerase
b. Reverse transcriptase
c. DNA ligase
d. RNA synthetase

Ans. (c) DNA ligase

381. Which of the following is associated with genetic engineering

a. Plastid
b. Plasmids
c. Mutations
d. Hybrid vigour

Ans. (b) Plasmids

382. In genetic engineering, for cutting DNA segment, which of the enzyme is used

a. Restriction nuclease
b. Ligase
c. ATPase
d. DNA polymerase

Ans. (a) Restriction nuclease

383. In *Rous sarcoma* virus, the flow of information is

a. DNA → RNA → Protein
b. DNA → Protein → RNA
c. RNA → DNA → RNA → Protein
d. RNA → DNA → Protein

Ans. (c) RNA → DNA → RNA → Protein

384. What is cDNA?

a. Circular DNA
b. Cloned DNA
c. DNA produced from reverse transcription of RNA
d. Cytoplasmic DNA

Ans. (c) DNA produced from reverse transcription of RNA

385. Teminism, i.e. the synthesis of DNA on RNA template was observed in

a. TMV
b. Rice dwarf virus
c. Reovirus
d. Rous sarcoma virus

Ans. (d) Rous sarcoma virus

386. Lac operon in *E. coli* consists of three structural genes. Out of these, one codes for transacetylase. The function of transacetylase is

a. To carry lactose into the cell
b. To convert lactose into glucose
c. To convert lactose into galactose
d. Not known

Ans. (d) Not known

387. In split genes, the coding sequence are called

a. Cistrons
b. Operons
c. Exons
d. Introns

Ans. (c) Exons

388. Restriction enzyme are used in genetic engineering because

a. They can cut DNA at specific base sequence
b. They are proteolytic enzymes which can degrade harmful proteins
c. They are nucleases that cut DNA at variable sites
d. They can join different DNA fragments

Ans. (a) They can cut DNA at specific base sequence

389. A piece of DNA, cut by a restriction enzyme, forms bonds with other DNA molecules which have

a. Been fragmented by the same restriction enzyme
b. Unpaired bases
c. Plasmid components
d. Methyl groups attached to them

Ans. (a) Been fragmented by the same restriction enzyme

390. It is preferable to use yeasts rather than bacteria as recipient cells for recombination of eukaryotic DNA because

a. Yeast can produce restriction enzymes
b. Yeast can excise introns from the RNA transcript
c. Yeast can remove methyl groups
d. Yeast can reproduce at a faster rate

Ans. (b) Yeast can excise introns from the RNA transcript

391. A bacterium modifies its DNA by adding methyl groups to the DNA. It does so to

a. Clone its DNA
b. Be able to transcribe many genes simultaneously
c. Turn its gene on
d. Protect its DNA from its own restriction enzymes

Ans. (d) Protect its DNA from its own restriction enzymes

392. The operon model of gene regulation and organization in prokaryotes was proposed by

a. Jacob and Monod
b. Beadle and Tatum
c. Meselson and Stahl
d. Wilkins and Franklin

Ans. (a) Jacob and Monod

393. Which site of a tRNA molecule hydrogen binds to an mRNA molecule?

a. Codon
b. Anticodon
c. 5′ end of the tRNA molecule
d. 3′ end of the tRNA molecule

Ans. (b) Anticodon

394. An environmental agent that triggers transcription from an operon is a

a. Derepressor   b. Inducer

c. Regulator   d. Controlling element

Ans. (b) Inducer

395. Alternative excision repair system is specialized for removal of thymine dimmers in

a. Human

b. Archaea

c. Saccharomyces pombe

d. Caenorhabditis elegans

Ans. (c) Saccharomyces pombe

396. Chromosome diminution in somatic cell can be displayed by

a. Yeast

b. Ascaris

c. Drosophila

d. Caenorhabditis elegans

Ans. (b) Ascaris

397. Vertebrates cells internalize insulin through

a. Facilitated diffusion

b. Receptor mediated endocytosis

c. Carriers

d. Simple diffusion

Ans. (b) Receptor mediated endocytosis

398. Which of the following statements is not correct?

a. Eukaryotic DNA replicates birectionally

b. Okazaki fragments of eukaryotes are larger than prokaryotes

c. Licencing factor must be attached at replication origin sites in eukaryotes before replication to occur

d. None of these

Ans. (b) Okazaki fragments of eukaryotes are larger than prokaryotes

399. 18 S RNA is synthesized by

a. RNA polymerase I

b. RNA polymerase II

c. RNA polymerase III

d. Both RNA polymerase I and III

Ans. (a) RNA polymerase I

400. Calmodulin, a calcium binding protein, is found in living organisms *except*:

a. Prokaryotes   b. Eukaryotes

c. Plant   d. Animals

Ans. (a) Prokaryotes

401. c-AMP has

a. Always positive control on lac operon

b. Always negative control on lac operon

c. No role in operon control

d. None of these

Ans. (a) Always positive control on lac operon

402. c-AMP is directly involved in regulation of

a. GTP   b. ATP

c. PFK   d. Protein kinase A

Ans. (d) Protein kinase A

403. Cancer drug vinblastin is obtained from

a. *Podophyllum*   b. *Taxus baccata*

c. *Catharanthus roseus*   d. Non of these

Ans. (c) *Catharanthus roseus*

404. Codominant markers, such as RFLPs, are useful for:

a. Marker assisted selection

b. Evolutionary studies

c. Linkage mapping

d. All of these

Ans. (d) All of these

405. The saturated molecular linkage maps initially developed in tomato. Potato and maize used which of the following molecular marker systems?

a. AFLP   b. RFLP

c. SNP   d. DAF

Ans. (b) RFLP

406. The first strategy used for molecular mapping was based on:

a. Recombinant inbred lines

b. Bulked segregant analysis

c. Near isogenic line

d. F2 population

Ans. (c) Near isogenic line

407. The first cloning of a gene and its expression in a foreign organism were achieved in:

a. 1972   b. 1971

c. 1973   d. 1969

Ans. (c) 1973

408. The same genome of the virus lambda when cleaved with the restriction endonuclease BstE II can be sued as DNA markers between the size of

a. 2 and 20 kb   b. 700 and 8 kb

c. 200 bases to 8 kb   d. None of these

Ans. (b) 700 and 8 kb

409. The first reported purification of chromosomal DNA was in:

a. 1943   b. 1944
c. 1945   d. 1946

Ans. (b) 1944

410. For most genetic engineering experiments which is most important:

a. Messenger RNA   b. Messenger DNA
c. D-RNAd.   C-DNA

Ans. (a) Messenger RNA

411. The human genome contain:

a. 10000–20000   b. 20000–30000
c. 30000–40000   d. 40000–50000

Ans. (c) 30000–40000

412. Which of the most critical in marker assisted Selection?

a. Their inherent repeatability
b. Map position
c. Linkage with economically important traits
d. All of these

Ans. (c) Linkage with economically important traits

413. Blood groups deciding antigens are:

a. Glycolipids   b. Glycoproteins
c. Phospholipids   d. Peripheral proteins

Ans. (a) Glycolipids

414. Button like points of intercellular contact that serve as anchoring sites of intermediate filaments and help to hold adjacent cells together are called

a. Cadherins   b. Desmosomes
c. Connection   d. Gap junction

Ans. (b) Desmosomes

415. Which one of the following is not an example of active transport?

a. Transcytosis
b. Transport through ion channel
c. Transport through ABC transporter
d. Transport of m-RNA from nucleus to cytosol

Ans. (b) Transport through ion channel

416. Ca+2 ATPase transports

a. Two Ca^{+2} from the inside of cells to the outside while returning two H+ from outside per ATP
b. Two Ca^{+2} from the inside of cells to the outside per ATP
c. One Ca^{+2} from the inside of cells to the outside while returning one H+ from outside per ATP
d. None of these

Ans. (a) Two Ca+2 from the inside of cells to the outside while returning two H+ from outside per ATP

417. Dominant markers supply as much information as codomiant marker in :

a. Doubled haploids
b. One of the two backcross population in coupling phase
c. RILs
d. All of these

Ans. (d) All of these

418. What is the order of the following steps in western blotting?

A. Protein denaturation
B. Hydrogen peroxide reduction
C. Primary antibody binding
D. Transfer onto membrane

a. A, D, C, B   b. A,B,C,D
c. A, C, D, B   d. B,C,D,A

Ans. (a) A, D, C, B

419. In *E.coli*, which of the following codons are reorganized by the release factor RF1?

a. UAG and UGA
b. UAA and UGG
c. UAG and UAA
d. UAG and UUA

Ans. (c) UAG and UAA

420. c-AMP has

a. Always positive control on lac operon
b. Always negative control on lac operon
c. No role in operon control
d. None of these

Ans. (a) Always positive control on lac operon

421. Which of the following statement is/are correct about leucine zipper motif?

A. A DNA binding motif
B. Homodimer or heterodimer
C. Present in transcription factors-Fos and Jun
D. Present in steroid receptors

a. A only   b. C only
c. A, B and C   d. None of these

Ans. (c) A, B and C

422. Cancer drug vinblastin is obtained from

a. Podophyllum
b. Taxus baccata
c. Catharanthus roseus
d. Non of these

Ans. (c) Catharanthus roseus

423. Caspases are involved in apoptosis. They are found in

a. Chloroplast
b. Mitochondria
c. ER lumen
d. Cytosol

Ans. (d) Cytosol

424. Which one of the following Transcription factor is involved in promoter recognition in eukayotes?

a. TFII F
b. TFII B
c. TFII D
d. TFII E

Ans. (c) TFII D

425. Cdc2 in cell cycle acts at

a. G 1-phase
b. G 2-phase
c. S-phase
d. M-phase

Ans. (d) M-phase

426. Cdk is a kinase which is important for

a. Cell division
b. Signal transduction
c. Transcription
d. Genetic engineering

Ans. (a) Cell division

427. How many loci can be detected from a single cross through AFLP?

a. > 25
b. >400
c. >70
d. >1000

Ans. (c) >70

428. The single primer amplification reaction is also called as:

a. MP-PCR
b. RAMP
c. SSLP
d. All of these

Ans. (d) All of these

429. The shine dalgarno sequence is responsible for:

a. Binding of RNA polymerase to gene during transcription
b. Binding of DNA polymerases to origin of replication during DNA replication
c. Binding of ribosomes to mRNA during initiation of translation
d. Binding of snurps during splicing

Ans. (c) Binding of ribosomes to mRNA during initiation of translation

430. Cell division primarily regulated at

a. G1- stage
b. G2-stage
c. S-stage
d. G0-stage

Ans. (a) G1- stage

431. Cell fusion is an essential phenomenon in development of

a. Nerve
b. Muscle
c. Spleend
d. Liver

Ans. (b) Muscle

432. Cell membrane is

a. A lipid bilayer
b. A protein bilayer sandwiched between two lipid layers
c. Protein in lipid is mosaic mixture
d. A lipid bilayer sandwiched between two protein layer

Ans. (a) A lipid bilayer

433. Cell size is determined by

a. Surface area: volume ratio
b. Volume: surface area ratio
c. Surface area: weight
d. Volume: weight ratio

Ans. (a) Surface area: volume ratio

434. Cell-cell recognition is achieved by

a. Glycoproteins
b. Phosphatidates
c. Glycolipids
d. Peripheral protein

Ans. (a) Glycoproteins

435. Cells uptake iron trough

a. Transcytosis
b. Phagocytosis
c. Receptor mediated endocytosis
d. None of these

Ans. (c) Receptor mediated endocytosis

436. β-1,4 glycosidic linkage is not found in

a. Sucrose
b. Fructose
c. Maltose
d. Lacose

Ans. (a) Sucrose

437. α-helix is stabilized through

a. Hydrogen bond
b. Hydrophobic bond
c. Ionic bond
d. None of these

Ans. (a) Hydrogen bond

438. Cellular proteins are degraded by

a. Cyclosomes
b. Chymotripsins
c. Proteasomes
d. Lysosomes

Ans. (c) Proteasomes

439. cellulose and hemicelluloses, which are the constituents of cell wall, are synthesized by

a. Lysosome
b. Golgi body
c. SER
d. RER

Ans. (b) Golgi body

440. Change from purine to pyrimidine or pyrimidine to purine is

a. Transversion
b. Transitition
c. Deletion
d. Frame-shift

Ans. (a) Transversion

441. Chiasmata are formed in meiosis

a. After metaphase I
b. Before metaphase I
c. During prophase I
d. During metaphase II

Ans. (b) Before metaphase I

442. Chitin is found in the exoskeleton of

a. Insect
b. Bryozoans
c. Echinoderms
d. Annelids

Ans. (a) Insect

443. Chitin occurs in cell wall of fungus. It is polymer of

a. Amino acid
b. Sucrose
c. Galactose
d. Glucose

Ans. (a) Amino acid

444. Cholera toxin causes diarrhea because it

a. Inhibits adenylate cyclase
b. Blocks conformational change in trimeric G- protein
c. Inhibits GTPase activity of Gá, by ADP ribosylation
d. None of these

Ans. (c) Inhibits GTPase activity of Gá, by ADP ribosylation

445. Cholesterol occurs in most of the membranes of organelles, except:

a. Endoplasmic reticulum
b. Golgi body
c. Inner membrane of mitochondria and chloroplast
d. Outer membrane of mitochondria and chloroplast

Ans. (c) Inner membrane of mitochondria and chloroplast

446. Chromosomal translocation and inversions are readily detectable in

a. Polytene chromosomes
b. Lampbrush chromosomes
c. B-chromosomes
d. All of the above

Ans. (a) Polytene chromosomes

447. Clathrin coated vesicles are usually involved in the

a. Transport of cargo form trans- Golgi to Lysosomes
b. Transport of cargo from ER to Golgi complex
c. Endocytosis
d. Both a and c

Ans. (d) Transport of cargo from ER to Golgi complex

448. Clathrin is a

a. Conserved coat protein
b. Variable coat protein
c. Virus coat protein
d. None of these

Ans. (a) Conserved coat protein

449. Coated vesicles in the cell gives rise to

a. Ribosome
b. Mitochondria
c. ER
d. Endosome

Ans. (d) Endosome

450. Which one of the following is the weakest bond found in protein?

a. Hydrogen bond
b. Ionic bond
c. Hydrophobic bond
d. Disulphide bond

Ans. (c) Hydrophobic bond

451. The 10 nm thick fibre of chromatin is called

a. Chromosome
b. Nucleosome
c. Nucleolus
d. Solenoid

Ans. (b) Nucleosome

452. The acidic environment of lysosome is regulated by?

a. B-type ATPase
b. V-type ATPase
c. P-type ATPase
d. F-type ATPase

Ans. (c) P-type ATPase

453. Which one of the following is not a second messenger?

a. PIP_3
b. Mn^{+2}
c. C-AMP
d. Ca^{+2}

Ans. (a) PIP_3

454. Which one of the following is not associated with eukaryotic transcription?

a. RNA polymerase-III
b. RNA polymerase-II
c. Poly (a) polymerase
d. None of these

Ans. (c) Poly (a) polymerase

455. Which one of the following is not the component of extra cellular matrix?

a. Major histocompatibilty complex
b. Glycoproteins
c. Proteoglycoans
d. Collagens

Ans. (a) Major histocompatibilty complex

456. The basic structural unit of the metaphase chromosome is

a. 10 nm filament   b. 50 nm filament
c. 300 nm filament   d. 30 nm filament

Ans. (d) 30 nm filament

457. The basis for the blocking action of the alkaloid colchicines on the division is

a. G_1 phase   b. S phase
c. M phase   d. G_0 phase

Ans. (c) M phase

458. The biologically active proteasome is

a. 20S   b. 30S
c. 26S   d. 50S

Ans. (c) 26S

459. The biologically predominant form of DNA is

a. Left handed B-DNA
b. Right handed A-DNA
c. Left handed A-DNA
d. Right handed B-DNA

Ans. (d) Right handed B-DNA

460. The protein complex 'dicer' is involved in

a. Gene silencing   b. Transcription
c. Translation   d. Protein sorting

Ans. (a) Gene silencing

461. The protein of Golgi complex which contain irregular cisternae and tubules is known as

a. Intercisternal golgi   b. Cis golgi
c. Trans golgi   d. Medial golgi

Ans. (d) Medial golgi

462. The region where RNA polymerase binds to promoter in prokaryotes is called

a. Hogness box
b. Homeo box
c. Pribnow box
d. Shine-dalgrano box

Ans. (c) Pribnow box

463. The shortening of eukaryotic chromosome during replication is prevented by

a. Telomerase
b. Ligase
c. Reverse transcriptase
d. RNA polymerase

Ans. (a) Telomerase

464. Which one of the following hormones binds to intracellular receptor?

a. Insulin   b. Estrogen
c. Glucagon   d. Growth hormone

Ans. (b) Estrogen

465. The Tm of DNA can be calculated using the formula: Tm = 69.1 + 0.41 (GC) where GC is the percent of guanine + cytosine. A double stranded DNA has 27% adenine. Its Tm is:

a. 79°C   b. 80.73°C
c. 95.50°C   d. 88°C

Ans. (d) 88°C

466. The type of intercellular signalling in which one cell can communicate with another over long distances is called

a. Autocrine   b. Paracrine
c. Juxtacrine   d. Endocrine

Ans. (d) Endocrine

467. The uptake of cholesterol by mammalian cells can be explained by

a. Pinocytosis
b. Phagocytosis
c. Transcytosis
d. Receptor mediated endocytosis

Ans. (d) Receptor mediated endocytosis

468. The Z-DNA helix

a. Tends to be found at the 3′ end of genes
b. Is favoured by an alternating GC sequence
c. Has fewer base pair per turn than the B-DNA
d. None of these

Ans. (b) Is favoured by an alternating GC sequence

469. Thymine dimmers in eukaryotes are repaired by

a. Mismatch repair mechanism
b. Nucleotide excision repair mechanism
c. Base excision repair mechanism
d. Direct repair mechanism

Ans. (b) Nucleotide excision repair mechanism

470. To achieve active conformation calmodulin protein binds minimum

a. Three Ca^{+2} ions   b. One Ca^{+2} ions
c. Six Ca^{+2} ions   d. Four Ca^{+2} ions

Ans. (b) One Ca^{+2} ions

471. which one of the following enzyme is involved in translation step in protein biosynthesis

a. RNA polymerase
b. Ribozyme
c. Reverse transcriptase
d. Aminoacyl–tRNA synthetase

Ans. (d) Aminoacyl–tRNA synthetase

472. Toll-like receptor play a central role in the signalling process which result is

a. Humoral immunity
b. Cell-mediated immunity
c. Innate immunity
d. Artificial passive immunity

Ans. (c) Innate immunity

473. Tonofilaments are the structural units of

a. Microfilaments
b. Intermediate filament
c. Micro tubules
d. Flagella

Ans. (b) Intermediate filament

474. Transcription coupled DNA repair is an example of

a. Mismatch repair   b. Excision repair
c. SOS response   d. Direct repair

Ans. (b) Excision repair

475. Which one of the following components of the plasma membrane of eukaryotic cells is not found in the membrane of prokaryotes?

a. Cholesterol
b. Glycoprotein
c. Sphingolipids
d. Glycerophospholipids

Ans. (a) Cholesterol

476. Transport of m-RNA from nucleus to cytosol is

a. Simple diffusion
b. Facilitated diffusion
c. Secondary active process
d. Primary active process

Ans. (d) Primary active process

477. Transport of sodium ions from outer side to the inner side of an eukaryotic cells is

a. Primary active
b. Facilitated diffusion
c. Simple diffusion
d. Secondary active

Ans. (b) Facilitated diffusion

478. Invice genome sequencing project, India contributed in sequencing

a. 12th chromosome
b. 8th chromosome
c. 11th chromosome
d. 6th chromosome

Ans. (c) 11th chromosome

479. Transport vesicles involved in retrograde transport are coated with

a. COP I   b. COP II
c. Clathrin   d. Caveolin

Ans. (a) COP I

480. Transposons cause mutation in plants, animal and bacteria. These are

a. Retroviruses
b. Mutagenic viruses
c. Infective protein molecule
d. Mobile genetic element

Ans. (d) Mobile genetic element

481. Trehalose is found in the exoskeleton of insects, it is

a. Polysaccharide
b. Disaccharide
c. Trisaccharide
d. Oligosaccharide

Ans. (b) Disaccharide

482. Two sisters chromatids are separated at anaphase by the action of

a. Seprarin   b. Cohesion
c. APC   d. MAD2

Ans. (a) Seprarin

483. Tyrosine kinase is activated by

a. Methylatioon   b. Acetylation
c. Dephosphorylation   d. Phosphorylation

Ans. (d) Phosphorylation

484. Ubiquitination of proteins is marked for all of the following *except*:

a. Chromatin remodelling
b. Protein degradation
c. Correct folding of protein
d. Endocytosis

Ans. (c) Correct folding of protein

485. UGA is a stop codon, but in mitochondrial genome it codes for

a. Trp   b. Met
c. Try   d. Asp

Ans. (a)

486. Under what thermodynamic conditions will a reaction proceed spontaneously?

a. "H < 0   b. "S < 0
c. "G < 0   d. "S = 0

Ans. (a) "H < 0

487. UV rays usually causes

a. Gene mutation   b. Genome mutation
c. Chromosome mutation   d. Both a and c

Ans. (d) Both a and c

488. Vascular ATPases are

a. Ca+2 pumps   b. K+ pumps
c. H+ pumps   d. Na+ pumps

Ans. (c) H+ pumps

489. Vertebrates achieved terrestrial habit due to presence of

a. Aminiotic egg
b. Vivipary
c. Thermoregulation
d. Internal fertilization

Ans. (a) Aminiotic egg

490. Viagra is used in the treatment of erectile dysfunction because

a. Inhibits NO synthase
b. Inhibits diesterase
c. Increase half-life of guanyly cyclase
d. Stimulates nitric oxide synthesis

Ans. (b) Inhibits diesterase

491. *Vibrio cholera* causes diahorrea by

a. Sestroys cells of intestinal lining
b. Closing absorption of water from gut epithelium
c. Constitutive expression of adenylate cyclase
d. Opening ion channel

Ans. (c) Constitutive expression of adenylate cyclase

492. Vinblastin is used as anticancerous drug because it

a. Causes cell death
b. Blocks cell division and functions as antimitotic drug
c. Promotes cell growth
d. Stimulates DNA synthesis

Ans. (b) Blocks cell division and functions as antimitotic drug

493. Vincristine is an anticancerious drug. It is obtained from

a. *Atropa*   b. *Colchicum*
c. *Catharanthus roseus*   d. *Taxus baccata*

Ans. (c) *Catharanthus roseus*

494. Viral encoded 'ras' oncogene transforms normal mammalian cells in to cancer cells. Viral Ras protein differs from its normal counterpart by

a. Diminished ATPase activity
b. Increased ATPase activity
c. Increased GTPase activity
d. Diminished GTPase activity

Ans. (d) Diminished GTPase activity

495. Viruses can cross biological membranes with the help of

a. Integral membrane proteins
b. Glycocalyx
c. Pores
d. Lipid bilayer

Ans. (b) Glycocalyx

496. What cellular connection is "leak-proof"?

a. Tight junction   b. Gap junction
c. Plasmodesmata   d. Anchoring junction

Ans. (a) Tight junction

497. What happens to the Cdk-cycA complex at metaphase?

a. Only cyclin A is degraded
b. Both cyclin A and Cdk remain under graded
c. Both cyclin A and Cdk are degraded
d. Only Cdk is degraded

Ans. (a) Only cyclin A is degraded

498. What is fate of most duplicated genes?

  a. Gene activation

  b. They become orthologous

  c. They are transferred to a new organism using lateral gene transfer

  d. Gain of a novel function through subsequent mutation

Ans. (d) Gain of a novel function through subsequent mutation

499. What is the maximum number of hydrogen bonds that can be formed by each molecule of water?

  a. 3   b. 5

  c. 4   d. 2

Ans. (c) 4

500. When a cell expands energy to move a solute across its membrane against a concentration gradient, the process is called

  a. Active transport

  b. Passive transport

  c. Facilitated duffusion

  d. Osmosis

Ans. (a) Active transport

501. When a mutation changes a termination codon in to codon specifying an amino acid, it is called

  a. Read through mutation

  b. Synonymous mutation

  c. Reverse nonsense mutation

  d. Back mutation

Ans. (a) Read through mutation

502. When bcl-2 gene is mutated it results in tumor, like chronic lymphoblastic leukemia (CLL). Normally this gene regulates

  a. Cell differentiation

  b. Cell division

  c. Programmed cell death

  d. Synthesis of growth factor

Ans. (c) Programmed cell death

503. When one amino acid is replaced by another by another owing to a mutation, it is called

  a. Silent mutation

  b. Missense mutation

  c. Frame shift mutation

  d. Synonymous mutation

Ans. (b) Missense mutation

504. When release factor binds to stop codon on m-RNA during translation, the synthesized peptide chain is transferred to

  a. H+   b. Water

  c. Amino acids   d. t-RNA

Ans. (b) Water

505. When repressor protein binds to operator of an operon which of the following process is regulated?

  a. Translation   b. Transcription

  c. Replication   d. None of the above

Ans. (b) Transcription

506. When the forces arise from the electrostatic attraction between the positively charged nucleus of one atom and the negatively charged electrons of the other it is called

  a. Hydrogen bonding   b. Stacking force

  c. Vanderwaals force d. Ionic bonding

Ans. (c) Vanderwaals force

507. Which element is present in diatoms

  a. Si   b. Ca

  c. Mg   d. Na

Ans. (a) Si

508. Which enzyme is exclusively involved in DNA repair mechanism

  a. DNA polymerase

  b. Photolyase

  c. RNA polymerase

  d. Restriction endonuclease

Ans. (b) Photolyase

509. Which group of bacteria on sporulation show cell coordination and social behaviour?

  a. Actino bacteria   b. Archaebacteria

  c. Myxobacteria   d. Bacillus species

Ans. (d) Bacillus species

510. Which GTPases regulates intracellular transport in mammalian cells through vesicle fusion?

  a. Rab   b. Ran

  c. Ras   d. Rho

Ans. (a) Rab

511. Which is crossing over suppressor?

  a. Translocation   b. Deletion

  c. Duplication   d. Inversion

Ans. (b) Deletion

512. Which is responsible for cytoplasmic streaming?

    a. Microtubules

    b. Endoplasmic reticulum

    c. Intermediate filament

    d. Microfilament

Ans. (a) Microtubules

513. Which is true for gap junction?

    a. It is made of connexion protein

    b. Allows free movement of large molecules across cells

    c. Made up of two subunit of connexions

    d. None of these

Ans. (a) It is made of connexion protein

514. Which of the following amino acids can easily be ionized at cellular pH?

    a. Histidine   b. Tryptophan

    c. Lysine   d. Arginine

Ans. (d) Arginine

515. Which one of the following components of cytoskeleton plays a crucial role in vesicular transport?

    a. Molecular motors   b. Microtubules

    c. Intermediate filaments d. Microfilaments

Ans. (b) Microtubules

516. Which of the following antibiotics causes misincorportation of amino acid in synthesizing polypeptide?

    a. Streptomycin   b. Polymixin B

    c. Chloramphenicol   d. Bacitracin

Ans. (a) Streptomycin

517. Which of the following antibiotic occasionally cause death when administered to persons who are allergic to them?

    a. Penicillin   b. Streptomycin

    c. Polymixin   d. Bacitracin

Ans. (a) Penicillin

518. Which of the following anticancerous drugs does not act on microtubules?

    a. Taxol   b. Methotrexate

    c. Thiabendazole   d. Colchicines

Ans. (b) Methotrexate

520. PCR was invented by:

    a. A. Kornberg (1952)   b. Nirenberg (1879)

    c. Kary mullis (1984)   d. Watson and crick (1953)

Ans. (c) Kary mullis (1984)

521. The temperature needed to denature DNA would also denature norma DNA polymerase. The polymerase used in PCR is:

    a. Taq DNA polymerase

    b. Pwo DNA polymerase

    c. RNA polymerase

    d. Both 'a' and 'b'

Ans. (d) Both 'a' and 'b'

522. Taq DNA Polymerse is isolated from:

    a. *Mycobacterium tuberculosis*

    b. *Bacillus thermophillus*

    c. *Thermos aquaticus*

    d. *Bacillus thermophillus*

Ans. (c) Thermos aquaticus

523. DNA sequencing method is:

    a. Kary mullis method

    b. Sanger dideoxy method

    c. Maxam gilbert method

    d. Both b and c

Ans. (d) Both b and c

524. Which of the following technique is used to separate the proteins?

    I. Ion exchange chromatograph

    II. Isoelectric focusing

    III. Gel electorphoresis

    IV. Gel filtration chromatography

    Choose the correct answer:

    a. I, II, III only   b. II and III only

    c. I and II only   d. I, II, III, IV

Ans. (d) I, II, III, IV

525. Protoplasm fusion can be achieved by which of the following method ?

    I. PEG

    II. Electric current

    III. Sandi virus

    IV. Ph and temperature shock

    a. III and IV only

    b. II and III only

    c. I and II only

    d. I, II, III and IV

Ans. (b) II and III only

526. Restriction endonuclease is ?

    a. Hind-III   b. EcoR-1

    c. Bamb-H_1 d. All of these

Ans. (d) All of these

527. pBR 322 is a:

a. Plasmid
b. Cosmid
c. Phage
d. Bacteriophage

Ans. (a) Plasmid

528. Edman's degradation technique is used for sequencing:

a. Fats
b. Proteins
c. Carbohydrates
d. Nucleic acids

Ans. (b) Proteins

529. The most commonly used to detected the presence of HIV is :

a. FIA
b. RIA
c. ELISA
d. HPLC

Ans. (c) ELISA

530. Template dependent enzyme is:

a. RNA polymerase
b. DNA- polymerase
c. DNA ligase
d. Oligonucleotide

Ans. (b) DNA- polymerase

531. Polymerase chain reaction is used for:

a. DNA-amplification
b. DNA recombination
c. DNA-repair
d. DNA identification

Ans. (a) DNA-amplification

532. Individual cells can be indentified by using:

a. Rate zonal centrifugation
b. Flow cytometry
c. Marker enzyme
d. Equilibrium density gradient centrifugation

Ans. (b) Flow cytometry

533. Biolistic PDS-1000 is:

a. An antibiotic
b. A gene therapy operation
c. An important cell fusion technique
d. An instrument used to transfer DNA to wide range of cells and tissues

Ans. (d) A gene therapy operation

534. The recognition site for EcoR-I a restricted endonuclease enzyme is :

a. 5′ GTT AAC 3′
b. 5′ AAG CTT 3′ 3′ CAA TTG 5′ 3′ TTC GAA 5′
c. 5′ GAA TCC 3′
d. l5′ CC GG 3′ 3′ CTT AAG 5′ 3′GG CCS 5′

Ans. (c) 5′ GAA TCC 3′

535. Polyacrylamide gel electrophoresis is used for :

a. Joining the two DNA fragments
b. Separation of fragments differing by a few base pairs
c. Separation of large DNA molecules (whole chromosomes)
d. Joining the two amino acids

Ans. (b) Separation of fragments differing by a few base pairs

536. PFGE stands for:

a. Pigment fragmented gel electrophoresis
b. Pulsed field gel electrophoresis
c. Poly fragment gel electrophoresis
d. Pulsed fragmented gel electrophoresis

Ans. (b) Pulsed field gel electrophoresis

537. RIA stands for:

a. Repeated Immuno Assay
b. Regulated Immuno Assay
c. Radio Immuno Assay
d. Regular Immuno Assay

Ans. (c) Radio Immuno Assay

538. NMR stand for:

a. Nuclear magnetic resonance
b. Nuclear mobidity rate
c. Nuclear management region
d. Nuclear material resource

Ans. (a) Nuclear magnetic resonance

539. CHEFE stands for:

a. Charged change homogeneous Electric Field Electrophoresis
b. Charged hanger electron field electrophoresis
c. Contour clamped homogeneous electric field electrophoresis
d. All of the above

Ans. (c) Contour clamped homogeneous electric field electrophoresis

540. DNA bands are blotted in:

a. Western blotting
b. Southern blotting
c. Northern blotting
d. PCR

Ans. (b) Southern blotting

541. Which of the following is not a cloning vector?

a. Ti-plasmid
b. pBR-322
c. Puc-8
d. EcoR-I

Ans. (d) EcoR-I

542. Which of the following set is related with cloning vector ?

    I. Charon-34, charon-35

    II. EMBL-3, EMBL-4

    III. λgt-10, gt-11

    IV. M-13, YACs, MP-13

    Choose the correct answer :

    a. I, II, III only   b. III and IV only

    c. I and II only   d. I, II, III and IV

Ans. (d) I, II, III and IV

543. RELPs stands for:

    a. Rapid Fragment length polymorphism

    b. Random fragment length polymorphism

    c. Restriction fragment length polymorphism

    d. Red fragment length polymorphism

Ans. (a) Rapid Fragment length polymorphism

544. RELPs, RAPD, VNTRs and SSRs are:

    a. Restriction exonucleases

    b. Restricition endonucleases

    c. Molecular markers

    d. Cloning vectors

Ans. (c) Molecular markers

545. Choose the incorrect statement:

    a. RAPD = Random amplified polymorphic DNA

    b. VNTRs = variable number of tandem repeats

    c. SSRs = Simple sequence repeats

    d. RAPD is also called minisatellites

Ans. (d) RAPD is also called minisatellites

546. Simple sequence repeats (SSRs) also called:

    a. Microsatellites

    b. Satellites

    c. Minisatellites

    d. Polymerase chain reaction

Ans. (a) Microsatellites

547. DIG based technique is used for the detection of certain known DNA in an animal cell. It is preferred over radio labeling techniques due to:

    I. Stability

    II. Easy handling

    III. Safety

    IV. Quick result

    Choose the correct answer :

    a. I, III   b. I, II, III

    c. I, II, III, IV   d. I, II

Ans. (c) I, II, III, IV

548. Gel filtration chromatography separates proteins on the basis of:

    a. Size   b. Charge

    c. Mass   d. Structure

Ans. (a) Size

549. Pregnancy can be detected with in very few days of conception by immune assaying urine for the presence of:

    a. Follicle stimulating hormone

    b. Lutinizing hormone

    c. HCGH

    d. Progesterone

Ans. (c) HCGH

550. DNA finger printing technique is a method of:

    a. Northern blotting   b. Southern blotting

    c. Eastern blotting   d. Western blotting

Ans. (b) Southern blotting

551. The method of detecting a very small sample of proteins by immune assay technique is called as:

    a. Southern blotting

    b. Eastern blotting

    c. Western blotting

    d. Northern blotting

Ans. (c) Western blotting

552. Sucrose gradient centrifugation method can be used to estimate the size of:

    a. Ribosomes   b. Proteins

    c. RNA molecules   d. All of these

Ans. (d) All of these

553. Ion exchange chromatography can be used to separate the protein mixture which differ in over all:

    a. Charge

    b. Structure

    c. Mass

    d. Molecular weight

Ans. (c) Mass

554. R-bands of chromosomes are visualized as green with the help of staining:

    a. Ninhydrin

    b. Cotton blue

    c. Safranin

    d. Acetocarmine

Ans. (a) Ninhydrin

555. Which of the following dye is used in-banding technique of chromosomes staining?

a. Acridine organe   b. Quinacrine

c. Giemsa   d. Acridine

Ans. (b) Quinacrine

556. Fuelgen stain is used for identification of:

a. Nucleolus

b. Chromosomes/DNA

c. Nucleus

d. Unicellular organisms

Ans. (b) Chromosomes/DNA

651. PCR based DNA amplification is an essential feature of which of the following combination of molecular markers?

a. RFLP, AFLP and SSR   b. AFLP, SSR and RAPD

c. RFLP, RAPD and SSR   d. RAPD, RFLP and SSR

Ans. (b) AFLP, SSR and RAPD

558. Biosensors are:

a. Devices that can convert biological or biochemical signal or response into a quantifiable electrical signal

b. Simple enzyme like proteinaceous substance

c. Chemical substances that used in pollution controlling

d. Substance that cause bioremediation

Ans. (a) Devices that can convert biological or biochemical signal or response into a quantifiable electrical signal

559. CsCI gradient centrifugation helps in separation of DNA fragments the basic principle involved is, that of:

a. DNA fragments can move and accumulated at a position where the density of the two (CsCI and DNA) is same

b. Only smaller fragments of DNA can bind with CsCl

c. DNA binds firmly to CsCl

d. CsCl degrades DNA

Ans. (a) DNA fragments can move and accumulated at a position where the density of the two (CsCI and DNA) is same

560. In electron microscope, the specimen has to be mounted in vacuum because :

a. Vacuum increase the size of specimen

b. Vacuum increases the power of electromagnetic lenses

c. Electrons can be absorbed by atoms in the air

d. None of these

Ans. (c) Electrons can be absorbed by atoms in the air

561. The resolution power of transmission electron microscope (TEM) is 0.10 nm whereas scanning electron microscope (SEM) is:

a. 100 fold less than that of TEM

b. 10 fold higher than that of TEM

c. 10 fold less that of TEM

d. 100 fold higher than that of TEM

Ans. (a) 100 fold less than that of TEM

562. SEM produce:

a. Three dimensional image of the specimen

b. Two dimensional image of the specimen

c. One dimensional image of the specimen

d. Four dimensional image of the specimen

Ans. (a) Three dimensional image of the specimen

563. Purines and pyrmidines are cleaved by:

a. Dimethly sulphate

b. Piperazine

c. Hydrazine

d. Dimethyl sulphates and hydrazine respectively

Ans. (d) Dimethyl sulphates and hydrazine respectively

564. The term cistorn, muton and recon were introduced by

a. Watson and crick   b. Benzer

c. Meselson   d. Morgan

Ans. (b) Benzer

565. The chemical used to prevent RNAase contamination during RNA isolation is

a. DEEPP   b. DEPCE

c. DCPPE   d. DEPC

Ans. (d) DEPC

566. Introduction of a gene or DNA fragment from one organism into another organism in such a form, so that it is maintained, replicated and expressed in the new host is known as

a. DNA fingerprinting   b. DNA cloning

c. RNA fingerprinting   d. RNA cloning

Ans. (b) DNA cloning

567. Adenine pairs with thymine with

a. Phosphodiester bond   b. Glycosidic bond

c. 4 hydrogen bond   d. 2 hydrogen bond

Ans. (d) 2 hydrogen bond

568. Guanine pairs with thymine with

    a. Phosphodiester bond   b. Glycosidic bond

    c. 3 hydrogen bond   d. 2 hydrogen bond

Ans. (c) 3 hydrogen bond

569. The DNA sequence which appear to have no function is called as

    a. Satellite DNA   b. Selfish DNA

    c. Palindrome DNA   d. Ct DNA

Ans. (b) Selfish DNA

570. Each strand in a chain of nucleotides are held together by

    a. Phosphodiester bonds   b. 2 hydrogen bond

    c. Glycosidic bond   d. 3 hydrogen bond

Ans. (a) Phosphodiester bonds

571. The set of bases in a t-RNA that pairs with a codon of a m-RNA is know as

    a. Cistron   b. Codon

    c. Exon   d. Anti-codon

Ans. (d) Anti-codon

572. The technique that is generally used for the identification of crinials from blood strains. Semen, etc. and for establishing parentage in case of dispute is called

    a. DNA fingerprinting   b. RNA fingerprinting

    c. DNA cloning   d. RNA cloning

Ans. (a) DNA fingerprinting

573. Purine and pyramidines are joined with de oxyribose by

    a. 2 hydrogen bond   b. 4 hydrogen bond

    c. Glycosidic bond   d. Phosphodiester bonds

Ans. (c) Glycosidic bond

574. All the reaction in the translational process from the formation of the first peptide bond to that of the last peptide bond of the polypeptide chain is called as

    a. Deformation   b. Elongation

    c. Transition   d. Transition

Ans. (b) Elongation

575. The enzyme that calalyses the covalent joining of okazaki fragments is called

    a. DNA polymerase   b. DNA ligase

    c. DNA helicase   d. DNA gyrase

Ans. (b) DNA ligase

576. The coding region of split genes is divided in to few to several small segments; each segment which is having the expressed sequences are called as

    a. Recon   b. Anti-codon

    c. Exons   d. Codon

Ans. (c) Exons

577. In eukaryotic transcription units, a conserved sequence located upstream of start point and recognized by a large group of transcriptional factors is called.

    a. TTAA box   b. TATA box

    c. CAAT box   d. CCTT box

Ans. (c) CAAT box

578. The DNA in which the base pair sequence can be read same in both the directions is called.

    a. Satellite DNA   b. Selfish DNA

    c. Ct DNA   d. Palindrome DNA

Ans. (d) Palindrome DNA

579. Which of the following is a mode of replication?

    a. Semiconservative   b. Dispersive

    c. Conservative   d. All of the above

Ans. (d) All of the above

580. The semi-conservative mechanism of replication was demonstrated by

    a. Watson and crick   b. Mendel

    c. Hershey and chase   d. Meselson and stahal

Ans. (d) Meselson and stahal

581. In meselson and stahl experiment, the E.coli cells were labelled with isotope of

    a. Nitrogen   b. Sulphur

    c. Uranium   d. Potassium

Ans. (a) Nitrogen

582. The modification of RNA polymerase in such a way that it does not recognize specific terminator sequences and continues transcription beyond the regular terminators is know is

    a. Termination   b. Annotation

    c. Bioconversion   d. Anti-termination

Ans. (d) Anti-termination

583. The point at which separation of the strands and synthesis of new DNA takes place is known as

    a. Initiation   b. Replication fork

    c. Origin   d. Template

Ans. (b) Replication fork

584. The enzyme that catalyses the formation of supercoils is

a. DNA ligase   b. DNA polymerase

c. DNA gyrase   d. DNA helicase

Ans. (c) DNA gyrase

585. The initiation of DNA replication within a replicon always occurs at a fixed point called as

a. Initiation   b. Origin

c. Template   d. Replication fork

Ans. (b) Origin

586. Among the following, the example for highly repetitive DNA is

a. Histone cluster

b. Dispersed repetitive DNA

c. DNA minisatelites

d. DNA microsatellites

Ans. (c) DNA minisatelites

587. The enzyme that can relieve super coiling in DNA by creating transitory breaks in sone or both strands of helicase backbone is called as

a. Topoisomerase   b. Gyrase

c. Helicase   d. Ligase

Ans. (a) Topoisomerase

588. The concept of central dogma was given by

a. Watson   b. Crick

c. Jones   d. Korenbeg

Ans. (a) Watson

589. The enzyme that is responsible for transcription is

a. Polynuclease   b. RNA polymerase

c. DNA polymerase   d. Endonuclease

Ans. (b) RNA polymerase

590. An enzyme that separate the two strand of a DNA duplex, usually using the energy from hydrolysis of ATP, is called

a. Ligase   b. Helicase

c. Gyrase   d. Topoisomerase

Ans. (b) Helicase

591. The sequence that consists of self complementary regions which from a stem loop/hairpin structure in RNA product is

a. Regulator   b. Terminator

c. CAAT box   d. TATA box

Ans. (b) Terminator

592. The enzyme that is responsible of heterogeneous nuclear RNA, the precursor of m-RNA is

a. DNA polymerase I   b. RNA polymerase I

c. RNA endonuclease   d. All of the above

Ans. (c) RNA endonuclease

593. Removal of the topological strain by inducting the negative super coiling, which is carried out by

a. DNA gyrase   b. DNA polymerase

c. RNA polymerase   d. RNA gyrase

Ans. (a) DNA gyrase

594. Genomic imprinting is a kind of epistasis which occurs due to

a. DNA polyI   b. DNA gyrase

c. DNA methylation   d. RNA polymerase

Ans. (c) DNA methylation

595. The strand that is used as a template to which ribonucleotides base pair for the synthesis of the RNA is called as

a. Sense strand

b. Antisense strand

c. Template strand

d. Both b and c

Ans. (d) Both b and c

596. The scientist, who had worked out fine structure of gene through cis- trans complementation test is

a. Fleming   b. Benzer

c. Jones   d. Shull

Ans. (c) Jones

597. The temperature at which of the *E.coli* RNA polymerase performs elongation reaction is

a. 37°C   b. 30°C

c. 40°C   d. 45°C

Ans. (a) 37°C

598. Reverse transcription enzyme was discovered by

a. Fleming and shull   b. Shull and jones

c. Watson and crick   d. Vilmorin and jones

Ans. (c) Watson and crick

599. A construct that joins the coding region of two open reading frames such that expression of the product results in a chimeric protein is called as

a. Gene cloning   b. Gene family

c. Gene fusion   d. Gene construct

Ans. (c) Gene fusion

600. The enzyme that can synthesize a new DNA strand on a template DNA strand is called

a. DNA pol III
b. DNA gyrase
c. DNA polymerase
d. All of the above

Ans. (c) DNA polymerase

601. DNA replicating enzyme in bacteria is called is

a. DNA gyrases
b. DNA poly III
c. DNA polymerase
d. DNA methylation

Ans. (b) DNA poly III

602. How many type of RNA polymerase were found in prokaryotes?

a. 4
b. 3
c. 2
d. 6

Ans. (b) 3

603. The distance between sites of initiation and termination by RNA polymerase is called as

a. Transcription unit
b. Transition unit
c. Transformation unit
d. Transduction unit

Ans. (a) Transcription unit

604. The DNA strand that is used as template during transcription is called as

a. Antisense RNA
b. Antisense DNA
c. CAT box
d. CPT box

Ans. (b) Antisense DNA

605. In eukaryotes, DNA methylation is mainly concerned with regulation of

a. Gene pairing
b. Gene amplification
c. Gene index
d. Genetic imprinting

Ans. (a) Gene pairing

606. The attachment point for the catabolite activator protein is called as

a. CAT box
b. CAC box
c. CAP box
d. CATT box

Ans. (c) CAP box

607. A series of DNA sequence fixed as distinct spots on a suitable solid support, such as a glass chip is called as

a. DNA array
b. DNA foot printing
c. DNA sequencing
d. All of the above

Ans. (a) DNA array

608. An RNA copy of a gene is described as

a. RNA replicase
b. RNA polymerase
c. RNA transcript
d. RNA splicing

Ans. (c) RNA transcript

609. The presence of a gene in multiple copies due to polyploidy, polytenic chromosomes, gene amplification, or chromosomal duplication is called

a. Gene redundancy
b. Gene splicing
c. Gene stacking
d. All of the above

Ans. (a) Gene redundancy

610. The removal of large non-coding sequence from the primary RNA transcript followed by rejoining of coding sequences to produce the functional m-RNA is called

a. RNA polymerase
b. RNA editing
c. RNA splicing
d. RNA transcript

Ans. (c) RNA splicing

611. A polymerase enzyme that catalyses self replication of single stranded RNA is called

a. RNA replicase
b. RNA ligase
c. RNA polymerase
d. DNA polymerase

Ans. (a) RNA replicase

612. The sequence 3′AAAAAAT5′ in sense strand of DNA is called as

a. Transcribed spacer
b. Transcriptional unit
c. Terminator sequence
d. Translational unit

Ans. (c) Terminator sequence

613. A genetic marker that is detected as differential mobility of a protein/DNA fragment is known as

a. Molecular marker
b. Molecular breeding
c. Molecular genetics
d. All of the above

Ans. (a) Molecular marker

614.The nucleotide sequence in DNA downstream of the of the termination codon of a gene which is transcribed and not translated is called as

a. Antitrailer
b. Transcribed spacer
c. Terminator sequence
d. Transcriptional unit

Ans. (a) Antitrailer

615. The labelling of a gene by a marker gene or specific DNA sequence closely kinked with the gene in question is called

a. Genetic code   b. Gene tagging

c. Gene therapy   d. Gene translation

Ans. (b) Gene tagging

616. A part of an RNA transcription unit, i.e. transcribed but discarded during maturation is called as

a. Transcribed spacer   b. Transcriptional unit

c. Terminator sequence   d. None of these

Ans. (a) Transcribed spacer

617. A group of gene that are related by sequence homologies usually are also related by their functions are called as

a. Multi-gene family

b. Multiple-cloning site

c. Multicistronic message

d. Multi locus probe

Ans. (c) Multicistronic message

618. The codon, usually but not exclusively 5′ AUG 3′ which indicates the point at which translation of an mRNA should begin is

a. Initiation complex

b. Initiation codon

c. Termination factor

d. Translation factor

Ans. (b) Initiation codon

619. The transfer or movement of a gene or gene fragment from the chromosomal location to another location is called

a. Gene translocation   b. Gene coding

c. Gene tagging   d. Gene therapy

Ans. (a) Gene translocation

620. The protein molecule that play an ancillary role in the initiation stage of translocation is called as

a. Initiation factor

b. Termination factor

c. Transcription factor

d. Translation factor

Ans. (a) Initiation factor

621. The protein required to obtain release of the newly synthesized polypeptide chain from t-RNA is called as

a. Termination factor

b. Initiation factor

c. Initiation codon

d. Initiation complex

Ans. (a) Termination factor

622. A region of DNA at one end of an operon that acts as a binding site for a specific repressor protein and so controls the functioning of adjacent cistrons is termed as

a. Operon   b. Promoter gene

c. Operator gene   d. Reporter gene

Ans. (c) Operator gene

623. A group of structural genes whose transcription is regulated by the coordinated action of a regulator gene, promoter, and operator elements is known as

a. Operon fusion   b. Operator gene

c. Operon   d. Reporter gene

Ans. (c) Operon

624. The largest element within a gene, which is a unit of function, is called

a. Exon   b. Recon

c. Muton   d. Cistron

Ans. (d) Cistron

625. In case of repressible operons, the repressor can bind DNA only when it is associated with the effector; in such cases, the effector is called

a. Operator   b. Reporter

c. Co-repressor   d. Terminator

Ans. (c) Co-repressor

626. The enzymes that produce internal cuts, called cleavage, in DNA molecules are called

a. Endonucleases   b. Kinases

c. Ligase   d. Galactase

Ans. (a) Endonucleases

627. When a single pre-mRNA molecule is processed in two or more ways to yield more than one type of mature m-RNA is called

a. Direct splicing   b. Alternative splicing

c. Destructive splicing   d. Alienation

Ans. (b) Alternative splicing

628. Premature aging due to loss a DNA repair enzyme, perhaps a ligase in human beings are the symptoms of the disease is called

a. Edward syndrome   b. Patau's syndrome

c. Progeria   d. Klinfelter syndrome

Ans. (c) Progeria

629. Nick translation is useful in labelling of molecules like

a. Protein sequence
b. Nucleotide sequence
c. ds-DNA molecules
d. None of these

Ans. (c) ds-DNA molecules

630. The chemical, which is used for breaking the plasma membrane during DNA isolation is known as

a. DNAase
b. Ligase
c. CTAB/SDS
d. Helicase

Ans. (c) CTAB/SDS

631. The absolute radical requirement for both RNA synthesis and DNA replication in the organisms is

a. Free 3'-CH4
b. Free 3'-OH
c. Free 5'-OH
d. Free 3'-H

Ans. (b) Free 3'-OH

632. A sequence of DNA nucleotide which codes for specific polypeptide chian is called as

a. Genome
b. Gene
c. Genetic code
d. Genetic marker

Ans. (b) Gene

633. The bond between sugar and nitrogenous base in case of DNA is known as

a. Hydrophobic bond
b. Glycosidic bond
c. Hydrogen bond
d. Wander wall bond

Ans. (b) Glycosidic bond

634. Restriction site for cloning should be

a. Palindromic in nature
b. Repeated sequence
c. Hexanucleotide
d. Tandemly tepeated

Ans. (d) Tandemly tepeated

635. GAATTC is restriction sequence of CTTAAG indicates

a. Bam HI
b. Sam I
c. Eco RI
d. Null

Ans. (c) Eco RI

636. For cloning Eukaryotic gene in prokaryotic, genes should be isolated from

a. Genomic library
b. Eukaryotic host
c. C-DNA library
d. None of these

Ans. (c) C-DNA library

637. Which enzyme play important role in reverse transcription?

a. Ribonuclease
b. DNA polymerase
c. RNA polymerase
d. Reverse transciptase

Ans. (d) Reverse transciptase

638. A term used to describe the excess DNA which is present in the genome beyond that required to encode protein is called as

a. Split gene
b. Active DNA
c. Junk DNA
d. Dead DNA

Ans. (c) Junk DNA

639. Micro-satellite are also known as

a. STRs
b. RAPDs
c. ISSR
d. RFLP

Ans. (a) STRs

640. Mini-satellites are also known as

a. RFLPs
b. RAPD
c. STS
d. VNTRs

Ans. (d) VNTRs

641. Protein involved for joining the DNA during replication is

a. Topoisomerase
b. Ligase
c. Gyrase
d. Helicase

Ans. (b) Ligase

642. The use of DNA marker for indirect selection of difficult to select traits like yield, etc. is known as

a. Marker assisted selection
b. Yield selection
c. DNA selection
d. RNA selection

Ans. (a) Marker assisted selection

643. The c-DNA libraries can be prepared by isolating

a. m-RNA
b. t-RNA
c. r-RNA
d. All of the above

Ans. (a) m-RNA

644. Actinomycin-D, rifampicin and 5-bromouracil are inhibitors to the synthesis of

a. t-RNA
b. m-RNA
c. r-RNA
d. all of the above

Ans. (b) m-RNA

645. A CsCl gradient will separate DNA molecule by

a. Resorption   b. Density

c. Adhesion   d. Absorption

Ans. (b) Density

646. Which of the following DNA structure forms left hand helix?

a. DNA B   b. DNA C

c. DNA Z   d. DNA A

Ans. (c) DNA Z

647. m-RNA usually is being extracted using

a. Poly T resin   b. RNase P

c. Poly A resin   d. None of the above

Ans. (a) Poly T resin

648. DNA is fit for making tools in case of nano-technology, which is due to

a. Small size of DNA

b. Flexibility in DNA conformation

c. Branching nature of DNA

d. All of the above

Ans. (d) All of the above

649. RFLP markers mapped in one species or genus can often be used to construct parallel gentic maps in related species or genera, which is called as

a. Reverse mapping   b. Parallel mapping

c. Targeted mapping   d. None of these

Ans. (b) Parallel mapping

650. Transgenic expression study can be done by

a. Transcription profiling

b. RT-PCR

c. Transcription profiling

d. All of the above

Ans. (d) All of the above

651. Gene, which have major effect on the expression of the concerned traits is called:

a. Oncogene   b. Oligogenes

c. Gene   d. None of these

Ans. (b) Oligogenes

652. A gene involved in tumour development, in case of Agrobacterium, genes specifying auxin and cytokinin biosynthesis is called:

a. Oligogenes   b. Oncogene

c. Luxury gene   d. Gene

Ans. (b) Oncogene

653. Those genes, which are expressed either in specialized cells or in response to an specific stimuli is called:

a. Oligogenes   b. Oncogene

c. Luxury gene   d. Gene

Ans. (c) Luxury gene

654. molecular marker pattern of an individual obtained by using highly polymorphic markers; used for unequivocal identification of strains, individuals, criminals etc., is called

a. DNA fingerprint   b. DNA finger printing

c. DNA footprinting   d. DNA sequencing

Ans. (a) DNA fingerprint

655. In enables identification of the site on a DNA molecule to which a protein, such as RNA polymerase, binds is called:

a. DNA fingerprint   b. DNA finger printing

c. DNA foot printing   d. DNA sequencing

Ans. (c) DNA foot printing

656. Determination of the base sequence of a DNA fragment is called:

a. DNA polymerase   b. DNA microarray

c. DNA footprinting   d. DNA sequencing

Ans. (d) DNA sequencing

657. A gene that gives rise to a product involved in the regulation of the expression of another gene; for example, a gene coding for a repressor protein is called:

a. Structural gene

b. Regulatory gene

c. Regulatory sequence

d. Reverse transcriptase

Ans. (b) Regulatory gene

658. Which varieties is the first variety in Indian developed by MAS?

a. Pusa Basmati I

b. Improved Pusa Basmati I

c. Pusa 1401

d. Pusa 1112

Ans. (b) Improved Pusa Basmati I

659. Pusa 1406 has which of the following genes transferred through MAS?

a. Xa21   b. Xa 13

c. Both a and b   d. None of these

Ans. (c) Both a and b

660. Primer designing for sequence tagged sites is based on

a. Random genomic DNA
b. Ends of large genomic DNA fragment
c. Sequences of cDNA
d. All of the above

Ans. (d) All of the above

661. Improved Pusa Basmati 1, the first variety in India developed through MAS, has been improved by transferring:

a. Vitamin A
b. QTLs for grain size
c. Disease resistance
d. Cooking quality

Ans. (c) Disease resistance

662. Which markers systems has been used for developing pusa 1460?

a. RFLP
b. STMS
c. ISSR
d. SCAR

Ans. (b) STMS

663. What would stop DNA replication in Bacteria?

a. Addition of a DNA polymerse inhibitor
b. Addition of dideoxyribonucleaotides
c. Both of these
d. None of these

Ans. (c) Both of these

664. Development of which of the following populations requires the greatest effort?

a. F_2
b. Backcross
c. RILs
d. NILs

Ans. (d) NILs

665. Once an RAPD marker linked to a trait of interest is found, it can be converted into a more reproducible PCR type assay by use of:

a. Allele specific ligation
b. Allele specific PCR
c. Sequence characterized amplified region
d. All of these

Ans. (d) All of these

666. Which is not correct about molecular markers?

a. The sequence tagged sites marker system has all the advantages of PCR technique
b. RFLP is the fist molecular marker that was developed in 1980s

c. RFLP marker are highly reproducible
d. None of these

Ans. (b) RFLP is the fist molecular marker that was developed in 1980s

667. Transgenic plants are easier to produce the transgenic animals because:

a. Plants can more easily be grown from single cultured cell into which foreign DNA has been introduced
b. Plant DNA is easier to clone
c. Plant cells can be transformed by bacterial infection
d. DNA passes more readily through the plant cell wass than through the animal cell membrane

Ans. (a) Plants can more easily be grown from single cultured cell into which foreign DNA has been introduced

668. A recombination dependent mechanism for repairing damaged DNA is:

a. SOS repair
b. Excision repair
c. Mismatch repair
d. Photo eactivation repair

Ans. (a) SOS repair

669. Group I introns are remarkable because

a. They are spliced by external RNA molecules with the help of protein
b. They are spliced by protein molecules in the absence of external RNA molecules they are autocatalytic
c. They are autocatalytic
d. They are only present in mitochondrial and chloroplast genomes

Ans. (c) They are autocatalytic

670. In 1923, the theory of QTL mapping was described by:

a. Stern
b. Sax
c. Mather
d. Galton

Ans. (b) Sax

671. Begining with 600 template DNA molecules, after 25 cycles of PCR, how many amplicons will be produced?

a. 2×10^{10}
b. 5×10^{10}
c. 10×10^{10}
d. 20×10^{10}

Ans. (a) 2×10^{10}

672. Which is not correct about cleaved Amplified polymorphic sequences

a. This marker captures some of the advantages of RFLP assay

b. It avoids the disadvantages of southern blot analysis

c. CAPS was initially developed for use in pea

d. CAPS detects DNA sequences variation in terms of the lengths of DNA fragments generated by the restriction digestion of PCR products

Ans. (c) CAPS was initially developed for use in pea

673. Which problem is associated with RAPD process?

a. It produces difficulties in reproducing RAPD patterns in different laboratories

b. RAPD patterns are not reproducible due to impurities in DNA preparation

c. RAPD patterns are not reproducible due to the use of small amount of DNA

d. Both a and b

Ans. (d) Both a and b

674. Mapping of disease resistance genes has been based on:

a. ISSR

b. RAPD

c. Microsatellite

d. All of the above

Ans. (d) All of the above

675. Human DNA is replicated in 5 hrs at a rate of 1 kb/min. The number off origins of replication utilized are:

a. 1

b. 300

c. 3000

d. 10000

Ans. (d) 10000

676. Which of the following reagents would be useful for labelling the oligodeoxyribo-nucleotide d(GGATATCC)?

a. [$Y^{-32}P$] ATP

b. Polynucleotide kinase

c. DNA dependent RNA polymerase

d. Both a and b

Ans. (d) Both a and b

677. A restriction enzyme with a four base recognition site would leave DNA with a statical frequency of one every:

a. 260 base pair

b. 256 base pair

c. 300 base pair

d. 500 base pair

Ans. (b) 256 base pair

678. In E.coli, attenuation and antitermination utilize which structure?

a. Stem loop structure in RNA

b. Stem loop structures in DNA

c. RNA/DNA hybrid

d. Differential protein folding

Ans. (a) Stem loop structure in RNA

679. A mixture containing two proteins having similar molecular mass but different oligomeric properties can be separated by:

a. SDS-PAGE analysis

b. Native PAGE analysis

c. Isoelectric focusing

d. Both b and c

Ans. (d) Both b and c

680. Selenocystein:

a. Only present in prokaryotes

b. Coded by UGA

c. Derives from cysteine

d. Forms post translationlally

Ans. (b) Coded by UGA

CHECK YOU GRASP

1. **Genetic engineering would not have been possible if one of these were absent**
   a. DNA polymerase
   b. Reverse transcriptase
   c. DNA ligase
   d. RNA synthetase

2. **Which of the following is associated with genetic engineering**
   a. Plastid
   b. Plasmids
   c. Mutations
   d. Hybrid vigour

3. **In proof reading during DNA replication**
   a. Wrong nucleotides are inserted
   b. Wrong nucleotides are taken out
   c. Wrong nucleotides are removes and correct ones inserted
   d. Mutations are prevented

4. **The idea that genes control the production of enzyme was given by**
   a. E.L. Tatum
   b. T.H. Morgan
   c. A.E. Garrod
   d. R.S. Kornberg

5. **One gene one enzyme theory (hypothesis) was proposed by**
   a. Beadle and Tatum
   b. Avery and McCarty
   c. Jacob and Monad
   d. Luria and Delburck

6. **Co-linearity between genes and polypeptides was established by**
   a. Linus pauling
   b. V. Ingram
   c. Yanofsky
   d. Brenner

7. **In DNA the histone responsible for higher order chromatin structure is**
   a. H1
   b. H2A
   c. H2B
   d. H3 AND H4

8. **In trimeric G protein GTPase activity is found in**
   a. Gs
   b. Gαs
   c. Gβs
   d. G$\alpha\beta$s

9. **In which of the following conformation of DNAs, there is no discernible major groove**
   a. Z-DNA
   b. B-DNA
   c. C-DNA
   d. None of these

10. **The region where RNA polymerase binds to promoter in prokaryotes is called**
    a. Hogness box
    b. Homeo box
    c. Pribnow box
    d. Shine-dalgrano box

11. **UGA is a stop codon, but in mitochondrial genome it codes for**
    a. Trp
    b. Met
    c. Try
    d. Asp

12. **What happens to the Cdk-cycA complex at metaphase?**
    a. Only cyclin A is degraded
    b. Both cyclin A and Cdk remain under graded
    c. Both cyclin A and Cdk are degraded
    d. Only Cdk is degraded

In case of less than 80% score, go through brief Review and Glance one again from chapter

Key: 1-c 2-b 3-c 4-c 5-a 6-c 7-a 8-b 9-a 10-c 11-a 12-a

3

Recombinant DNA Technology

1. **Which of the following is not true about restriction endonuclease?**

   a. Restriction enzymes work in presence of Mg^{2+}

   b. Type II restriction endonucleases do not require ATP for restriction activities

   c. It is present in both eukaryotes and prokaryotes

   d. Each restriction enzyme only recognizes the same palindromic sequences regardless of source of DNA

Ans. (c) It is present in both eukaryotes and prokaryotes

2. **A restriction enzyme *AluI* with a 4- bp recognition site produces restriction fragments that should have average size of**

   a. 4096 bp   b. 256 bp

   c. 16 bp   d. 436 bp

Ans. (b) 256 bp

3. **Identify the mismatch**

   a. Alkaline phosphatise   1. Remove phosphate group present at 5'end of DNA

   b. DNA polymerase I   2. Nick translation

   c. S1 endonuclease   3. Cleaves only single strand DNA

   d. DNAase 1   4. Cleaves only dsDNA

Ans. (d) DNAase 1   4. Cleaves only dsDNA

4. **Restriction enzyme digestion of a 4 kb pst–digested DNA molecule with EcoRI yields two fragments of 1 kb and 3 kb each. Digestion of the same molecule with HindIII yields fragments of 1.5 kb and 2.5 kb. Finally, disgestion with EcoRI and HindIII together yields fragments of 0.5kb, 1kb and 2.5 kb. Based on this information, the 0.5kb fragment is flanked by which of the following enzyme sites**

   a. PstI-HindIII   b. EcoRI-HindIII

   c. EcoRI   d. EcoRI-pstI

Ans. (b) EcoRI-HindIII

5. **A linear DNA fragment is (100%) labeled at one end and has 3 restriction sites for EcoRI. If it is partially digested by EcoRI so that all possible fragments are produced, how many of these fragments will be labeled and how many will not be labeled?**

   a. 4 labeled; 6 unlabeled

   b. 4 labeled; 4 unlabeled

   c. 3 labeled; 5 unlabeled

   d. 3 labeled; 3 unlabeled

Ans. (a) 4 labeled ; 6 unlabeled

6. **Restriction endonucleases hydrolyzes poly-nucleotide from**

   a. Only the 5'end

   b. From either terminal

   c. At an internal phosphodiester bond

   d. A phosphodiester bond within a specific sequence

Ans. (d) A phosphodiester bond within a specific sequence

7. **Bacteria protect themselves from viruses by fragmenting viral DNA upon entry with**

   a. Methtylase

   b. Endonucleases

   c. Ligases

   d. Exonucleases

Ans. (b) Endonucleases

8. **Which of the following tools of recombinant DNA technology is incorrectly paired with its use?**

   a. Restriction enzyme-production of RFLPs

   b. DNA ligase-enzyme that cuts DNA, creating the sticky ends of restriction fragments

   c. DNA polymerase-used in a polymerase chain reaction to amplify section of DNA

   d. Reverse transcriptase-production of cDNA from mRNA

Ans. (b) DNA ligase-enzyme that cuts DNA, creating the sticky ends of restriction fragments

9. Match list I (Enzyme) with list II (Characteristic/ activity) and select the correct using the codes given below the lists

   a. Terminal transferases , 1. Stable above 90°C

   B. Polynucleotide kinases 2. Cleave the ends of linear DNA

   c. Taq DNA polymerases 3. Adds phosphate to 5'OH end of DNA or RNA

   D. Exonucleases 4. Adds a number of nucleotides to 3'end of DNA/RNA

Ans. (A-4, B-3, C-1, D-2)

10. Restriction endonuccleases are

    a. Used for vitro DNA synthesis

    b. Synthesized by bacteria as part of their defense mechanism

    c. Present in mammalian cells for degradation of DNA when the cells dies

    d. Used in genetic engineering for ligating two DNA molecules

Ans. (b) Synthesized by bacteria as part of their defense mechanism

11. Which of the following sequences along a double–stranded DNA molecule may be recognized as a cutting site for a particular restriction enzyme?

    a. A A G G   b. A G T C
       T T C C   T C A G
    c. G G C C   d. A C C A
       C C G G   T G G T

Ans. (c) G G C C, C C G G

12. Restriction-modification systems of bacteria exists to

    a. Protect bacteria from invading foreign DNA

    b. Promote conjugation

    c. Help the bacterial chromosome to replicate

    d. Encourage recombination of new genetic material

Ans. (a) Protect bacteria from invading foreign DNA

13. Which of the following processes require energy?

    a. Ligation

    b. Transformation

    c. Restriction digestion

    d. Hybridization

Ans. (a) Ligation

14. The restriction endonuclease Eco521 recognizes the sequence C/GGCGG and cuts between the first C and the first G, indicated by the slash. DNA cut by which of the following enzymes (given with their recognition sequences and cut sites) could be cloned into a plasmid digested with Eco521?

    a. EcoRI (G/AATTC)

    b. XmaIII (C/GGCGG)

    c. SmaI (CCC/GCG)

    d. SacII (CCGC/GG)

Ans. (b) XmaIII (C/GGCGG)

15. T4 polynucleotide kinase is used for

    a. Labelling 3'ends of DNA

    b. Labeling 5'ends of DNA

    c. Creating blunt ends of DNA

    d. Dephosphorylation of DNA

Ans. (b) Labeling 5'ends of DNA

16. You have cut the genome of a double –stranded viral genome with a restriction endonuclease and electrophoresed the products on an agarose gel. You observe only one band on the gel, equivalent to the size of the genome. This is because

    a. There are no introns in the genome

    b. The introns contain the recognition sites and have already been spliced out

    c. All of restriction fragments are too small to detect

    d. Restriction endonucleases do not cut RNA, and this virus has a dsRNA genome

Ans. (d) Restriction endonucleases do not cut RNA, and this virus has a dsRNA genome

17. A southern transfer of E.coil DNA after complete digestion with EcoRI was probed with labeled cDNA probe of a gene which occurs only once in the E.coil genome. If the gene contains one EcoR1 cleavage site near its center, the number of radioactive bands you are most likely to find on autoradiography would be

    a. 0   b. 1
    c. 2   d. 3

Ans. (c) 2

18. The substrate for restriction enzyme is

    a. Single stranded RNA

    b. Partially double stranded RNA

    c. Cell wall proteins

    d. Double stranded DNA

Ans. (d) Double stranded DNA

19. **If you discovered a bacterial cell that contained no restriction enzymes, which of the following would you expect to happen?**

    a. The cell would be unable to replicate its DNA

    b. The cell would create incomplete plasmids

    c. The cell would be easily infected and lysed by bacteriophages

    d. The cell would become an obligate parasite

Ans. (c) The cell would be easily infected and lysed by bacteriophages

20. **Mung bean nuclease could be used for**

    a. DNA synthesis

    b. Nucleotide hydrolysis

    c. Trimming single stranded region in DNA

    d. Removal of phosphate groups from the end of the DNA

Ans. (c) Trimming single stranded region in DNA

21. **DNA of a bacterium is not cleaved by its own restriction enzymes the recognition DNA sequences are**

    a. Methylated

    b. Deleted

    c. Bound by inhibitory proteins

    d. Not accessible to restriction enzymes

Ans. (a) Methylated

22. **Two restriction enzymes A and B have eight and four base pairs as their recognition sites respectively .The ratio of the number of fragments that they will generate on restriction digestion of a genomic DNA of E. coli is approximately**

    a. 4 : 8   b. 8 : 4

    c. 1 : 64   d. 1 : 256

Ans. (d) 1 : 256

23. **Restriction endonucleases are enzymes that**

    a. Cleave the 5'terminal nucleotides from duplex DNA molecules

    b. Make sequence-specific cuts in both strands of duplex DNA molecules

    c. Promote circularization of the duplex DNA molecule by removal of the 5' terminal nucleotides

    d. Generate 3'-hydroxyl and 5'- phosphate ends in the cut DNA strands

Ans. (b) Make sequence-specific cuts in both strands of duplex DNA molecules

    (d) Generate 3'-hydroxyl and 5'- phosphate ends in the cut DNA strands

24. **Correct statements regarding the enzyme reverse transcriptase include which of the following?**

    a. It requires a primer

    b. It requires an RNA template

    c. It synthesizes an RNA - DNA hybrid molecule

    d. It can be extracted from retroviruses

Ans. (a, b, c, d)

25. **If the liner double stranded genomic DNA of bacteriophage T4 is heated and cooled, one gets both liner and circular molecule because**

    a. All liner DNA on heating and cooling attain circular shape

    b. The DNA molecule are circularly permuted

    c. The DNA molecule has cohesive terminal ends

    d. The RNA component of the genomes gets hydrolyzed to result in the circularization

Ans. (c) The DNA molecule has cohesive terminal ends

26. **Terminal transferase is used**

    a. To add base at the 3' end of the DNA

    b. To add base at the 5' end of the DNA

    c. To carry out nick translation

    d. To transfer phosphate at the 3' end of the DNA

Ans. (a) To add base at the 3' end of the DNA

27. **Which statement about restriction enzymes are false?**

    a. Restriction enzymes cut DNA at specific sequence called recognition sites

    b. A restriction enzymes always cut DNA to leave the same sequence at the ends

    c. Some restriction enzymes cut the two DNA strands at slightly different points within their recognition site to make a 'sticky' end

    d. Restriction enzymes are exonucleases rather than endonucleases

Ans. (d) Restriction enzymes are exonucleases rather than endonucleases

28. **If a transcript of a given gene is degraded when mixed with DNA encoding the same gene, one could conclude that the RNA solution is contaminated with**

    a. RNAse A

    b. RNAse T

    C. RNAse H

    d. DNAse III

Ans. (c) RNAse H

29. A gene that does not contain introns has an EcoRI site just down stream of the translational termination codon in the 3' untranslated region . The size of the gene is 4 Kbp. The length of 3'UTR is 2 k bp, the 5' UTR is 1 Kbp and that the open reading frame is 1 Kbp. Upon probing a southern blot of an Eco RI digested genomic DNA with the radioactively labeled fragment containing only the open reading frame the size of the band detected by hybridization would be

   a. 1 Kbp   b. > 2 Kbp
   c. 0.5 Kbp   d. 1.5 Kbp

Ans. (b) > 2 Kbp

30. Which of the following sequences is most likely to be a restriction enzyme recognition site?

   a. CGGCTT   b. CGCCGC
   c. GTAATG   d. GTCGAC

Ans. (d) GTCGAC

31. You are attempting to clone a gene .you cut a vector with the restriction enzyme EcoRI .You mix your cleaved plasmid with an EcoRI fragment carrying the gene of interest , carry out a ligation reaction ,transform the ligation mix, and plate the bacteria. When you examine plasmids from individual colonies what do you primarily find?

   a. Plasmids that contain the EcoRI
   b. Plasmids that contain concatamers of the EcoRI fragment carrying the gene (i.e. multiple copies of the gene)
   c. Plasmids that do not contains the EcoRI fragment carrying the genes
   d. Plasmid dimers held together by the EcoRI fragment carrying the gene

Ans. (c) Plasmids that do not contains the EcoRI fragment carrying the genes

31. To be cloning vector, a plasmid does not require

   a. An origin of replication
   b. An antibiotic resistance marker
   c. A restriction site
   d. To have a high copy number

Ans. (d) To have a high copy number

32. In recombinant DNA methods, the term vector refers to

   a. The enzyme that cuts DNA into restriction fragments
   b. The sticky of a DNA fragment
   c. Plasmid used to transfer DNA into a living cell
   d. A DNA probe used to identify a particular gene

Ans. (c) Plasmid used to transfer DNA into a living cell

33. Which of the following is a desirable characteristic for a cloning plasmid?

   a. A site at which replication can be initiated
   b. One or more unique restriction endonuclease sites
   c. One or more antibiotic-resistance or drug resistance genes
   d. All of the above

Ans. (d) All of the above

34. A multiple cloning copies of a cloned gene

   a. Contains many copies of a cloned restriction enzymes for cloning
   b. Allows flexibility in the choice of restriction enzymes for cloning
   c. Allows flexibility in the choice of organism for cloning
   d. Contains many copies of the same restriction enzyme site

Ans. (b) Allows flexibility in the choice of restriction enzymes for cloning

35. Many plasmids have ampicillin marker this implies

   a. The plasmids contain genes for ampicillin biosynthesis
   b. Ampicillin is required for bacterial growth after transformation
   c. The plasmid contains the gene encoding β-lactamase
   d. Ampicillin is essential for cell survival

Ans. (c) The plasmid contains the gene encoding β-lactamase

36. BAC, which can be used to clone large DNA fragments, is derived from

   a. CoIE plasmid   b. F plasmid
   c. 2µ plasmid   d. Mu phage

Ans. (b) F plasmid

37. A cloning vector consisting of cos site inserted in a plasmid, used to clone DNA fragments of lambda phage is

   a. Phagemid   b. Cosmid
   c. Plasmid   d. YAC

Ans. (b) Cosmid

38.Which of the following is not component of yeast artificial chromosome?

   a. Centromere   b. Telomere
   c. Origin of replication   d. Cos site

Ans. (d) Cos site

39. Indentify the incorrect statement for cosmids

a. Cosmids are hybrid between a phage DNA and bacterial plasmid
b. Cosmids are basically a plasmid that carries a cos site
c. Cosmids can be used to clone DNA of 30-40 Kb
d. Cosmids produce plaques

Ans. (d) Cosmids produce plaques

40. Bacterial artificial chromosomes (BACs), cosmids phage plasmids, and yeast artificial chromosomes (YACs) are all commonly used cloning vectors that differ in their cloning capacities with a range from approximately 100 bp to 3000 kb. which of the following is the proper order for these vector in terms of increasing cloning capacity?

a. BAC, cosmid, phage, plasmid, YAC
b. YAC, BAC, cosmid, phage, plasmid
c. Plasmid, phage, cosmid, BAC, YAC
d. Plasmid, cosmid, phage, BAC, YAC

Ans. (c) Plasmid, phage, cosmid, BAC, YAC

41. Choose the mismatch

a. Phagemid	1. Part of M13 genome with plasmid DNA
b. P1 -derived artificial chromosome	2. Combine features of P1 vector and BACs
c. Shuttle vector	3. Yeast episomal plasmids
d. Ti plasmid	4. *Agrobacterium rhizogenes*

Ans. (d) Ti plasmid

42. Match list I (cloning vector) with list II (character) and select the correct answer using the codes given below the lists

List I (cloning vector)	List II (character)
A. yeast episomal plasmid (YE$_P$)	1. Integrates with host chromosome for replication
B. Yeast integrative plasmid (YI$_P$)	2. Carries a chromosomal origin of replication
C. Yeast replication plasmid (YR$_P$)	3. Carries origin of replication of the 2μ plasmid

Ans. (a-3, b-1, c-2)

43. pBR322 which is frequently used as a vector for cloning gene in *E.coli* is

a. An original bacterial plasmid
b. A modified bacterial plasmid
c. A viral genome   d. A transposon

Ans. (b) A modified bacterial plasmid

44. Phage T7 promoter containing plasmids are used for over expression of cloned genes because of

a. Their convennient size
b. Their single stranded nature
c. Exquisite specificity of T7 RNA polymerase to phage promoters
d. T7 infects *E.coli* and lysogenizes the cell

Ans. (c) Exquisite specificity of T7 RNA polymerase to phage promoters

45. Yeast artificial chromosomes (YAC) is used for

a. Cloning large segments genomic of DNA
b. Cloning only yeast genomic sequences
c. Cloning of only cDNA sequences
d. All DNA except plant DNA sequences

Ans. (a) Cloning large segments genomic of DNA

46. For cloning a DNA fragment larger than 100 Kb, which of the following vector system would be suitable?

a. Plasmid
b. Cosmid
c. Yeast artificial chromosome
d. Lambda bacteriophage

Ans. (c) Yeast artificial chromosome

47. Expression vector contain a sequence, not normally found in other vector that is known as

a. A ribosome-binding site
b. An ori site
c. A multiple-cloning site
d. An antibody-resistant marker

Ans. (a) A ribosome-binding site

48. What is the difference between a PAC and a BAC?

a. One has ampicillin and another has kanamycin resistance marker
b. One is plasmid-based vector and the other is derived a yeast chromosome
c. One is derived from the E. coli F-plasmid and other is derived from bacteriophage P1
d. One is derived from bacteriophage P1 and other is derived from bacteriophage

Ans. (c) One is derived from the E. coli F-plasmid and other is derived from bacteriophage P1

49. For a plasmid to be a cloning vector, the minimum numbers of elements required are

a. Origin of replication, multiple cloning site, selection marker
b. Origin of replication, multiple cloning site, selection marker, promoter

c. Origin of replication, multiple cloning site, selection marker, translation start site

d. Origin of replication, multiple cloning site, promoter

Ans. (a) Origin of replication, multiple cloning site, selection marker

50. **What is the most logical sequence of steps for splicing foreign DNA into a plasmid and inserting the plasmid into a bacterium?**

    a. Transform bacteria with recombinant DNA molecule

    b. Cut the plasmid DNA using restriction enzymes

    c. Extract plasmid DNA from bacterial cells

    d. Hydrogen–bond the plasmid DNA to nonplasmid DNA fragments

    e. Use ligase to seal plasmid DNA to nonplasmid DNA

Ans. (c, b, d, e, a)

51. **Eukaryotic genes may not function properly when cloned into bacteria because of**

    a. Inability to excise introns

    b. Destruction by native endonucleases

    c. Failure of promoter to be recognized by bacterial RNA polymerase

    d. All of the above

Ans. (a) Inability to excise introns

52. **The presence of a plasmid in a bacterial culture is usually determined by**

    a. Blue- white screening

    b. Growth in the presence of an antibiotic

    c. A restriction enzyme digests

    d. Agarose gel electrophoresis

Ans. (b) Growth in the presence of an antibiotic

53. **Blue–white selection is used**

    a. To test for the presence of a plasmid in bacteria

    b. To reveal the identity of a cloned DNA fragment

    c. To express the product of a cloned gene

    d. To test for the presence of a cloned insert in a plasmid

Ans. (d) To test for the presence of a cloned insert in a plasmid

54. **Infection of *E.coli* by bacteriophage λ is normally detected by**

    a. Resistance of the bacteria to an antibiotic

    b. The growth of single bacterial colonies on an agar plate

c. The appearance of areas of lysed bacteria on an agar plate

d. Restriction digest of the bacterial DNA

Ans. (c) The appearance of areas of lysed bacteria on an agar plate

55. **Which of the following statements givens a correct explanation for the use of vectors containing drug resistance genes in the cloning of recombinant DNA (cDNA) molecules?**

    a. The products of the drug resistance genes protect the cDNA from destruction by the host cells

    b. The drug resistance genes provide additional base sequences that enable the vector to accommodate larger inserts of cDNA

    c. Entry of the vector containing the DNA and the drug resistance genes into the host cell renders the later identifiable as it is now resistance to antibiotic drugs

    d. The cloned cDNA imparts drug resistance upon any cellular system with which it is used

Ans. (c) Entry of the vector containing the DNA and the drug resistance genes into the host cell renders the later identifiable as it is now resistance to antibiotic drugs

56. **What is the approximate length of DNA between two COS sites that can be packed by a lambda packing extract?**

    a. 10 Kb

    b. 15 Kb

    c. 25 Kb

    d. 45 Kb

Ans. (d) 45 Kb

57. **Which statement correctly describes sequential steps in cDNA in DNA cloning?**

    a. Reverse transcription of mRNA, second strand synthesis, cDNA end modification, ligation to vector

    b. mRNA preparation, cDNA synthesis using reverse transcription, second strand synthesis using terminal transferase, ligation to vector

    c. mRNA synthesis using RNA polymerase ,reverse transcription of mRNA, second strand synthesis ligation to vector

    d. Double stranded cDNA synthesis, restriction enzyme digestion, addition of linkers, ligation to vector

Ans. (a) Reverse transcription of mRNA, second strand synthesis, cDNA end modification, ligation to vector

58. The PCR is used to

a. Amplify a small amount of DNA
b. Cleave bacteria plasmids
c. Seal sticky ends
d. Identify target plasmids

Ans. (a) Amplify a small amount of DNA

59. The polymerase enzyme used in PCR is

a. DNA polymerase I   b. Taq polymerase
c. Reverse transciptase   d. DNA polymerase

Ans. (b) Taq polymerase

60. The first step in the PCR is

a. Denaturation   b. Primer extension
c. Annealing   d. Cooling

Ans. (a) Denaturation

61. Polymerase chain reaction is considered as a revolutionary because all of the following, *except*:

a. It enables an unlimited production of a DNA fragment in vitro
b. It is a highly sensitive technology
c. Its experimental protocol is simple
d. It enables the direct production of a synthetic gene that did not exist before

Ans. (d) It enables the direct production of a synthetic gene that did not exist before

62. PCR amplification cycle involves

a. Template denaturation
b. Primer annealing
c. DNA polymerization
d. Reaction mixture containing target DNA, prime, thermostable DNA polymerase and dNTP

Ans. (a, b, c, d)

63. The amplification product of a PCR reaction is defined by the sequence of the PCR primers. Several general rules follow to design primer. Select the following rules commonly used to design primers

a. Length of primers
b. Tm of both primers
c. G + C content of both primers
d. Complementarity between the primers

Ans. (a, b, c, d)

64. Choose the correct statements (s) about thermostable DNA polymerase used in PCR

a. Taq Pol has no proof reading ability
b. Taq Pol has 5′ → 3′ exonuclease activity

c. *pfu* pol has 3′ → 5′ exonuclease activity
d. T*li* Pol has no 3′ → 5′ exonuclease activity

Ans. (a, b, c)

65. Which of the following would be eliminated by hot start PCR?

a. Aerosol contamination from the barrel of pipetors
b. Addition of a nucleotide to the terminal end of PCR products
c. Infidelity of DNA copying by Taq DNA polymerase
d. Formation of primer–dimers

Ans. (d) Formation of primer–dimers

66. The annealing temperature, at which the primers attach to the template, can be calculated by determining the melting temperature (Tm)of the primer template hybrid .What will be Tm of the primer 5′-AGACTCAGAGAGAACCC-3′

a. 50°C   b. 52°C
c. 102°C   d. 43°C

Ans. (b) 52°C

67. Efficient expression of a heterologous protein product is influenced by

a. Transcriptional efficiency
b. Copy number of the plasmid
c. Codon bias
d. All of the above

Ans. (d) All of the above

68. Which of the following is not a potential problem associated with expressing a eukaryotic, protein coding nuclear gene in prokaryotic cells?

a. Lack of an intron-splicing mechanism in prokaryotes
b. Differences in the translation intiation codons used by eukaryotic cells and prokaryotic cells
c. Stability of mRNA in prokaryotic cells
d. Differences in transcriptional signals between eukaryotic cells and prokaryotic cells

Ans. (b) Differences in the translation intiation codons used by eukaryotic cells and prokaryotic cells

69. Which of the following conditions prevent efficient expression of foreign gene cloned in *E.coli*?

a. The foreign gene might contain introns
b. Foreign gene might contain sequence that act as termination signals in *E.coli*
c. Codon bias
d. Nature of nitrogenous bases in nucleotides

Ans. (a, b, and c)

70. A reporter gene

    a. A acts as repressor

    b. Allows gene expression to be readily measured

    c. Enhances mRNA stability

    d. Interacts with RNA polymerase

Ans. (b) Allows gene expression to be readily measured

71. Most common reporter whose product can be directly visualized in transformed cells is

    a. NPTII (Neomycim phosphotransferase)

    b. CAT (choramphniol acetyl transferase)

    c. β-galactosidase

    d. GFP (green fluorescent protein)

Ans. (c) β-galactosidase

72. Which of the following statement is false about reporter genes?

    a. Replace the coding region of a gene of interest with a coding region that is easily assayed

    b. Replace the promoter region of a gene of interest with a promoter region that is easily assayed

    c. Can be used to measure the activity of a promoter

    d. Can be used to determine when and where a promoter is active

Ans. (b) Replace the promoter region of a gene of interest with a promoter region that is easily assayed

73. Which of the following is incorrect about reporter gene?

    a. Gene whose phenotype can be assayed in a transformed organism

    b. β-galactosidase gene is an example of reporter gene

    c. Test gene that is fused to the upstream region of the cloned gene

    d. None

Ans. (d) None

74. The principle behind the yeast two-hybrid system is

    a. The detection of protein and DNA interaction from yeast hydrid strains

    b. The detection of protein-protein interactions by assembling a functional transcription factor from two fusion proteins

    c. The detection of protein-protein interaction by studying the hybridization of two cDNA sequence

    d. The detection of protein-protein interactions in a pair of hybrid yeast strains

Ans. (b) The detection of protein-protein interactions by assembling a functional transcription factor from two fusion proteins

75. Shotgun approach is used for the construction of

    a. cDNA   b. Genomic library

    c. Both   d. None

Ans. (b) Genomic library

76. Which one of the following statements about genomic libraries are false?

    a. Genomic libraries are made from cDNA

    b. Genomic libraries must be representative if they are to contain all the genes in an organism

    c. Genomic libraries must contain a minimum number of recombinants if they are to contain all the genes in an organism

    d. The DNA must be fragmented to an appropriate size for the vector that is used

Ans. (a) Genomic libraries are made from cDNA

77. The term cDNA library means

    a. Colloction of cDNA clones by an individual researcher

    b. Compilation of cDNA sequences in the database

    c. Pool of cDNA generated from a specific tissue inserted into an appropriate vector that can be used as a source of the cDNA of interest

    d. It is manual for cDNA research

Ans. (c) Pool of cDNA generated from a specific tissue inserted into an appropriate vector that can be used as a source of the cDNA of interest

78. A gene cannot be isolated from a human genomic DNA library by functional complementation in *E.coli* because of

    a. Non-functional promoter

    b. The absence of splicing machinery

    c. Coupled transcription and translation

    d. Codon bias

Ans. (b) The absence of splicing machinery

79. What clones should a eukaryotic cDNA library contain?

    a. Clones that represent every fragment of DNA in approximately equal frequencies

    b. Clones that represent one copy of every coding region

    c. Clone representing transcribed DNA in approximately equal frequencies

    d. Clones representing transcribed DNA in frequencies that reflect their level of expression

Ans. (d) Clones representing transcribed DNA in frequencies that reflect their level of expression

80. Identify the incorrect statement for the model plant *Arabidopsis thaliana*

a. Its mutants can be easily produced and characterized

b. Its genome sequence is known

c. All genes encompassing its genome have already been identified

d. The molecular genetic of its flowering has been extensively studied

Ans. (c) All genes encompassing its genome have already been identified

81. *Agrobacterium tumefaciens* is often used as vehicle to introduce foreign DNA into plants. The agrobacterial T-DNA in plant cells can be found as

a. Anautonomously replicating nuclear plasmid

b. A mitochondrial plasmid

c. A chloroplast plasmid

d. Integrated into the plant genome

Ans. (d) Integrated into the plant genome

82. The following are useful to introduce genes into crop plants *except*:

a. Ti plasmid　　　　b. Particle gun

c. Breeding　　　　　d. Auxin

Ans. (d) Auxin

83. Which one of these statements about the applications of gene cloning is false?

a. A large amounts of recombinant protein can be produced by gene cloning

b. DNA fingerprinting is used detect proteins to DNA

c. Cloned genes can be used to detect carriers of disease–causing genes

d. Gene therapy attempts to correct a disorder by delivering a good copy of a gene to a patient

Ans. (b) DNA fingerprinting is used detect proteins to DNA

84.

GROUP -1	GROUP-2
a. Biolistic	1. Gene pulser
b. Agrobacterium	2. PDS1000 He
c. Electroporation	3. Micromanipulator
d. Microinjection	4. Vir operons 6Crol C

Ans. (a-2, b-4, c-1, d-3)

85. The length of each boarder sequence in Ti–plasmid is about

a. 25 million base pairs　　b. 200 kilo base pairs

c. 25 kilo base pairs　　　d. 25 base pairs

Ans. (d) 25 base pairs

86. The essential component of Ti plasmid required for integration into plant genome is

a. Origin of replication

b. Tumor inducing gene

c. Nopaline utilization gene

d. All of the above

Ans. (b) Tumor inducing gene

87. *Agrobacterium tumefaciens* is an effective vector for use with

a. Corn　　　　　b. Rice

c. Wheat　　　　d. Soyabean

Ans. (d) Soyabean

88. What role do opines play in crown gall diseases?

a. Source of carbon nitrogen and energy for the *Agrobacterium*

b. Transfer of T-DNA to plant cells

c. Attachment of *Agrobacterium* to the plants

d. Induction of the expression of vir genes

Ans. (a) Source of carbon nitrogen and energy for the *Agrobacterium*

89. A plant genetic engineer wishes to transfer and express a gene from sunflower into beans. Which of the following would be the vector of choice?

a. Lambda phage　　　b. pBR plasmid

c. Ti plasmid　　　　　d. Maize streak virus

Ans. (c) Ti plasmid

90. Genetically engineered male sterile crop plants may be produced by inserting

a. BT toxin gene　　　b. Barnase gene

c. Lectin gene　　　　d. Chitinase gene

Ans. (b) Barnase gene

91. The term *tumefaciens* refers to which of the following?

a. Synthesis of mRNA from a DNA template

b. Synthesis of protein based on an mRNA sequence

c. Introduction of foreign DNA into a cell

d. The process by which a normal cell becomes malignant

Ans. (c) Introduction of foreign DNA into a cell

92. This of the following methods for the production of transgenic mice involves the initial creation of a cell chimera (a mixture of cells from distinct s sources?)

a. Pronuclear microinjection

b. Retroviral transduction

c. Transfection of ES cells

d. All of the above

Ans. (c) Transfection of ES cells

93. **Which of the following methods for studying loss of gene function does not involve any modification of the genome?**

    a. RNA interference by injection of double stranded RNA

    b. Expression of an integrated antisense transgene

    c. Gene knockout by homologous recombination

    d. None of the above

Ans. (a) RNA interference by injection of double stranded RNA

94. **The major difference between transgenic mice and knockout mice is that**

    a. Transgenic mice always employ the use of cloned genes derived from other species

    b. Transgenic mice have foreign that integrate at targeted loci through homologous recombination

    c. Transgenic mice have a functional foreign gene added to their genome

    d. Knockout mice always have a unique phenotype

Ans. (c) Transgenic mice have a functional foreign gene added to their genome

95. **Match the gene of interest for various aspects of crop improvement Gene insert Aspects of crop improvement**

a. Bar	1. Tolerance to heavy metals
b. vip 3A	2. Nutritional improvement with increased vitamin A
c. β-lac	3. Insect resistance
d. gsh-II	4. Herbicide resistance

Ans. (a-4, b-3, c-2, d-1)

96. **Dideoxy DNA sequence exclusively depends on one of the followings**

    a. Termination

    b. b.ATP

    b. Plasmid vector

    c. Vector primer

Ans. (a) Termination

97. **The genome sequencing of rice is important because**

    a. The rice genome is very unique and contains genes not found in other plants

    b. The rice genome is very large compared to the DNA of other grains and so more genes will be identified

c. It can identify genes associated with disease resistance, growth capacity, etc

d. It has a rapid life cycle and has many identifiable mutations

Ans. (c) It can identify genes associated with disease resistance, growth capacity, etc

98. **An analysis of chromosomal DNA, using the southern blot technique, involves the following five major steps**

    a. Autoradiography   b. Blotting

    c. Cleavage   d. Electrophoresis

    e. Hybridization

    Which of the following sequence of steps best illustrates this technique?

Ans. (c, d, b,e, a)

99. **Which is not a step in the blotting procedure?**

    a. Ligation of the DNA into a vector

    b. Separation of the DNA fragments on a gel

    c. Transfer of the DNA fragments to a nitrocellulose membrane

    d. Hybridization of the membrane with a labelled probe

Ans. (a) Ligation of the DNA into a vector

100. **Which of the following types of information cannot determined from the traditional northern blotting technique?**

    a. The size of an mRNA species

    b. The half-life of an mRNA species

    c. The strand of DNA that is transcribed into mRNA

    d. The amino acid sequence of the protein coded by an mRNA species

Ans. (d) The amino acid sequence of the protein coded by an mRNA species

101. **Which of the following would not be possible to address using a Northern Blot?**

    a. Location of restriction sites in a particular gene

    b. Spatial expression of a particular gene

    c. Temporal expression of a particular gene

    d. mRNA size

Ans. (a) Location of restriction sites in a particular gene

102. **Choose the mismatch**

a. Reporter molecule	1. Acts as shuttle vector
b. Maxam-gilbert method	2. Chemical modification of bases
c. Dideoxy terminators	3. Sanger method
d. Biotin	4. non-radioactive label

Ans. (a) Reporter molecule   1. Acts as shuttle vector

103. **There are two different ways to determining the nucleotide sequence of a nucleic acid: the chemical sequencing (Maxam-Gilbert) method and the enzymatic sequencing (Sanger) method. The basic principle/advantage of the Sanger method is**

    a. The differential interaction of the bases with particular dyes
    b. Extension of a synthetic primer and reliable termination of DNA repair synthesis
    c. The correlation of restriction sites with the end-label of the DNA
    d. The ability to 'sequence' both strands of the DNA duplex simultaneously

Ans. (d) **The ability to 'sequence' both strands of the DNA duplex simultaneously**

104. **In agarose gel electrophoresis**

    a. DNA migrates toward the negative electrode
    b. Supercoiled plasmids migrate slower than their nicked counterparts
    c. Larger molecules migrate faster than smaller molecules
    d. Ethidium bromide can be used to visualize the DNA

Ans. (d) **Ethidium bromide can be used to visualize the DNA**

105. **Which of the following are not valid methods of labeling duplex DNA?**

    a. 5'-end labeling with polynucleotide kinase
    b. 3'-end labeling with polynucleotide kinase
    c. 3'-end labeling with terminal transferase
    d. Nick translation

Ans. (b) **3'-end labeling with polynucleotide kinase**

106. **Which of the following methods would give you the most precise and accurate information about where and when a given gene is expressed?**

    a. In situ hybridization
    b. DNA microarray
    c. Protein microarray
    d. Reporter gene fusion including introns

Ans. (d) **Reporter gene fusion including introns**

107. **Which of the following methods can not be used to introduce a specific mutation at a predetermined site in a DNA sequence?**

    a. Primer extension on a single stranded template using a primer that incorporates a base mismatch
    b. Primer extension on a single stranded template using an error-prone DNA polymerase

    c. PCR amplification using a double template with one primer incorporating a base mismatch
    d. None of the above

Ans. (b) **Primer extension on a single stranded template using an error-prone DNA polymerase**

108. **Which of the following is/are useful marker(s) for genetic or physical mapping of human chromosomes?**

    a. Restriction fragment length polymorphisms
    b. Expressed sequence tags
    c. Short tandem repeat polymorphisms
    d. Sequence tagged sites

Ans. (a, b, c, d)

109. **Which of the following type(s) of polymorphism are commonly detected by using the polymerase chain reaction (PCR) and specific oligonucleotide primers?**

    a. Restriction fragment length polymorphism
    b. Expressed sequence tags
    c. Short tandem repeat polymorphisms
    d. Sequence tagged sites

Ans. (b, c, d)

110. **A certain purified DNA sample was cut with two restriction endonucleases E1 and E2. The following result were obtained from agarose gel electrophoresis Sample cut with E1 alone: two bands of size 35 kb and 15kb Sample cut with E2 alone: two bands of size 40 kb and 10kb Sample cut simultaneously with E1 and E2: three bands of size 35 kb, 10 kb, and 5 kb**

    a. Two sites for E1 and one site for E2
    b. One sites for E1 and two sites for E2
    c. One site each for E1 and E2
    d. Three sites for E1 and one site for E2
    The different in the restriction maps between two individuals of one species

Ans. (c) **One site each for E1 and E2**

111. **In order to identify the person who committed a crime. Forensic experts will need to extract DNA from the tissue sample collected at the crime scene, and conduct one of the folloeing procedures for DNA finger-printing analysis**

    a. Cut the DNA and hybridize with specific micro-satellite probes
    b. Cut the DNA and subclone the fragments
    c. Determine the sequence of the subclones
    d. b followed by c

Ans. (a) **Cut the DNA and hybridize with specific micro-satellite probes**

112. The DNA fingerprinting process involves

a. Chain terminators

b. Degenerate oligonucleotides

c. VNTR loci

d. RFLPs

Ans. (c) VNTR loci

113. Restriction fragment length polymorphism (RFLP) is

a. The technique used to fingerprint patterns of inheritance

b. The different in the restriction maps between the two alleles in a diploid cell

c. The different in the restriction maps between two individuals of one species

d. The different in the restriction maps between four individuals of one species

Ans. (c) The different in the restriction maps between two individuals of one species

114. Which of the following could not possibly give rise to restriction fragment length polymorphism (RFLP)?

a. A missense mutation within the protein coding region of a gene

b. A silent mutation within the protein coding region of a gene

c. A single base change within the intron sequence of a gene

d. An error in RNA splicing that mistakenly removes an exon during RNA processing

Ans. (d) An error in RNA splicing that mistakenly removes an exon during RNA processing

115. RFLP analysis can be used to distinguish between alleles based on differences in

a. Restriction enzyme recognition sites between the alleles

b. The amount of DNA amplified from the alleles during PC R

c. The ability of the alleles to be replicated in bacterial cells

d. The proteins expressed from the alleles

Ans. (a) Restriction enzyme recognition sites between the alleles

116. Positional cloning refers to

a. Using a selection procedure to clone a cDNA

b. Isolating a gene by PCR using primers from another species

c. Isolating a gene from a specific tissue in which it is being expressed

d. Mapping a gene to a chromosomal region and then identifying and cloning a genomic copy of the gene from the region

Ans. (d) Mapping a gene to a chromosomal region and then identifying and cloning a genomic copy of the gene from the region

117. Which of the following gene is defective in patients suffering from severe combined immunodeficiency syndrome (SCID)

a. CFTR

b. Adenosine deaminase

c. Ribonucleotide reductase

d. α2-microoglobin

Ans. (b) Adenosine deaminase

118. A mouse in which one particular gene has been replaced by its inactivated from generated in vitro is called

a. Transgenic mouse

b. Knockout mouse

c. Nude mouse

d. Mutant mouse

Ans. (b) Knockout mouse

119. The principle of the yeast two-hybrid system is

a. The detection of protein-protein interactions by assembling a functional factor from twob detection proteins

b. The detection of protein-protein interactions in a pair of hybrid yeast strains

c. The detection of protein-protein interactions by studying the hybridization of two cDNA sequence

d. The detection of protein-protein interactions between phage coat protein and target proteins

Ans. (a) The detection of protein-protein interactions by assembling a functional factor from twob detection proteins

120. Which of the following is not one of the objectives of the Human Genome project?

a. Create a detailed genetic map of every human chromosome, with an average of 2–5% recombination frequency between markers

b. Obtain a detailed physical map of every human chromosome, based on overlapping recombinant DNA molecules cloned as yeast artificial chromosomes

c. Determine the sequence of all expressed human genes by cDNA cloning and sequencing

d. Determine the complete DNA sequence of each human chromosome

e. All

Ans. (e) All

121. Which of the following is not tool of genetic engineering?

a. Vectors　　　　　b. Enzymes

c. Foreign DNA　　　d. GMO

Ans. (d) GMO

122. In recombinant DNA technology a plasmid vector is cleaved by

a. Modified DNA ligase

b. A heated alkaline solution

c. The same enzyme that cleave the donor DNA

d. The different enzyme other than that cleave the donor DNA

Ans. (c)　The same enzyme that cleave the donor DNA

123. The most common plasmid vector used in genetic engineering is

a. PBR 328　　　　b. PBR 322

c. PBR 325　　　　d. PBR 330

Ans. (b) PBR 322

124. Eco RI is an

a. Ligase　　　　　b. Polymerase

c. Restriction enzyme　d. Gyrase

Ans. (c)　Restriction enzyme

125. The transgenic plant flavr savr tomato carries an artificial gene for

a. Delay ripening process

b. Longer shell life

c. Added flavours

d. All of these

Ans. (d) All of these

126. Hirudin is obtained from the transgenic plant

a. *Brassica napus*　　b. *Hibiscus rosasinesis*

c. *Raphanus sativus*　d. *Vinca rosea*

Ans. (a)　*Brassica napus*

127.　Bt Cotton is

a. Cloned plant　　　b. Transgenic plant

c. Hybrid plant　　　d. Mutated plant

Ans. (b) Transgenic plant

128.　Dolly sheep was genetically similar to

a. The mother from which nucleated fertilized egg was taken

b. The mother from which nuclear DNA of udder cell was taken

c. The surrogate mother

d. Both surrogate mother and nuclear donor mother

Ans. (b) The mother from which nuclear DNA of udder cell was taken

129.　Genome is

a. Genes on nuclear DNA

b. Nuclear DNA + mitochondrial DNA

c. Nuclear DNA + chloroplast DNA

d. Nuclear DNA + Mitochondrial DNA + Chloroplast DNA

Ans. (d) Nuclear DNA + Mitochondrial DNA + Chloroplast DNA

130. A technique of using very small metal particles coated with desired gene in the gene transfer is called

a. Electroporation　　b. Microinjection

c. Liposome　　　　d. Biolistics

Ans. (d) Biolistics

131.　The complete set of chromosomal and extra-chromosomal genes of an organisms is called

a. Genome　　　　b. Gene pool

c. Gene bank　　　d. Gene library

Ans. (a)　Genome

132.　The study of all the proteins coded by the genome is called

a. Proteome　　　　b. Proteomics

c. Genome　　　　d. Protein formation

Ans. (b) Proteomics

133.　Sequencing of genomic DNA is included under

a. Structural genomics

b. Functional genomics

c. Proteomics

d. Transgenesis

Ans. (a)　Structural genomics

134.　Gene expression, regulation and phenotype production are studied in second phase of genome analysis called

a. Structural genomics　b. Functional genomics

c. Proteomics　　　d. Transmeiosis

Ans. (b) Functional genomics

135. In forensic science which of the following is used?

a. Bacterial cloning
b. DNA foot printing
c. DNA fingerprinting
d. DNA cloning

Ans. (c) DNA fingerprinting

136.DNA fingerprinting is based on

a. Occurance of VNTR's
b. Knowledge of human karyotype
c. Cloned DNA
d. Recombinant DNA

Ans. (a) Occurance of VNTR's

137. VNTRs represnets

a. New terminal regions in DNA
b. Functional genes in the DNA
c Split genes in the sample DNA
d. Specific non-coding sequences with unique tandem repeats

Ans. (d) Specific non-coding sequences with unique tandem repeats

138. Which ones produce androgenic haploids in anther cultures?

a. Anther wall
b. Tapetal layer of anther wall
c. Connective tissue
d. Young pollengrains

Ans. (d) Young pollengrains

139. Variations observed during tissue culture of some plants are known as

a. Clonal variations
b. Somatic variations
c. Somaclonal variations
d. Tissue culture variations

Ans. (c) Somaclonal variations

140. Virus free plants can be obtained through

a. Anitibiotic treatment
b. Bordeaux micture
c. Root tip culture
d. Shoot tip culture

Ans. (d) Shoot tip culture

141. To raising of plants from a small tissue in culture is known as

a. Macroproduction
b. Micropropagation
c. Tissue culture
c. Mass production

Ans. (b) Micropropagation

142. Callus is

a. Tissue that forms embryo
b. An insoluble carbohydrate
c. Unorganised actively dividing mass of cells maintained in culture
d. Tissue that growth to form embryoid

Ans. (c) Unorganised actively dividing mass of cells maintained in culture

143. Biopatents are_____.

a. Right to use invention
b. Right to use biological entities
c. Right to use products
d. Right to use process

Ans. (b) Right to use biological entities

144. African plant Pentadiplandra is used as_____.

a. Low calories sweetner
b. 2000 times sweeter agent
c. Sweetner for diabetic patients
d. All of these

Ans. (d) All of these

145. Which organism was used as bioweapon derived from_____.

a. Clostridium
b. Yerstsinia pestis
c. Fusarium species
d. Green algae

Ans. (c) Fusarium species

146. A set standards used to regulate own or community activity in relation to biological world is

a. Biopotency
b. Biopiracy
c. Biowar
d. Bioethics

Ans. (d) Bioethics

147. Biopiracy means

a. Use of biopatents
b. Thefts of plants and animals
c. Stealing of bioresources
d. Exploitation of bioresources without authentic permission

Ans. (d) Exploitation of bioresources without authentic permission

148. Bioethics is related to

a. Preventing biopiracy
b. Regulation of unethical activities likegene cloning in animals
c. Preventing theft of living materials
d. Moral guidance to the problems in biology

Ans. (b) Regulation of unethical activities likegene cloning in animals

149. Which of these restriction enzymes produce blunt ends?

a. SaII
b. EcoRV
c. XhoI
d. HindIII

Ans. (b) EcoRV

150. The RP13 gene of chromosome 17 codes for a protein _____ .

a. Involved in glucose transport
b. That is a component of hair and nails
c. Involved in eye development
d. Involved in the determination of personality

Ans. (c) Involved in eye development

151. Introduction of foreign genes for improving genotype is:

a. Tissue culture
b. Immunisation
c. Biotechnology
d. Genetic engineering

Ans. (d) Genetic engineering

152. Genetic engineering means:

a. Meiotic division of cells
b. Nucleotide transfer
c. Deletion and repair mechanism
d. None of these

Ans. (c) Deletion and repair mechanism

153. Isoschizomers recognize

a. Same recognition sequence but different recognition site
b. Same recognition site and recognition sequence
c. Same recognition site and different recognition sequence
d. Different recognition site and different recognition sequence

Ans. (b) Same recognition site and recognition sequence

154. A set of techniques that enables DNA from different sources to be identified, isolated and recombined so that new characteristics can be introduced into an organism is called

a. RDT
b. Genetic engineering
c. Molecular biology technique
d. All of these

Ans. (d) All of these

155. Restriction enzymes are named for

a. The person who discovered
b. The bacterium they are derived from
c. The viral DNA that they attack
d. Bone of the above

Ans. (b) The bacterium they are derived from

156. The recombinant DNA technique was engineered by:

a. Stanley norman cohen
b. Herbert bayer
c. Both of these
d. None of these

Ans. (c) Both of these

157. Which of these genes codes for a protein that plays a role in white blood cell function?

a. DCP1   b. MPO
c. GLUT4   d. RP13

Ans. (b) MPO

158. Phosphatediester bond of DNA and RNA involves:

a. 2°C and 1°C   b. 5°C and 3°C
c. 5°C and 2°C   d. 3°C and 1°C

Ans. (b) 5°C and 3°C

159. When populations are small, gene frequencies can change from generation to generation and some alleles may become fixed in a population. This is called _____ .

a. Assortative mating
b. Inbreeding
c. Heterosis
d. Genetic drift

Ans. (d) Genetic drift

160. Production of RDT and its transfer into a suitable host for multiplication/expression of the RDT. The recombinant DNA may or may not become integrated into the most genome is called:

a. Genetic engineering
b. Genetic transformation
c. Genetic material
d. Genetic resource

Ans. (a) Genetic engineering

161. Genetic engineering was born on:

a. 1971   b. 1973
c. 1984   d. 1985

Ans. (b) 1973

162. Sum total of all the genes and their alleles present in a species and its wild relatives is called:

a. Genetic engineering
b. Genetic metabolism
c. Genetic material
d. Genetic resource

Ans. (d) Genetic resource

163. Which of the following is correct in terms of determination of location of genetic traits?

a. Known protein coding sequences are too far apart to allow linkage determination for most new genes
b. Restriction sites allow DNAs to be digested
c. Protein-coding genes are always associated with a restriction pattern
d. None of the above

Ans. (a) Known protein coding sequences are too far apart to allow linkage determination for most new genes

164. Introduction of DNA or Recombinant DNA into a suitable cell/organism is called:

a. Genetic engineering
b. Genetic metabolism
c. Genetic material
d. Genetic resource

Ans. (b) Genetic metabolism

165. In gel electrophoresis, DNA molecules migrate from _____ to _____ ends of the gel.

a. Negative ... positive
b. Basic ... acidic
c. Long ... short
d. Positive to negative

Ans. (a) Negative ... positive

166. Restriction enzymes

a. Protect bacteria from viral infection
b. Cut DNA in a staggered fashion
c. Cut DNAs producing a blunt end
d. All of the above

Ans. (d) All of the above

167. A DNA molecule created in the laboratory by ligation of two or more different pieces of DNA is called:

a. Recombinant DNA
b. Recombinant clone
c. Genetic counselling
d. Genetic diversity

Ans. (a) Recombinant DNA

168. A bacterial clone containing a recombinant DNA molecules is called:

a. Recombinant DNA
b. Recombinant clone
c. Genetic counselling
d. Genetic diversity

Ans. (b) Recombinant clone

169. First discovered, Type II restriction endonuclease was

a. Hinf I
b. Eco K
c. Hind II
d. EcoRI

Ans. (c) Hind II

170. Which of the following techniques can be used to determine the defective gene and for developing cancer?

a. Western blot
b. Southern blot
c. Northern blot
d. Eastern blot

Ans. (b) Southern blot

171. Educating perspective parents, either suffering from or suspected to be heterogynous for some genetic disease, on the risk of their children genetic disease, on the risk of their children suffering from the same diseases is called:

a. Recombinant DNA
b. Recombinant clone
c. Genetic counselling
d. Genetic diversity

Ans. (c) Genetic counselling

172. The variability present within a species, between individual of a population or different population groups of the same species for one or a group of traits is called:

a. Recombinant DNA
b. Recombinant clone
c. Genetic counselling
d. Genetic diversity

Ans. (d) Genetic diversity

173. The transfer of antibiotic-resistant genes from genetically engineered bacteria to disease-causing bacteria _____ .

a. Would be of no concern if it occurred.
b. Has occurred
c. Can never occur
d. Seems unlikely

Ans. (d) Seems unlikely

174. Some genetic diseases cannot be diagnosed by changes in restriction sites. Some of these can be detected by allele-specific oligonucleotide probes. These are

a. Copies of the gene with an altered sequence so that a restriction site is inserted
b. Mutagenized copies of a gene
c. Short sequences that will hybridize only to a specific base sequence
d. PCR-amplified variable numbers of tandem repeats (VNTRs)

Ans. (c) Short sequences that will hybridize only to a specific base sequence

175. Origin or genetic variation in a relatively high frequency, usually, much higher than that ascribales to spontaneous mutation is called

   a. Genetic instability
   b. Recombinant clone
   c. Genetic counselling
   d. Genetic diversity

Ans. (a) Genetic instability

176. In order to insert a foreign gene into a plasmid, both must _____.

   a. Have identical DNA sequences
   b. Originate from the same type of cell
   c. Be cut by the same restriction enzyme
   d. Be of the same length

Ans. (d) Be of the same length

177. The DNA segment to be cloned is called

   a. DNA ligase
   b. DNA insert
   c. DNA array
   d. DNA methylation

Ans. (b) DNA insert

178. A gene construct in which the gene is located in antisense coientation so that the natural sense strand of the gene is now transcribed to produce antisense RNA; used is antisense RNA technology is called

   a. Antisense gene construct
   b. Antisense RNA technology
   c. Both a and b
   d. None of these

Ans. (a) Antisense gene construct

179. Which of the following genetic diseases would be amenable to genetic engineering?

   a. Down's syndrome
   b. Muscular dystrophy
   c. Cystic fibrosis
   d. Cri du Chat

Ans. (c) Cystic fibrosis

180. The process of an antisense construct of the target gene is integrated into the genome to suppress the concerned endogenous genes is called:

   a. Antisense gene construct
   b. Antisense RNA technology
   c. Both a and b
   d. None of these

Ans. (b) Antisense RNA technology

181. X-rays cause

   a. The formation of thymine dimmers
   b. Ionization of water in the cell
   c. Heat
   d. None of the above

Ans. (b) Ionization of water in the cell

182. The antigenic peptides bind within the cleft of MHC I or MHC II molecules and are displayed on the surface of antigen processing cells is called

   a. Antigen presentation   b. Antisense orientation
   c. Antisense strand   d. None of these

Ans. (a) Antigen presentation

183. Reverse orientation of a gene in relation to its promoter; the promoter is now located at the 5' end of the antisense strand so that the natural sense is now transcribed is called

   a. Antigen presentation   b. Antisense orientation
   c. Antisense strand   d. None of these

Ans. (b) Antisense orientation

184. The order for the construction of a cDNA fragment from mRNA is to

   a. Bind oligo-dT, treat with reverse transcriptase, digest with RNase, add G residues to the 3' end, bind oligo-dC, treat with DNA polymerase
   b. Treat with reverse transcriptase, digest with RNase, add G residues to the 3' end, bind oligo-dC, treat with DNA polymerase and bind oligo-dT
   c. Digest with RNase, add G residues to the 3' end, treat with reverse transcriptase, add G residues to the 3' end and treat with DNA polymerase
   d. Bind oligo-dC, treat with reverse transcriptase, digest with RNase, add G residues to the 3' end, bind oligo-dT and treat with DNA polymerase

Ans. (a) Bind oligo-dT, treat with reverse transcriptase, digest with RNase, add G residues to the 3' end, bind oligo-dC, treat with DNA polymerase

185. The strand of a native gene, which is used by RNA polymerase as template to genetrate its complementary copy of RNA; this RNA ultimately function as measenger RNA; the promoter sequence is, as a rule, located at the 3' end of the antisense strand is called

   a. Antigen presentation
   b. Antisense orientation
   c. Antisense strand
   d. None of these

Ans. (c) Antisense strand

186. The TP53 gene of chromosome 17 codes for a protein _____ .

    a. That plays a role in the digestive process
    b. Involved in glucose transport
    c. Involved in the regulation of the cell cycle
    d. That is like a white blood cell protein

Ans. (c) Involved in the regulation of the cell cycle

187. Colonies from a master plates are either lifted or replica plates onto a nitrocellulose filter, cells are lysed, DNA is denatured and hybridised with radioactive probe to detect the colonies having DNA/RNA sequence complementary to the probe is called;

    a. Colony hybridization
    b. Northern hybridization
    c. Southern hybridization
    d. None of these

Ans. (a) Colony hybridization

188. Why is golden rice pale yellow in color?

    a. It is rich in chlorophyll *a*.
    b. It is rich in beta-carotene
    c. It is rich in chlorophyll *b*
    d. It is rich in phycobilins

Ans. (b) It is rich in beta-carotene.

189. An enzyme that seals nicks in DNA strand catalysing the formation of phospodiester bond between the contiguous nucleotides is called:

    a. DNA ligase   b. DNA insert
    c. DNA array   d. DNA methylation

Ans. (a) DNA ligase

190. Which type of restriction enzymes do not usually require ATP?

    a. Type I   b. Type II
    c. Type III   d. Type IV

Ans. (b) Type II

191. RNA sample is subjected to gel electrophoresis, RNA transferred from the gel onto a nylon membrane, immobilized and hybridized with a single stranded radioactive probe; autoradiography revers the RNA and hybridized to the probe, used for detection of transcription of transgenes is called;

    a. Colony hybridization
    b. Northern hybridization
    c. Southern hybridixation
    d. Somatic hybridization

Ans. (b) Northern hybridization

192. production of hybrid plants via protoplast fussion; feasible in sexuality incompatible combinations, is sterile/non flowering species, etc. by:

    a. Southern blotting   b. Northern blotting
    c. Both a and b   d. None of these

Ans. (d) None of these

193. An example of a restriction fragment length polymorphism is

    a. An Eco RI cuts DNA at a different sequence than Hind III
    b. Different length fragments of DNA resulting from loss or gain of a restriction site
    c. Cystic fibrosis results from a three base deletion in most cases but in other cases, other mutations are involved
    d. All of the above

Ans. (b) Different length fragments of DNA resulting from loss or gain of a restriction site

194. The characteristics two dimensional pattern formed by the separation of a mixture of peptides resulting from partial hydrolysis of a protein is known as;

    a. Genetic map   b. Peptide mapping
    c. Peptide map   d. None of these

Ans. (b) Peptide mapping

195. A series of DNA sequence fixed as distinct spots on a suitable solid support, like glass chip; basically two types, spotted DNA array and printed oligonucleotide chips is called:

    a. DNA ligase   b. DNA insert
    c. DNA array   d. DNA methylation

Ans. (b) DNA insert

196. Addition of methyl residues, chiefly to C residues, usually, located in CG or CNG sequence, after they are incorporated in DNA is called

    a. DNA ligase   b. DNA insert
    c. DNA array   d. DNA methylation

Ans. (d) DNA methylation

197. Knockout mice are created by

    a. Mutagenizing a mouse and selecting for mutant offspring
    b. Creating a chimera by fusing cells from two different cell lines
    c. Infecting the mouse with a retrovirus
    d. Transfecting embryonic stem cells with an altered gene sequence

Ans. (d) Transfecting embryonic stem cells with an altered gene sequence

198. The biotin labelled mRNA from non stressed cell is called

a. Driver m RNA   b. c- DNA

c. Both a and b   d. None of these

Ans. (a) Driver m RNA

199. A plasmid

a. Is a circular DNA molecule

b. Always contains an origin of replication

c. Usually contains one or more restriction sites

d. All of the above

Ans. (d) All of the above

200. The copy of DNA or complementary DNA produced y using RNA as tempelate; produced by rerverse transcriptase enzyme is called;

a. Driver m-RNA   b. c-DNA

c. BOTH a and b   d. None of these

Ans. (b) c- DNA

201. RNA produced by transcription of the antisense stand of a gene; in case of structure genes encoding protein, it usually means m-RNA is

a. Driver m-RNA   b. c-DNA

c. BOTH a and b   d. None of these

Ans. (c) BOTH a and b

202. A diagram showing the relative sequence and position of specific genes along a chromosome is called:

a. Genetic map

b. Genetic information

c. Genetic code

d. Gene expression

Ans. (a) Genetic map

203. A molecular technique in which DNA sequences between two oligonucleotide primers can be amplified is known as

a. Southern blotting

b. Northern blotting

c. Polymerase chain reaction

d. DNA replication

Ans. (c) Polymerase chain reaction

204. The Southern blotting technique depends on

a. Similarities between the sequences of probe DNA and experimental DNA

b. Similarities between the sequences of probe RNA and experimental RNA

c. Similarities between the sequences of probe protein and experimental protein

d. The molecular mass of proteins

Ans. (a) Similarities between the sequences of probe DNA and experimental DNA

205. The hereditary information contained in a sequence of nucleotide bases in chromosomal DNA or RNA is known as:

a. Genetic map   b. Genetic information

c. Genetic code   d. Gene expression

Ans. (b) Genetic information

206. In genetic engineering, a chimera is

a. An enzyme that links DNA molecules

b. A plasmid that contains foreign DNA

c. A virus that infects bacteria

d. A fungi

Ans. (a) An enzyme that links DNA molecules

207. The set of triplet code words in DNA coding for the amino acid of proteins is known as:

a. Genetic map   b. Genetic information

c. Genetic code   d. Gene expression

Ans. (c) Genetic code

208. The deliberate modifications of an organism's genetic information by directly changing its nucleic acid content is a subject matter of

a. Genetic engineering

b. Population genetics

c. Microbiology

d. Protein engineering

Ans. (a) Genetic engineering

209. Transcription and in the case of proteins, translation to yield the product of a gene a gene is expressed when its biological product is present and active is known as

a. Genetic map   b. Genetic information

c. Genetic code   d. Gene expression

Ans. (d) Gene expression

210. Electroporation is

a. The process of separating charged molecules through a gel maintained in an electric field

b. The process of combining foreign DNA to an electrically charged vector molecule

c. The application of high voltage pulses

d. The process of multiplication of the cells

Ans. (c) The application of high voltage pulses

211. What is the normal role of restriction endonucleases in bacterial cells?

a. To degrade the bacterial chromosome into small pieces during replication

b. To degrade invading phage DNA

c. To produce RNA primers for replication

d. All of the above

Ans. (b) To degrade invading phage DNA

212. Recombination between two DNA molecules of similar sequence, occurring in all cells; occurs during meiosis and mitosis in eukaryotes is called:

a. Homologous Genetic Recombinatioin

b. Recombinant DNA

c. Recombinational DNA repair

d. Recombination

Ans. (a) Homologous Genetic Recombinatioin

213. Peptide mapping is also known as:

a. Peptide fingerprinting

b. DNA fingerprinting

c. DNA footprinting

d. None of the above

Ans. (a) Peptide fingerprinting

214. A short molecule containing 2–20 nucleotide is

a. Oligonucleotide   b. Plasmid

c. Vector   d. Mononucleotide

Ans. (a) Oligonucleotide

215. Charged molecules are separated based on varying rates of migration through a solid matrix when subjected to an electric field. This technique is known as

a. Photoreactivation

b. Gel electrophoresis

c. Autoradiography

d. Blotting

Ans. (b) Gel electrophoresis

216. The transfer of genetic information from one cell to another by means of a viral vector is called

a. Transmination   b. Transcription

c. Transduction   d. Transformation

Ans. (c) Transduction

217. Introduction of an exogenous DNA into a cell, causing the cell to require a new phenotype is called:

a. Transmination   b. Transcription

c. Transduction   d. Transformation

Ans. (d) Transformation

218. For gene probes to be useful they must

a. Be large enough to contain gene-specific sequences

b. Be labeled in some manner to allow detection

c. Both a and b

d. None of these

Ans. (c) Both a and b

219. A genomic library is

a. A database where the sequence of an organism's genome is stored

b. A collection of many clones possessing different DNA fragments from the same organisms bound to vectors

c. A book that describes how to isolate DNA from a particular organism

d. A place where the information of the genetic organization of organisms are kept.

Ans. (b) A collection of many clones possessing different DNA fragments from the same organisms bound to vectors

220. The process in which the genetic information present in an mRNA molecule specifies the sequence of amino acids during protein synthesis is called

a. Translation   b. Transcription

c. Transduction   d. Transformation

Ans. (a) Translation

221. The movement of gene or set of genes from one site in the genome to another is called:

a. Transmination   b. Transcription

c. Transduction   d. Transformation

Ans. (b) Transcription

222. A DNA sequence at which RNA polymerase may bind, leading to initiation of transcription is called;

a. Transamination

b. Transcription

c. Promoter

d. Transformation

Ans. (c) Promoter

223. DNA formed by the joining of genes in tow new combination is called:

a. Recombinant DNA

b. Recombination

c. Recombinational DNA repair

d. None of these

Ans. (a) Recombinant DNA

224. Which of the variation of PCR aims to enhance specificity?

a. Anchored PCR   b. Hotatart PCR
c. Touchdown PCR   d. Both a and b

Ans. **(b) Hotatart PCR**

225. Which *E. coli* vectors yields single stranded copies of cloned DNA?

a. p-UC18/19
b. λ-Phage vectors
c. Phage M13 vector
d. Cosmid ectros

Ans. **(c) Phage M13 vector**

226. Which bacteria has at least two circular chromosomes in its genome?

a. Bacillus
b. Pseudomonas
c. Vibrio chlerae
d. Mycoplasma genitalium

Ans. **(c) Vibrio chlerae**

227. Which is not correct about DNA?

a. Double helix model of DNA was produced by Watson and Crick
b. DNA molecule ordinarily consist of two polynucleotide chains
c. DNA double helix is stabilized by hydrogen bonds
d. Two strands of a DNA molecule are oriented antiparallel to each other

Ans. **(c) DNA double helix is stabilized by hydrogen bonds**

228. Which is not correct?

a. If the base sequence of one DNA strand is known, the base sequence of its other strand can be easily deduced
b. The formation of hydrogen bonds between adenine and thymine, and between guanine and cytosine is known as complementary base pairing
c. Usually, B-DNA molecule has righe handed coiling
d. Hydrophobic interaction are important in transcription

Ans. **(d) Hydrophobic interaction are important in transcription**

229. Multiple copies of a gene can be obtained by:

a. Gene cloning
b. Polymerase chain reaction
c. Combination of PCR with chemical synthesis
d. All of the above

Ans. **(d) All of the above**

230. DNA polymerase III serves which type of function?

a. DNA repair
b. DNA replication
c. Initiation of DNA replication
d. All of the above

Ans. **(b) DNA replication**

231. Which is not correct about DNA replication?

a. The presence of replication fork in *E.coli* chromosome was first demonstrated by chain in 1953
b. DNA replication always proceed in the 5'–3' direction
c. Both strands of DNA replicate continuously
d. DNA replication of DNA replication synthesis of a small RNA primer

Ans. **(c) Both strands of DNA replicate continuously**

232. Which enzyme is called molecular scissor?

a. DNA ligase
b. DNA gyrase
c. Restriction endonuclease
d. Topoisomerase

Ans. **(c) Restriction endonuclease**

233. A class of enzymes which cleaves DNA only within or near those sites that have specific base sequence is called

a. Type I endonuclease
b. Type II endonuclease
c. Type III endonuclease
d. Exonuclease

Ans. **(c) Type III endonuclease**

234. Which scientist was awarded Nobel Prize in 1978 for the discovery of endonucleases?

a. Smith   b. Nathans
c. Arber   d. All of these

Ans. **(d) All of these**

235. Near isogenic lines can be developed by:

a. Single seed descont   b. Mutagenesis
c. Backcross method   d. Continued inbreeding

Ans. **(c) Backcross method**

236. Which is an example of type I restriction endonuclease?

a. Eco K   b. Hinf III
c. Hind II   d. Bgl II

Ans. **(a) Eco K**

237. IRGSP stand for:

a. International Rice Genome Sequencing Project
b. International Rice and Groundnut Sequencing Project
c. International Research on Groundnut, sorghum and Pigeonpea
d. Indian Rice genetic resources programme

Ans. (a) International Rice Genome Sequencing Project

238. Most of the type II restriction endonucleases have recognition site of how much length?

a. 4 bp
b. 5 bp
c. 6 bp
d. 4–6 bp

Ans. (d) 4–6 bp

239. Which restriction enzymes produces blunt ends?

a. Bam H1
b. Alu I
c. Pst I
d. Hind III

Ans. (b) Alu I

240. Which one has the largest number of genes?

a. Arabidopsis
b. Yeast
c. Caenorhabditis
d. Drosophila

Ans. (a) Arabidopsis

241. Identification of protein using antibodies may be done by:

a. Enzyme linked immunosorbant assay
b. Western blotting
c. Precipitation and electrophoresis
d. All of the above

Ans. (d) All of the above

242. Which scientist isolated ribolomal RNA gene in 1965?

a. Maxam and Gilbert
b. Wallace and Birnstiel
c. Sanger and Southern
d. Brown and Gilbert

Ans. (b) Wallace and Birnstiel

243. Which has the smallest genome size

a. Mycoplasma genitalium
b. Saccharomyces cerevisiae
c. E. coli
d. Caenorhabditis elegans

Ans. (a) Mycoplasma genitalium

244.The l genome contains:

a. Origin of replication
b. Genes for head and tail protein
c. Proteins involved in lysogeny
d. All of these

Ans. (d) All of these

245. Which population are used for linkage mapping?

a. F₂ population
b. Backcross population
c. Recombinant inbred lines
d. All of these

Ans. (d) All of these

246. Restrictive polyacrylamide gels are used for:

a. Viroid test
b. Analysis of point mutations
c. DNA sequencing
d. All of these

Ans. (d) All of these

247. During DNA isolation, if bacterial cell extract has a heavy load of proteins, it is treated with?

a. Proteinase K
b. Trypsin
c. Pronase
d. Both a and c

Ans. (d) Both a and c

248. Which is the least likely to accumulate property folded proteins encoded by an eukaryotic transgene?

a. Animal cell
b. Saccharomyces
c. E. coli
d. Pichia

Ans. (c) E. coli

249. Which one has the largest genome size?

a. Arabidopsis
b. Yeast
c. Caenorhabditis
d. Drosophila

Ans. (d) Drosophila

250. In general, which is used for initial cloning?

a. B. Subtilis
b. Agrobacterium
c. E. coli
d. B.thuringiensis

Ans. (c) E. coli

251. Use of an antibiotic resistance and the lac Za in a vector, eliminates the need for:

a. Planting on the antibiotic containing
b. Peplica planting
c. Planting on a second seclection medium
d. Both B and c

Ans. (d) Both B and c

252. AFLP may arise due to:

a. A difference in restriction site

b. Deletions and insertion within the amplified restriction fragments

c. Mutatioin beyond the restriction sites that affect complementarity with the selection

d. All of these

Ans. (d) All of these

253. In case of linkage maps, the distance, between the markers are measured in terms of:

a. Recombination frequency

b. Mutation frequency

c. Angstroms

d. Nucleotide numer

Ans. (a) Recombination frequency

254. Which of the following cleaves both the DNA strands at random sites?

a. DNase I   b. SI nuclease

c. Eco R I   d. Hind III

Ans. (a) DNase I

255. Which one has smallest genome size?

a. Arabidopsis   b. Yeast

c. Caenorhabditis d. Drosophila

Ans. (b) Yeast

256. Which of the following enzymes is used for converting protruding ends into blunt ends?

a. Polynucleotide kinase

b. S1 nuclease

c. Klenow fragment of E. Coli DNA polynuclease I

d. Both B and C

Ans. (d) Both B and C

257. Which is the preferred strategy for converting potruding ends in to blunt end ?

a. Polynucleotide kinase

b. S1 nuclease

c. Klenow fragment of E. Coli DNA polynuclease I

d. Both b and c

Ans. (c) Klenow fragment of E. Coli DNA polynuclease I

258. DNA fingerprinting is used for:

a. Identification of varieties

b. Resolving disputed parentages

c. Identification of criminals

d. All of these

Ans. (d) All of these

259. ARMS PCR achieves differential amplification of allele due to:

a. Primer sequence

b. Annealing temperature

c. Ion concentration

d. Specific PCR protocol

Ans. (a) Primer sequence

260. In most PCR product, a single nucleotide overhang is of:

a. A at the 3'-end

b. A at the 5'-end

c. C at the 3'-end

d. T at the 5'-end

Ans. (a) A at the 3'-end

261. The genome of eukaryotes was first to be sequenced:

a. Arabidopsis   b. Yeast

c. Caenorhabditis d. Drosophila

Ans. (b) Yeast

262. Which of the following enzyme is used to covalently bond foreign DNA to a vector plasmid?

a. DNA polymerase

b. Restriction endonuclease

c. DNA ligase

d. DNA helicase

Ans. (c) DNA ligase

263. Bacterial cells protect their own DNA from degradation by restriction endonucleases by

a. Methylating the DNA at the sites that the enzyme recognizes

b. Deleting all recognition sites from the genome

c. Not producing any restriction endonucleases

d. Having anti restriction endonucleases

Ans. (a) Methylating the DNA at the sites that the enzyme recognizes

264. The piece of equipment, that introduces DNA into cells via DNA-coated microprojectiles is known as

a. Inoculating needle

b. Gene gun

c. DNA probe

d. Laser

Ans. (b) Gene gun

265. Which is not an example of insertion vector?

a. λgt 10   b. λgt 11

c. λgt 12   d. zap 11

Ans. (b) λgt 11

266. Identification of protein using antibodies may be done by:

a. Enzyme linked immunosorbant assay
b. Precipitation and electrophoresis
c. Western blotting
d. All of these

Ans. (d) All of these

267. Replacement vector, λ ENBLA can be used to c lone DNA of upto which size?

a. 10 kb
b. 20 kb
c. 10 kb
d. 45 kb

Ans. (b) 20 kb

268. Bacterial cell are usually multiply in:

a. Jensson medium
b. Luria betani medium
c. YE medium
d. Ganberg medium

Ans. (a) Jensson medium

269. Pulsed field gel electrophoresis is able to separate chromosome of:

a. Yeast
b. Bacteria
c. Protoson
d. All of these

Ans. (d) All of these

270. Who developed pBR 322

a. Boliver Rodrigues
b. Berg Rosenberg
c. Benfy Ris
d. Bonner Riggs

Ans. (a) Boliver Rodrigues

271. Which vector has been constructed for use in two different hosts?

a. Shuttle vectors
b. Cosmids
c. Phasmids
d. Phagemids

Ans. (a) Shuttle vectors

272. DNA marker can be used for:

a. Preparation of linkage map
b. Map based cloning of genes
c. Mapping of quantitative traits loci
d. All of these

Ans. (d) All of these

273. Which is not correct about RNA?

a. RNA molecules ordinarily consist of a single polyribonucleotide strand
b. RNA molecules contain uracil in the place of cytosine

c. Phosphodiseter bonds are formed between ribonuceotides in the same manner as in the case of deoxyribonucleotides
d. RNA was, most likely, the first genetic material, it was much later replaced by DNA

Ans. (b) RNA molecules contain uracil in the place of cytosine

274. Isozyme markers behave like:

a. Recessive
b. dominant
c. Co dominant
d. Over dominant

Ans. (c) Co dominant

275. An animal, that has gained new genetic information from the acquisitior of foreign DNA, is considered as

a. A chimera
b. A transgenic animal
c. A vector
d. An enzyme that links DNA molecules

Ans. (b) A transgenic animal

276. The advantage of using DNA polymerases from thermophilic organisms in PCR is that

a. The DNA polymerases of these bacteria are much faster than those from other organisms
b. The DNA polymerases of these bacteria can withstand the high temperatures needed to denature the DNA strands
c. The DNA polymerases of these bacteria never make mistakes while replicating DNA
d. All of the above

Ans. (d) All of the above

277. Difference between λ gt 10 and λ gt 11 vectors is that

a. λ gt 11 is an expression vector
b. λ gt 10 is an expression vector
c. λ gt 10 is a replacement vector
d. λ gt 11 is a repl cement vector

Ans. (a) λ gt 11 is an expression vector

278. λ ZAP vector is an example of

a. Phage
b. Cosmid
c. Plasmid
d. Phagemid

Ans. (d) Phagemid

279. λ gt 10 and λ gt 11 vectors can propagate cloned fragments up to

a. 6–7 kb
b. 16–17 kb
c. 26–27 kb
d. 30–40 kb

Ans. (a) 6–7 kb

CHECK YOU GRASP

1. Blue–white selection is used

a. To test for the presence of a plasmid in bacteria
b. To reveal the identity of a cloned DNA fragment
c. To express the product of a cloned gene
d. To test for the presence of a cloned insert in a plasmid

2. pBR322 which is frequently used as a vector for cloning gene in *E.coli* is

a. An original bacterial plasmid
b. A modified bacterial plasmid
c. A viral genome
d. A transposon

3. Choose the correct statements (s) about thermostable DNA polymerase used in PCR

a. Taq Pol has no proof reading ability
b. Taq Pol has $5' \rightarrow 3'$ exonuclease activity
c. *pfu* pol has $3' \rightarrow 5'$ exonuclease activity
d. T*li* Pol has no $3' \rightarrow 5'$ exonuclease activity
e. a, b, c, all

4. If a transcript of a given gene is degraded when mixed with DNA encoding the same gene, one could conclude that the RNA solution is contaminated with

a. RNAse A   b. RNAse T
c. RNAse H   d. DNAse III

5. The length of each boarder sequence in Ti-plasmid is about

a. 25 million base pairs   b. 200 kilo base pairs
c. 25 kilo base pairs   d. 25 base pairs

6. For cloning a DNA fragment larger than 100 Kb, which of the following vector system would be suitable?

a. Plasmid
b. Cosmid
c. Yeast artificial chromosome
d. Lambda bacteriophage

7. Which of the following sequences is most likely to be a restriction enzyme recognition site?

a. CGGCTT
b. CGCCGC
c. GTAATG
d. GTCGAC

8. Which of the following is not component of yeast artificial chromosome?

a. Centromere
b. Telomere
c. Origin of replication
d. Cos site

9. BAC, which can be used to clone large DNA fragments, is derived from

a. CoIE plasmid
b. F plasmid
c. 2μ plasmid
d. Mu phage

In case of less than 80% score, go through brief Review and Glance one again from chapter

Key: 1-d   2-b   3-e   4-c   5-d   6-c   7-d   8-d   9-b

4

Plant Tissue Culture and Genetic Transformation

1. The scientist, who has first tested the invitro selection for diseases resistance of wild fire disease of tobacco is

a. Watson   b. Carlson

c. Waldeyer   d. Fleming

Ans. (b) Carlson

2. High ration of cytokinin to Auxin in growth medium favours

a. Shoot formation   b. Leaf formation

c. Root formation   d. Callus formation

Ans. (a) Shoot formation

3. The deletion of genes governing Auxin and cytokinin production from T-DNA of a Ti plasmid is known as

a. Addition   b. Deletion

c. Disarming   d. Cohesion

Ans. (c) Disarming

4. Most commonly used medium for tissue culture is

a. BS medium   b. MS medium

c. LS medium   d. B6 medium

Ans. (b) MS medium

5. The culture of whole plants and organ is has been termed as

a. Protoplast culture

b. Callus culture

c. Non organised culture

d. Organised culture

Ans. (d) Organised culture

6. The presence of the following phytohormones in the medium is generally essential for embryo initiation

a. Cytokinin   b. Auxin

c. Kinetin   d. All of the above

Ans. (b) Auxin

7. Factors contributing to produce somaclones are

a. Explants source

b. Genotype

c. Duration of cell culture

d. All of the above

Ans. (d) All of the above

8. Scarlet is a disease resistance variety of the crop called

a. Radish   b. Tomato

c. Sweet potato   d. Turnip

Ans. (c) Sweet potato

9. The molecules, which can stimulate the production of secondary metabolites in plant cell is called

a. Repressor   b. Elicitors

c. Promoter   d. Adapter

Ans. (b) Elicitors

10. A bead of gel containing a somatic embryo needed for the development of a complete plantlet from the enclosed somatic embryo or shoot bud is called

a. Calcitrant seed   b. Bio seed

c. Artificial seed   d. Natural seed

Ans. (c) Artificial seed

11. A natural genetic engineer in genetic is

a. Trigoderma

b. Ppseudomonas

c. Agrobacterium

d. Fusarium

Ans. (c) Agrobacterium

12. A chemical that is added to rooting media to prevent/eradicate the root inhibiting agent is

a. Gibberellins

b. Ethylene

c. Activated charcoal

d. None of these

Ans. (c) Activated charcoal

13. Introduction of a viral genome in to plant cells by placing it within the T-DNA of a Ti plasmid is called

    a. Lipoinfection   b. Agroinfection
    c. Reconinfection   d. Vector infection

Ans. (b) Agroinfection

14. The process in which the young embryos are removed from developing seeds and are placed on suitable nutrient medium to obtained seedling is called as

    a. Callus culture   b. Embryo culture
    c. Meristem culture   d. Stem culture

Ans. (b) Embryo culture

15. The process of a prolonged exposure to low temperature followed by shoot tip culture to eliminate the virus is called as

    a. Heliothrapy   b. Cryotherapy
    c. Thermotherapy   d. None of these

Ans. (b) Cryotherapy

16. Preservation of cell, tissues and organs in liquid nitrogen at −196°C is called as

    a. Thermopreservation
    b. Cryopreservation
    c. Hydropreservation
    d. Helopreservation

Ans. (b) Cryopreservation

17. Introduction of a tobacco mosaic virus transgene in to plants in 1986 was used to demonstrate a process called as

    a. Cross protection   b. Co-transfection
    c. Co-transformation   d. Co-suspension

Ans. (a) Cross protection

18. The technique of grafting of shoot tips onto young rootstock seedling grown *in vitro* allowing the recovery of complete shoots from the them is called

    a. Micropropagation   b. Microprotoplast
    c. Mobilization   d. Micrografting

Ans. (d) Micrografting

19. The mass production of clonal progeny through tissue culture is called

    a. Micropropagation
    b. Micrografting
    c. Microprotoplast
    d. None of these

Ans. (a) Micropropagation

20. The cell to cell transfer of an otherwise non conjugative plasmid in the presence of a conjugative plasmid inside the same cell as the former is called as

    a. Mobilization   b. Micropropagation
    c. Microprotoplast   d. Micrografting

Ans. (a) Mobilization

21. Use of diploids in breeding of crops like potato offers which of the following advantage?

    a. A lesser efficiency of selection
    b. Much easier hybridization with diploid wild species. Which offers many genes of great value.
    c. Both a and b
    d. None of these

Ans. (b) Much easier hybridization with diploid wild species. Which offers many genes of great value.

22. Gametoclonal variation may occur due to which of the following?

    a. Gene amplification
    b. Gene mutation
    c. Residual heterozygosity
    d. All of the above

Ans (d) All of the above

23. The phenomenon of a natural cell reverting to meristematic state and forming a dedifferentiated callus tissue is called as

    a. Organogenesis   b. Rhizogenesis
    c. Caulogenesis   d. Dedifferentiation

Ans. (d) Dedifferentiation

24. Which of the following is correct about anther culture?

    a. Anther are generally cultured in the light at 25–30°C, but regenerated plantlets are transferred to dark
    b. Low concentration 1–2% of sucrose is essential for androgenesis.
    c. In *barssica compestris*, pretreatment of anthers at 30–45°C gives better induction.
    d. All of the above

Ans. (c) In barssica compestris, pretreatment of anthers at 30–45°C gives better induction.

25. A type of organogenesis by which only adventitious shoot bud initiation takes place in callus tissue is called as

    a. Organogenesis   b. Caulogenesis
    c. Rhizoenesis   d. Dedifferentiation

Ans. (b) Caulogenesis

26. Match the column A and B and select the correct option from those listed below them.

   A. Transgene   I. PEG
   B. Probe   II. Gene isolation
   C. Meristem   III. Transgenic
   D. Fusogen   IV. Micropropagation

   a. A-III, B-II, C-IV, D-I   b. A-II, B-III, C-IV, D-I
   c. A-III, B-I, C-IV, D-III   d. A-I, B-II, C-IV, D-III

   Ans. (a) A-III, B-II, C-IV, D-I

27. The process by which cell and tissues are forced to undergo change which lead to the production of a unipolar structure namely shoot/root primordium is called as

   a. Rhizogenesis   b. Organogenesis
   c. Caulogenesis   d. None of these

   Ans. (b) Organogenesis

28. The type of organogenesis by which only adventitious initiation takes place in callus tissue is called

   a. Rhizogenesis   b. Organogenesis
   c. Dedifferentiation   d. Caulogenesis

   Ans. (a) Rhizogenesis

29. In 1922, Blakeslee and co-workers, for the first time, reported occurrence of haploids in Datura due to which of the following process?

   a. Mutagenesis   b. Parthenogenesis
   c. Androgenesis   d. Gynogenesis

   Ans. (d) Gynogenesis

30. Which of the following is correct about haploid production?

   a. Androgenic induction is only possible with immature anthers, containing immature pollen.
   b. The early or mid uninucleate stage of microspore development is the most responsive stage in most of the species.
   c. In 1964, Guha and Maheshwari reported *in vitro* production of haploids through anther culture.
   d. All of the above

   Ans. (b) The early or mid uninucleat stge of microspore development is the most responsive stage in most of the species.

31. An amorphous mass of parenchyma cells arising from the proliferation cells of the parent tissue is called as

   a. Explants   b. Medium
   c. Callus   d. Stock plant

   Ans. (c) Callus

32. A piece of plant tissue placed in an environment free from microorganisms supplemented with balanced diet of chemical is called as

   a. Medium   b. Callus
   c. Explants   d. Stock plant

   Ans. (c) Explants

33. During distant hybridization, problem of endosperm abortion can be overcome by which of the following?

   a. Callus culture   b. Anther culture
   c. Embryo culture   d. All of the above

   Ans. (c) Embryo culture

34. Which of the following are the characteristic of cytokinin?

   a. Induce flowering in long day plant
   b. Promote *in vitro* shoot regeneration
   c. Initiate callus division
   d. All of the above

   Ans. (b) Promote *in vitro* shoot regeneration

35. The plant from which the explants is removed is called as

   a. Explant   b. Stock plant
   c. Medium   d. Callus

   Ans. (b) Stock plant

36. Mixture of certain chemicals to from a nutrient rich gel/liquid for growing cultures is referred to as

   a. Medium
   b. Callus
   c. Explants
   d. All of the above

   Ans. (a) Medium

37. In plant tissue culture ABA may effect which of the following?

   a. Enhance root differentiation
   b. Promote somatic embryo maturation
   c. Induce somatic embryo conversion
   d. All of the above

   Ans. (b) Promote somatic embryo maturation

38. Plants with gametic chromosome number are termed as which of the following?

   a. Dihaploid   b. Monoploid
   c. Haploid   d. None of these

   Ans. (c) Haploid

39. Micropropagation can be achieved through which of the following?

a. Production of adventitious shoot buds
b. Enhanced axillary branching
c. Somatic embryogenesis
d. All of the above

And. (d) All of the above

40. The chemical that induces cell division and formation of adventitious roots is

a. Cytokinin
b. Agar
c. Auxin
d. Diphenyl urea

Ans. (c) Auxin

41. A seaweed derivative which act as the most popular solidifying agent is called as

a. Cytokinin
b. Agar
c. Auxin
d. Diphenyl urea

Ans. (b) Agar

42. The important growth regulator for induction of embryogenesis is called as

a. Abscissic acid
b. IAA
c. Gibberellic acid
d. IBA

Ans. (a) Abscissic acid

43. How many types of synthetic seed have been proposed?

a. Encapsulated, hydrated somatic embryos
b. Dehydrated somatic shoot bud with a gel
c. Both a & b
d. None of these

Ans. (a) Encapsulated, hydrated somatic embryos

44. Which of the following are characteristics of an Auxin?

a. Prevents apical bud dominance
b. Involve differentiation of phloem
c. Basipetal translocation
d. All of the above

Ans. (c) Basipetal translocation

45. Higher the agar concentration in the medium, the binding of water will be

a. Stronger
b. Lower
c. Weaker
d. Higher

Ans. (b) Lower

46. Tissues injured during explants excision from the stock plant causes release of compounds like

a. Sulphur exudates
b. Polyphenol oxidase
c. Oxalate
d. Hydrocynates.

Ans. (b) Polyphenol oxidase

47. Culture of isolated plant organs is called as

a. Cell culture
b. Callus culture
c. Organ culture
d. All of the above

Ans. (c) Organ culture

48. Progress in haploid and dihaploid production is still slow due to which of the following bottlenecks?

a. Genetic instability
b. Low level of albinism
c. High frequency of plantlet regeneration.
d. All of the above

Ans. (a) Genetic instability

49. Which of the following hydrogels have been used for encapsulation of hydrated somatic embryos?

a. Carageenan and gel-rite
b. Sodium pectate and agar
c. Sodium and potassium alginate
d. All of the above

Ans. (d) All of the above

50. Which of the following are characteristic of gibbrellic acid?

a. Induces bud dormancy
b. Enhance genetic and physiological dwarfism
c. In tissue culture, elongation of shoot
d. All of the above

Ans. (c) In tissue culture, elongation of shoot

51. Culture of a diferential tissue from explants which is allowed to dedifferentiate *in vitro* is called as

a. Cell culture
b. Callus culture
c. Organ culture
d. None of these

Ans. (b) Callus culture

52. Somaclonal variation occurs due to which of the following ?

a. Activation of silent genes in multigene families
b. Methylation and demethylation in the promoter region of gene
c. Non-reciprocal mitotic recombination and activation of transposable elements.
d. All of the above

Ans. (d) All of the above

53. Among the given hydrogels, which one s the most perfected?

a. Agarose   b. Potassium aliginate

c. Sodium aliginate   d. Agar

Ans. (c) Sodium aliginate

54. Which of the following is correct about bulbosum technique of haploid production?

a. It is based on chromosome elimination during early embryo development.

b. Embryo culture is essential for obtaining haploid plants form the crosses between *Triticum aestivum* and *H.bulbosum*.

c. This method was reported by kasha and kao in 1970

d. All of the above

Ans. (d) All of the above

55. Survival of encapsulated somatic embryo has often been reported to be lower than that of the non-capsulated one probably due to which of the following?

a. Poor photosynthesis

b. Poor storage of food material

c. Poor respiration under the almost anaerobic condition within the capsule.

d. All of the above

Ans. (c) Poor respiration under the almost anaerobic condition within the capsule.

56. The process of formation of a bipolar structure containing the shoot and root meristem from the explants or from cell callus culture is called as

a. Somatic embryogenesis

b. Androgenetic analysis

c. Parthogenetic embryo

d. All of the above

Ans. (a) Somatic embryogenesis

57. Anther culture is used for the production of

a. Diploid plants   b. Haploid plants

c. Polyploidy plant   d. All of the above

Ans. (d) All of the above

58. The scientist, who was able to obtain callus from isolated pollen culture of gymnosperms is

a. O.Hertwig

b. Sunderland

c. Tulecke

d. Haberlandt

Ans. (d) Haberlandt

59. Ethylene promotes which of the following?

a. Ageing of stem

b. Activity of chlorophyllase

c. Activity of cell wall promoting enzyme

d. All of the above

Ans. (b) Activity of chlorophyllase

60. Guha and Maheshwari produced haploids from anther culture of which of the following?

a. Solenum esculantum

b. Nicotana

c. Datura

d. Ginkgo

Ans. (c) Datura

61. Somaclonal variation generally serves the same purpose as which of the following?

a. Test cross breeding   b. Hybrid sorting

c. Mutation breeding   d. None of the above

Ans. (c) Mutation breeding

62. A Ti plasmid having a functional *vir* region but lacking the T-DNA region, including the border sequence is known as

a. Binary vector   b. Helper plasmid

c. Helper T-cell   d. All of the above

Ans. (b) Helper plasmid

63. Virus free plant can be obtained by

a. Pollen culture   b. Ovary culture

c. Meristem culture   d. Shoot tip culture

Ans. (c) Meristem culture

64. Which of the following is correct about ethylene?

a. It is a natural product of ripening fruit.

b. It is phytogerontological hormone

c. Ethylene treatment increases the number of female flowers in cucumber

d. All of the above

Ans. (d) All of the above

65. Culturing of unfertilized ovaries to obtained haploid plant from egg cell or other haploid cells of the embryo sac is called

a. Meristem culture

b. Anther culture

c. Ovary culture

d. Stem culture

Ans. (c) Ovary culture

66. **Synthetic seeds are**

    a. Somatic embryo   b. Somaclone
    c. Cybrids   d. Protoplast

Ans. (a) **Somatic embryo**

67. **Which of the following is not correct about Abscissic acid?**

    a. Precursor of ABA is malic acid
    b. It is a naturally occurring growth inhibitor
    c. It destroyed the effect of GA and promotes dormancy in buds and seeds.
    d. It is synthesis in leaves

Ans. (a) **Precursor of ABA is malic acid**

68. **Which phytohormones is used for development of synthetic seeds?**

    a. GA   b. ABA
    c. Auxin   d. Ethylene

Ans. (b) **ABA**

69. **The approach of isolating pollen grains and culturing in vitro, giving rise to haploid embryos is called as**

    a. Ovary culture   b. Meristem culture
    c. Pollen culture   d. Stem culture

Ans. (c) **Pollen culture**

70. **Which of the following scientists first reported interspecific hybridization through protopast fusion in two species of Nicotiana?**

    a. Power and co-worker
    b. Miller and co-worker
    c. Carson and co-worker
    d. None of these

Ans. (c) **Carson and co-worker**

71. **Use of which of the following minimizes the risk of variation during in vitro conservation of germplasm?**

    a. Somatic embryo   b. Root apices
    c. Zygotic embryo   d. All of the above

Ans. (c) **Zygotic embryo**

72. **Which of the following factors is responsible for the loss of plant genetic resources?**

    a. Urbanization and industrialization
    b. Modern farming practices
    c. Extension for farming into wild habitates
    d. All of the above

Ans. (d) **All of the above**

73. **Success in germplasm storage is determined by which of the following factor?**

    a. Storage method and condition used
    b. Initial quality of material stored
    c. Both a and b
    d. None of these

Ans. (c) **Both a and b**

74. **Pusa jai kisan (bio-902) is a somaclonal variety of which of the following crops?**

    a. Indian pumpkin
    b. Indian mustard
    c. Indian rice
    d. Indian groundnut

Ans. (b) **Indian mustard**

75. **Which of the following material is conserved as germplasm?**

    a. Parents of hybrids, mutants and cytogenetic stocks
    b. Normal variety and wild cultivars
    c. Wild texa related to animal species
    d. All of the above

Ans. (a) **Parents of hybrids, mutants and cytogenetic stocks**

76. **Which of the following variety was developed from somaclona variation?**

    a. Delgold   b. A.C. Chang
    c. Sigma   d. All of the above

Ans. (c) **Sigma**

77. **Which of the following requirement must be fulfilled by any tissue culture technique that is used for conservation of germplasm**

    a. Plant virus elimination from the stored tissues/organ
    b. Genetic variability of the material to be preserved should be guaranteed.
    c. Well defined protocol which guarantees a high percentage of plant recovery form stored tissue
    d. All of the above

Ans. (c) **Well defined protocol which guarantees a high percentage of plant recovery form stored tissue**

78. **Which of the following steps are involved in conservation of plant genetic resources?**

    a. Data storage and retrieval
    b. Conservation and evaluation of germplasm
    c. Utilization, training and global coordination
    d. All of the above

Ans. (d) **All of the above**

79. The national research center on plant biotechnology is located at which of the following place?

    a. Mumbai
    b. Dehradun
    c. New Delhi
    d. Bangalore

Ans. (c) New Delhi

80. Which of the following is thermolabile?

    a. IBA
    b. ABA
    c. GA
    d. IAA

Ans. (b) ABA

81. Most commonly used method for transformation of plants is

    a. Protoplast method
    b. Agrobacterium mediated transformation
    c. Microinjection
    d. Protoplast method

Ans. (b) Agrobacterium mediated transformation

82. In tissue culture, regeneration of shoot and root occurs by manipulating the balance of

    a. Auxin and cytokinin
    b. Cytokinin and ABA
    c. ABA and ethylene
    d. Auxin and ABA

Ans. (a) Auxin and cytokinin

83. In 1998, the concept of traitor gene is given by a company called

    a. Pioneer seeds
    b. Indo American hybrids
    c. Vaibhav seeds
    d. Monsanto campany USA

Ans. (b) Indo American hybrids

84. Cryopreservation is based on which of the following?

    a. Liquid ammonia
    b. Liquid nitrogen
    c. Liquid carbon di oxide
    d. None of these

Ans. (b) Liquid nitrogen

85. Which of the following scientist is regarded as father of plant tissue culture?

    a. Aristotal
    b. Gottlieb Harberlandt
    c. Jean P. Nitsch
    d. Fleming

Ans. (b) Gottlieb Harberlandt

86. Which of the following is thermolaible?

    a. Cytokinin
    b. Pectinnase
    c. Lectinase
    d. Protease

Ans. (b) Pectinnase

87. The technique of embryo culture can be used to obtain which of the following?

    a. Propagation of orchid
    b. Interspecific hybrids
    c. Overcoming dormancy and to shorten breeding cycle
    d. All of these

Ans. (d) All of these

88. For long term storage of germplasm, which of the following is used?

    a. Liquid nitrogen
    b. Carbon di-oxide
    c. Liquid ammonia
    d. Mineral oil

Ans. (a) Liquid nitrogen

89. Which of the following is correct about alloplasmic lines?

    a. Used for production of allopolyploidy
    b. Produced by hybridization
    c. Production of cybridization/repeated backcrossing
    d. None of these

Ans. (c) Production of cybridization/repeated backcrossing

90. Which of the following enzyme is used for obtaining protoplasts?

    a. Catalase
    b. Protease
    c. Pectinase
    d. None of these

Ans. (c) Pectinase

91. Somatic embryo maturation is not promoted by which of the following?

    a. Auxin
    b. Cytokinin
    c. GA
    d. Abscissic acid

Ans. (b) Cytokinin

92. In general, callus culture are subculture after which of the following periods?

    a. 5–10 weeks
    b. 6–12 weeks
    c. 4–6 weeks
    d. 10–12 days

Ans. (c) 4–6 weeks

93. In general, suspension culture are subculture after which of the following periods?

    a. 4–6 weeks
    b. 3–10 days
    c. 10–20 days
    d. None of these

Ans. (b) 3–10 days

94. The technique of cryopreservation involves which of the following?

    a. Freezing and reculture
    b. Freezing and subculture

c. Thawing and reculture

d. All of these

Ans. (c) Thawing and reculture

95. Among the given Auxin, which one is the most frequently used in plant tissue culture?

a. ABA
b. IBA
c. NAA
d. 2,4-D

Ans. (d) 2,4-D

96. The term somaclonal variation was coined by which of the following scientists?

a. Skirvin and karp
b. Larkin and Scowcroft
c. Fleming and Watson
d. None of the above

Ans (b) Larkin and Scowcroft

97. Protoplast fusion is induced by which of the following treatments?

a. PEG
b. High voltage electric pulse
c. High pH and high calcium concentration
d. All of the above

Ans. (d) All of the above

98. Pusa jai kisan (Bio-902) somaclonal of Indian mustard was isolated from which of the following varieties?

a. Pusa 288
b. Kranti
c. Karuna
d. Varuna

Ans. (d) Varuna

99. Meristem culture can be used for which of the following purposes?

a. Cybrid formation
b. Germplasm collection
c. Germplasm exchange and conservation
d. All of the above

Ans. (c) Germplasm exchange and conservation

100. Delgold and A.C.Change, developed through somatic hybridization are cultivars of which of the following?

a. *Brassica compristis*
b. *Phenoxy dectyliferus*
c. *Nicotiana rustica*
d. *Nicotiana tabacum*

Ans. (d) Nicotiana tabacum

101. Among the given varieties of tobacco, which one was developed through haploid phase?

a. F 330
b. F211
c. GSM331
d. None of these

Ans. (b) F211

102. Among the given compound which one is the most commonly used as cryoproectant?

a. Glycerol
b. Methanol
c. DMSO
d. Toluene

Ans. (c) DMSO

103. Sugarcane somaclone Ono, isolated from the parental variety pindar, is resistance to a disease caused by which of the following?

a. Virus
b. Fungus
c. Bacteria
d. All of these

Ans. (a) Virus

104. In which of the following tree species, embryo culture is used to overcome dormancy?

a. *Iris*
b. *Prunus*
c. *Taxus*
d. All of the above

Ans. (d) All of the above

105. Scarlet is somaclone of which of the following?

a. Soybean
b. Wheat
c. Sweet potato
d. All of the above

Ans. (c) Sweet potato

106. The first plant from a mature plant cell was regenerated by which of the following?

a. Yellow
b. Braun
c. White
d. Haberlandt

Ans. (b) Braun

107. Among the given agents, which one is used as cryoprotectants?

a. DMSO, glycerol and formic acid
b. DMSO, proline and acotinic acid
c. DMSO, glycerol and proline
d. None of these

Ans. (c) DMSO, glycerol and proline

108. During gynogenesis, haploid plants cell was regenerated by which of the following?

a. Polar cell
b. Egg cell
c. Synergids cell
d. None of these

Ans. (b) Egg cell

109. Delgold is a variety of which of the following?

a. Chewing tobacco
b. Flue-cured tobacco
c. Both a and b
d. None of these

Ans. (b) Flue-cured tobacco

110. Somatic hybridization has been the most successful in which of the following?

a. Poaceae   b. Malvaceae

c. Solanaceae   d. Euphorbiaceae

Ans. (c) Solanaceae

111. In which of the following, somaclonal variation can occurs?

a. Direct adventitious shoot regeneration

b. Suspension culture

c. Direct somatic embryogenesis

d. All of the above

Ans. (d) All of the above

112. Evergreen is a somaclone of which of the following?

a. Tomato   b. Blackberry

c. Potato   d. Radish

Ans. (b) Blackberry

113. Among the given supplements/additives, which is an example of complex organic supplement/additive?

a. Coconut milk and tomato juice

b. Corn milk and malt extract

c. Yeast extract and casein hydrolysate

d. All of the above

Ans. (d) All of the above

114. Tobacco culture A.C. Change is resistant to which of the following?

a. White rust   b. Black rot

c. YMV   d. TMV

Ans. (b) Black rot

115. Among the given surface sterilizing agents, which one gives the best result?

a. Silver iodide   b. Sodium hypochlorite

c. Sodium chloride   d. Bromine water

Ans. (b) Sodium hypochlorite

116. Somaclone scarlet has improvement in which of the following traits?

a. Disease resistance   b. Skin colour

c. Herbicide resistance   d. None of these

Ans. (b) Skin colour

117. Slow growth shoot culture protocols protocols have been developed for which of the following?

a. Coconut and citrus   b. Ginger and banana

c. Sweet potato and garlic   d. Both b & c

Ans. (d) Both b & c

118. The cultivar A.C. Chang and delgold were released for commercial cultivation in which of the following countries?

a. New delhi   b. Canada

c. Japan   d. China

Ans. (b) Canada

119. Hyperhydracity of culture may not be reduced by which of the following?

a. Gibberellic acid   b. Growth retardants

c. Agar hydrolyate   d. All of the above

Ans. (a) Gibberellic acid

120. For long term *in vitro* storage of plant germplasm, which of the following is in practical use?

a. Lyophilizaton   b. Cryoperservation

c. Mobilization   d. None of these

Ans. (b) Cryoperservation

121. Among the given variety of rice, which was developed through haploid phase?

a. ICPH-8   b. IR-8

c. IR-20   d. Shin shu

Ans. (d) Shin shu

122. In protoplast isolation and culture , ionic osmoticum is not preferred because of which of the following?

a. It reduces protoplast fusion

b. It reduces protoplast yield

c. It reduces protoplast survival

d. It inhibits cell wall regeneration

Ans. (d) It inhibits cell wall regeneration

123. Andro is a somaclone of which of the following?

a. Potato   b. Tomato

c. Apple   d. Flax

Ans. (d) Flax

124. Bio-13 is a somaclone of which of the following?

a. *Glycin max*   b. *Zea maize*

c. *Citronella java*   d. None of the above

Ans. (c) *Citronella java*

125. PEG induced protoplast fusion is enhanced by which of the following?

a. Low pH PEG treatment medium

b. High Ca^{+2} culture medium

c. High pH PEG treatment medium

d. All of the above

Ans. (c) High pH PEG treatment medium

126. Which of the following steps are not involved in cryopreservation?

a. Thawing
b. Encapsulation
c. Preculture
d. Freezing

Ans. **(b) Encapsulation**

127. Among the given varieties of wheat, which one is of the following traits?

a. PBW 373
b. HUW 206
c. Jinghua I
d. Halna

Ans. **(c) Jinghua I**

128. Intergeneric hybrids from which of the following crsses have been recovered through embryo culture?

a. *Hordeum vulgareX triticum aestivum*
b. *Triticum aestivum X secale cereal*
c. *Brasica compristis X brasica nigra*
d. All of the above

Ans. **(b) *Triticum aestivum X secale cereal***

129. Somaclone andro has improvement in which of the following?

a. Wilt resistance
b. Disease resistance
c. Rust immunity
d. All of the above

Ans. **(c) Rust immunity**

130. Anther culture ordinary yields which of the following?

a. Diploid plant
b. Haploid plant
c. Polyploidy plant
d. None of these

Ans. **(b) Haploid plant**

131. Sugarcane variation arises due to which of the following?

a. Cos 771
b. Co 1188
c. Pindar
d. Co 1148

Ans. **(c) Pindar**

132. Somaclonal variation arises due to which of the following?

a. Change in chromosome number
b. Gene mutation
c. Gene amplification
d. All of the above

Ans. **(d) All of the above**

133. Stirred tank reactor can be used as which of the following?

a. Air bubble reactor
b. Feed batch reactor
c. Batch reactor
d. Immobilized reactor

Ans. **(c) Batch reactor**

134. Which of the following is not an example of alkaloid?

a. Codeine
b. Morphine
c. Camphor
d. Berberine

Ans. **(c) Camphor**

135. New alleles of known gene and even new mutation of genes not known so far have been recovered through which of the following?

a. Hybridization
b. Somaclonal variation
c. Cybrdization
d. Embryo rescue

Ans. **(b) Somaclonal variation**

136. Somatic hybridization produces which of the following?

a. Symmetric hybrid
b. Asymmetric hybrid
c. Both a and b
d. None of the above

Ans. **(c) Both a and b**

137. Which of the following is not correct about taxol?

a. It is obtained from trichosanthes species
b. It acts on spindle like colchicines
c. It is used for treatment of breast cancer
d. It is used for the treatment of ovarian cancer

Ans. **(a) It is obtained from trichosanthes species**

138. Somatic hybrids are also called which of the following?

a. Somatic hybrid
b. Cytoplasmic hybrid
c. Vybrids
d. Both b and c

Ans. **(b) Cytoplasmic hybrid**

139. Which of the following is not correct about Micropropagation?

a. Suitable techniques of Micropropagation are available for all valuable sp.
b. Somaclonal variation may arise during *in vitro* culture
c. Vitrificaton may be a problem in some Micropropagation
d. All of the above

Ans. **(a) Suitable techniques of Micropropagation are available for all valuable sp.**

140. Conventional *in vitro* environment used for Micropropagation has which of the following feature?

a. High sugar concentration and growth
b. Low photosynthesis photon flux density
c. Constant temp. and high relative humidity
d. All of the above

Ans. **(d) All of the above**

141. Secondary metabolite include which of the following compound?

a. Alkaloid   b. Phenylpropanoids

c. Terpinoids   d. All of the above

Ans. (d) All of the above

142. Which of the following is not correct about biotransformation?

a. Arbutin is produced commercially by biotransformation

b. Products generated by biotransformation are more useful or valuable than the precursors used

c. Biotransformation reactions are catalyzed by enzymes present in cells

d. Low rate of biotransformation prevents commerce exploitation of the very large number of bio-conversions known for the plant cell.

Ans. (a) Arbutin is produced commercially by bio-transformation

143. Which of the following is correct about taxol?

a. It is obtained from trichosanthes sp.

b. It promote dissolution of microtubules in to tubulin molecules

c. It is used for the treatment of breast cancer

d. Both b & c

Ans. (d) Both b & c

144. Which of the followings not correct about asymmetric hybrids?

a. Asymmetric hybrids can be produced by fusion of cytoplasts of a species with irradiated protoplast of another species.

b. Several asymmetric hybrids have been produced in *Nicotiana*, *Brassica*, etc.

c. Asymmetric hybrids can be produced by fusion of cytoplasts of a species with irradicated protoplasts of another species.

d. All of the above

Ans. (a) Asymmetric hybrids can be produced by fusion of cytoplasts of a species with irradiated protoplast of another species.

145. Which of the following is not a feature of Somaclonal variation?

a. Somaclonal variation occurs or very low frequency.

b. A very effective selection can be practised at the cell level for several traits

c. Use of Somaclonal variation may reduce the time required for the release of new variety as compared to mutation breeding

d. Their chromosome number may be doubled to obtained homozygous lines is at least 6-8 times as efficient as that among segregating population

Ans. (a) Somaclonal variation occurs n very low frequency

146. Which of the following plant species, bio-transforms hydroquinone into arbutin?

a. *Datura innoxia*   b. *Rauwofia serpentine*

c. *Catharanthus roseus*   d. All of the above

Ans. (d) All of the above

147. A spin filter bioreactor is a good example of which of the following?

a. Air lift bioreactor

b. Continues flow reactor

c. Fed batch reactor

d. Fluidized bed reactor

Ans. (b) Continues flow reactor

148. Micropropagation of woody trees presents which of the following problems?

a. Difficulties in rooting   b. Poor growth *in vitro*

c. Browning of medium   d. All of the above

Ans. (d) All of the above

149. Which of the following advantage is correct about micropropation?

a. Extremely low multiplication rates

b. Limited to a particular season.

c. Plant of desired sex can be selectively multiplied

d. Plant can not be maintained *in vitro* in a pathogen free state

Ans. (c) Plant of desired sex can be selectively multiplied

150. Symmetric hybrid produced through protoplast fusion provides which of the following opportunities n crop improvement programmes?

a. Widening of genetic base of an allopolyploid

b. Generation of noval material for scientific studies

c. Creation of superior hybrid

d. All of the above

Ans. (d) All of the above

151. Protoplasts can be used for genetic transformation by which of the following technique?

a. Liposome mediated delivery

b. PEG mediated DNA uptake

c. Electorporation

d. All of the above

Ans. (d) All of the above

152. Which of the following limitation are associated with haploid production?

a. In many crops, large number of haploid can be easily obtained

b. A sophisticated tissue culture laboratory and a dependable greenhouse are essential for success

c. Low frequency of albinos are produced n anther cultures of monocots especially cereals

d. Occurrence of sporophitic variation may limit the usefulness of pollen embryo for genetic transformation.

Ans. (b) A sophisticated tissue culture laboratory and a dependable greenhouse are essential for success

153. It is desirable to preserve which of the following tissue to minimise the risk of genetic instability

a. Root tip
b. Shoot tip
c. Zygotic embryo
d. Both b & c

Ans. (b) Shoot tip

154. Which of the following are the characteristic feature of batch bioreactors?

a. Continuous in growth rate
b. Constant level of cellular waste
c. Continuous change in the composition of cells
d. None of the above

Ans. (c) Continuous change in the composition of cells

155. For rapid development of homozygous lines, haploids can be produced by which of the following approaches?

a. Anther culture
b. Interspecific hybridization
c. Ovary culture
d. All of the above

Ans. (d) All of the above

156. Which of the following element is essential for plant cell and tissue culture?

a. Co   b. Cl
c. Ni   d. P

Ans. (d) P

157. Which of the following problems are correct about large scale culture of plant cells?

a. The longer fermentation time decrease the risk of contamination

b. Characterstics of a cell population may change during culure, and prolonged continuous culture may be desirable

c. In case of biochemical production growth may enhance biochemical formation and vice-versa

d. Small reactor and short formation time required

Ans. (b) Characteristics of a cell population may change during culure, and prolonged continuous culture may be desirable

158. Which of the following is used as growth retardant?

a. TIBA and paclobutrazole
b. Daminozide
c. ABA and chlormequat
d. All of the above

Ans. (d) All of the above

159. Which of the following chemicals interferes with virus multiplication?

a. Chloroamphinicol
b. Raffinose
c. Actinomycin D
d. None of these

Ans. (c) Actinomycin D

160. In case of slow growth culture, high osmotic concentration are created by which of the following?

a. Fructos   b. Mannose
c. Sorbitol   d. Galactose

Ans. (c) Sorbitol

161. Cryoprotactant reduce cryoinjury by which of the following?

a. Enhance the cellular dehydration
b. Reduced ice crystal formation
c. Enhance the dislocation of structural water.
d. All of these

Ans. (b) Reduced ice crystal formation

162. Which of the following cryoprotactant acts through withdrawal of cellular water?

a. Glycerol
b. Tyrosine
c. Proline
d. DMSO

Ans. (a) Glycerol

163. Cryoinjury results from which of the following?

a. Dislocation of structural water
b. Toxic solution effect
c. Ice crystal formation
d. All of the above

Ans. (d) All of the above

164. **Which of the following are the features of a spin-filter bioreactor?**

    a. The culture s aerated by a sparger
    b. A stirrer plate magnetically coupled to the central shaft provides continuous stirring
    c. The central shaft of bioreactor houses a spinning filter
    d. All of the above

Ans. (d) All of the above

165. **Cryoprotection is done at which of the following temperature?**

    a. 5°C
    b. 0°C
    c. 15°C
    d. 25°C

Ans. (b) 0°C

166. **Partial desiccation step can be combined with cryopreservation of which of the following?**

    a. Cryoprotection
    b. LN refrigerator
    c. Controlled freezing
    d. All of the above

Ans. (c) Controlled freezing

167. **Which of the following is not correct?**

    a. Dividing cells are more likely to survive cryopreservation than nondividing cells.
    b. Partial desiccation of tissues reduces cryoinjury
    c. Cryoprotectants minimise loss of structural water
    d. Meristematic cells suffer from less cryoinjury than differentiated cells

Ans. (a) Dividing cells are more likely to survive cryopreservation than nondividing cells.

168. **Partial desiccation step can be combined with cryopreservation of which of the following?**

    a. Zygotic embryo
    b. Encapsulated somatic embryos
    c. Vitrified somatic embryo
    d. None of the above

Ans. (b) Encapsulated somatic embryos

169. **Which of the following is correct about cryo-protectant?**

    a. Fructose in non permeable
    b. Glycerol is highly permeable
    c. Sucrose is highly permeable
    d. PEG is highly permeable

Ans. (b) Glycerol is highly permeable

170. **Which of the following techniques used for cell cloning are used for protoplast culture as well?**

    a. Somaclone method
    b. Microdrop method
    c. Filter paper raft tissue
    d. Microchamber technique

Ans. (b) Microdrop method

171. **Which of the following vitamins s essential for plant tissue culture?**

    a. Pyridoxine
    b. Formic acid
    c. Thiamine
    d. Inositole

Ans. (c) Thiamine

172. **In case of shoot regeneration, GRs are required during which of the following?**

    a. Developmental determination phase
    b. Morphogenic competence acquisition phase
    c. Bothe a and b
    d. None of these

Ans. (c) Bothe a and b

173. **Which of the following was the first to be achieved?**

    a. Pollen culture
    b. Embryo culture
    c. Embryogenesis
    d. Somatic hybridization

Ans. (b) Embryo culture

174. **A batch culture has which of the following feature?**

    a. Progressive nutrient depletion
    b. Typical Sigmoidal growth curve
    c. Limitation culture duration
    d. All of the above

Ans. (d) All of the above

175. **Which of the following chemicals has been used to eliminate viruses from plant?**

    a. Penicillin
    b. Riboflavin
    c. Actinomycn D
    d. None of the above

Ans. (c) Actinomycn D

176. **A high Auxin concentration is required during which of the following?**

    a. SE transformation
    b. SE induction
    c. SE maturation
    d. SE conversion

Ans. (b) SE induction

177. Which of the following is the limitation of artificial seed?

a. Difficult large scale production
b. Low production cost
c. Difficulties in storage
d. All of the above

Ans. (c) Difficulties in storage

178. GRs are not used during which of the following stages of Micropropagation?

a. Shooting
b. Rooting
c. Culture establishment
d. Multiplication

Ans. (c) Culture establishment

179. In Micropropagation, *in vitro* hardening is achieved by which of the following?

a. Use of *pseudomonas* culture
b. Cooling of culture vessels at bottom
c. PEG in medium
d. All of the above

Ans. (d) All of the above

180. Virus free plants produced by various *in vitro* techniques can be used for which of the following?

a. Commercial cultivation
b. Breeding programmes
c. For germplasm exchange
d. Both b & c

Ans. (d) Both b & c

181. Certain biochemicals are produced by specialized cells present in organized structures. Which of the following culture systems will be useful for production of such compounds?

a. Embryo culture
b. Callus culture
c. Organ culture
d. Suspension culture

Ans. (c) Organ culture

182. Genetic erosion is the consequence of which of the following?

a. Enhanced the genetic variability among cultivated variety
b. Extinctions of wild relatives of crop species
c. Enhanced the genetic variability within the species
d. None of these

Ans. (b) Extinctions of wild relatives of crop species

183. Which of the following is a sweetening agent?

a. Shikonin
b. Digitoxin
c. Pyrethrini
d. Thaumatin

Ans. (d) Thaumatin

184. Which of the following can serve as elicitors?

a. Some glycosidic protein
b. Cell wall pectins
c. Chitosan
d. None of these

Ans. (c) Chitosan

185. Shikonin production by cultured cells of *Lithospermum erythrorhizon* is suppressed by which of the following?

a. NAA
b. 2, 4-D
c. Kinetin
d. IBA

Ans. (c) Kinetin

186. Which of the chemical promotes shikonin production by cultured cells of *L. Erythrorhizon*?

a. NH_4^+
b. Cu^{+2}
c. 2,4-D
d. Thiamine

Ans. (b) Cu^{+2}

187. Which of the following is a steroid?

a. Shikonin
b. Dioxgenin
c. Pyrethrin
d. Thaumatin

Ans. (b) Dioxgenin

188. Which of the following has insecticidal activity?

a. Shikonin
b. Digitoxin
c. Pyrethrin
d. Thaumatin

Ans. (c) Pyrethrin

189. Biochemical accumulation by cultured plant cells is affected by which of the following?

a. Inoculum size
b. Light quality
c. Chemical composition of medium
d. All of the above

Ans. (d) All of the above

190. Which of the following breeding procedure applicable to only autopolyploid crop species?

a. Somaclonal breeding
b. Analytical breeding
c. Hybrid sorting
d. Both b and C

Ans. (d) Both b and C

191. In most species, cells become committed to gametophytic development after which of the following stages?

a. Binucleate pollen
b. Somatic mother cell
c. Trinucleat pollen
d. Uninucleat pollen

Ans. (a) Binucleate pollen

192. Which of the following involves in haploid production?

a. Somaclonal breeding
b. Analytical breeding
c. Hybrid sorting
d. Both b & C

Ans. (d) Both b & C

193. In which of the following, dihaploids are used for breeding, while tetraploids are used as commercial varieties?

a. Tobacco
b. Tomato
c. Potato
d. Soybean

Ans. (c) Potato

194. In which of the following plant species, YY males are used to produce all male population?

a. *Asparagus*
b. *Coccinia*
c. *Trichosanthes*
d. None of these

Ans. (a) *Asparagus*

195. Which of the following stresses are known to promote androgenesis?

a. Drought treatment
b. IBA
c. Heat treatment
d. NAA

Ans. (c) Heat treatment

196. Which of the following have been shown to prevent precocious germination of cultured embryos?

a. Lactine hydroysate
b. ABA
c. NAA
d. Low score levels

Ans. (b) ABA

197. Which of the following have been used as selection agents for cells selections to develop disease resistance Somaclonal variant?

a. Pathogen
b. Toxins
c. Culture filterate
d. All of the above

Ans. (d) All of the above

198. Somatic hybridization can be resorted to only when which of the following criteria are satisfied?

a. Totipotancy of the isolated protoplasts
b. Availability of the effective strategy for selection of hybrid cells
c. Isolation protoplast in large quantities
d. Both b and c

Ans. (d) Both b and c

199. Match the columns A and column B

A. Absisic acd	I. IAA
B. Synthetic seed	II. Dormin
C. Ethylene	III. IBA
D. Natural Auxin	IV. Ethrel

a. A-II, B-III, C-IV, D-I
b. A-II, B-I, C-IV, D-III
c. A-III, B-II, C-IV, D-I
d. A-II, B-III, C-I, D-IV

Ans. (a) A-II, B-III, C-IV,D-I

200. The instrument that is used to measure the growth of plants is called as

a. Gulconometer
b. Auxanometer
c. Algometer
d. Anemometer

Ans. (b) Auxanometer

201. The smallest viable unit which can grow, multiply and from a plant in tissue culture

a. Chromosome
b. Cell
c. Tissue
d. Nucleus

Ans. (b) Cell

202. Micropropagation is

a. Raising of plants from a small tissue in culture
b. Multiplication of small plant
c. Propagation of small parts of organisms
d. Indefinite maintenance of an organ or tissue

Ans. (a) Raising of plants from a small tissue in culture

203. Tissue culture is

a. Growth and multiplication of cell on artificial medium
b. Growth of specific plant structure on artificial medium
c. Maintenance, growth and differentiation of cell, tissue and organs on artificial medium
d. None of the above

Ans. (c) Maintenance, growth and differentiation of cell, tissue and organs on artificial medium

204. Part of plant used for culturing is called

a. Stock
b. Explants
c. Scion
d. Callus

Ans. (b) Explants

205. Tissue culture technique was first attempted by

a. Nobecourt
b. Hanning
c. Haberlandt
d. Gautheret

Ans. (c) Haberlandt

206. Tissue culture technique was first performed successfully by

a. White
b. Harberlandt
c. Nobecourt
d. Gautheret

Ans. (a) White

207. The structure employed by white for first successful tissue culture was

a. Root of carrot
b. Root of tomato
c. Leaf cells
d. Apical meristem

Ans. (b) Root of tomato

208. Callus is

a. Tissue that forms embryo
b. Tissue that grows to form embryoid
c. Unorganised actively dividing mass of cells maintained in culture
d. None of the above

Ans. (c) Unorganised actively dividing mass of cells maintained in culture

209. Callus formation is promoted by

a. Proper light and subculturing
b. Excess of NAA
c. Absence of cell
d. Darkness and subculturing

Ans. (d) Darkness and subculturing

210. Differentiation of callus into plant part is

a. Embryogenesis
b. Morphogenesis
c. Totipotency
d. Embryoid formation

Ans. (b) Morphogenesis

211. Who discovered that morphogenesis in culture medium is controlled by hormones

a. Skoog and miller
b. Muir at al
c. Vasil and hilderbrandt
d. Helperin and wetherell

Ans. (a) Skoog and miller

212. Embryo culture technique was discovered by

a. Skoog and miller
b. Muir at al
c. Vasil and hilderbrandt
d. Steward

Ans. (d) Steward

213. Embryoid is

a. A miniature embryo
b. Non-zygotic embryo formed *in vitro* culture
c. Embryo raised in culture medium
d. Cellular aggregate similar to embryo in appearance

Ans. (b) Non-zygotic embryo formed *in vitro* culture

214. The concept of cellular totipotency was given by

a. Skoog and miller
b. Steward
c. Vasil and hilderbrandt
d. Helperin and wetherell

Ans. (c) Vasil and hilderbrandt

215. Ramet is

a. Clone
b. Cell aggregate
c. Callus
d. Individual of clone

Ans. (d) Individual of clone

216. Guha and Maheshwari are famous for

a. Protoplast culture
b. Pollen culture
c. Shoot tip culture
d. None of the above

Ans. (b) Pollen culture

217. The technique of protoplast fusion was developed by

a. Skoog and miller
b. Muir at al
c. Vasil and hilderbrandt
d. Carlson et al

Ans. (c) Vasil and hilderbrandt

218. Explants is required to be disinfectant before placing in culture. This done by

a. Autoclaving
b. Ultraviolet rays
c. Clorax or hyprochlorite
d. X-rays

Ans. (c) Clorax or hyprochlorite

219. Aseptic culture means

a. Presence of bacteria
b. Absence of other organism like microbes
c. Parthenogenetic development
d. None of the above

Ans. (b) Absence of other organism like microbes

220. Abnormal growth of a plant organ is

a. Teratoma
b. Tumour
c. Witches broom
d. Callus

Ans. (b) Tumour

221. Crown gall is caused by

    a. *Aspergillus*

    b. *Agrobacterium tumefaciens*

    c. *Bacillus stolonifer*

    d. *Rhizopus stolonifer*

Ans. (b) *Agrobacterium tumefaciens*

222. TIP is

    a. Tuber inducing protein

    b. Tuber inducing principle

    c. Tumour inducing protein

    d. Tumour inducing principle

Ans. (d) Tumour inducing principle

223. Root knots are generally due to

    a. Symbiotic bacteria

    b. Symbiotic cyanobacteria

    c. Nematodes

    d. Insect larvae

Ans. (c) Nematodes

224. Teratoma is

    a. Abnormal swelling

    b. Formation of a number of shoots from a tumour

    c. Development of a number of close branches

    d. Secretion of tumour inducing principle

Ans. (b) Formation of a number of shoots from a tumour

225. Witches broom is characterised by

    a. Hypertrophy

    b. Typotrophy

    c. Teratoma

    d. A number of close branches

Ans. (d) A number of close branches

226. Variation appearing suddenly in culture

    a. Somatic variation   b. Somaclonal variation

    c. Mutation   d. Aberration

Ans. (b) Somaclonal variation

227. Abnormal growth can be due to

    a. Infection   b. Injury

    c. Hybridization   d. All of the above

Ans. (d) All of the above

228. Virus free plants can be obtained through

    a. Shoot tip culture   b. Root tip culture

    c. Haploid culture   d. Embryo culture

Ans. (a) Shoot tip culture

229. What additional treatment is required by protoplast fusion in plant

    a. PEG and sodium nitrate

    b. Coconut milk and glycine

    c. Cellulose and pectinase

    d. All of the above

Ans. (c) Cellulase and pectinase

230. Protoplast fusion result in

    a. Genetic hybridization

    b. Male sterility

    c. Abundant seeds of rare plants

    d. Parasexual/somatic hybridization

Ans. (d) Parasexual/somatic hybridization

231. Pollen culture produces

    a. Haploid plant where every gene can excess its effect

    b. Homozygous diploid plant

    c. Abundant seed of rare plant

    d. Abundant pollen in male sterile plant

Ans. (a) Haploid plant where every gene can excess its effect

232. An androgenic plant can be converted in to homozygous diploid plant through the application of

    a. Nitrogen mustard   b. Nitrous acid

    c. Colchicines   d. Acridine orange

Ans. (c) Colchicines

233. The enzyme required to obtained wall free/naked protoplast are

    a. Cellulase and proteinase

    b. Cellulase and pectinase

    c. Cellulase and amylase

    d. Amylase and pectinase

Ans. (b) Cellulase and pectinase

234. Which technique can be helpful in overcoming hybridisation barrier

    a. Shoot tip culture   b. Embryo rescue

    c. Protoplast fusion   d. Both b and c

Ans. (d) Both b and c

235. Two protoplast can be made to fuse through the application of

    a. Electrofusion   b. PEG

    c. Sodium nitrate   d. All of the above

Ans. (d) All of the above

236. Who developed the technique of nurse tissue to show cellular totipotency

a. Hilderbrandt
b. Steward
c. Muir
d. Konar

Ans. (c) Muir

237. Pollen embryoids were discovered by

a. Konar and Nataraja
b. Guha and maheshwari
c. Skoog and miller
d. Heparin and wetherell

Ans. (b) Guha and maheshwari

238. Which of the following can yield a completely haploid plant

a. Root tip
b. Anther
c. Carpel
d. Stem apical meristem

Ans. (b) Anther

239. Cellular totipotency was demonstrated by

a. Theodore schwann
b. A.V. Leeuwenhoek
c. F.C. Steward
d. Robert hooke

Ans. (c) F.C. Steward

240. A totipotency cell means

a. An undifferentiated cell capable of developing in to a system or entire plant
b. An undifferentiated cell capable of developing into an organ
c. An undifferentiated cell capable of developing in to complete embryo
d. Cell which lacks the capability to differentiate in to an organ or system

Ans. (a) An undifferentiated cell capable of developing in to a system or entire plant

241. Micropropagation refer to

a. Mature stage of endosperm
b. The phenomenon of manufacture of hormones
c. Germination of seed where cotyledons come above the soil
d. A technique to obtain new plants by culturing cell or tissue in culture medium

Ans. (d) A technique to obtain new plants by culturing cell or tissue in culture medium

242. A major use of embryo culture is in

a. Induction of Somaclonal variation
b. Overcoming hybridisation barriers
c. Production of alkaloids
d. Clonal propagation

Ans. (b) Overcoming hybridisation barriers

243. On culturing the young anther of a plant a botanist got a few diploid plant along with haploid plants. Which of the following might have given the diploid plant?

a. Exine of pollen grain
b. Vegetative cell of pollen
c. Cells of anther wall
d. Generative cell of pollen

Ans. (c) Cells of anther wall

244. Which one produce androgenic haploids in anther cultures

a. Anther cell
b. Tapetal layer of anther wall
c. Connective tissue
d. Young pollen grain

Ans. (d) Young pollen grain

245. In tobacco callus, which one shall induce shoot differentiation in combination of Auxin and cytokinin

a. Higher concentration cytokinin and lower concentration of Auxin
b. Lower concentration cytokinin and higher concentration of Auxin
c. Only cytokinin and no Auxin
d. Only Auxin and no cytokinin

Ans. (a) Higher concentration cytokinin and lower concentration of Auxin

246. In callus culture, roots can be induced by the supply of

a. Auxin and no cytokinin
b. Higher concentration cytokinin and lower concentration of Auxin
c. Lower concentration cytokinin and higher concentration of Auxin
d. None of the above

Ans. (c) Lower concentration cytokinin and higher concentration of Auxin

247. After demonstration of cellular totipotency, a botanist wishes to raise identical plants. The tissue or part likely to yield haploid embryo are

a. Stem apices
b. Root tips
c. Young anther
d. Young leaves

Ans. (c) Young anther

248. Who could grow tomato roots successfully and developed the technique of tissue culture for the first time

a. Hilderbrandt   b. P.R. white

c. W.H. muir   d. F.C. Steward

Ans. (b) P.R. white

249. Plant tumour/ crown gall/ abnormal growth is caused by

a. Agrobacterium   b. Azotobactor

c. Nostoc   d. *E.coli*

Ans. (a) Agrobacterium

250. Which of the following plant cells will show totipotency

a. Sieve tubes

b. Xylem vessels

c. Meristem

d. Cork cell

Ans. (c) Meristem

251. Variations observing during tissue culture of some plant are known as

a. Clonal variation

b. Somaclonal variation

c. Somatic variation

d. Tissue culture variation

Ans. (b) Somaclonal variation

252. Virus free plants can be obtained by

a. Antibiotic treatment   b. Bordeaux mixture

c. Root tip culture   d. Shoot tip culture

Ans. (d) Shoot tip culture

253. Tissue culture technique can be produce in definite number of new plants from a small parental tissue. The economic importance of the technique is in raising

a. Variants through picking up Somaclonal variation

b. Genetically uniform population of an elites species

c. Homozygous diploid plants

d. Development of new species

Ans. (b) Genetically uniform population of an elites species

254. Haploid plant culture are got from

a. Leaves

b. Root tip

c. Pollen grain

d. Buds

Ans. (c) Pollen grain

255. Somaclonal variation are the ones

a. Caused by mutagens

b. Produced during tissue culture

c. Induced during sexual embryogeny

d. Caused by gamma rays

Ans. (b) Produced during tissue culture

256. Parasexual hydridisation means fusion of

a. Male gamete with female gametes

b. Male gamete with synergid

c. Somatic protoplasts

d. Male gamete with somatic cell

Ans. (c) Somatic protoplasts

257. Application of embryo culture is in

a. Clonal propagation

b. Overcoming hybridization barrier

c. Production of alkaloids

d. Formation of Somaclonal variation

Ans. (b) Overcoming hybridization barrier

258. Plants developed *in vitro* culture from pollen grains are

a. Androgenic haploid   b. Pollen plant

c. Male plant   d. Sterile plant

Ans. (a) Androgenic haploid

259. In tissue/bacterial culture glassware and nutrients are sterilised through

a. Water bath at 200°C

b. Dry air oven at 200°C

c. Dehumidifier

d. Autoclave

Ans. (d) Autoclave

260. Development of shoot and root in tissue culture is determined by

a. Cytokinin and Auxin ratio

b. Enzymes

c. Temperature

d. Plant nutrient

Ans. (a) Cytokinin and Auxin ratio

261. Plant raised from single germinating pollen grain under culture condition would be

a. Diploid

b. Haploid

c. Triploid

d. Tetraploid

Ans. (b) Haploid

262. Plant medium used widely in preparation of culture medium is got from

    a. *Cycas revolute*

    b. *Cocus nucifera*

    c. *Pinus roxburghii*

    d. *Borassus flabellifera*

Ans. (b) *Cocus nucifera*

263. Clonal cell lines are got from

    a. Tissue culture

    b. Tissue fractionation

    c. Tissue homogenisation

    d. Tissue system

Ans. (a) Tissue culture

264. Auxenic culture is

    a. Culture of tissue

    b. Culture of genes

    c. Pure culture without contamination

    d. Pure culture of microbes without any external nutrient

Ans. (c) Pure culture without contamination

265. A cell from leaf is made to grow into complete plant under culture conditions. It shows cellular

    a. Cloning   b. Totipotency

    c. Hybridization   d. All of the above

Ans. (b) Totipotency

266. Use of Agrobacterium T-DNA, transposons etc., for identification and/or isolation of a gene by first integrating it into the concerned gene and isolating mutants so produced is known as:

    a. Gene tagging   b. Gene silencing

    c. Gene expression   d. Gene modification

Ans. (a) Gene tagging

267. Multiplication of plants via asexual reproduction, e.g. via micropropagation, vegetative propagation, etc. is called

    a. Clonal deletion   b. Clonal propagation

    c. Clonal selection   d. None of these

Ans. (b) Clonal propagation

268. Growth in such culture shows a typical sigmoid curve, and they require subculture/termination after a specific period of time in:

    a. Assay culture   b. Batch culture

    c. Cell culture   d. Root culture

Ans. (b) Batch culture

269. *In vitro* culture of single or relatively small groups of cells, e.g. suspension culture, this term is often used for callus culture as well as:

    a. Assay cuture   b. Cell culture

    c. Root culture   d. None of these

Ans. (b) Cell culture

270. Evergreen is a somaclone of:

    a. Cucumber   b. Carrot

    c. Potato   d. Blackberry

Ans. (d) Blackberry

271. Among the given surface which is best sterilizing agents is?

    a. Silver nitrate

    b. Carbemide

    c. Calcium or sodium hypochlorite

    d. Bromine water

Ans. (c) Calcium or sodium hypochlorite

272. Somaclone scarlet has improvement in:

    a. Skin colour   b. Insect resistance

    c. Yield   d. Disease resistance

Ans. (a) Skin colour

273. Which variety of rice was developed through haploid phase?

    a. Sindhu   b. Shin shu

    c. IR8   d. Pragati

Ans. (b) Shin shu

274. Andro is a somaclone of:

    a. Apple   b. Radish

    c. Flax   d. Maize

Ans. (c) Flax

275. Anther culture ordinarily yields:

    a. Haploid plants

    b. Disomic plants

    c. Polyploidy plants

    d. Double haploid plants

Ans. (a) Haploid plants

276. Somaclonal variation arises due to:

    a. Change in chromosome number

    b. Deletion/duplication

    c. Gene mutation/gene amplification

    d. All of these

Ans. (d) All of these

277. Sugar cane somaclone one was isolated from:

a. CO1148   b. Pindar
c. BO 54   d. COS 176

Ans. (a) CO1148

278. Somatic hybrid are also called:

a. Parasexual hybrids
b. Cytoplasmic hybrids
c. Vybrids
d. Both a and b

Ans. (a) Parasexual hybrids

279. Which element is not essential for plant cells and tissue culture?

a. Ni   b. Mg
c. K   d. Ca

Ans. (a) Ni

280. A spin filter bioreactor is a good example of:

a. Air lift bioreactor
b. Batch reactor
c. Continuous flow bioreactor
d. None of these

Ans. (a) Air lift bioreactor

281. Micropropagation of woody trees presents whic problems?

a. Browning in medium
b. Difficulties in rooting
c. Poor growth *in vitro*
d. All of these

Ans. (d) All of these

282. Protoplasts can be used for genetic transformation by:

a. PEF mediated DNA uptake
b. Liposome mediated delivery
c. Electroporation
d. All of these

Ans. (d) All of these

283. In case of slow growth culture, high osmotic concentrations as created by:

a. Mannitol   b. Sorbitol
c. Sucrose   d. All of these

Ans. (d) All of these

284. Cryoprotectants reduce cryoinjury by:

a. Reduction in cellular dehydration
b. Reduced ice crystal formation

c. Reduced dislocation of structural water
d. All of these

Ans. (d) All of these

285. Vitrification/encapsulation eliminated the need during cryopreservation:

a. Controlled freezing   b. Cryoproetctant
c. LN refrigerator   d. Both a and b

Ans. (a) Controlled freezing

286. Which vitamins is essential for plant tissue culture?

a. Thiamine   b. Pyridoxine
c. M-Inositol   d. Nicotinic acid

Ans. (a) Thiamine

287. Which was the first to be achieved?

a. Embryo culture   b. Anther culture
c. Somatic hybridization   d. Embryogenesis

Ans. (c) Somatic hybridization

288. Which following techniques used for cell cloning are used for protoplast culture as well?

a. Microchamber technique
b. Filter paper raft nurse tissue
c. Microdrop method
d. Bergman's planting technique

Ans. (c) Microdrop method

289. High auxin concentration is required during:

a. SE induction   b. SE development
c. SE maturation   d. SE conversion

Ans. (a) SE induction

290. GA_3 has a beneficial effect during:

a. SE induction   b. SE development
c. SE maturation   d. SE conversion

Ans. (a) SE induction

291. ABA is generally promotive during:

a. SE induction   b. SE development
c. SE maturation   d. SE conversion

Ans. (c) SE maturation

292. Biochemical accumulatioin by cultured plant cells is affected by:

a. Chemical composition of medium
b. Light quality
c. Inoculums size
d. All of these

Ans. (c) Inoculums size

293. Which have been shown to prevent precocious germination of cultured embryos?

a. High sucrose levels
b. ABA
c. Casein hydrolysate
d. All of these

Ans. (d) All of these

294. Which of the following is a evergreen temperate plant?

a. Apricot   b. Chilgoza
c. Plum   d. Almond

Ans. (a) Apricot

295. Which of the following is a very dwarf root stock for propagation of apple?

a. M-27   b. M-12
c. M-13   d. None of these

Ans. (a) M-27

296. Which of the following chemical is used to enhances rootings in cuttings?

a. IAA   b. IBA
c. NAA   d. All of these

Ans. (d) All of these

297. Which of the following hormone is used for fast rootings in cutting?

a. Seredix-A   b. Vitamin A
c. Vitamin E   d. None of these

Ans. (a) Seredix-A

298. The rooting of cuttings can be induced by cutting before planting in:

a. IAA   b. GA
c. ABA   d. Zn solution

Ans. (a) IAA

299. Exchange of germplasm is carried mostly through shoot tips because it is:

a. Cheap
b. Small and handy
c. Virus free
d. Genetically stable

Ans. (c) Virus free

300. The gynophores of groundnut is commonly referred to as the:

a. Perinth   b. Peg
c. Ovate   d. Monadelph

Ans. (b) Peg

301. The rice variety containing "Dee gee woo gen" gene is:

a. Indrasan   b. Basmati
c. Tilak   d. IR 8

Ans. (d) IR 8

302. Which varieties developed through somatic hybridization followed by back cross?

a. Delgold   b. Sigma
c. A.C. Change   d. Both a and c

Ans. (b) Sigma

303. The technique of embryo culture can be used to obtain:

a. Interspecific hybrids
b. Propagation of orchids
c. Dormancy and to shorten breeding cycle
d. All of these

Ans. (d) All of these

304. In general, callus cultures are subcultured after:

a. 4–6 days   b. 4–6 weeks
c. 8–10 days   d. 8–10 weeks

Ans. (b) 4–6 weeks

305. Somatic embryo maturation is not promoted by:

a. Cytokinin   b. High sucrose
c. Partial desiccation   d. Abscissic acid

Ans. (a) Cytokinin

306. The term somaclonal variation was coined by

a. Freezing and storage   b. Larkin and scowcroft
c. Skirvin and Karp   d. Evans and sharp

Ans. (b) Larkin and scowcroft

307. The first plant from a mature plant cell was regenerated by:

a. Braun   b. Haberlandt
c. Cocking   d. White

Ans. (a) Braun

308. During gynogenesis, haploid plants generally originated from:

a. Synergids   b. Antipodal cells
c. Egg cell   d. Polar nuclei

Ans. (c) Egg cell

309. Somatic hybridization has been the most successful in:

a. Malvaceae
b. Leguminosae

c. Graminae

d. Solanaceae and crucifereae

Ans. (d) Solanaceae and crucifereae

310. The green revolution was a product of:

a. Hybrids

b. Conventional plant breeding

c. Selection breeding

d. None of these

Ans. (b) Conventional plant breeding

311. Protoplasts can be produced from suspension cultures, callus tissues or intact tissues by enzymatic treatment with

a. Cellulotyic enzymes

b. Pectolytic enzymes

c. Both cellulotyic and pectolytic enzymes

d. Proteolytic enzymes

Ans. (c) Both cellulotyic and pectolytic enzymes

312. Which of the following is considered as the disadvantage of conventional plant tissue culture for clonal propagation?

a. Multiplication of sexually derived sterile hybrids

b. Less multiplication of disease free plants

c. Storage and transportation of propagates

d. Both (b) and (c)

Ans. (c) Storage and transportation of propagates

313. What is meant by 'Organ culture'?

a. Maintenance alive of a whole organ, after removal from the organism by partial immersion in a nutrient fluid

b. Introduction of a new organ in an animal body with a view to create genetic mutation in the progenies of that animal

c. Cultivation of organs in a laboratory through the synthesis of tissues

d. The aspects of culture in community which are mainly dedicated by the need of a specified organ of the human body

Ans. (a) Maintenance alive of a whole organ, after removal from the organism by partial immersion in a nutrient fluid

314. Which method of plant propagation involves the use of girdling?

a. Grafting

b. Cutting

c. Layering

d. Micropropagation

Ans. (c) Layering

315. Which of the following is used in the culture of regenerating protoplasts, single cells or very dilute cell suspensions?

a. Nurse medium

b. Nurse or feeder culture

c. Both (a) and (b)

d. None of the above

Ans. (c) Both (a) and (b)

316. In a callus culture

a. Iincreasing level of cytokinin to a callus induces shoot formation and increasing level of auxin promote root formation

b. Increasing level of auxin to a callus induces shoot formation and increasing level of cytokinin promote root formation

c. Auxins and cytokinins are not required

d. Only auxin is required for root and shoot formation

Ans. (a) Iincreasing level of cytokinin to a callus induces shoot formation and increasing level of auxin promote root formation

317. Which breeding method uses a chemical to strip the cell wall of plant cells of two sexually incompatible species?

a. Mass selection

b. Protoplast fusion

c. Transformation

d. Transcription

Ans. (b) Protoplast fusion

318. The phenomenon of the reversion of mature cells to the meristematic state leading to the formation of callus is known as

a. Redifferentiation

b. Dedifferentiation

c. Both a and b

d. None of the above

Ans. (b) Dedifferentiation

319. Cell fusion method includes the preparation of large number of

a. Plant cells stripped of their cell wall

b. Cells from different species

c. Single plant cell stripped of their cell wall

d. Plant cells with cell wall

Ans. (c) Single plant cell stripped of their cell wall

320. Subculturing is similar to propagation by cuttings because

a. It separates multiple microshoots and places them in a medium

b. It uses scions to produce new microshoots

c. They both use *in vitro* growing conditions

d. All of the above

Ans. (a) It separates multiple microshoots and places them in a medium

321. When plated only in nutrient medium, how much time is required for the protoplast to synthesize new cell wall?

a. 2–5 days　　　　　b. 3–5 days
c. 5–10 days　　　　d. 10–15 days

Ans. (c) 5–10 days

322. Agrobacterium based gene transfer is efficient

a. Only with dicots
b. Only with monocots
c. With both monocots and dicots
d. With majority monocots and few dicots

Ans. (a) Only with dicots

323. Which of the following is an ethylene biosynthesis inhibitor?

a. Citric acid
b. Succinic acid
c. Activated charcoal
d. Silver thiosulphate

Ans. (d) Citric acid

324. Nitrogen in the plant cell culture media is provided by either ammonia or nitrate salt. In the media

a. Utilization of ammonium cause culture pH to drop while utilization of nitrate cause culture pH to rise
b. Utilization of nitrate cause culture pH to drop while utilization of ammonium cause culture pH to rise
c. Utilization of both ammonium and nitrate result in rise in pH
d. Utilization of both ammonium and nitrate result in drop in pH

Ans. (a) Utilization of ammonium cause culture pH to drop while utilization of nitrate cause culture pH to rise

325. Which of the following growth regulator is added for short initiation during plant regeneration from callus?

a. Auxins　　　　　b. Cytokinins
c. Gibberellins　　　d. Brassinosteroids

Ans. (b) Cytokinins

326. Which of the following growth regulator is used to stimulate embryo or shoot development?

a. Auxins
b. Cytokinins
c. Gibberellins
d. Brassinosteroids

Ans. (c) Gibberellins

327. Which of the following growth regulator cause plant cells to grow?

a. Auxins　　　　　b. Cytokinins
c. Gibberellins　　　d. Brassinosteroids

Ans. (a) Auxins

328. Silver thiosulphate is added to culture medium as it helps to

a. Maintain the pH
b. Remove toxic phenolics from plant cells
c. Prevent the gaseous plant hormone, ethylene dioxide from accumulating to detrimental condition
d. All of the above

Ans. (c) Prevent the gaseous plant hormone, ethylene dioxide from accumulating to detrimental condition

329. In plant cell culture media, auxins and cytokinins are used in the range of

a. 1–50 μM　　　　b. 15–50 μM
c. 20–50 μM　　　　d. 40–50 μM

Ans. (a) 1–50 μM

330. Concentration of sucrose generally used in plant cell culture media is

a. 10–15 g/l　　　　b. 20–30 g/l
c. 25–45 g/l　　　　d. 10–65 g/l

Ans. (b) 20–30 g/l

331. Which is/are the naturally occurring plant auxins?

a. IBA
b. NAA
c. IAA
d. None of the above

Ans. (b) NAA

332. Which is/are the disadvantage/(s) of using IAA in plant cell culture media?

a. It is unstable in solution
b. Gets easily oxidized
c. Conjugated to inactive form by plant cells
d. All of the above

Ans. (d) All of the above

333. To maintain the pH of the culture

a. Organic acid such as citric, fumaric, malic and succinic acid is used
b. Synthetic buffers such as Tris, MES or HEPS are used
c. Both (a) and (b)
d. Ammonium salts are used

Ans. (c) Both (a) and (b)

334. Which of the following is not a cytokinin?

a. 2,4-dichlorophenoxyacetic acid

b. 6 benzylaminopurine

c. Zeatin

d. Kinetin

Ans. (a) 2,4-dichlorophenoxyacetic acid

335. Which of the following is not true about nurse or conditioned medium?

a. It is liquid removed from the suspension of fast growing cells

b. It contains uncharacterized growth factor released by growing cells

c. It is used in the culture of regenerating protoplast

d. It is removed aseptically from the culture and is autoclaved before use

Ans. (d) It is removed aseptically from the culture and is autoclaved before use

336. What is 'nurse' or conditioned medium?

a. It is the media full of growth factors used for the growth of cells

b. It is the medium added to nurse the callus culture

c. Both (a) and (b)

d. None of these

Ans. (c) Both (a) and (b)

337. Neutralized activated charcoal is occasionally added to young regenerating cultures to

a. Remove toxic phenolics produced by the stressed plant cell

b. Help to remove plants growth regulators introduced at an earlier stage

c. Both (a) and (b)

d. Maintain the pH of the medium

Ans. (c) Both (a) and (b)

338. Virulence trait of *Agrobacterium tumefaciens* is borne on

a. Chromosomal DNA

b. Tumour inducing plasmid DNA

c. Both chromosomal and plasmid DNA

d. Cryptic plasmid DNA

Ans. (b)

339. The size of the virulent plasmid of *Agrobacterium tumefaciens* is

a. 40–80 kb   b. 140–235 kb

c. 100–135 kb   d. 200–235 kb

Ans. (b) 140–235 kb

340. Which of the following is not true about the helper plasmids?

a. These can replicate in *Agrobacterium*

b. These help in the mediating conjugation of intermediate vectors

c. These can't replicate in *Agrobacterium*

d. All of the above

Ans. (a) These can replicate in *Agrobacterium*

341. Which technique is used to introduce genes into dicots?

a. Electroporation

b. Particle acceleration

c. Microinjection

d. Ti plasmid infection

Ans. (d) Ti plasmid infection

342. In a plant tumour cell

a. Complete Ti plasmid is incorporated in plant nuclear DNA

b. Different parts of the Ti-plasmid are incorporated

c. Only a small specific segment of callus T DNA is incorporated

d. May vary from plant to plant

Ans. (c) Only a small specific segment of callus T DNA is incorporated

343. Co-integrating transformation vectors must include a region of homology in

a. The vector plasmid

b. The Ti-plasmid

c. Between vector plasmid and Ti-plasmid

d. None of these

Ans. (c) Between vector plasmid and Ti-plasmid

344. Integrated nopaline T-DNA occurs as

a. Single segment

b. Two segments

c. Three segments

d. None of these

Ans. (a) Single segment

345. Opines are

a. Amino acid derivatives found in tumor tissues

b. Amino acid derivatives found in normal tissues

c. Amino acid derivatives found in both normal as well as tumor tissues

d. None of the above

Ans. (a) Amino acid derivatives found in tumor tissues

346. Which of the following is true about *Agrobacterium tumefaciens*?

 a. It causes crown gall disease of plants

 b. It infects gymnosperms

 c. It infects dicotyledonous angiosperms

 d. All of the above

Ans. (d) All of the above

347. Advantage of microprojectile method over microinjection method for gene transfer in plants include

 a. Intact cells are used

 b. Method is universal in its application irrespective of all shape, size, type and presence or absence of cell wall

 c. Gene can be transferred to many cells simultaneously

 d. All of the above

Ans. (d) All of the above

348. On Ti-plasmid T-region or T-DNA is flanked by a direct repeat of

 a. 12 bp   b. 32 bp

 c. 25 bp   d. 45 bp

Ans. (c) 25 bp

349. *Agrobacterium tumefaciens* is a

 a. Gram (+) bacteria   b. Gram (–) bacteria

 c. Both a and b   d. None of these

Ans. (b) Gram (–) bacteria

350. Which of the following genes are constitutively expressed and control the plant induced activation of other vir genes?

 a. *vir* A and *vir* G   b. *vir* T and *vir* G

 c. *vir* D and *vir* A   d. *vir* A and *vir* C

Ans. (a) *vir* A and *vir* G

351. Integrated octopine T DNA occurs as

 a. Single segment   b. Two segment

 c. Third segment   d. Five segment

Ans. (b) Two segment

352. Which of the following plant signal molecules regulate the expression of vir B, C, D and E in case of tobacco?

 a. Acetosyringone

 b. α-hydroxy syringone

 c. Both a and b

 d. None of these

Ans. (c) Both a and b

353. Intermediate vectors containing T-DNA are conjugation deficient. Thus conjugation is mediated in presence of which of the following plasmid?

 a. pRK 2013

 b. pRN 3

 c. Either (a) or (b)

 d. None of these

Ans. (c) Either (a) or (b)

354. Which of the following is true about T DNA?

 a. Integration of T DNA can occur at many different, apparently random, sites in the plant nuclear DNA

 b. Integration of T DNA occurs only at one specific sites in the plant nuclear DNA

 c. Integration of T DNA occurs at two specific sites in the plant nuclear DNA

 d. Integration of T DNA occurs at one site that may be random in the plant nuclear DNA

Ans. (a) Integration of T DNA can occur at many different, apparently random, sites in the plant nuclear DNA

355. Which of the following is not true about the direct repeats flanking T-DNA?

 a. They are conserved between nopaline and octopine Ti-plasmids

 b. These repeats are transferred intact to the plant genome

 c. These are important in integration mechanism

 d. All of these

Ans. (b) These repeats are transferred intact to the plant genome

356. The left segment of octopine T-DNA (TL) is necessary for

 a. Enzymes for agropine biosynthesis

 b. Tumour formation

 c. Conjugative transfer

 d. None of these

Ans. (b) Tumour formation

357. Which of the following is not true for microinjection technique that involves transfer of DNA into protoplast?

 a. It is carried out with the help of micromanipulator

 b. The recipient cells are immobilized on artificial support or artificially bound to substarate

 c. It employs needle with diameter greater than cell diameter

 d. All of these

Ans. (c) It employs needle with diameter greater than cell diameter

358. Virulent strains of Agrobacterium contain large Ti-plasmids, which are responsible for the DNA transfer and subsequent disease symptoms. It has been shown that Ti-plasmids contain

a. One set of sequence necessary for gene transfer
b. Two sets of sequence necessary for gene transfer
c. Three sets of sequence necessary for gene transfer
d. Four sets of sequence necessary for gene transfer

Ans. (b) Two sets of sequence necessary for gene transfer

359. The direct repeats flanking the T-DNA of *Agrobacterium tume-faciens* are known as

a. Cos site
b. Flanking sequences
c. Border sequences
d. Transfer sequences

Ans. (c) Border sequences

360. T-DNA transfer and processing into plant genome requires products of which of the following genes?

a. *vir* A,B
b. *vir* G,C
c. *vir* D,E
d. All of these

Ans. (d) *vir* G,C

361. Because of large size of Ti-plasmid, intermediate vectors (IV) are developed in which T DNA has been subcloned into

a. pBR 322 based plasmid vector
b. pRK 2013
c. pRN 3
d. All of these

Ans. (a) pBR 322 based plasmid vector

362. Which of the following are used as selection marker for the cells transformed with *Agrobacterium*?

a. Neomycin phosphotransferase
b. Streptomycin phosphotransferase
c. Hygromycin phosphotransferase
d. Any of the above

Ans. (d) Any of the above

363. Vir genes required for the T-DNA transfer and processing are located

a. On the T-DNA
b. Outside the T-DNA region
c. On the plant genome
d. All of the above

Ans. (b) Outside the T-DNA region

364. Plant transformation vectors based on *Agrobacterium* can generally be divided into

a. Two vectors
b. Three vectors
c. Four vectors
d. Five vectors

Ans. (a) Two vectors

365. The tumour phenotype, which can be maintained indefinitely in tissue culture, results from the expression of genes on the

a. T-DNA
b. c-DNA
c. r-DNA
d. m-RNA

Ans. (a) T-DNA

366. Synthetic seeds are

a. Artificially synthesized seeds
b. Somatic embryos encapsulated in suitable matrix
c. Seeds of plants modified genetically
d. None of these

Ans. (b) Somatic embryos encapsulated in suitable matrix

367. Somatic embryoids are

a. Identical with zygotic embryos and without seed coats
b. Identical with zygotic embryos and with seed coats
c. Non-identical with zygotic embryos and without seed coats
d. Non-identical with zygotic embryos and with seed coats

Ans. (a) Identical with zygotic embryos and without seed coats

368. The production of high quality and uniform embryos has been limited to only

a. Carrot
b. Alfalfa
c. Both (a) and (b)
d. None of these

Ans. (c) Both (a) and (b)

369. The preserved embryoids are termed as

a. Synthetic seeds
b. Semi-synthetic seeds
c. Natural seeds
d. Fermented seeds

Ans. (a) Synthetic seeds

370. Encapsulation is necessary to produce and protect synthetic seeds. The encapsulation is carried out by various types of hydrogels, which are

    a. Soluble in water

    b. Soluble in organic solvents

    c. Insoluble in water

    d. Insoluble in organic solvents

Ans. (a) Soluble in water

371. Recalcitrant seeds are

    a. Resistant to drying and freezing temperature

    b. Killed by drying and freezing temperature

    c. Both (a) and (b)

    d. None of above

Ans. (b) Killed by drying and freezing temperature

372. The encapsulation of somatic embryos can be carried out by

    a. Automatic encapsulation process

    b. Gel complexation

    c. Both (a) and (b)

    d. Coating proteins

Ans. (c) Both (a) and (b)

CHECK YOU GRASP

1. **A spin filter bioreactor is a good example of which of the following?**
   a. Air lift bioreactor
   b. Continues flow reactor
   c. Fed batch reactor
   d. Fluidized bed reactor

2. **Micropropagation of woody trees presents which of the following problems?**
   a. Difficulties in rooting
   b. Poor growth in vitro
   c. Browning of medium
   d. All of the above

3. **Culturing of unfertilized ovaries to obtained haploid plant from egg cell or other haploid cells of the embryo sac is called**
   a. Meristem culture   b. Anther culture
   c. Ovary culture   d. Stem culture

4. **Synthetic seeds are**
   a. Somatic embryo   b. Somaclone
   c. Cybrids   d. Protoplast

5. **Preservation of cell, tissues and organs in liquid nitrogen at -196°C is called as**
   a. Thermopreservation   b. Cryopreservation
   c. Hydropreservation   d. Helopreservation

6. **Introduction of a tobacco mosaic virus transgene in to plants in 1986 was used to demonstrate a process called as**
   a. Cross protection   b. Co-transfection
   c. Co-transformation   d. Co-suspension

7. **Most commonly used medium for tissue culture is**
   a. BS medium   b. MS medium
   c. LS medium   d. B6 medium

8. **The culture of whole plants and organ is has been termed as**
   a. Protoplast culture
   b. Callus culture
   c. Non organised culture
   d. Organised culture

9. **Which of the following variety was developed from somaclona variation?**
   a. Delgold   b. A.C.Chang
   c. Sigma   d. All of the above

10. **Which of the following requirement must be fulfilled b any tissue culture technique that is used for conservation of germplasm**
    a. Plant virus elimination from the stored tissues/ organ
    b. Genetic variability of the material to be preserved should be guaranteed.
    c. Well defined protocol which guarantees a high percentage of plant recovery form stored tissue
    d. All of the above

11. **Which of the following involves in haploid production?**
    a. Somaclonal breeding
    b. Analytical breeding
    c. Hybrid sorting
    d. Both b & C

In case of less than 80% score, go through brief Review and Glance one again from chapter

Key: 1-b 2-d 3-c 4-a 5-b 6-a 7-b 8-d 9-c 10-c 11-d

5

Genomic and Proteomics

1. **The proportion of coding to non coding sequence in a genome is known as**
   a. Exon to intron ratio
   b. Heterochromatin/Euchromatin ratio
   c. p/q ratio
   d. Signal to noise ratio

   Ans. (d) Signal to noise ratio

2. **the sequence that helps to identify the starting point of a gene is known as**
   a. Kozak sequence
   b. TATA box
   c. CAAT box
   d. Shine-dalgarno sequence

   Ans. (a) Kozak sequence

3. **Which of the following sequence is conserved at the start point of a m-RNA?**
   a. CCGCAUGG
   b. GGCCAUGC
   c. CGGGUAAG
   d. CCCGAUGC

   Ans. (a) CCGCAUGG

4. **One of the major landmarks for identification of human gene from the sequence data is**
   a. Alu sequence
   b. CpG islands
   c. Retrotransposon sequence
   d. EcoRI restriction sites

   Ans. (b) CpG islands

5. **The amount of DNA occupied by coding exon in human genome is about**
   a. 4%
   b. 5%
   c. 3%
   d. 7%

   Ans. (c) 3%

6. **Size of X174 genome is**
   a. 3000 nt
   b. 6542 nt
   c. 5386 nt
   d. 4523 nt

   Ans. (c) 5386 nt

7. **Recombinant DNA technology was developed in the year**
   a. 1983
   b. 1984
   c. 1977
   d. 1972

   Ans. (d) 1972

8. **Term genomics was coined by**
   a. P. Berg
   b. T. Roderick
   c. F. Sanger
   d. T.B. Lee

   Ans. (b) T. Roderick

9. **Technique of two dimensional gel electrophoresis for protein separation was developed by**
   a. P.H.O. farrell
   b. F. Sanger
   c. E.M. Southern
   d. H. Temin

   Ans. (a) P.H.O. farrell

10. **In 2DE, separation is done on the basis of**
    a. Charge
    b. Mass
    c. Both charge and mass
    d. None of these

    Ans. (c) Both charge and mass

11. **For first dimensional separation in 2DE, the gels used include**
    a. Polyacrylamide with IPG
    b. Polyacrylamide with SDS
    c. Normal poilyacrylamide
    d. None of these

    Ans. (a) Polyacrylamide with IPG

12. **Genome of the smallest bacterium, Mycoplasma genitelium codes for**
    a. 498 protein
    b. 456 protein
    c. 1022 protein
    d. 479 protein

    Ans. (d) 479 protein

13. Which of the following genomics technology is being used extensively in diagnostics?

a. Gradient PCR

b. qRT-PCR

c. Automated sequencing

d. None of these

Ans. (b) qRT-PCR

14. The private company that produced human genome sequence is

a. Genetic computer group

b. Affymetrix

c. Celera genomics

d. Applied Biosystem

Ans. (c) Celera genomics

15. Draft sequence of human genome was published in

a. 2000

b. 2001

c. 2002

d. 2003

Ans. (a) 2000

16. Sequencing technique used by Celera Genomics for rapid genome sequencing was

a. End sequencing

b. Map based cloning

c. Pyrosequencing

d. Shotgun sequencing

Ans. (d) Shotgun sequencing

17. Draft genome of human was published by

a. Celera genomics

b. National institute of helth

c. None of these

d. Both a and b

Ans. (c) None of these

18. Sequencing of Drosophila genome was done by

a. Celera benomics

b. Berkeley Drosophila genome project

c. None of these

d. Bothe a and b

Ans. (d) Bothe a and b

19. The genome sequence of the fruit fly was published in the journal

a. Science

b. Nature

c. Genome

d. Genomics

Ans. (a) Science

20. Shotgun sequencing strategy was developed by

a. A. Maxam

b. F. Sanger

c. S. Cohen

d. J. C.Venter

Ans. (d) J. C.Venter

21. The concept of expressed sequence tags was developed by

a. S. Cohen

b. J.C.Venter

c. F. Sanger

d. None of these

Ans. (b) J.C.Venter

22. EST are

a. Cloned c-DNA molecule

b. Cloned c-RNA molecule

c. Partially sequenced cloned c-DNA molecule

d. None of these

Ans. (c) Partially sequenced cloned c-DNA molecule

23. ESTs libraries are sources of

a. Coding regions

b. Non coding regions

c. Unique genes

d. None of these

Ans. (a) Coding regions

24. First automated sequencing machine was marketed by

a. Bio rad

b. Applied biosystems

c. Perkin-elmer

d. Invitrogen

Ans. (b) Applied biosystems

25. The person credite for development of automated sequencer is

a. L. Hood

b. J.c.venter

c. F. Sanger

d. None of these

Ans. (a) L. Hood

26. Nobel prize in chemistry in 1980 was received by

a. P. Berg

b. F. Sanger

c. W. gilbert

d. All of these

Ans. (d) All of these

27. The scientist who received Nobel prize in chemistry in 1958 as well as 1980 was

a. F. Sanger

b. P.berg

c. W.gilbert

d. N one of these

Ans. (a) F. Sanger

28. F. Sanger received Nobel prize in chemistry for developing.

a. DNA sequencing methods

b. Protein sequencing

c. Both a and b

d. None of these

Ans. (c) Both a and b

29. Draft sequence of mouse genome was published by

a. Celera genomics

b. National institute of health

c. Department of energy

d. None of these

Ans. (a) Celera genomics

30. Bacterium having anti-tumorigenic activity that has been sequenced recently is

a. Clostridium novyi

b. Bacillus subtilis

c. Xanthomonas campestris

d. None of these

Ans. (a) Clostridium novyi

31. Restriction enzymes was first isolated by

a. H. Smith   b. M. Meselson

c. S. Luria   d. D. Baltimore

Ans. (b) M. Meselson

32. First type II restriction enzyme was isolated from

a. E. coli   b. S.aureus

c. H. influenzae   d. None of these

Ans. (c) H. influenzae

33. Credit for discovery of first type II restriction enzyme goes to

a. S. Luria   b. H. smith

c. B. hohn   d. W. arber

Ans. (b) H. smith

34. The plasmid vector used for development of first recombinant DNA molecule was

a. Puc19   b. Psc101

c. pBR 322   d. Puc18

Ans. (b) Psc101

35. Type II restriction enzyme that was isolated first

a. Eco RI   b. Sma I

c. HindIII   d. Hind II

Ans. (d) Hind II

36. Host controlled restriction modification was discovered in

a. E. coli   b. Sma I

c. H. influnzae   d. S. aureus

Ans. (a) E. coli

37. Phenomenon of restriction modification was reported by

a. W. Arber   b. D. Nathans

c. J.lederberg   d. H. Smith

Ans. (a) W. Arber

38. Type I restriction enzymes are

a. ATP independent

b. Methylation sensitive

c. Used in genetic engineering

d. Artificially designed

Ans. (b) Methylation sensitive

39. EcoRI was discovered by

a. J. Hedgepeth, H.M. Goodman and H.W.Boyer

b. S.cohen and H.W.Boyer

c. W. Arber and D. Nathans

d. None of these

Ans. (a) J. Hedgepeth, H.M. Goodman and H.W.Boyer

40. The restriction enzyme used by cohen and boyer to create recombinant DNA molecule was

a. Hind III   b. Hind II

c. Sma I   d. Eco RI

Ans. (d) Eco RI

41. Sma 1 is a

a. Sticky end hexacutter

b. Blunt end hexacutter

c. Sticky end tetracutter

d. Blunt end tetracutter

Ans. (b) Blunt end hexacutter

42. Taq 1 is a

a. Sticky end tetracutter   b. Blunt end hexacutter

c. Blunt end tetracutter   d. Sticky end hexacutter

Ans. (a) Sticky end tetracutter

43. Which of the following restriction enzyme is methylation insensitive?

a. Sma 1   b. Eco RI

c. Sau 3A   d. Hind III

Ans. (c) Sau 3A

44. As carrier host for cloned DNA fragment, a bacterium should be

a. Fast growing

b. Auxotroph

c. Restriction deficient

d. Resistant to antibiotics

Ans. (c) Restriction deficient

45. Nobel prize physiology or medicine in 1978 was awarded for

    a. Development of DNA sequencing methods
    b. Discovery of restriction endonucleases
    c. Discovery of transposons
    d. Construction of recombination

Ans. (b) Discovery of restriction endonucleases

46. Nobel prize in physiology or medicine in 1978 was awarded

    a. W. Arber   b. H. Smith
    c. D. Nathans   d. All of them

Ans. (d) All of them

47. Which of the following vector system is specific for plant?

    a. TAC   b. BAC
    c. MAC   d. YAC

Ans. (a) TAC

48. Which of the following vector is extensively used for chromosome physical mapping

    a. Plasmid   b. YIP
    c. BAC   d. MAC

Ans. (c) BAC

49. Lac Z is used as a

    a. Reporter gene
    b. Promoter sequence
    c. Selectable marker
    d. Helper plasmid

Ans. (a) Reporter gene

50. pUC vectors have been developed in

    a. University of florida
    b. University of california
    c. University of louisiana
    d. University of copenhagen

Ans. (b) University of california

51. A multiple cloning site is present in

    a. pBR327   b. pUC19
    c. pBR322   d. RSF 2124

Ans. (b) pUC19

52. The number of antibiotic resistance gene present in Pbr322 is

    a. 2   b. 3
    c. 4   d. 5

Ans. (a) 2

53. Which of the following is a common expression vector?

    a. pUC 18   b. pUC 327
    c. pBR322   d. λ gt11

Ans. (d) λ gt11

54. Which of the following is a replacement vector?

    a. Charon-40   b. λgt15
    c. λgt11   d. pBR322

Ans. (a) Charon-40

55. A stuffer fragment is present in

    a. Insertion vector   b. Replacement vector
    c. Both of these   d. None of these

Ans. (b) Replacement vector

56. In vitro DNA packaging is observed in

    a. BAC   b. YAC
    c. MAC   d. Cosmid vector

Ans. (d) Cosmid vector

57. Which of the following is a phagemid vector?

    a. pBR322   b. λgt11
    c. λ-ZAP11   d. pUC19

Ans. (c) λ-ZAP11

58. Cosmids can clone up to

    a. 10 kb DNA   b. 30 kb DNA
    c. 40 kb DNA   d. 50 kb DNA

Ans. (d) 50 kb DNA

59. Which of the yeast based vector are present in high copy number?

    a. YEps   b. YRPs
    c. YAC   d. Yips

Ans. (a) YEps

60. Which of the yeast based vector can carry very large DNA segment?

    a. YAC   b. BAC
    c. MAC   d. Cosmid

A ns. (a) YAC

61. A yeast shuttle vector can be cloned in

    a. Yeast only
    b. *E.coli* only
    c. Both of these
    d. None of these

Ans. (c) Both of these

62. λ-ZAP vector can clone about

 a. 20 kb DNA b. 10 kb DNA
 c. 30 kb DNA d. 40 kb DNA

Ans. (b) 10 kb DNA

63. Baculovirus vectors are

 a. ds DNA b. ss DNA
 c. ds RNA d. ss RNA

Ans. (a) ds DNA

64. SV 40 vector are

 a. ds DNA b. ds RNA
 c. ss DNA d. ss RNA

Ans. (a) ds DNA

65. Retroviral vectors are

 a. ds RNA b. ss DNA
 c. ds DNA d. ss RNA

Ans. (a) ds RNA

66. Vectors based on BPV have plasmid components of

 a. Cosmid vectors b. pBR322
 c. pUC vector d. pBluescript vector

Ans. (b) pBR322

67. Which of the following is a retroviral vector used in animal cloning?

 a. MLV b. EBV
 c. BPV d. SV 40

Ans. (a) MLV

68. Gag and pol genes are present in

 a. Adenoviral vectors b. Retroviral vectors
 c. Both of these d. None of these

Ans. (b) Retroviral vectors

69. Which of the following virus uses reverse transcription?

 a. HIV b. BPV
 c. Baculovirus d. None of these

Ans. (a) HIV

70. Which of the following vectors are used widely in plant genetic transformation?

 a. Cosmid vector
 b. Plasmid vector
 c. Bacteriophage vector
 d. BAC vector

Ans. (b) Plasmid vector

71. Which of the following measure is most widely used to construct a genetic map

 a. Chromosome mutation
 b. Non independent segregation
 c. Chromosomal exchange
 d. Physical demarcation on chromosome

Ans. (b) Non independent segregation

72. In human, distance between two loci and recombination frequency show

 a. Linear relationship for long distance
 b. Logarithuic relationship for long distances
 c. Curvilinear relationship for long distance
 d. Inverse relationship for long distance

Ans. (c) Curvilinear relationship for long distance

73. One of the common techniques for human genetic analysis is

 a. Hybridization and segregation analysis
 b. Pedigree analysis
 c. Both of these
 d. None of these

Ans. (c) Both of these

74. For indirect estimation of linkage in human, which method is most common?

 a. Monte carlo simulations
 b. Maximum likelihood
 c. Expectation maximization
 d. None of these

Ans. (b) Maximum likelihood

75. Lod score is used for

 a. Gene identification b. Genetic mapping
 c. Physical mapping d. Gene sequencing

Ans. (b) Genetic mapping

76. A lod score of 3 indicates

 a. No linkage
 b. Low probability linkage
 c. Independent segregation during meiosis
 d. High probability of linkage

Ans. (d) High probability of linkage

77. A map where markers are placed in their most likely position is known as a

 a. Saturated map
 b. Gene map
 c. Comprehensive map
 d. Approximate map

Ans. (c) Comprehensive map

78. **A map where individual loci are placed in such a way so that each loci is linked to another with lod score of at least 3 is known as**
    a. Comprehensive map
    b. Framemwork map
    c. Inclusive map
    d. Approximate map

Ans. **(b) Framemwork map**

79. **Which of the following banding technique should be used to located r-RNA gene?**
    a. C-banding
    b. N-banding
    c. G-banding
    d. R-banding

Ans. **(b) N-banding**

80. **Chromosome banding is widely used in**
    a. Tumor cell diagnosis
    b. Detection of somatic cell hybrid
    c. Karyotype construction
    d. All of these

Ans. **(d) All of these**

81. **Chromosome bancding technique was first discovered by**
    a. J.G.Gall
    b. M. L.pardue
    c. T. Casperson
    d. All of them

Ans. **(c) T. Casperson**

82. **In R-banding, the stain used is**
    a. Rhodamine red
    b. Texas red
    c. Quinacrine mustard
    d. Giemsa

Ans. **(d) Giemsa**

83. **Q-banding, was discovered by**
    a. T. Casperson
    b. R.Feulgen
    c. J.G.Gall
    d. M. L . Pardue

Ans. **(a) T. Casperson**

84. **Concept of chromosome walking was developed by**
    a. W. Bender
    b. E. Lander
    c. D. Botstein
    d. D. C. Schwart

Ans. **(a) W. Bender**

85. **It the distance between two loci is large, recombination frequency and map distance follows**
    a. Normal distribution
    b. Poisson distribution
    c. Binomial distribution
    d. None of these

Ans. **(b) Poisson distribution**

86. **The concept of mapping function was developed by**
    a. K. Pearson
    b. R. A. Fisher
    c. J.B.S. Haldane
    d. S. Wright

Ans. **(c) J.B.S. Haldane**

87. **Human-rodent somatic cell hybridization is a technique of**
    a. Production of transgenic rodent
    b. Somatic cell line identification
    c. Assigning of gene to chromosome
    d. Comparative genome

Ans. **(c) Assigning of gene to chromosome**

88. **Common fusion agent used in somatic cell hybridization of human and rodent is**
    a. Calcium phosphate
    b. Sendai virus
    c. Electric shock
    d. Magnesium sulphate

Ans. **(b) Sendai virus**

89. **The number of fragments generated by a restruction enzyme depends on**
    a. The nature of the restriction enzyme
    b. The length of the recognition sequence
    c. The GC content of the fragment
    d. All of these

Ans. **(d) All of these**

90. **In situ hybridization is used for**
    a. Genetic mapping
    b. Physical mapping
    c. Both of these
    d. None of these

Ans. **(b) Physical mapping**

91. **Radioactivity is used in**
    a. GISH
    b. FISH
    c. mcFISH
    d. Chromosome painting

Ans. **(a) GISH**

92. **Which of the fluorescing agent produce red color?**
    a. FITC
    b. AMCA
    c. Rhodamine
    d. None of these

Ans. **(c) Rhodamine**

93. **The color produced by FITC is**
    a. Green
    b. Yellow
    c. Orange
    d. Red

Ans. **(a) Green**

94. In situ hybridization is performed on

a. Metaphase chromosome
b. Interphase chromosome
c. Both of these
d. None of these

Ans. (c) Both of these

95. Which of the following is a common vector used for large scale human genome sequencing?

a. BAC
b. MAC
c. YAC
d. PAC

Ans. (a) BAC

96. ESTs are generated from

a. Gene sequence
b. mRNA sequence
c. Protein sequence
d. None of these

Ans. (b) mRNA sequence

97. FISH can be used for mapping

a. YAC clones
b. Repetitive sequences
c. Centromeric regions
d. All of these

Ans. (d) All of these

98. Physical mapping of a gene avoiding lage intron region can be achieved by

a. Chromosome jumping
b. Chromosome walking
c. Chromosome painting
d. Fiber FISH

Ans. (a) Chromosome jumping

99. Which of the following is not a physical mapping procedure?

a. Positional cloning
b. Chromosome banding
c. Radiation hybrid mapping
d. HAPPY mapping

Ans. (a) Positional cloning

100. In FISH, probes are labelled with

a. FITC
b. AMCA
c. Biotin
d. Texas red

Ans. (c) Biotin

101. Which of the following is not a labeling agent for probe in FISH?

a. Biotin
b. Digoxigenin
c. AMCA
d. None of these

Ans. (c) AMCA

102. A hapten is a

a. Staining agent
b. Clearing agent
c. Reporter molecule
d. Conjugative antibody

Ans. (c) Reporter molecule

103. Which of the following is a hapten?

a. Biotin
b. FITC
c. Saponin
d. Pheny mercuric acetate

Ans. (a) Biotin

104. In chromosome painting, biotin is used for labelling for detection of

a. Texas red
b. FITC
c. Both of these
d. None of these

Ans. (a) Texas red

105. In chromosome painting, digoxigenin is used for labelling for detection of

a. Texas red
b. FITC
c. Both of these
d. None of these

Ans. (b) FITC

106. For separation of individual chromosomes which of the following method can not be used?

a. Somatic cell hybridization
b. Radiation Hybridization
c. FACS
d. None of these

Ans. (b) Radiation Hybridization

107. Somatic cell hybridization is performed by

a. Polyethylene glycol
b. Sendai virus
c. Both of these
d. None of these

Ans. (c) Both of these

108. Common selection system for identification of human-mouse hybrid cell is

a. Resistance to 8-Azaguanine
b. Mutation in hypoxanthine phosphoribosyl transferase
c. Mutation in thymidine kinase
d. All of these

Ans. (d) All of these

109. HAT medium, a medium for selection of hyman-mouse hybrid cell contain

a. Hypersensitive adenine and thymidine
b. Hypoxanthine, aminopterin and thymidine
c. Hypoxanthine, Auxin and tetracycline
d. None of these

Ans. (b) Hypoxanthine, aminopterin and thymidine

110. Radiation hybrid mapping was first described by

a. S.J. Goss and H. Harris
b. N.R.Carter et al
c. T.R. Chen
d. G. Pontecorvo

Ans. (a) S.J.Goss and H. Harris

111. Technique of reverse chromosome painting was described by

a. S.J.Goss and H. Harris
b. N.R.Carter et al
c. T.R. Chen
d. G. Pontecorvo

Ans. (b) N.R.Carter et al

112. The technique of muticolor FISH was developed by

a. S.J. Goss and H. Harris
b. N.R. Carter et al
c. T.R. Chen
d. P.M. Nederlof et al.

Ans. (d) P.M. Nederlof et al.

113. The concept of in situ hybridization was developed by

a. S.J.Goss and H.Harris
b. N.R.Carter et al
c. T.R. Chen
d. M.L. Pardue and J.G. Gall

Ans. (d) M.L. Pardue and J.G. Gall

114. T-Banding technique was developed by

a. Sumner
b. Pardue and gall
c. Dutrillaux
d. Casperson

Ans. (c) Dutrillaux

115. Which of the following banding pattern is reverse to G-Banding?

a. T-banding
b. R-banding
c. C-banding
d. Q-banding

Ans. (b) R-banding

116. The terminator used in sanger sequencing method is

a. 3′, 4′-dideoxynucleotide riphosphate
b. 2′, 3′- dideoxynucleotide triphosphate
c. 1′, 4′-dideoxynucleotide riphosphate
d. 3′, 6′-dideoxynucleotide riphosphate

Ans. (b) 2′, 3′- dideoxynucleotide triphosphate

117. The vector used in sanger sequencing method is

a. Phage M13
b. Phage T2
c. Coliphage P1
d. Bacteriophage λ

Ans. (a) Phage M13

118. Most widely used automated non-sanger method of DNA sequencing is

a. Pyrosequencing
b. Sequencing by Chemical modification
c. Both of these
d. None of these

Ans. (a) Pyrosequencing

119. Sanger sequencing method use

a. Antibody detection
b. Conjugate detection
c. Radioactive detection
d. Fluorescent detection

Ans. (c) Radioactive detection

120. Automated sequencing method use

a. Antibody detection
b. Fluorescent detection
c. Radioactive detection
d. Conjugate detection

Ans. (b) Fluorescent detection

121. Technique of pyrosequencing was described first by

a. F. Sanger5
b. A.R. Coulson
c. D.J. Harrison
d. E. D. Hyman

Ans. (c) D.J. Harrison

122. Idea of capillary array electrophoresis for sequencing was developed by

a. F. Sanger
b. A.R. Coulson
c. D.J. Harrison
d. E. D. Hyman

Ans. (c) D.J. Harrison

123. In pyrosequencing, light energy is released by the action of

a. ATP sulfurylase
b. Luciferase
c. Both of these
d. None of these

Ans. (c) Both of these

124. Which of the following is true

a. It involves chain termination method
b. It can sequencing large DNA fragments
c. It involves chain extension by DNA polymerase
d. Pyrosequencing uses a fluorescent detection process

Ans. (c) It involves chain extension by DNA polymerase

125. RNAi was first reported in

a. A. thaliana
b. D. melanogaster
c. C. elegans
d. Human

Ans. (c) C. elegans

126. The technique of radioimmunoassay was developed by

a. R.S. Yalow and S.A. Berson
b. E. Engvall and P. Periman
c. Both of them
d. None of these

Ans. (a) R.S. Yalow and S.A. Berson

127. ELISA technique was developed by

a. R.S.Yalow and S.A. Berson
b. E. Engvall and P. Periman
c. Both of them
d. None of these

Ans. (b) E. Engvall and P. Periman

128. The term transcriptome was coined by

a. F. Crick
b. D. Baltimore
c. S. Brenner et al.
d. V.E.Veculescu et al.

Ans. (d) V.E.Veculescu et al.

129. Gene chip is a microarray system marketed by

a. Promega
b. Sigma
c. Affymetrix
d. bioRad

Ans. (c) Affymetrix

130. The microarray system that do not require cloning is

a. C-DNA microarray
b. Oligo-nt microarray
c. Both of these
d. None of these

Ans. (b) Oligo-nt microarray

131. MIAME stands for

a. Mining information about a microarray experiment
b. Major information About a Microarray experiment
c. Minimum information about a Microarray experiment
d. None of these

Ans. (c) Minimum information about a Microarray experiment

132. The guideline of MIAME was proposed to share microarray data by

a. Gene expression omnibas
b. NHGRI
c. Array express
d. Micro array gene expression data society

Ans. (d) Micro array gene expression data society

133. SAGE technique was invented by

a. R.S. Yalow and S.A. Berson
b. E. Engvall and P.Periman
c. V. E. Veculescu et al.
d. None of these

Ans. (c) V. E. Veculescu et al.

134. The length of ESTs used in SAGE is about

a. 5–10 nt
b. 20–25 nt
c. 9–14 nt
d. 10–20 nt

Ans. (c) 9–14 nt

135. Global expression profiling was accomplished first in

a. Maize
b. Yeast
c. Drosophila
d. Arabidopsis

Ans. (b) Yeast

136. Technique of DNA synthesis on microarray chip was developed by

a. R.S. Yalow and S.A. Berson
b. E. Engvall and P.Periman
c. S. Fodor et al.
d. Both a and b

Ans. (c) S. Fodor et al.

137. An Affymetrix gene chip can handle............ probes per square cm.

a. 64000
b. 22000
c. 37000
d. 32000

Ans. (a) 64000

138. Higher specific hybridization I sobserved in

a. Spotted microarray
b. Oligo microarray
c. Both of these
d. None of these

Ans. (a) Spotted microarray

139. In silico chip designing is possible in

a. Spotted microarray
b. Oligo microarray
c. Both of these
d. None of these

Ans. (b) Oligo microarray

140. MPSS technique was developed by

a. R.S.Yalow and S.A. Berson
b. E. Engvall and P.Periman
c. Brenner et al.
d. None of these

Ans. (c) Brenner et al.

141. Fluorescence based sequencing is used in
   a. MPSS
   b. SAGE
   c. ELISA
   d. RNA dot blot

Ans. (a) MPSS

142. Tags and anti-tags are used in
   a. SAGE
   b. MPSS
   c. Two hybrid system
   d. None of these

Ans. (b) MPSS

143. The enzyme used in homomeric tailing is
   a. Terminal transferase
   b. Deoxymucleotidyl transferase
   c. Reverse transcriptase
   d. DNA polymerase

Ans. (b) Deoxymucleotidyl transferase

144. In which of the processes specific and different primers are used for IInd strand PCR amplification?
   a. Homomeric tailing
   b. Adapter ligation
   c. Template switching
   d. None of these

Ans. (b) Adapter ligation

145. Which of the following technique can not be used or analysis of whole Transcriptome at a time?
   a. Template switching
   b. Adapter ligation
   c. Homomeric tailing
   d. Multiplex-PCR

Ans. (d) Multiplex-PCR

146. Which of the following gene expression technique is quicker to perform?
   a. MPSS
   b. SAGE
   c. AP-PCR
   d. DNA microarray

Ans. (c) AP-PCR

147. The length of the signature sequence of MPSS is
   a. 12 nt
   b. 15 nt
   c. 17 ntd.
   19 nt

Ans. (c) 17 ntd.

148. The technique which does not require any previous knowledge about cellular RNA sequence is
   a. SAGE
   b. MPSS
   c. Both of these
   d. None of these

Ans. (b) MPSS

149. The length of tag in SAGE is about
   a. 14 nt
   b. 15 nt
   c. 17 nt
   d. 10 nt

Ans. (a) 14 nt

150. Yeast two hybrid assay for proteome analysis was developed by
   a. R.S. Yalow and S.A. Berson
   b. E. Engvall and P. Periman
   c. S. Fields and O. Song
   d. C. Sandchez et al.

Ans. (c) S. Fields and O. Song

151. The term interactome is related to
   a. Protein-protein interaction
   b. DNA-RNA interaction
   c. DNA-DNA interaction
   d. DNA-protein interaction

Ans. (a) Protein-protein interaction

152. Term interactome was coined by
   a. R.S. Yalow and S.A. Berson
   b. E. Engvall and P. Periman
   c. C. Sanchez et al.
   d. None of these

Ans. (c) C. Sanchez et al.

153. What is the most sensitive method for protein staining in electrophoresis
   a. Silver staining
   b. Staining with fluorescent molecule
   c. Staining with bromopenol blue
   d. None of these

Ans. (a) Silver staining

154. Technique of peptide mass fingerprinting was developed by
   a. D. J. Pappin et al.
   b. S. Brenner et al.
   c. F. Sanger
   d. None of these

Ans. (a) D. J. Pappin et al.

155. Protein sequencing method was developed by
   a. F. Sanger
   b. S. Brenner et al
   c. D.J. pappin et al
   d. None of these

Ans. (a) F. Sanger

156. Technique of 2-DE was developed by
   a. P. H. O'farrell
   b. F. Sanger
   c. D. J. Fappin et al.
   d. None f these

Ans. (a) P. H. O'farrell

157. A carrier ampholyte is used in
   a. 2-DE
   b. NMR spectroscopy
   c. Mass spectroscopy
   d. Protein sequencing

Ans. (a) 2-DE

158. The function of carrier ampholyte is

a. Denature protein
b. Create pH gradient
c. Stain protein bands
d. Used as loading mixture

Ans. (b) Create pH gradient

159. In first dimensional analysis of 2-DE proteins migrate to

a. The end of the gel
b. Starting point of the gel
c. The isoelectric point of the protein
d. Do not migrate at all

Ans. (c) The isoelectric point of the protein

160. Immobilized pH gradient is used in

a. 2-DE   b. Mass spectroscopy
c. NMR spectroscopy   d. Protein sequencing

Ans. (a) 2-DE

161. In 2-DE protein get separated on the basis of

a. Isoelectric point   b. Molecular weight
c. Both of these   d. None of these

Ans. (c) Both of these

162. Pelation between TOF and molecular weight can be expressed as

a. TOF = k v(m/z)   b. TOF = k v(z/m)
c. TOF = k v(m-z/z)   d. TOF = k v(z-m/z)

Ans. (a) TOF = k v(m/z)

163. MALDI technique was developed by

a. P. H. O' Farrell
b. M. Karas and F. Hillenkamp
c. Both a and b
d. None of these

Ans. (b) M. Karas and F. Hillenkamp

164. PIR stands for

a. Protein internet resource
b. Protein information resource
c. Protein information report
d. None of these

Ans. (b) Protein information resource

165. Which of the following database is not related to protein sequence characterization?

a. Uniport   b. Swiss port
c. Array express   d. PIR

Ans. (c) Array express

166. GMP is a regulatory system developed by

a. WHO   b. WTO
c. FAO   d. UN

Ans. (a) WHO

167. GMP stands for

a. Genetically modified protein
b. Gross modification of property
c. Good manufacturing practice
d. Good marketing potential

Ans. (c) Good manufacturing practice

168. GMP regulation is applicable to

a. Agrochemical industry
b. Pharmaceutical industry
c. Biotechnology industry
d. Food industry

Ans. (b) Pharmaceutical industry

169. The term franken food is applied by some NGO to describe

a. Genetically modified food
b. Transgenic animal
c. Transgenic plant
d. Harmful elements in food

Ans. (a) Genetically modified food

170. Which of the following gene is not considered desirable in genetically modified foods?

a. Luciferase reporter gene
b. Antibiotic marker gene
c. Gus reporter gene
d. Beta-Calactosidase marker gene

Ans. (b) Antibiotic marker gene

171. Chance of gene escape from plants is higher through

a. Recombination
b. Asexual propagation
c. Intake of food
d. Pollen dispersal

Ans. (d) Pollen dispersal

172. Super bug is

a. Genetically modified bug
b. Supervirulent pathogenic organism created by genetic modification
c. Both a and b
d. None of these

Ans. (b) Supervirulent pathogenic organism created by genetic modification

173. For temporal isolation of transgenic corn, minimum difference in planting days should be

a. 21 days   b. 11 days
c. 15 days   d. 19 days

Ans. (a) 21 days

174. Environment protection act in India came into effect from

a. 1976   b. 1986
c. 1996   d. 2006

Ans. (b) 1986

175. The guidelines for research in transgenic crops in India was published in

a. 1998   b. 1988
c. 1977   d. 1966

Ans. (a) 1998

176. Recombinant DNA guidelines in India was published in

a. 1980   b. 1990
c. 2000   d. 1988

Ans. (b) 1990

177. National containment facility for testing transgenic plants is available in

a. BARC, Mumbai   b. IISC, Bangalore
c. CCMB, Hyderabad   d. NBPGR, New Delhi

Ans. (d) NBPGR, New Delhi

178. Genetically modified seeds with_____technology is banned in India

a. Electroporation   b. GURT
c. Antibiotic transfer   d. None of these

Ans. (b) GURT

179. GURT stands for

a. Genetic use regulation technology
b. Genetic use regulation treaty
c. Genetic use restriction technology
d. Gene use regulation technology

Ans. (c) Genetic use restriction technology

180. A biosafety protocol in the montreal convention on biological Diversity was developed in the Year

a. 1988
b. 1998
c. 1999
d. 2000

Ans. (b) 1998

181. A guideline of safety in biotechnological application in 1986 was developed by

a. Organization of economic cooperation and development
b. Convention on biological diversity
c. World health organization
d. Food and agricultural organization

Ans. (a) Organization of economic cooperation and development

182. The international protocol on biosafety of living modified organisms developed by CBD is popularly known as

a. Kyoto protocol
b. Geneva protocol
c. Cartagena protocol
d. Nairobi protocol

Ans. (c) Cartagena protocol

183. The guidelines for research on transgenic plants has been developed by

a. Department of science and technology
b. Department of biotechnology
c. Ministry of Health
d. Ministry of Environment and forestry

Ans. (b) Department of biotechnology

184. Which of the following category of transgenic plant research has higher rsik as defined by the DBT guideline?

a. Category I
b. Category II
c. Category III
d. Category IV

Ans. (c) Category III

185. The authority of importing transgenic plants in India lies with

a. National research centre on biotechnology
b. Ministry of environment and forestry
c. National bureau of plant genetic resources
d. None of these

Ans. (b) Ministry of environment and forestry

186. Guidelines on protection of transgenic plant variety is provided in

a. Plant variety protection and farmers' right act
b. Environment protection act
c. Recombinant DNA guidelines
d. Guidelines for research in transgenic crops

Ans. (a) Plant variety protection and farmers' right act

187. **A transgenic plant is**
    a. A new variety
    b. An old variety with new gene
    c. An essentially derived variety
    d. Does not have variety status

Ans. (c) An essentially derived variety

188. **The apex regulatory body on GMO in India is**
    a. Recombinant DNA advisory committee
    b. Review committee on genetic manipulation
    c. Department of Biotechnology
    d. Genetic engineering approval committee

Ans. (d) Genetic engineering approval committee

189. **Secretariat of GEAC is associated with**
    a. Ministry of health and family welfare
    b. Ministry of environment and forestry
    c. Ministry of science and technology
    d. None of these

Ans. (b) Ministry of environment and forestry

190. **Secretariat of GCGM is associated with**
    a. Ministry of health and family welfare
    b. Ministry of environment and forestry
    c. Ministry of science and technology
    d. Department of biotechnology

Ans. (d) Department of biotechnology

191. **Regulation on quality of transgenic food is defined by**
    a. Environment protection act
    b. Prevention of food adulteration act
    c. Guidelines for research in transgenic crops
    d. Recombinant DNA guidelines

Ans. (b) Prevention of food adulteration act

192. **According to hierarchy, the regulatory committees can be arranged as**
    a. GEAC > IBSC > RCGM
    b. GEAC > RCGM > IBSC
    c. IBSC > GEAC > RCGM
    d. None of these

Ans. (b) GEAC > RCGM > IBSC

193. **The approval for production of GMO by GEAC is valid up to**
    a. 1 year
    b. 2 year
    c. 3 year
    d. 4 year

Ans. (d) 4 year

194. **Field trials on transgenic plants should get approval from**
    a. RCGM
    b. IBSC
    c. SBCC
    d. GEAC

Ans. (a) RCGM

195. **Controversy on toxicity of Bt-maize is related to**
    a. Danaus plexippus
    b. Agrotis ipsilon
    c. Papileo demolius
    d. None of these

Ans. (a) Danaus plexippus

196. **Primary host of monarch butterfly is**
    a. Grassy weed
    b. Milkweed
    c. Convolvulus sp.
    d. Phalaris sp.

Ans. (b) Milkweed

197. **The toxicity of transgenic Bt maize to Lepidoptoran pests is due to**
    a. Cry toxin
    b. Zein
    c. Tab toxin
    d. Thuringienin

Ans. (a) Cry toxin

198. **Undesirable incorporation of genes in a gene pool is known as**
    a. Genetic pollution
    b. Genetic load
    c. Genetic erosion
    d. None of these

Ans. (a) Genetic pollution

199. **First regulatory guideline on rDNA technology was developed by**
    a. National institute of health, USA
    b. Food and agricultural organization
    c. World health organization
    d. Organization for economic cooperation and development

Ans. (a) National institute of health, USA

200. **The transgenic maize variety that persisted in the seed chain as admixture even four years after withdrawal in USA is**
    a. Roundup ready
    b. Star link
    c. Boll guard
    d. Yield guard

Ans. (b) Star link

201. **The multinational company that released GM cotton in india is**
    a. Novartis
    b. ProAgro
    c. Aventis
    d. Monsanto

Ans. (d) Monsanto

202. First Indian partner Monsanto in India for release of GM cotton was

a. MAHYCO b. Rasi

c. ProAgro d. None of these

Ans. (a) MAHYCO

203. The Indian company that had highest share in GM cotton business in India in 2006 is

a. Pro agro b. MAHYCO

c. Rasi seeds d. None of these

Ans. (c) Rasi seeds

204. The Cartagena protocol on Biosafety was developed under the framework of

a. Environment protection Act

b. Convention on biological diversity

c. Food and agricultural organization

d. World health organization

Ans. (b) Convention on biological diversity

205. First patent for GURT technology was given to

a. Syngenta b. Aventis

c. Monsanto d. Delta and pine Co.

Ans. (d) Delta and pine Co.

206. RAFI stands for

a. Rural and farmers' international

b. Rural and advancement foundation international

c. Rural and foundation international

d. Rural agricultural farmers' international

Ans. (b) Rural and advancement foundation international

207. The terminator technology was coined by

a. Syngenta b. Monsanto

c. RAFI d. None of these

Ans. (c) RAFI

208. The promoter used in terminator technology was

a. LEA b. SV 40

c. TA 29 d. CaMV 35S

Ans. (a) LEA

209. Access factor for E.coli K12 is

a. 10^{-3} b. 10^{-2}

c. 10^{-1} d. 10^{-4}

Ans. (a) 10^{-3}

210. Which of the following is not true for GLSP?

a. Host should be non pathogenic

b. The vector should not have resistance marker

c. The carrier organism should be non pathogenic

d. Shuttle vector can not be used

Ans. (d) Shuttle vector can not be used

211. Which of the following experiments are exempted from detailed biosafety analysis?

a. Self cloning experiments

b. Experiments involving plant pathogens

c. Experiments involving animal pathogens

d. Agrobacterium mediated transformation

Ans. (a) Self cloning experiments

212. Cloning of GRAS organisms fall in the

a. Category I experiment

b. Category II experiment

c. Category III experiment

d. None of these

Ans. (a) Category I experiment

213. Field testing of transgenic crop for release as a variety is done by

a. ICAR b. DBT

c. GEAC d. MoEF

Ans. (a) ICAR

214. The Indian company not involved in Bt-cotton variety production

a. Ankur seeds

b. Indoi-American Hybrid Seed Company

c. Mayhco

d. Rasi Seeds

Ans. (b) Indoi-American Hybrid Seed Company

215. Rooty locus of T-DNA codes for

a. Tryptophan monooxygenase

b. Indoleacetamide hydrolase

c. Indole pentenyl transferase

d. Nopaline synthase

Ans. (c) Indole pentenyl transferase

216. Shooty locus of T-DNA indicate genes

a. iaaH b. iaaM

c. Both of these d. None of these

Ans. (c) Both of these

217. Number of genes prescent in vir region of T-DNA is

a. 25 b. 20

c. 15 d. 10

Ans. (a) 25

218. Size of Ti-plasmid is about

a. 100 bp b. 100 kb
c. 200 kb d. 200 bp

Ans. (c) 200 kb

219. Hairy root phenotype is caused by

a. A. Rhizogenes b. A. Tumefaciens
c. Both of these d. None of these

Ans. (a) A. Rhizogenes

220. Better expression of vir genes takes place at

a. Alkaline pH b. Acidic pH
c. Neutral pH d. None of these

Ans. (b) Acidic pH

221. Octopine is converted by Agrobacterium to produce

a. Pyruvate and arginine
b. Glucose and Alanine
c. Sucrose and nopaline
d. Glucose and arginine

Ans. (a) Pyruvate and arginine

222. In binary plasmid for T-DNA transfer, the direct repeats of T-DNA

a. Are trans to vir region
b. Are absent
c. Are about 50 bp
d. Are present in duplicate copies

Ans. (a) Are trans to vir region

223. During infection, the Agrobacterium cell show

a. Phototropic movement
b. Nastic movement
c. Chemotactic movement
d. No movement

Ans. (c) Chemotactic movement

224. During transfer T-DNA remains as

a. Naked, single stranded
b. Naked double stranded
c. SsDNA –Protein complex
d. dsDNA-protein complex

Ans. (c) SsDNA –Protein complex

225. Acetpsuromgpme at lower concentration acts as

a. Regulator of operon
b. Chemoattractant
c. Inhibitor of host-Agrobacterium ecognition
d. Inducer of T-DNA excision

Ans. (b) Chemoattractant

226. Technique of floral dip for transformation was developed by

a. S.J. clough and A.F. Bent
b. J.R. Kikkert
c. Both of these
d. None of these

Ans. (a) S.J. clough and A.F. Bent

227. Acetosyringone at higher concentration acts as

a. Inhibitor of host-Agrobacterium recognition
b. Chemoattractant
c. Regulator of chromosomal operon
d. Inducer of T-DNA excision

Ans. (d) Inducer of T-DNA excision

228. Nopaline is converted by Agrobacterium to produce

a. Glucose and arginine
b. Glutamine and Alanine
c. U-ketoglutarate and agrinine
d. Glutamate and Pyruvate

Ans. (c) U-ketoglutarate and agrinine

229. Site specific endonucleases are encoded by

a. Ipt b. Vir D
c. Vir G d. Vir A

Ans. (b) Vir D

230. Size of T-DNA in nopaline type Ti-plasmid is

a. 28 kb
b. 30 kb
c. 25 kb
d. 50 kb

Ans. (c) 25 kb

231. The agrolistic method of transformation was developed by

a. J. R. Kikkert
b. G.Hansen and M.D. Chilton
c. J. C. Sanford
d. None of these

Ans. (b) G.Hansen and M.D. Chilton

232. Vacuum infiltration method of transformation was developed by

a. J. R. Kikkert
b. G.H ansen and M.D. Chilton
c. J. C. Sanford
d. N. Bechtold et al.

Ans. (d) N. Bechtold et al.

233. Concept of biolistic transformation was given by

a. J. R. Kikkert

b. G.Hansen and M.D. Chilton

c. J. C. Sanford

d. None of these

Ans. (c) J. C. Sanford

234. The method of pollen tube transformation was developed by

a. J. R. Kikkert

b. G.Hansen and M.D. Chilton

c. Z. X. Luo and R. Wu

d. None of these

Ans. (c) Z. X. Luo and R. Wu

235. Pollen tube transformation was first reported in

a. Wheat

b. Rice

c. Brassica

d. Arubulopsis

Ans. (b) Rice

236. A. Rhizogenes infects

a. Monocots only

b. Gymnosperms

c. Dicots only

d. Both a and c

Ans. (c) Dicots only

237. The gene expressing hairy root phenotype in A. Rhizogenes is

a. ipt

b. ocs

c. rol

d. nos

Ans. (c) rol

238. A gene of A. Rhizogenes that can induce male sterility is

a. rolC

b. rolA

c. rolB

d. ocs

Ans. (a) rolC

239. The techniqye of liposome mediated transformation in plant was developed by

a. A. Deshayes et al

b. A. Crossway et al.

c. I. Potrykus

d. J. D. Liu

Ans. (a) Deshayes et al

240. During Electroporation the potential of electric current passed is

a. 2–5 kv

b. 10–20 kv

c. 20–30 kv

d. None of these

Ans. (a) 2–5 kv

241. More number of stable transformants can be obtained by

a. Lipofection

b. Electroporation

c. Laser beam

d. Agrobacterium

Ans. (d) Agrobacterium

242. Diameter of gene guns are about

a. 2000–4000 nm

b. 200–400 nm

c. 20–40 nm

d. 2–4 nm

Ans. (a) 2000–4000 nm

243. Silicon carbide fiber was used for gene delivery in plants by

a. H. F. Kaeppler et al.

b. A. Deshayes et al.

c. J. C. sanfrd

d. None of these

Ans. (a) H. F. Kaeppler et al.

244. Technique of microinjection for genetic transformation in plant was first used by

a. G. Neuhaus

b. R. L. Brinster et al.

c. M. R. Capecchi

d. All of them

Ans. (a) G. Neuhaus

245. The plant that was transformed first using micro-injection was

a. Arabidopsis

b. Acetabularia

c. Chlamydomonas

d. Alfalfa

Ans. (b) Acetabularia

246. Laser beam mediated gene delivery in plant cell was performed

a. G. Neuhaus

b. R. L. Brinster et al.

c. M. R. Capecchi

d. G. Weber

Ans. (d) G. Weber

247. The concept of lipofection was developed by

a. G. Neuhaus

b. R. L. Brinster et al.

c. M. R. Capecchi

d. P. L. Felgner

Ans. (d) P. L. Felgner

248. Leaf disc transformation technique by Agro-bacterium was developed by

a. R. B. Horsch et al.

b. N. Grimsley et al.

c. Both of them

d. None of these

Ans. (a) R. B. Horsch et al.

249. The technique of agroinfection was invented by

a. G. Neuhaus

b. R. L. Brinster et. al.

c. M. R. Capecchi

d. N. Grimsley et. al.

Ans. (d) N. Grimsley et. al.

250. Which of the following detection technique involves antibody?
a. Western blotting   b. Northern blotting
c. Southern blotting   d. None of these

Ans. (a) Western blotting

251. Stable transformation is not required for
a. Transient gene expression assay
b. Development of stable transformation
c. Generation of genetically modified crops
d. None of these

Ans. (a) Transient gene expression assay

252. The concept of transgenic plant vaccine was pioneered by
a. C. arntgen   b. S. Cohen
c. I. Potrykus   d. A. Dutta

Ans. (a) C. arntgen

253. Genetic transformation was first performed in the plant
a. Wheat   b. Rice
c. Tobacco   d. Tomato

Ans. (c) Tobacco

254. Macroinjection was first performed in
a. Secale   b. Rice
c. Tobacco   d. Arabidopsis

Ans. (a) Secale

255. Golden rice was developed by
a. I. Potrykus
b. P.beyer
c. Both of these
d. None of these

Ans. (c) Both of these

256. Higher provitamin A containing golden rice has been developed by the biotech company
a. Invitrogen
b. Syngenta
c. Monsanto
d. PPL Therapeutics

Ans. (b) Syngenta

257. Technique of plastid transformation was perfected by
a. P. Beyer   b. P. Maliga
c. A. Dutta   d. C. Arntgen

Ans. (a) P. Beyer

258. First transgenic crop developed in india is
a. Potato   b. Tomato
c. Rice   d. Brassica

Ans. (a) Potato

259. Nutritional enhancement of potato by engineering high protein synthesizing gene was achieved by
a. P. Beyer   b. P. Maliga
c. A. Dutta   d. None of these

Ans. (c) A. Dutta

260. The gene used for genetic engineering of potato for high protein content was obtained from
a. Soybean   b. Amaranthus
c. Groundnut   d. Mungbean

Ans. (b) Amaranthus

261. Bacillus thuringiensis is a
a. Gram positive motile bacteria
b. Gram positive spore forming bacteria
c. Gram negative motile bacteria
d. Gram negative spore forming bacteria

Ans. (b) Gram positive spore forming bacteria

262. Toxic activity of the delta-endotoxin is present in the
a. C-terminal end of the protein
b. N-terminal end of the protein
c. Amino terminal end of the protein
d. At both end of the protein

Ans. (c) Amino terminal end of the protein

263. Which of the following enzyme can cleave protoxin?
a. Endonuclease   b. EPSP synthase
c. Trypsin   d. None of these

Ans. (c) Trypsin

264. Which of the following subspecies of Bt was used most for transgenic crop development?
a. Bt subsp. Kurstaki
b. Bt. Subsp. Finitimus
c. Bt. Subsp. Dendrohmus
d. None of these

Ans. (a) Bt subsp. Kurstaki

265. The cry gene are coded in Bt
a. Plasmid
b. Nuclear DNA
c. Both of these
d. None of these

Ans. (c) Both of these

266. First Bt transgenic tobacco was produced by

a. Plant genetic system
b. Bayer
c. Syngenta
d. Monsanto

Ans. (a) Plant genetic system

267. First reported of transgenic plant development through engineering of a plant gene was published by

a. G. Neuhaus
b. R. L. Brinster et al.
c. M. R. Capecchi
d. V. A. Hilder et al.

Ans. (d) V. A. Hilder et al.

268. The gene that was first transformed from a plant origin was

a. Tomato inhibitor II
b. Delta endotoxin
c. Alpha-amylase
d. Cow pea trypsin inhibitor

Ans. (d) Cow pea trypsin inhibitor

269. The gene CpTI provides resistance against insects of order

a. Coleopteran
b. Orthoptera
c. Lepidoptera
d. All of these

Ans. (d) All of these

270. Which of the following transgenic crop is grown in India

a. Soybean
b. Rice
c. Cotton
d. Maize

Ans. (c) Cotton

271. Transgenic rice is being grown in

a. Iran
b. Spain
c. USA
d. Paraguay

Ans. (a) Iran

272. Which of the following country in Europs does not grow GM crop?

a. Czech republic
b. Germany
c. Spain
d. United kingdom

Ans. (d) United kingdom

273. The number of countries that grow GM crop (till 2006) is

a. 20
b. 21
c. 22
d. 24

Ans. (b) 21

274. Which of the following gene was engineered in transgenic cotton released in India?

a Cry 1 Ac
b. Cry II a
c. Cry 1 Aa
d. None of these

Ans. (a) Cry 1 Ac

CHECK YOU GRASP

1. The promoter used in terminator technology was
   a. LEA
   b. SV 40
   c. TA 29
   d. CaMV 35S

2. SAGE technique was invented by
   a. R.S.Yalow and S.A. Berson
   b. E. Engvall and P.Periman
   c. V. E. Veculescu et al.
   d. None of these

3. The length of ESTs used in SAGE is about
   a. 5–10 nt
   b. 20–25 nt
   c. 9–14 nt
   d. 10–20 nt

4. The vector used in sanger sequencing method is
   a. Phage M13
   b. Phage T2
   c. Coliphage P1
   d. Bacteriophage ë

5. HAT medium, a medium for selection of hyman-mouse hybrid cell contain
   a. Hypersensitive adenine and thymidine
   b. Hypoxanthine, aminopterin and thymidine
   c. Hypoxanthine, Auxin and tetracycline
   d. None of these

6. Which of the following banding technique should be used to located r-RNA gene?
   a. C-banding
   b. N-banding
   c. G-banding
   d. R-banding

7. Lod score is used for
   a. Gene identification
   b. Genetic mapping
   c. Physical mapping
   d. Gene sequencing

8. In R-banding, the stain used is
   a. Rhodamine red
   b. Texas red
   c. Quinacrine mustard
   d. Giemsa

9. Retroviral vectors are
   a. ds RNA
   b. ss DNA
   c. ds DNA
   d. ss RNA

10. Vectors based on BPV have plasmid components of
   a. Cosmid vectors
   b. pBR322
   c. pUC vector
   d. pBluescript vector

In case of less than 80% score, go through brief Review and Glance one again from chapter

Key: 1-a 2-c 3-c 4-a 5-b 6-b 7-b 8-d 9-a 10-b

6

Biosafety, IPR and Bioethics

1. Physical containment relates to which of the following?

a. Special procedures

b. Containment equipment

c. None of these

d. Both a and b

Ans. (d) Both a and b

2. Which of the following is considered as primary physical containment?

a. Containment equipment

b. Special procedures

c. Laboratory design

d. Both a and c

Ans. (d) Both a and c

3. Consider the options given in Q. 2 and pick the correct option that lists the secondary physical containment?

a. Special procedures

b. Laboratory design

c. Laboratory technique

d. None of these

Ans. (a) Special procedures

4. It is freared that transgenic plants, may lead to which of the following?

a. Transfer of their transgenic feature to weeds.

b. May themseleves become weeds.

c. Degrade the environment.

d. All of the above

Ans. (d) All of the above

5. Which of the following statements are correct?

a. Intellectual property is an idea, a design, an invention, a manuscript, etc. Which can ultimately give rise to a useful product/application

b. The first law on patent was passed in venice in 1547

c. The first law on patent was passed in venice in 1647

d. All of the above

Ans. (a) Intellectual property is an idea, a design, an invention, a manuscript, etc. Which can ultimately give rise to a useful product/application

6. Which of the following statements are correct about intellectual property rights?

a. The main from of IPR protection are trade secret, patent, copyright, plant breeder,s right, trade mark and geographical indication

b. Intellectual property may be a design, an idea, an invention, a manuscript, etc.

c. Both a and b

d. None of these

Ans. (c) Both a and b

7. Trade secret related to which of the following?

a. Formulae

b. Processes

c. Certain material, e.g. bacterial strains

d. All of the above

Ans. (d) All of the above

8. Which of the following is not correct about patent?

a. It is granted by the Government of a country to the applicant for an unlimited period of time.

b. When a patent is granted, the inventor becomes the owner of the patent like any other from of property.

c. Patents are granted for an invention, innovation/ improvent in an invention, process/ product of an invention and a concept.

d. All of the above

Ans. (a) It is granted by the Government of a country to the applicant for an unlimited period of time.

9. In the area of biotechnology, which of the following material can be kept as trade secret?

a. Production process

b. Strains of microorganism

c. Cell lines

d. All of the above

Ans. (d) All of the above

10. In the early 1970s which of the following were considered as the possible potential health hazards of cloning recombinant DNA molecules?

a. Hybrid organisms could be created with biological activities of an unpredictable nature

b. Hybrid organisms may escape from the laboratory with unpredictable consequence

c. None of the above

d. Both a and b

Ans. (d) Both a and b

11. Consider the following activities:

a. Hazard analysis   b. Risk determination

c. Consequence analysis   d. Hazard identification

e. Risk evaluation

Ans. (a) Hazard analysis

12. A transgenic variety of which of the following crops had to be withdrawn from cultivation following deaths due to allergy?

a. Soybean   b. Tomato

c. Maize   d. Potato

Ans. (a) Soybean

13. Which of the following is not correct about NIH guidelines?

a. The guidelines were revised after two year

b. NIH guidelines were more liberal than the recommendation of the asilomar conference.

c. In 1977, NIH prepared an Environmental impact statement.

d. The first NIH guidelines were prepared

Ans. (b) NIH guidelines were more liberal than the recommendation of the asilomar conference.

14. Which of the following is the chief requirements for the grant of a patent?

a. Not novelty

b. Usefulness is not required

c. Inventiveness

d. All of the above

Ans. (c) Inventiveness

15. Trade secret offers which of the following advantage?

a. Low cost of maintaining the secret.

b. The risk of innovation by someone else is minimized.

c. Not effective for unlimited duration

d. All of the above

Ans. (b) The risk of innovation by someone else is minimized.

16. Trade secrets suffer from which of the following disadvantage?

a. Maintaining a trade secret itself is costly

b. It offers protection from independent innovation/invention.

c. It can be applied to many inventions.

d. All of these

Ans. (a) Maintaining a trade secret itself is costly

17. Which of the following statements are correct about patents?

a. The subject matter must be ordinary

b. In 1985, the Ammerican Supreme court ruled that a live, human made microorganism can be patented under the American patent law as a manufacture or composition of matter

c. In 1980, the Ammerican Supreme court ruled that a live, human made microorganism can be patented under the American patent law as a manufacture or composition of matter

d. None of these

Ans. (c) In 1980, the Ammerican Supreme court ruled that a live, human made microorganism can be patented under the American patent law as a manufacture or composition of matter

18. Trade secret can not be applied for which of the following invention?

a. Cell lines

b. Strain of microorganism

c. Plant varieties

d. All of the above

Ans. (c) Plant varieties

19. The concerns given as the options of Q.5 were examined by a committee of national academy of Sciences (USA) in 1974; it made which of the following recommendation.

1. NIH, USA be requested to set up an advisory committee on recombinant DNA to oversee experimental programmes to develop procedures to minimize hazards and devise guidelines.

2. Use of caution in experiments linkage animal DNAs to bacterial, phage or plasmid DNAs.

3. Certain types of experiments, e.g., cloning of genes for bacterial toxins, etc., be deferred

4. Human cloning experiments can be exempted from scrutiny

Option:

a. 3, 2, 1   b. 1, 2, 3,4

c. 2, 3, 4, 1   d. 1, 4, 3

Ans. (a) 3, 2, 1

20. In February 1975, a historic intermationa meeting was convened about cloning of recombinant DNA molecule at Asilomar California; it reached which of the following conclusion?

a. Certain experiments should be deferred

b. Most of the work on recombinant DNA could proceed with appropriate safety measures.

c. Potential risks were assigned to different types of experiments.

d. Suck bacterial and plasmids that could not survive in the environment, it they escaped from the laboratory should be developed.

e. All of the above

Ans. (e) All of the above

21. Which of the following terms is not used as synonym of planned introduction?

a. Contained use

b. Deliberate introduction

c. Deliberate release

d. Field testing

Ans. (a) Contained use

22. Which of the following is not correct about NIH guidelines?

a. In USA, the NIH guidelines are followed by all federal agencies that fund research on recombinant DNA.

b. Experiments that were previously prohibited, were changed to category requiring review and approval by NIH.

c. In the revision, the containment levels were made more stringent

d. A major revision of the guidelines was effected in 1982

Ans. (c) In the revision, the containment levels were made more stringent

23. For bio safety consideration, modern biotechnology includes which of the following?

a. RDT

b. Direct injection of nucleic acids in to cell of organelles

c. Fusion of cells beyond the taxonomic family that overcomes natural physiological, reproductive or recombination barriers.

d. All of the above

Ans. (d) All of the above

24. Which of the following statements are correct about plant breeder,s right?

a. A person holding PBR title to a variety can not authorize other interested persons/organizations to produce and sell the propagating material of that variety.

b. These are the right s granted by the government to a plant vreeder, or owner of a variety to exclude others for producing or commercializing th propagating material of that variety.

c. Both a and b

d. None of these

Ans. (b) These are the right s granted by the government to a plant vreeder, or owner of a variety to exclude others for producing or commercializing th propagating material of that variety.

25. Which of the following is not correct about breeder's exemption?

a. The PBR for a new variety evolved from the initial variety will be of the breeder who developed the new variety and of the holder of PBR title of the initial variety as well

b. Under the UPOV 1978 Act, all new varieties evolved using a protected variety were exempted from protection under this provision.

c. The use of a protected variety for the development of new varieties is exempted from protection.

d. All of the above

Ans. (a) The PBR for a new variety evolved from the initial variety will be of the breeder who developed the new variety and of the holder of PBR title of the initial variety as well

26. Which of the following is correct about an essentially derived variety?

a. It is a variety produced by mutation or transfer of gene through backcross method in to another variety.

b. It will be covered under the PBR title granted to the initial variety

c. The breeder of such a variety will be required to obtain permission from PBR title holder of the initial variety.

d. All of the above

Ans. (d) All of the above

27. Which of the following is correct about farmer's rights?

a. It should not be obligatory and should be relegated as privilege.

b. The key question relating to farmer's right remain as to whom to reward, to what extent and in what manner.

c. Both of these

d. None of these

Ans. (b) The key question relating to farmer's right remain as to whom to reward, to what extent and in what manner.

28. **Which of the following people are considered under farmer's rights for sharing the profit earned from the development of high yielding varieties evolved from the use of raw materials/plant genetic resources?**

    a. Urban communities

    b. Non traditional farming families

    c. Tribal people

    d. All of the above

Ans. (c) Tribal people

29. **An otherwise excellent transgenic variety of which of the following crops developed during 1990s could not be released due to IPR problems?**

    a. Nicotiana tobaccm   b. Solanum tubrosum

    c. Solanum esculantum   d. Brassica napus

Ans. (c) Solanum esculantum

30. **India has created a National Biodiversity Authority with headquarters at which of the following?**

    a. Mumbai   b. Chennai

    c. Kolkata   d. Delhi

Ans. (b) Chennai

31. **Which of the following intellectual properties can be protected by copyright?**

    a. Computer hardware   b. DNA chip

    c. DNA Sequence   d. None of the above

Ans. (c) DNA Sequence

32. **The copyright of a book may be held by which of the following?**

    a. Author's

    b. Printer's

    c. Both

    d. None of the above

Ans. (a) Author's

33. **Which of the following steps are involved in the procedure of patenting?**

    a. In case a patent is not challenged, the patent is awarded immediately after the expiry of the specified period.

    b. If it is found suitable for patenting the invention along with adequate details of the desired patent is published for the information of all concerned.

c. Anyone can challenge the award of patent within a specified period of time.

d. All of the above

Ans. (d) All of the above

34. **The NIH, USA guidelines specify the practices for constructing and handling which of the following?**

    a. Products obtained from organisms and viruses containing RDT

    b. Organism and viruses containing RDT

    c. Recombinant DNA molecules

    d. Both b and c

Ans. (d) Both b and c

35. **The bio safety guidelines and developed to ensure and adequate level of protection during which of the following activities of modern biotechnology?**

    a. Safe transfer   b. Use of GMOs

    c. Handling   d. All of the above

Ans. (d) All of the above

36. **In case of which of the following products, an empirical approach based on data obtained through experimentation about the source of potential hazards has proved satisfactory?**

    a. Drugs   b. Vaccines

    c. Pesticides   d. All of the above

Ans. (d) All of the above

37. **In risk assessment, a lack of scientific knowledge or scientific consensus should not necessarily be interpreted as indicating which of the following?**

    a. Absence of risk   b. Acceptable risk

    c. None of the these   d. Both a and b

Ans. (d) Both a and b

38. **The assessment of risk during laboratory research is usually done in which of the following steps?**

    a. Initial risk assessment

    b. Advanced risk assessment

    c. Comprehensive risk assessment

    d. Both a and c

Ans. (d) Both a and c

39. **The chief objectives of risk assessment during laboratory research are to decide about which of the following of the proposed research?**

    a. Laboratory procedures

    b. Biological containment

    c. Physical containment

    d. All of the above

Ans. (d) All of the above

40. On the basis of their potential effects on a healthy adult human, organisms can be classified in to which of the following?

a. Risk group 1   b. Risk group 2
c. Risk group 3   d. Risk group 4
e. All of the above

Ans. (e) All of the above

41. In which of the following risk group, agents are not associated with disease in heathy humans?

a. Risk group 1
b. Risk group 2
c. Risk group 3
d. Risk group 4

Ans. (a) Risk group 1

42. In USA which of the following systems are available for protection of IPRs related to palnts?

a. The plant patents Act (1945)
b. The plant variety protection Act of 1975
c. The plant patents Act 1930
d. All of the above

Ans. (c) The plant patents Act 1930

43. Which of the following is the most powerful and the most expansive in scope of coverage for protection of IPRs related to palnts?

a. The plant patents Act 1930
b. The plant variety protection Act of 1970
c. The utility patent Act 1985
d. All of the above

Ans. (c) The utility patent Act 1985

44. Which of the following is correct?

a. A patent act to provide patents on plants was first introduced in Germany in 1960
b. A patent act to provide patents on plants was first introduced in Germany in 1866
c. In 1995, UPOV had 20 member states
d. All of the above

Ans. (b) A patent act to provide patents on plants was first introduced in Germany in 1866

45. Which of the following is correct about farmer's privilege?

a. Under UPOV 1978 Act, there was explicit provision for farmer's privilege.
b. PBR systems generally allow the farmers to use the seeds of protected varieties produced by themselves.
c. It is very important provision for countries like India, where over 90% of the total cropped area is sown by seed produced by the farmers themselves.
d. All of the above

Ans. (d) All of the above

46. The copyright suffers from which of the following limitation?

a. It prevents another person from using either the idea or the information contained in a copyright material.
b. It does not provide protection for a specific period and only from reproduction as such of the copyright material.
c. In case of DNA sequence, one may get around this protection by designing an alternative sequence to encode the same protein.
d. All of the above

Ans. (c) In case of DNA sequence, one may get around this protection by designing an alternative sequence to encode the same protein.

47. Which of the following is correct?

a. The UPOV 1991 Act has not strengthened the PBR in comparison to the UPOV 1978 Act
b. The UPOV 1978 Act is now revised as UPOV 1991 Act
c. The PPVFR Act 2001 is not similar to UPOV Act 1978 in some respects, has not same features of UPOV Act 1991 and is unique in respect to some of its other feature
d. All of the above

Ans. (b) The UPOV 1978 Act is now revised as UPOV 1991 Act

48. PPVFR Act 2001 is similar to UPOV Act 1978 with respect to which of the following?

a. The duration of protection is 5 year
b. Provision for farmer privilege
c. The duration of protection is 8 year
d. All of the above

Ans. (b) Provision for farmer privilege

49. PPVFR Act 2001 is comparable to UPOV Act 1991 with respect to which of the following?

a. Protection extended to commercial use of all the material of the protected variety.
b. Requirement of novelty, distinctiveness, uniformity and stability for registration of a variety.
c. Essentially-derived varieties being subjected to PBR protection granted to the concerned initial varieties.
d. Both b and c

Ans. (d) Both b and c

50. **PPVFR Act 2001 has which of the following unique features which of the following unique features which are not provided for the UPOV Act (1978,1991)?**
    a. Registration of extant varieties
    b. Registration of farmer's varieties
    c. It permits farmers to exchange share or sell their farm produce, including seed, except as branded seed.
    d. All of the above

Ans. (d) All of the above

51. **Under the provisions of UPOV Act 1991, a plant variety must satisfy which of the following criteria for protection?**
    a. Distinctiveness   b. Not novel
    c. Not stable   d. Not uniform

Ans. (a) Distinctiveness

52. **Which of the following risk group is associated with such serious or lethal human diseases for which preventive or therapeutic interventions may be available?**
    a. Risk group 1   b. Risk group 2
    c. Risk group 3   d. Risk group 4

Ans. (c) Risk group 3

53. **Which of the following risk group agent is concerned with organisms, which cause serious or lethal disease for which preventive or therapeutic invention are not usually available?**
    a. Risk group 1   b. Risk group 2
    c. Risk group 3   d. Risk group 4

Ans. (b) Risk group 2

54. **Which of the following risk group agent is concerned with organisms, which cause serious or lethal disease for which preventive or therapeutic invention are not usually available?**
    a. Risk group 1   b. Risk group 2
    c. Risk group 3   d. Risk group 4

Ans. (d) Risk group 4

55. **Which of the following is not correct about Biosafety Guidelines in India?**
    a. Initially, the Indian Recombinant DNA safety Guidelines and Regulations were prepared in 1990 by Recombinant DNA Advisory Committee, Deptt. Of Biotechnology, New Delhi.
    b. The Indian Recombinant DNA safety Guidelines and Regulations were revised in 1994.

c. Field trials, in India, using transgenic plants began in 1995
    d. Canada becomes the first country to begin commercial use of virus resistant transgenic tobacco and tomato in the early 1990

Ans. (d) Canada becomes the first country to begin commercial use of virus resistant transgenic tobacco and tomato in the early 1990

56. **Which of the following statements is correct about comprehensive risk assessment?**
    a. The level of containment appropriate for an experiment is decided on the basis of comprehensive risk assessment.
    b. The containment level for the experiment amy, in the end, be comparable to that of the risk group of the agent or it may be raised or lowered as a result of the comprehensive risk assessment.
    c. It is done after the initial risk assessment.
    d. All of the above

Ans. (d) All of the above

57. **Risk assessment in case of planned release of transgenic crops may take into account which of the following?**
    I. Nature of marker genes
    II. The characteristics of promoters in terms of whether they are organ-specific or constructive
    III. Location and proximity of related crops in relation to isolation distance needed for prevention for pollination
    IV. Proximity of wild relatives and the distance of inter pollination with such relatives
    a. I, II, III   b. I, II, III, IV
    c. I, III, IV   d. I, II, IV

Ans. (b) I, II, III, IV

58. **In case of transgenic plants, which o the following are the main concerns related to their planned introduction?**
    a. Virus resistance genes may provide opportunities for evolution of newer virulent strains by recombination
    b. Insect resistant plants, would be cultivated on a large scale; this may lead to evolution of resistant insect biotypes.
    c. Transgenic plants may affect the flora and fauna of their phyllosphere and rhizosphere.
    d. The products of transgenes may pose health hazards
    e. All of the above

Ans. (e) All of the above

59. Which of the following countries has 30 years protection for inbred lines of maize and for clovers and a few grasses?

a. India
b. France
c. USA
d. Australia

Ans. (b) France

60. PPVFR Act 2001 aims to provide for the establishment of suitable systems for which of the following?

a. Development of new breeds of animals
b. Protection of plant breeder
c. Implementing plant breeder's rights
d. All of the above

Ans. (c) Implementing plant breeder's rights

61. Which of the following are the main considerations for the development of PBR systems?

a. Private sectors are not invest in the plant breeding and seed industry.
b. It is encourages plant breeding activities
c. Both a and b are correct
d. None of these

Ans. (b) It is encourages plant breeding activities

62. Which of the following statements are correct about historical development of intellectual property rights in India?

a. In 1855, the act of protection of invention was introduced
b. In 1875, patents and designs protection Act was passed.
c. In 1872, patents and designs protection Act was passed
d. None of these

Ans. (c) In 1872, patents and designs protection Act passed

63. Which of the following is not correct about historical development of intellectual property rights in India?

a. The Indian copyright Act 1957, amended in 1999, is comparable to international standards
b. Trademark protection is in force since August 1947 under the 1950 Act
c. The Indian patents Act 1970 was introduced in the parliament in 1965
d. Protection of designs is covered by the Indian Patent and design Act 1911 with subsequent amendments

Ans. (b) Trademark protection is in force since August 1947 under the 1950 Act

64. Which of the following is not correct about international harmonization of patent laws?

a. The Paris convention also allows inventors to claim in all the member countries by filing a patent application initially in one of the member states.
b. The Paris convention has 50 member states; India joined the convention on July 15, 1995.
c. The Paris convention established equal protection of industrial IPR under the laws of ember countries for both nationals and residents of other member countries of the convention.
d. All of the above

Ans. (d) All of the above

65. Government of India has now established the PPVFR Authority with headquarters at which of the following place?

a. Mumbai
b. New Delhi
c. Kolkata
d. Chennai

Ans. (b) New Delhi

66. Which of the following is not correct about international harmonization of patent laws?

a. TRIPs became effective on January 1, 1998
b. WIPO operates by asking member states to ratify a convention and to introduce the agreed basic principles in to their national laws.
c. IPRs are administered but not enforced, by the world Intellectual property Organization, Geneva.
d. The Trade Related Intellectual Property Rights agreement is the most comprehensive multilateral agreement on IPR.

Ans. (a) TRIPs became effective on January 1, 1998

67. Which of the following is not correct?

a. The member countries of WTO have been given a period of 5 year to suitable amend their IPR law according to TRIPs.
b. Each member country has the option to frame its own patent laws within the broad framework defined in the GATT agreement.
c. The provision of GATT are administered and enforced by WTO, Geneva.
d. None of these

Ans. (d) None of these

68. It is feared that genetically engineered microorganisms may disturb the ecosystem and its processes, in which of the following ways?

a. They may transfer genes related to virulence or pathogenesis in to the native bacterial population
b. They may cause unexpected health hazards

c. They may rapidly multiply and out complete the native microbes.

d. Both a and c

Ans. (d) Both a and c

---

69. Genetically modified plants could pose biological and ecological risks that may be summed up as which of the following?

a. Production of toxic or allergenic metabolites

b. Transmission of new traits to related sexually compatible weed species.

c. Unexpected new susceptibilities to pathogens

d. The ecosystems may be disturbed by their dispersal, persistence or altered reaction to parasites, symbionts or competitor.

e. All of the above

Ans. (e) All of the above

---

70. During assessment of risk on a case-by-case basis, which of the following factors should be considered?

a. The biological characteristics of the recipient organisms.

b. Genetic characteristics of the DNA insert, the function it specifies and/or characteristics of the modification introduced

c. Characteristics of the vector, including its origin, source and host range.

d. Taxonomic status and the relevant biological characteristics of the donor organisms.

e. All of the above

Ans. (e) All of the above

---

71. During assessment of risk for food obtained from transgenic varieties of crops, which of the following is evaluated?

a. The potential for introduced DNA to encode harmful substances

b. The fold crop that has been modified

c. Proof that known plant toxicants and important nutrients are within acceptable levels in the new variety.

d. The safety of proteins encoded by transgenes

e. All of the above

Ans. (e) All of the above

---

72. Which of the following is correct about GM foods?

a. GM food includes foods and additives obtained from genetically modified organisms.

b. European Union has adopted legislation requiring mandatory labelling of all GM food.

c. Japan has announced mandatory evaluation of GM food for potential health risk

d. US food and Drug Administration requires the food to be labelled as genetically modified only if the changes introduced through genetic engineering have an impact on the safety or nutrition of the food itself.

e. All of the above

Ans. (e) All of the above

---

73. Which of the following is not correct?

a. Oral exposure to transgenic tomato containing cry protein poses no additional risk to human and animal health

b. Cowpea trypsin inhibitors do show some adverse affects on rats in nutritional studies

c. In general, the quality of produce from Cry gene carrying transgenic crops is regarded different from that from the nontransgenic plants of the same variety

d. Significant hypertrophy of small intestine and altered enzyme activities in brush border cells occur due to wheat germ agglutinin

Ans. (c) In general, the quality of produce from Cry gene carrying transgenic crops is regarded different from that from the nontransgenic plants of the same variety

---

74. The α-amylase inhibitor from phaseolus vulgaris caused allergy when expressed in which of the following by Australian Scientists?

a. Maize   b. Peas

c. Soybean   d. Tomato

Ans. (b) Peas

---

75. The α-amylase inhibitor gene described in Q-40 was transferred to modify which of the following traits?

a. Insect resistance

b. Amino acid balance

c. Food digestibility

d. Both a and c

And. (a) Insect resistance

---

76. In case of biological containment, initially, NIH guidelines required the use of *E.coli* strains and vectors that were severely debilitated, so that they could not infect humans, survive and spread outside the laboratory, and transfer the introduced foreign genes readily in to other organisms. These objectives can be achieved using which of the following?

a. Plasmid vectors that are non-self transmissible and non-mobilizable

b. Autotrophic mutants of *E.coli*

c. Rec A-strain

d. Both a and c

Ans. (d) Both a and c

---

77. The host vector system for prokaryotes are grouped in to which of the following?

a. Host vector 1 system

b. Host vector 3 system

c. Host vector 2 system

d. Both a and c

Ans. (d) Both a and c

---

78. In case of *E.coli* the host for any HVI system is which of the following?

a. Strain K-12   b. Strain chi 1140

c. Strain K-17   d. Strain K-1777

Ans. (a) Strain K-12

---

79. The vector under host-vector I system includes which of the following?

a. Variants of vacteriophages

b. Nonconjugative plasmids

c. Derivative of nonconjugative plasmid

d. All of the above

Ans. (d) All of the above

---

80. Which of the following is correct?

a. Under 'mail box provision' a country will accept patent applications for products related to pharmaceuticals and agricultural chemicals from January 1, 1995 and keep them for consideration after the patent laws are suitably amended.

b. The member countries are required to guarantee exclusive marketing right for 5 year to each invention.

c. Both a and b

d. None of these

Ans. (c) Both a and b

---

81. Which of the following is correct about TRIPs in relation to India?

a. India is required to change its patent laws as per the broad framework of TRIPs latest by 2008.

b. India was given time till April 1999 to meet the basic commitment to TRIPs, failing which USA could call for appropriate sanctions.

c. In 2000, USA complained to WTO that India has failed to meet the basic commitments to TRIPs.

d. All of the above

Ans. (b) India was given time till April 1999 to meet the basic commitment to TRIPs, failing which USA could call for appropriate sanctions.

---

82. In India which of the following is correct?

a. Product patent are not allowed

b. A provision for grant of exclusive marketing rights has been made up to July 15, 2000.

c. A provision for grant of exclusive marketing right has been made up to December 31, 2004.

d. All of the above

Ans. (c) A provision for grant of exclusive marketing right has been made up to December 31, 2004.

---

83. The PPVFR Act 2001 recognizes the farmer's rights in which of the following respects?

a. Registrations of farmer's varieties are not allowed.

b. Freedom of farmers to save, use, sow, resow, exchange, share or sell their own farm produces, including seed.

c. Reward for the farmers engaged in the conservation of genetic resources provided that the material have been used as donors of genes in varieties registered under PPVFR Act.

d. Both b and c

Ans. (d) Both b and c

---

84. Which of the following features are concerned with protection of plant varieties and farmers Rights Act, 2001?

a. Any variety involving any technology, which is injurious to life or health of human beings, animals or plants ay be registered

b. Registration of farmer's are not allowed

c. Variety that has been 'essentially' derived' from an initial variety can be registered as a new variety.

d. All of the above

Ans. (c) Variety that has been 'essentially' derived' from an initial variety can be registered as a new variety

---

85. Which of the following features are concerned with the PPVFR Act 2001?

a. Freedom to use any registered variety for research and for creation of new varieties, except essentially derived varieties.

b. Registration of variety confers an exclusive right to produce, sell, market, distribute, import or export the varieties.

c. Compulsory license may be granted after 3 years of registration of a variety if seed of the variety is not available to the public.

d. All of the above

Ans. (d) All of the above

86. Which of the following biotechnological invention can be patented?

   a. DNA sequence and the proteins encoded, if any, by them.
   b. Micro-organism, cell lines, plant lines obtained through biotechnological approach.
   c. Bothe a and b
   d. None of these

Ans. (c) Bothe a and b

87. Which of the following feature is not concerned with the PPVFR Act 2001?

   a. Application for registration of a variety may be made in India within 2 years from the date of application for registration of the same plant variety made in the convention country.
   b. The right of PBR holder shall not be deemed infringed by a farmer who was not aware of the existence of such right'.
   c. Citizens of convention countries will have the same rights as citizens of India under the Act.
   d. The Central Govt. Is to constitute a National Gene fund.

Ans. (a) Application for registration of a variety may be made in India within 2 years from the date of application for registration of the same plant variety made in the convention country.

88. Which of the following biotechnology related matters can be patented?

   a. Process of production
   b. Process material.
   c. Application of material
   d. Any of the above

Ans. (a) Process of production

89. Methods for which of the following can be patented?

   a. Method of production
   b. Treatment of diseases
   c. Prevention of diseases
   d. Diagnosis of disease

Ans. (a) Method of production

90. In case of PPVFR Act 2001, the gene fund shall be used for which of the following?

   a. Conservation of genetic resources.
   b. Sustainable use of genetic resources
   c. Paying compensation to communities for their contributions to the development of a variety
   d. All of the above

Ans. (d) All of the above

91. Effective dissemination of plant-associated microorganisms beyond the green house can be prevented by using which of the following?

   a. Organisms which require another organisms for their survival.
   b. Organisms whose natural mode of transmission requires injury to the host.
   c. Both a and b
   d. None of these

Ans. (b) Organisms whose natural mode of transmission requires injury to the host.

92. The type of regulation necessary during field trials should depend on which of the following?

   a. Ability of the modified plants to survive in nature
   b. Their ability for dispersal and reproduction
   c. Their ability to hybridize with crop and weed plants.
   d. All of the above

Ans. (d) All of the above

93. Which of the following is correct about transmission of transgenes from one crop species to another?

   a. If male sterility is introduced in to transgenic cross-pollinated crops, it can check the movement of transgenes through pollen gratin
   b. In case of cross-pollinated species, isolation by distance is rarely sufficient to prevent inter-population mating.
   c. Both a and b
   d. None of these

Ans. (c) Both a and b

94. Which of the following is not correct about Cry proteins?

   a. The cry protein present in the soil become associated with soil clay/ humus, and become prone to microbial degradation
   b. Cry protein are rapidly degraded by the stomach juices o vertebrates
   c. They could have harmful effects on non target insect species
   d. None of the above

Ans. (a) The cry protein present in the soil become associated with soil clay/ humus, and become prone to microbial degradation

95. The survival of GEMs in nature, and gene transfer from them to native bacterial population can be minimized by which of the following strategies?

   a. Use of auxotroph mutant
   b. Use of *Rec A* strains.

c. Integration of the transgene in to the bacterial chromosome

d. Use of appropriate lethal genes to limits the survival of GEMs to the specified

e. All of the above

Ans. (e) All of the above

96. Which of the following is not correct?

a. *Rec A⁻* strain lack recombination

b. Auxotrophic mutants can survive in nature

c. Transgenes integrated in to plansmids may be transferred to other bacteria

d. Transposon vectors lacking transposase gene are not able to transpose to other bacteria

Ans. (b) Auxotrophic mutants can survive in nature

97. The *gef* containment system is based on which of the following elements?

a. The regulator gene lac I linked to the promoter pm.

b. The structural gene *gef* driven by *E.coli* promoter *Plac.*

c. Both of these

d. None of these

Ans. (c) Both of these

98. First recombinant micro-organism (Tn5- containing strain of pseudomonas fluorescens) was released in which of the following countries?

a. India

b. Australia

c. Germany

d. Netherland

Ans. (d) Netherland

99. Most of the recombinant microorganism released in the environment consisted of only a simple inactivation of genes by which of the following?

a. Genetic tagging of bacteria with specific marker.

b. Transposon insertion

c. Deletion of genes by molecular genetic procedure *in-vitro*

d. All of the above

Ans. (d) All of the above

100. Which of the following non-infectious illnesses is associated with endotoxin production?

a. Hypotension

b. Hypertension

c. Ferminization of male

d. Both b an c

Ans. (d) Both b an c

101. Which of the following non-infectious illnesses is associated with endotoxin production?

a. Hepatitis
b. Asthma

c. Flu symptoms
d. Dermatitis

Ans. (c) Flu symptoms

102. Which of the following hazards is associated with operation of bioreactor fermentation?

a. Aerosols from reactor

b. Effluent contamination of gases

c. Spillage

d. All of the above

Ans. (d) All of the above

103. Non-infections illnesses like allergic asthma and dermatitis are associated with which of the following production processes?

a. Non antibiotic
b. Brewing

c. Single cell protein
d. Antibiotic

Ans. (c) Single cell protein

104. Which of the following is correct about guidelines and regulation of bio-safety?

a. A licensing may be imposed on the export of genetically manipulated organisms.

b. A voluntary code of conduct, i.e., an international agreement between industry and governments on various biotechnological products and processes, may be promoted.

c. Appropriate legislation should be promoted in those countries that lack them.

d. All of the above

Ans. (d) All of the above

105. Which of the following standard micro-biological practices are concerned with bio-safety level 1 experiments with microorganism?

a. Access to the laboratory is restricted at the discretion of principle investigator, when the experiments are in progress.

b. All contaminated liquid or solid wastes are decontaminated before disposal.

c. Mouth pipetting is prohibited

d. All of the above

Ans. (d) All of the above

106. Which of the following is correct about parenting of genes and DNA sequences isolated from naturally occurring organisms?

a. Patents are allowed in Australia

b. The first patent was for the protein Cry A

c. The first patent was for the gent aro A

d. Patent are allowed in India

Ans. (c) The first patent was for the gent aro A

107. Which of the following is correct about gene Xa21?

a. The gene was isolated first by Dr. V. Kurian

b. Dr G.S.Khush transferred it into Oryza Sativa, named it as Xa21 and located it on chromosome 11

c. A.G.Tensely identified the molecular markers flanking Xa21

d. All of the above

Ans. (b) Dr G.S.Khush transferred it into Oryza Sativa, named it as Xa21 and located it on chromosome 11

108. Which of the following forms can not be patented in India under the provisions of Indian patents Act 1970?

a. Animals

b. DNA sequence

c. Microorganism obtained through biotechnological approach

d. All of the above

Ans. (a) Animals

109. Patent activity is the lowest in which of the following?

a. India

b. Japan

c. USA

d. Europe

Ans. (a) India

110. Which of the following is concerned with broad patents in biotechnological?

a. Patent listed in item I was challenged and the US PTO revoked it in December 1994 as a consequence of its re-examination.

b. A similar patent to Agracetus was granted in India in 1991, but it was revoked in 1994.

c. The final position of this revocation will be clear only after Agracetus has exhausted all the opportunities of appeal.

d. All of the above.

Ans. (d) All of the above.

111. Column A lists the names of companies and column B lists names of technologies/ processes for which broad patents were granted. Match both the columns carefully and select the correct option from those listed below them.

A. Enzo Biochemm, Inc.   I. Gene gun method of genetic engineering of soybean

B. Mycogen corp   II. Any method of modifying the cry gene of B. Thuringiensis

C. W.R. Grace & Co.   III. Antisense 'RNA technology'

a. A-III, B-II, C-I   b. A-II, B-III, C-I

c. A-I, B-II, C-III   d. A-III, B-I, C-II

Ans. (a) A-III, B-II, C-I

112. Column A lists the names of the companies and column B lists the traits for which broad patents were granted. Match both the columns carefully and select the correct option from those given below them.

A. Pioneer Hi-Bred   I. Insect resistance (cry. Gene)

B. Dekalb genetic crop   II. Low level of saturated fatty acids

C. Plant genetic system   III. Increased lysine content

a. A-II, B-III, C-I

b. A-III, B-II, C-I

c. A-I, B-II, C-III

d. A-III, B-I, C-III

Ans. (a) A-II, B-III, C-I

113. Column A lists the names of companies and column B lists names of the transgenic plants for which broad patents were granted. Match both the columns carefully and select the correct option from those listed below them.

A. W.R.Grace & Co.   I. Brassica family

B. DNA plant technology   II. Pepper

C. Calgene, Inc.   III. Cotton, soybean

a. B-III, A-II, C-I

b. A-III, B-II, C-I

c. A-I, B-II, C-III

d. A-II, B-III, C-I

Ans. (b) A-III, B-II, C-I

114. Which of the following is correct about the convention on biological diversity?

a. CBD recognizes the sovereign rights of nations over their genetic rsources

b. India was a signatory to the International Undertaking on Plant Genetic Resources developed by the FAO in 1983.

c. On December 29, 1993, India and 172 other nations singed this.

d. All of the above

Ans. (d) All of the above

115. Which of the following technologies and raw material were used to develop Endless Summer tomato by DNA plant Technology?

a. Antisense RNA technology and Agrobacterium tumefaciens mediated genetic transformation

b. Selectable marker hpt II

c. Both of these

d. None of these

Ans. (a) Antisense RNA technology and Agrobacterium tumefaciens mediated genetic transformation

116. Which of the following laboratory facilities are concerned with BL 1 experiments with micro-organisms?

a. Laboratory furniture must be sturdy and spaces between benches, cabinets and equipments must be accessible for cleaning.

b. Each laboratory must have a sink for hand washing

c. Bench tops must be impervious to water, and resistant to acids, alkalis, organic solvents and moderate heat.

d. All of the above

Ans. (d) All of the above

117. Which of the following standard microbiological practices are concerned with BL1 experiments with micro-organism?

a. All procedures must be performed carefully so that a mminimum of aerosols are created

b. Eating, drinking, smoking and applying cosmetics are not permitted in the laboratory premises

c. None of these

d. Both a and d

Ans. (d) Both a and d

118. In case of experiments with micro-organisms, BL2 differs from BL1 with respect to which of the following?

a. Spills and accidents involving organisms containing recombinant DNA molecules are immediately reported to the institutional bio safety committee and higher bodies concerned with bio safety

b. Access to the to the laboratory is limited when the experiment are in progress

c. Both a and b

d. None of these

Ans. (c) Both a and b

119. In case of experiments with microorganisms, BL3 has which of the following additional chief safety measures over BL2?

a. Laboratory personnel have specific training in handling pathogenic and potentially lethal agents.

b. All procedures involving the manipulation of infectious material are conducted with biological safety cabinets.

c. Both a and b

d. None of these

Ans. (c)

120. In case of experiments with microorganisms, which of the following is related to BL4?

a. Biological materials to be removed from class III cabinets in a viable state are transferred in to non-breakable sealed primary and secondary containers.

b. Entry in the laboratory is limited to only those who work in the area.

c. Personnel enter and exit the facility only through the clothing change and shower rooms.

d. All of the above

Ans. (d) All of the above

121. In case of experiments with animals, which of the following procedures is followed at all biosafety levels?

a. Animal carcass is disposed off to avoid its use as food.

b. A permanent record is maintained of the experimental use and disposal of each animal

c. Only b is correct

d. Both a and b is correct

And. (d) Both a and b is correct

122. Which of the following is correct about biosafety level 1 for animals?

a. Access to the containment area shall be limited or restricted when experimental animals are being held

b. The containment area shall not be monitored at frequent intervals

c. The animals shall not be confined to security fenced areas

d. All of the above

Ans. (a) Access to the containment area shall be limited or restricted when experimental animals are being held

123. Biosafety level 3 for animals differs from BL-2N in which of the following respects?

a. Animals room doors shall be kept closed when experiment are in progress

b. The work surfaces of containment equipment shall be decontaminated when work with organisms containing recombinant DNA is finished.

c. All animals shall be euthanized at the end of their experimental usefulness.

d. Special procedures and IBC approval shall be requied to transfer specimens to a low biosafety level area.

e. All of the above

Ans. (e) All of the above

124. In which of the following respects, BL4 for animals represents greater stringency than BL-3-N?

a. All waste from the animal rooms and laboratories shall not be decontaminated before disposal

b. The animal shower entrance exit area shall not be equipped with an chemical disinfectant shower.

c. Individuals under 16 years of age shall not be allowed entry.

d. All of the above

Ans. (c) Individuals under 16 years of age shall not be allowed entry.

125. Which of the following are related to biosafety level 2 for animals?

a. Appropriate steps should be taken to prevent exposure of laboratory personnel.

b. Eating, drinking, smoking and applying cosmetic shall be prohibited.

c. Viable biological materials are removed from the containment as in the case of BL-4 plants.

d. All of the above

Ans. (d) All of the above

126. Which of the following is correct about biosafety guidelines in India?

a. Every organization involved in research and development using recombinant DNA is required to set up an University Biosafety committee

b. The DBT has a review committee for genetic manipulation which reviews all the approvals of ongoing projects on GMOs.

c. The minority of environment and forestry has an international committee, called the Genetic Engineering Approval committee.

d. All of the above

Ans. (b) The DBT has a review committee for genetic manipulation which reviews all the approvals of ongoing projects on GMOs.

127. Which of the following is related to biosafety guidelines in India?

a. The guidelines recognise three levels of risk in the case of experiments with microorganisms.

b. Four different biosafety levels are recognised and containment facilities for each level are recommended for necessary safeguard.

c. Biological containment consists of the use of vectors and hosts in such way so that it limits the host vector survival in the environment.

d. All of the above

Ans. (d) All of the above

128. According to biosafety guidelines of India, physical containment envisages to limit the spread of dangerous microorganism by which of the following?

a. Laboratory design and facilities

b. Safety equipment

c. Both a and b

d. None of these

Ans. (c) Both a and b

129. According to biosafety guidelines of India, experiments with microorganism, plants and animals are grouped into which of following categories?

a. Category requiring intimation of initiation to competent authority

b. Category requiring review and approval by the competent authority.

c. Both of the correct

d. None of these

Ans. (c) Both of the correct

130. Which of the following is related to biosafety guidelines of India?

a. Application for recognition of research facility to carry out genetic manipulation should be made to the department of Environment before the commencement of work

b. All products obtained using recombinant DNA technology shall be subject to the general regulations normally applicable for such products.

c. The controlled release of GMOs should be done under appropriate containment facilities.

d. Pre-release tests of GMOs in agriculture should include elucidation of requirements for vegetative growth and persistence and stability in small plots and experimental fields.

e. All of the above

Ans. (e) All of the above

131. Risk assessment for transgenic plants takes into account which of the following?

a. Diagram of the expression cassette to describe fully the marker genes used.

b. Cell lines used for shuttling and amplification of the cassette.

c. None of these

d. Only a is correct

Ans. (d) Only a is correct

132. Crop yield can be stabilized by introducing which of following genes in transgenic varieties?

a. Genes for better tolerance/resistance to biotic and/or abiotic stresses

b. Genes for herbicide resistance

c. Genes for improved nutritional quality.

d. All of the above

Ans. (a) Genes for better tolerance/resistance to biotic and/or abiotic stresses

133. The PPVFR Authority began registration of plant varieties in which of the following years?

a. 2004

b. 2000

c. 2007

d. 2010

Ans. (c) 2007

134. In order to survive in an IPR hungry world, systematic, effective and continued effort must be made to train Indian scientists and technologists to enable to provide technical support for which of the following?

a. Defending patents.

b. Identifying infringements.

c. Writing 'world-class' patent based on their innovation.

d. All of the above

Ans. (d) All of the above

135. Which of the following is offered by PBR?

a. Disincentive to private companies to invest in plant breeding activities

b. Decreased competition among various organization engaged in plant breeding

c. Access to varieties developed in other countries and protected by IPR laws

d. All of the above

Ans. (c) Access to varieties developed in other countries and protected by IPR laws.

136. In order to survive in an IPR hungry world, efforts must be made to bring about which of the following in India?

a. Modernisation of Indian parliament office

b. Drastic reform of educational system to produce vibrant, innovative, committed and motivated individuals

c. Introduction of IIA in curriculum

d. Creation of Logitech data of our national resources

Ans. (b) Drastic reform of educational system to produce vibrant, innovative, committed and motivated individuals

137. IPR management involves which of the following?

a. Transfer of the IPR appropriately and at optimum value.

b. Renewal of patents and designs periodically.

c. Monitoring infringements and enforcing IPRs.

d. All of the above

Ans. (d) All of the above

138. Which of the following benefits is offered by IPRs?

a. It discourage and not safe intellectual and artistic creations

b. It enables the dissemination of new ideas and technology quickly and widely

c. Discourage investments in R & D efforts

d. None of these

Ans. (b) It enables the dissemination of new ideas and technology quickly and widely

139. Which of the following may be associated with PBR?

a. Polipolies in genetic materials for specific traits

b. Lower than the demand of seed production in order to achieve more profits

c. Decrease cost of seed

d. Higher than the demand of seed production in order to achieve more profits

Ans. (b) Lower than the demand of seed production in order to achieve more profits

140. Which of the following is an example of geographical indications?

a. Scotch whiskey

b. California whiskey

c. Champagne whiskey

d. Champion wine

Ans. (a) Scotch whiskey

141. Which of the following may be the consequence of IPR regime?

a. Adverse effects on biological diversity and ecological balance.

b. Detrimental to the livelihood of poor in developing countries.

c. Threat to food security.

d. All of the above

Ans. (d) All of the above

142. Geographical indication includes which of the following?

a. Natural products
b. Bad for handicraft
c. Not good for agriculture
d. Artificial products.

Ans. (a) Natural products

143. In the first instance, PPVFR began registration of varieties in how many of the crops?

a. 10   b. 12
c. 15   d. 20

Ans. (b) 12

144. Which of the following is not correct about geo-graphical indication?

a. The GIs do not cover manufactured products and even food products
b. India has enacted the Geographical indication Act (1999) to claim GI for a variety of goods, including 'Basmati rice'
c. Once enforced by legislation, GIs exclude others from using a GI as trademark
d. The chief requirements for GI protection is that a given quality, reputation or some other characteristic of the product be essentially attributable to the locality of its origin

Ans. (a) The GIs do not cover manufactured products and even food products

145. PPVFR Act (2001) allows registration of which of the following?

a. Breeder varieties   b. Wild varieties
c. Farmer varieties   d. All of the above

Ans. (c) Farmer varieties

146. Monitoring and tackling the IPR aspects of inventions has which of the following features?

a. May act as a disincentive for R & D efforts.
b. Enhances cost
c. Demands time
d. All of the above

Ans. (d) All of the above

147. GM food may differ from those prepared from the conventionally developed varieties with respect to which of the following?

a. A metabolic product generated by the transgene products
b. Altered levels of natural toxins and important nutrients

c. Both of the above
d. None of these

Ans. (c) Both of the above

148. The potential risk from novel DNA sequences used during transgenic development may be summed up as which of the following?

a. Protein products of transgenes or products generated by them may be toxic
b. The transgene product may be allergenic
c. Antibiotic resistance genes may be taken up by human intestinal microflora. Which, as a consequence, become resistant to these antibiotics?
d. All of the above

Ans. (d) All of the above

149. Transgenic plants could serve as vectors for transgene dissemination through which of the following?

a. DNA released form debris of transgenic plant
b. Stigma
c. Flower
d. All of the above

Ans. (a) DNA released form debris of transgenic plant

150. Which of the following is not correct?

a. Volunteers are not likely to pose problems in crops like rapeseed and mustard
b. All foods that contain more than 1% GMOs related to the different ingredients have to be labelled
c. In case of organic farming, utilization and presence of GMOs is excluded
d. In European Union, the maximum permissible limit for GMO content in conventional food products and food ingredients is 1% at the marketing stage

Ans. (a) Volunteers are not likely to pose problems in crops like rapeseed and mustard.

151. The rate of gene flow is affected by which of the following factors?

a. Mode of seed dispersal
b. Mode of pollination
c. Mode of pollution
d. Both a and b

Ans. (d) Both a and b

152. Which of the following is not correct about lectins?

a. They are involved in defence mechanism of plants
b. They are polysaccharides

c. Several lectins have been identified as food allergens.

d. None of the above

Ans. (b) They are polysaccharides

153. The international life science institute advocates which of the following criteria for assessing whether a protein poses no risk of allergy?

a. Known to cause allergies

b. It is not expressed at low levels

c. Lack of amino acid sequence similar to that of known allergens

d. All of the above

Ans. (c) Lack of amino acid sequence similar to that of known allergens.

154. In the assessment of allergenicity, the source of transgene is the first consideration; the transgene may be obtained from which of the following?

a. Less commonly allergenic food

b. Commonly allergenic food

c. Both of these

d. None of these

Ans. (c) Both of these

155. Which of the following toxic effects is associated with proteinase inhibitor?

a. Hypoplasia   b. Weight loss

c. Hyperplasia   d. None of the above

Ans. (c) Hyperplasia

156. Which of the following compounds is associated with toxic effects and is also involved in plant defence reaction/mechanism?

a. Phytoalexins   b. Alcohol

c. Thiamine   d. Thyroxin

Ans. (a) Phytoalexins

157. Which of the following is known to be a food allergen?

a. Wheat germ agglutinin b. Tryptophan inhibitor

c. Tyrosin inhibitor   d. None of the above

Ans. (a) Wheat germ agglutinin

158. Which of the following is correct about wheat germ agglutinin?

a. It is effective against insects at concentration of 10 mg/kg body weight

b. It produces cytotoxic effects in rats at a lower concentration

c. Safe food has it only at 0.3 mg/kg

d. All of the above

Ans. (d) All of the above

159. Which of the following is not correct?

a. Acute toxic effect depends on the concentration of the compound in question

b. Any outstanding insect resistant whose biochemical basis is not known should be considered as the prime candidate for toxicological evaluations

c. Transgene isolation from a food crop guarantees the food safety of the transgene product

d. None of the above

Ans. (c) Transgene isolation from a food crop guarantees the food safety of the transgene product.

160. Which of the following is not correct about bromoxynil?

a. It is toxic to fish and may cause cancer in humans.

b. It causes birth defects in laboratory animals.

c. It is a non-biodegradable herbicide.

d. Bromoxynil is absorbed through the skin.

Ans. (c) It is a non-biodegradable herbicide.

161. Transgenic crops are perceived by many to pose which of the following threats to the environment?

a. Insect resistant transgenic crops may affect target species

b. They have no adverse impact on biodiversity

c. They may alter the composition of rhizosphere and phyllosphere microflora

d. None of the above

Ans. (c) They may alter the composition of rhizosphere and phyllosphere microflora

162. Which of the following techniques can be used for minimising pollen-mediated gene flow from transgenic varieties of crops?

a. Gene tagging

b. Integration of transgene in to the chloroplast

c. Female sterility

d. All of the above

Ans. (b) Integration of transgene in to the chloroplast

163. For minimising pollent-mediated gene flow from transgenic varieties of *solanum tuberosum*, how many meters of isolation distance is recommended?

a. 50   b. 20

c. 40   d. 70

Ans. (b) 20

164. Which of the following can be used to minimise transgene transfer from transgenic varieties of crops?

a. Apomixes   b. Polyploidy

c. Cleistogamy d. Trisomy

Ans. (c) Cleistogamy

165. Seed sterility can be reduced by using which of the following technique?

    a. Recoverable block of function
    b. Cleistogamy
    c. Apomixes
    d. Transgenic mitigation

Ans. (a) Recoverable block of function

166. Strategy of temporal and tissue specific expression for preventing transgene transfer from transgenic varieties of crops is based on which of the following techniques?

    a. Inducible promoters allow expression only when the inducer is present
    b. Tapetum-specific promoters allow expression only when the suppressor is present
    c. Terminator technology
    d. Recoverable block of function

Ans. (a) Inducible promoters allow expression only when the inducer is present

167. Which of the following concerns has been expressed about the agriculture performance of transgenic varieties?

    a. Unstable transgene expression over environment product.
    b. Genetic vulnerability due to large scale cultivation of single varieties
    c. Yield drag
    d. All of the above

Ans. (d) All of the above

168. Roundup ready transgenic variety of soybean showed, on an average, how much yield decrease as compared to the non transgenic parent varieties in USA, in a comparison based on field trials at 8,200 different location?

    a. 10 %   b. 20%
    c. 5%   d. 8%

Ans. (c) 5%

169. The risk assessment in relation to transgenic crop varieties should include which of following considerations?

    a. Occurrence of wild relatives of the concerned crop in the area where transgenic varieties are to be cultivated
    b. The degree of pollinator insect activity
    c. The pest diversity of the given crop and their relative economic importance
    d. All of the above

Ans. (d) All of the above

170. In India, it is insisted upon that field trials with transgenic plants observe which of he following?

    a. Within the isolation distance, nontransgenic varieties of the crop should be planted to assess the extent and distance of pollen transfer from the transgenic plants.
    b. The isolation distance recommended for the foundation seed crop of the concerned crop be maintained.
    c. Both a and b
    d. None of these

Ans. (c) Both a and b

171. In India, it is insisted upon that field trials with transgenic plants observe which of the following?

    a. All the vegetative plants and leftover seed be destroyed by burning after the experiment.
    b. The experimental field be visited by the company authorised personnel only.
    c. Full account of transgenic seeds produced be maintained and no transgenic seed be transacted or further propagated without authorization.
    d. All of the above

Ans. (d) All of the above

172. The European Patent Convention excludes from patent protection such inventions that are contrary to the public order of morality is under the act of:

    a. Article 53 (A)   b. Article 53 (B)
    c. Article 54 (A)   d. Article 54 (B)

Ans. (a) Article 53 (A)

173. The European patent convention excludes from patent protection

    1. Plant and animal varieties
    2. Essential biological processes for the production of plants and animals under the act of
    a. Article 53 (A)
    b. Article 53 (B)
    c. Article 54 (A)
    d. Article 54 (B)

Ans. (b) Article 53 (B)

174. Intellectual property is categories into:

    a. Industrial property
    b. Artistic and Literary property
    c. Both a and b
    d. None of these

Ans. (c) Both a and b

175. The deals with protection of the expression of an idea; however it does not protect the idea itself is called:

a. Copy right
b. Industrial design
c. Geographical indication
d. Trade mark

Ans. (a) Copy right

176. The TRIPs agreement came is:

a. 1994
b. 1995
c. 1996
d. 1997

Ans. (b) 1995

177. The patent Act, 1970 was amended first time in the year of:

a. 1999
b. 1996
c. 1995
d. 1991

Ans. (a) 1999

178. The patent Act, 1970 was amended second time in the year of:

a. 1999
b. 2000
c. 2001
d. 2002

Ans. (d) 2002

179. The patent Act, 1970 was amended third time in the year of:

a. 1999
b. 2002
c. 2004
d. 2005

Ans. (d) 2005

180. The time period accorded for protection of the invention has been set uniformly for all categories of inventions at:

a. 18 year
b. 19 year
c. 20 year
d. 22 year

Ans. (c) 20 year

181. An 'invention' as a new product or process involving an inventive step and capable of industrial application under:

a. Section 2(1) (j)
b. Section 3(j)
c. Section 2(1) (ja)
d. Section 3(ja)

Ans. (a) Section 2(1) (j)

182. Patentability requirements as per the Indian patents act are:

a. It should be new
b. It should involve an inventive step

c. It should be capable of industrial application
d. All of these

Ans. (d) All of these

183. Essentially biological process falls under the exclusion of patentability under the section of the Indian Patent Act:

a. Section 2(1) (j)
b. Section 2(1) (ja)
c. Section 3(j)
d. Section 3(ja)

Ans. (c) Section 3(j)

184. The genes are not patentable when they are in the:

a. *In-situ*
b. *Ex-situ*
c. Both a and b
d. None of these

Ans. (a) *In-situ*

185. The 2001 utility examination guidelines follow the 1999 revised interim Utility Guidelines in adopting the structure of:

a. Specific, substantial and credible utility test
b. Well established utility test
c. Both a and b
d. None of these

Ans. (c) Both a and b

186. Under both 1999 and 2001 guidelines establish that a substantial utility is one that defines a:

a. Subject matter claimed
b. Real world use
c. DUS test
d. Novelty

Ans. (b) Real world use

187. A US patent (US5, 972,609) has been awarded in 1999 for a utrophin gene promoter that they may be used to control of:

a. Transcription of heterologous sequence
b. PPVFR act 2001
c. Distinctiveness
d. Uniformity

Ans. (a) Transcription of heterologous sequence

188. Indian chose to opt for a Sui generis System for protection of plant and plant varieties by enacting the:

a. Transcription of Heterologous sequence
b. PPVFR act 2001
c. Distinctiveness
d. Uniformity

Ans. (b) PPVFR act 2001

189. There has been a decreasing intellectual property activity in the area of biotechnology since:

a. 2000
b. 2001
c. 2002
d. 2003

Ans. (c) 2002

190. Which Indian organisation is more active in the are of patenting

a. ICAR
b. CSIR
c. ICMR
d. BARC

Ans. (b) CSIR

191. Some of the Indian companies active in the area of intellectual property right are:

a. Ranbaxy
b. Dabur
c. Ayur
d. All of these

Ans. (d) All of these

192. The institution of CSIR active in the area of intellectual right are:

a. NBRI
b. IICT
c. CIMAP
d. All of these

Ans. (d) All of these

193. The utility patents and the plant protection patents are granted by:

a. USPTO
b. PVTO
c. Both a and b
d. None of these

Ans. (a) USPTO

194. The plant variety protection act is granted by:

a. Plant variety protection officer
b. Plant Breeder
c. Plant protection officer
d. All of these

Ans. (a) Plant variety protection officer

195. In India, animals in whole and any part thereof are not patentable under section of PATENT Act:

a. Section 2(1) (j)
b. Section 2(1) (ja)
c. Section 3 (j)
d. Section 3(1) (j)

Ans. (c) Section 3 (j)

196. In biotechnological components that are also patentable:

a. Transformation vectors
b. Selectable marker gene
c. Reporter gene
d. All of these

Ans. (d) All of these

197. The first patent of a life form was issued on:

a. March 31, 1980
b. March 31, 1981
c. March 31, 1982
d. March 31, 1983

Ans. (c) March 31, 1982

198. Trade secret related to:

a. Certain material, e.g. bacterial strain
b. Processes
c. Formulae
d. Any of the above

Ans. (d) Any of the above

199. In the area of biotechnology, which material can be kept as trade secret?

a. Strains of microorganism
b. Cell lines
c. Production process
d. All of these

Ans. (d) All of these

200. Indian has created a National Biodiversity authority with headquarters at:

a. Chennai
b. New Delhi
c. Kolkata
d. Mumbai

Ans. (a) Chennai

201. In USA, which systems are available for protection of IPRs related to plants?

a. The plant patents Act (1930)
b. The plant variety protection act (1970)
c. The utility patents act (1985)
d. All of the above

Ans. (d) All of the above

202. Government of India has now established the PPVFR Authority with headquarters at:

a. Chennai
b. Kolkata
c. New Delhi
d. Hyderabad

Ans. (c) New Delhi

203. Which biotechnology related matters can be patented?

a. Method/process of production
b. Products
c. Application
d. Any of these

Ans. (d) Any of these

204. Monitoring and tackling the IPR aspects of invention has

    a. Demand time

    b. Enhances cost

    c. May act as a distinctive for R&D effort

    d. All of these

Ans. (d) All of these

205. PPVFR act (2001) allows registration of:

    a. Farmer's varieties

    b. Extant varieties

    c. New varieties

    d. All of these

Ans. (d) All of these

CHECK YOU GRASP

1. **Which of the following are the chief requirements for the grant of a patent?**
   a. Not novelty
   b. Usefulness is not required
   c. Inventiveness
   d. All of the above

2. **Trade secret offers which of the following advantage?**
   a. Low cost of maintaining the secret.
   b. The risk of innovation by someone else is minimized.
   c. Not effective for unlimited duration
   d. All of the above

3. **Trade secrets suffer from which of the following disadvantage?**
   a. Maintaining a trade secret itself is costly
   b. It offers protection from independent innovation/invention.
   c. It can be applied to many inventions.
   d. All of these

4. **Which of the following statements are correct about patents?**
   a. The subject matter must be ordinary
   b. In 1985, the American Supreme court ruled that a live, human made microorganism can be patented under the American patent law as a manufacture or composition of matter
   c. In 1980, the American Supreme court ruled that a live, human made microorganism can be patented under the American patent law as a manufacture or composition of matter
   d. None of these

5. **Trade secret can not be applied for which of the following invention?**
   a. Cell lines
   b. Strain of microorganism
   c. Plant varieties
   d. All of the above

6. **PPVFR Act (2001) allows registration of which of the following?**
   a. Breeder varieties
   b. Wild varieties
   c. Farmer varieties
   d. All of the above

7. **Monitoring and tackling the IPR aspects of inventions has which of the following features?**
   a. May act as a disincentive for R & D efforts.
   b. Enhances cost
   c. Demands time
   d. All of the above

8. **In case of which of the following products, an empirical approach based on data obtained through experimentation about the source of potential hazards has proved satisfactory?**
   a. Drugs
   b. Vaccines
   c. Pesticides
   d. All of the above

9. **In risk assessment, a lack of scientific knowledge or scientific consensus should not necessarily be interpreted as indicating which of the following?**
   a. Absence of risk
   b. Acceptable risk
   c. None of the these
   d. Both a and b

10. **The assessment of risk during laboratory research is usually done in which of the following steps?**
    a. Initial risk assessment
    b. Advanced risk assessment
    c. Comprehensive risk assessment
    d. Both a and c

In case of less than 80% score, go through brief Review and Glance one again from chapter

Key: 1-c   2-b   3-a   4-c   5-c   6-c   7-d   8-d   9-d   10-d

7

General Biochemistry and Metabolism

1. In beta vulgaris, the storage product of photo-synthesis is:

a. Glucose　　　　b. Lactose

c. Sucrose　　　　d. Starch

Ans. (c) Sucrose

2. Malt sugar consists of two molecules of:

a. Sucrose

b. Maltose

c. Glucose

d. Fructose

Ans. (c) Glucose

3. Examples of neutral amino acid are:

a. Lysine, Argenine, Valine

b. Proline, Lucine, Isolucine

c. Argentine, Aspatate, Alanine

d. Alanine, glycine, Valine

Ans. (d) Alanine, glycine, Valine

4. The precursor of nicotinamide and IAA is:

a. Alanine

b. Tryptophan

c. Proline

d. Glycine

Ans. (b) Tryptophan

5. Adenosine comprises:

a. Adenine and sugar

b. Adenine and phosphate

c. Adenine and tyrosine

d. None of these

Ans. (a) Adenine and sugar

6. Which vitamin is a constituent of FMN?

a. Tocoferol

b. Nicotinic acid

c. Riboflavin

d. Nicotinamide

Ans. (c) Riboflavin

7. Nocotinamide-ribose phosphate-adenine are the components of:

a. NAD　　　　b. NADH

c. NADP　　　　d. FADH2

Ans. (c) NADP

8. An organelle rich in Mn is:

a. SER　　　　b. Mitochondria

c. RER　　　　d. Ribosome

Ans. (b) Mitochondria

9. Enzyme requiring ATP essentially require:

a. Na　　　　b. Mg

c. B　　　　d. K

Ans. (b) Mg

10. A polysaccharide made up of arabinose, galactose and galacturonic acid is:

a. Pectin　　　　b. Cellulose

c. Hemicelluloses　　　　d. None of these

Ans. (c) Hemicelluloses

11. An element essential for the biosynthesis of protein is:

a. Mg　　　　b. Fe

c. N　　　　d. K

Ans. (a) Mg

12. What type of starch grains are found in wheat?

a. Simple and centric

b. Compound and centric

c. Compound and eccentric

d. All of these

Ans. (b) Compound and centric

13. Algin is a:

a. Mucoprotein　　　　b. Mucopolypeptide

c. Mucopolysacchaide　　　　d. None of these

Ans. (c) Mucopolysacchaide

14. The most abundant protein found in the biosphere is met within:

   a. Cytosol
   b. Cytoplasm
   c. Chloroplast
   d. Legumes

Ans. (c) Chloroplast

15. The most abundantly met organic compound in the biosphere is:

   a. Protein
   b. Fat
   c. Carbohydrate
   d. Cellulose

Ans. (d) Cellulose

16. Highest percentage of cellulose is found in the fibres of:

   a. Flax
   b. Wood
   c. Cotton
   d. Linter

Ans. (c) Cotton

17. An ayurvedic medicine isabgol is obtained from:

   a. Root
   b. Leaves
   c. Seeds
   d. Stem

Ans. (c) Seeds

18. Which one of the following is a water-soluble vitamin?

   a. K
   b. D
   c. C
   d. E

Ans. (c) C

19. A vitamin carotenoid in nature is:

   a. C
   b. B
   c. A
   d. K

Ans. (c) A

20. The protein part of the holoenzyme is called:

   a. Isoenzyme
   b. Ribozyme
   c. Apoenzyme
   d. Coenzyme

Ans. (c) Apoenzyme

21. A co-factor of cytochrome oxidase is:

   a. Mg
   b. Co
   c. Cu
   d. Fe

Ans. (d) Fe

22. Which of the following are coenzymes?

   a. ATP, NAD, TPP
   b. NAD, ATP, NADP
   c. FAD, FADH, AMP
   d. None of these

Ans. (a) ATP, NAD, TPP

23. A coenzyme constituent of cristae of mitochondria is:

   a. Ferredoxin
   b. Plastocynin
   c. Cytochrome
   d. NADP

Ans. (c) Cytochrome

24. An enzyme that entirely consists of mitochondria is:

   a. Amylase
   b. Catalase
   c. Carboxylase
   d. Phosphatise

Ans. (a) Amylase

25. Kinase belongs to which group of enzyme?

   a. Lyases
   b. Transferases
   c. Hydrolase
   d. Reductase

Ans. (b) Transferases

26. Enzymes which are regularly required throughout the life-time are called?

   a. Ligases
   b. Transferases
   c. Constitutive enzymes
   d. Metabolic enzymes

Ans. (c) Constitutive enzymes

27. A rare enzyme that does not contain protein is:

   a. Transferase
   b. Lyases
   c. Hydrolase
   d. Ribozyme

Ans. (d) Ribozyme

28. An enzyme that brings about rearrangement of molecular structure and forms a compound of the same molecular weight is referred to as:

   a. Protease
   b. Lipase
   c. Ligase
   d. Isomerise

Ans. (d) Isomerise

29. Blocking of active site of an enzyme is a kind of:

   a. Feed-back inhibition
   b. Non-competitive inhibition
   c. Competitive inhibition
   d. None of these

Ans. (c) Competitive inhibition

30. Which one of the following is correct in respect to competitive inhibition:

   a. ES + I = ESI
   b. E + I = EI + S = ESI
   c. E + I = EI
   d. None of these

Ans. (c) E + I = EI

31. **The best evidence of enzyme action to support lock and key theory is that:**
    a. All enzymes are made up of protein
    b. Enzymes speed up certain reaction
    c. Occurrence of competitive inhibitor
    d. Enzymes determine the direction of a reaction

Ans. (c) Occurrence of competitive inhibitor

32. **Enzyme lipase acts upon:**
    a. Fat
    b. Lipid
    c. Amino acid
    d. Carbohydrate

Ans. (a) Fat

33. **Which of the following is not an enzyme?**
    a. Papain
    b. Ptylin
    c. Zeatin
    d. Bromelain

Ans. (c) Zeatin

34. **Nitrite is formed from nitrate in plant cell during nitrogen metabolism. This process is mediated by:**
    a. Nitrate reductase
    b. Nitrate oxidase
    c. Nitrite reductase
    d. Nitrite oxidase

Ans. (c) Nitrite reductase

35. **An allosteric enzyme has**
    a. An active and one allosteric site
    b. Two active sites
    c. One active site
    d. One active site and two type of allosteric sites

Ans. (d) One active site and two type of allosteric sites

36. **The enzyme catalysing break-down without addition of water are called:**
    a. Ligases
    b. Lyases
    c. Lipase
    d. Oxidoreductase

Ans. (d) Oxidoreductase

37. **Which one of the following is a constituent of coenzyme?**
    a. Thiamine
    b. Cytosine
    c. Inulin
    d. Insulin

Ans. (a) Thiamine

38. **Carbohydrates, esterases, proteases phosphatises, sucrose, amylase and invertase belong to how many groups of enzymes?**
    a. Five
    b. Four
    c. Two
    d. One

Ans. (d) One

39. **An example of conjugated protein enzyme is:**
    a. Protease
    b. Urease
    c. Amylase
    d. All of the above

Ans. (b) Urease

40. **Which enzyme is required to digest the reserve food material found in castor?**
    a. Ligase
    b. Lipase
    c. Diastase
    d. Protease

Ans. (b) Lipase

41. **Which process is inhibited by ribozyme?**
    a. Transcription
    b. Translation
    c. Replication
    d. Translocation

Ans. (a) Transcription

42. **Non-competitive inhibitor of enzyme?**
    a. Changes enzyme structure
    b. Is a protein
    c. Block synthesis of enzyme
    d. None of these

Ans. (a) Changes enzyme structure

43. **The coenzyme FMN and FAD incorporate a vitamin in its structure which is:**
    a. Vit. C
    b. Vit. A
    c. Vit. B_2
    d. Vit. K

Ans. (c) Vit.B_2

44. **Which of the following is a Fe-porphyrin coenzyme?**
    a. FADH
    b. NAD
    c. FAD
    d. Cytochrome

Ans. (d) Cytochrome

45. **Coenzyme is often a:**
    a. Fats
    b. Lipids
    c. Protein
    d. Vitamin

Ans. (d) Vitamin

46. **Which enzyme has the efficient activity at pH = 2?**
    a. Trypsin
    b. Lysine
    c. Pepsin
    d. Ligase

Ans. (c) Pepsin

47. **The enzyme concerned with CO_2 assimilation in sugarcane is:**
    a. PEPMO
    b. PEPCO
    c. PPO
    d. PPCA

Ans. (b) PEPCO

48. What amount of light falling on earth is utilized in photosynthesis by plants?

a. 2%   b. 4%

c. 0.2%   d. 0.3%

Ans. (c) 0.2%

49. Who proposed that impure air is purified in the presence of light and green plants?

a. Priestly   b. Fleming

c. De saussure   d. None of these

Ans. (a) Priestly

50. The ration between chlorophyll a and b in most plant is:

a. 1:1   b. 2:3

c. 3:1   d. 2:4

Ans. (c) 3:1

51. Photophosphorylation process was discovered by:

a. Calvin   b. Blackman

c. Arnon   d. Emerson

Ans. (c) Arnon

52. Calvin worked on

a. Paramecium   b. Euglena

c. Spirogyra   d. Scenedesums

Ans. (d) Scenedesums

53. The main function of carotenoids in plants is:

a. Protection from photo-oxidation

b. Precursor of vit.b

c. Precursor of vit.c

d. Precursor of ABA

Ans. (a) Protection from photo-oxidation

54. Discovery of Emerson effect revealed the presence of:

a. Light and Dark reaction

b. Photorespiration

c. Photophosphorylation

d. Two photochemical reaction

Ans. (d) Two photochemical reaction

55. The main difference between Chl. a and b is that chlorophyll a:

a. Has methyl group whereas chl. b has CHO group

b. Is more oxidised from

c. Is more reduced from

d. Is linear whereas Chl.b is branched

Ans. (a) Has methyl group whereas chl. b has CHO group

56. Which colour of light is absorbed maximum in photosynthesis?

a. Red   b. Yellow

c. Orange   d. Blue

Ans. (d) Blue

57. Chlorella was first used in photosynthesis by:

a. Hill   b. Blackman

c. Warburg   d. Calvin

Ans. (c) Warburg

58. Chlorophyll b is found in:

a. Prokaryotes   b. Eukaryotes

c. Bacteria   d. None of these

Ans. (b) Eukaryotes

59. Chlorophylls are:

a. Tetrapyrroles b. Steroids

c. Vitamin   d. Chromoproteins

Ans. (a) Tetrapyrroles

60. DCPIP(dichlorophenol indophenols)is used to demonstrate:

a. Photolysis is water   b. Calvin cycle

c. Cori cycle   d. Hill reaction

Ans. (d) Hill reaction

61. The net product/s of non-cyclic electron flow in photosynthesis is /are:

a. ATP   b. O_2

c. $NADH_2$ d. All of these

Ans. (d) All of these

62. In cyclic flow of electrons during photosynthesis, the electrons from ferredoxin are accepted by:

a. Ferrodoxin   b. Plastoquinone

c. Cytochromes   d. Plastocyanin

Ans. (b) Plastoquinone

63. In photosynthesis, the energy released by the protons when they diffuse across the thylakoid membrane in to the stroma is used to produce:

a. NAD   b. $NADH_2$

c. ATP   d. AMP

Ans. (c) ATP

64. The highest amount of protein in the biome is:

a. Rubisco   b. Zein

c. Phytochrome   d. Gliadin

Ans. (a) Rubisco

65. Photolysis of water occurs in association of :
   a. PSII   b. PSI
   c. Both PSI andPSII   d. Stroma

Ans. (a) PSII

66. ADP from ATP and NADP from NADPH are regenerated in:
   a. Blackman reaction   b. Hill reaction
   c. Calvin cycle   d. None of these

Ans. (c) Calvin cycle

67. The first photochemical reaction in the process of photosynthesis is.
   a. Photolysis of water
   b. Photorespiration
   c. Excitation of chlorophylld
   d. Liberation of oxygen

Ans. (c) Excitation of chlorophylld

68. Ferredoxin is a component of:
   a. PSII   b. PSI
   c. Matrix   d. Cristae

Ans. (b) PSI

69. In photosynthesis, the conversion of PGA in to PGAL requires:
   a. NADP   b. $NADPH_2$
   c. ATP   d. Both b and c

Ans. (d) Both b and c

70. The efficiency of photosynthesis is about:
   a. 25%   b. 30%
   c. 35%   d. 40%

Ans. (d) 40%

71. PSI in photosynthesis plays an important role in:
   a. Reduction of $NADPH_2$
   b. Reduction of NADP
   c. Release of O_2 from water
   d. None of these

Ans. (b) Reduction of NADP

72. Which elements play important role in photolysis of water?
   a. Mg and Cl
   b. Mg and Mo
   c. Mn and Cl
   d. Fe and Mg

Ans. (c) Mn and Cl

73. In photosynthetic bacteria, the electron donor is:
   a. H_2O b. H_2S
   c. O_2 d. Ferredoxin

Ans. (b) H_2S

74. The assimilatory power in photosynthesis are:
   a. ATP
   b. ADP
   c. $NADPH_2$ and ATP
   d. $NADPH_2$ and ADP

Ans. (c) $NADPH_2$ and ATP

75. Which colour of light is absorbed during bacterial photosynthesis?
   a. Orange   b. Far red
   c. Red   d. Blue

Ans. (b) Far red

76. The CO_2 acceptor in chlorella or C_3 plant is:
   a. PGA   b. RuBP
   c. PEPCO   d. None of these

Ans. (b) RuBP

77. The first stable compound formed during photosynthesis in C_3 plant is:
   a. PEP   b. PCAL
   c. RuBP   d. PGA

Ans. (d) PGA

78. A process which involves more than one organelle is:
   a. Translation
   b. Transcription
   c. Photorespiration
   d. Photosynthesis

Ans. (c) Photorespiration

79. How many turns of Calvin cycle are taken to produce one hexose molecule?
   a. 3   b. 4
   c. 5   d. 6

Ans. (d) 6

80. In C_4 plants, calvin cycle occurs in:
   a. Stroma of bundle sheath chloroplast
   b. Mesophyll of chloroplast
   c. Grana of bundle sheath chloroplast
   d. None of these

Ans. (a) Stroma of bundle sheath chloroplast

81. **For the synthesis of one glucose molecule, how many ATP and NADPH₂ molecule are required?**

    a. 12 and 18   b. 6 and 12
    c. 12 and 6   d. 18 and 12

Ans. (d) 18 and 12

82. **The inhibitory effect of oxygen on the rate of photosynthesis is called**

    a. Blackman effect   b. Hill effect
    c. Warburg effect   d. Emerson effect

Ans. (c) Warburg effect

83. **The first limiting factor in nature for photosynthesis is:**

    a. H_2O b. CO_2
    c. O_2 d. Light

Ans. (b) CO_2

84. **The most efficient light for photosynthesis is:**

    a. Orange   b. Red
    c. Blue   d. Yellow

Ans. (b) Blue

85. **The ratio of photosynthesis to respiration during day time remains:**

    a. 1:5   b. 1:9
    c. 10:1   d. 10:12

Ans. (c) 10:1

86. **The law of limiting factor in photosynthesis was proposed by:**

    a. F. Blackman
    b. R. hill
    c. H. Kerb
    d. None of these

Ans. (a) F. Blackman

87. **Substrate for photorespiration is**

    a. Malic acid   b. Formaic acid
    c. Glycolate   d. Oxaloacetate

Ans. (c) Glycolate

88. **How many ATP molecules are used during synthesis of one hexose molecule in C_4 plant?**

    a. 20   b. 30
    c. 40   d. 18

Ans. (b) 30

89. **In C_4 plant, NADPH₂ are produced in:**

    a. Mesophyll chloroplast
    b. Collenchymas
    c. Bundle sheath chloroplast
    d. Both a and c

Ans. (c) Bundle sheath chloroplast

90. **Kranz type of anatomy is found in the leaves of:**

    a. Most C_4 plant
    b. Most C_3 plant
    c. Both C_3 and C_4 plant
    d. None of these

Ans. (a) Most C_4 plant

91. **In most succulent plants, CO_2 is fixed by the activity of:**

    a. PEP carboxylase
    b. RuBP carboxylase
    c. PEP oxygenase
    d. RuBP oxygenase

Ans. (a) PEP carboxylase

92. **The CO_2 acceptor in sugarcane is:**

    a. Phosphoglycolic acid
    b. Oxaloacetate
    c. PEP
    d. RuBP

Ans. (c) PEP

93. **Dimorphic chloroplast are found in:**

    a. Sugarcane   b. Rice
    c. Wheat   d. Sugarbeat

Ans. (a) Sugarcane

94. **PEPCO has an advantage as compared to RUBISCO. It is that**

    a. RUBISCO fixes CO_2 only in C_3 plants whereas pepco does it both in C_3 and C_4 plant.
    b. PEPCO is found in all chlorophyllous cells but rubisco is not
    c. RUBISCO is subjected to photorespiration but PEPCO is not
    d. None of these

Ans. (c) RUBISCO is subjected to photorespiration but PEPCO is not

95. **Tropical grasses like sugar cane show high efficiency of CO_2 fixation because of**

    a. Calvin cycle
    b. Double calvin cycle
    c. Hatch and slack cycle
    d. Warburg effect

Ans. (c) Hatch and slack cycle

96. The ratio of CO_2 reduced and oxygen release during photosynthesis is:

a. 1:1
b. 1:2
c. 1:3
d. 1:4

Ans. (a) 1:1

97. The number of quanta energy required for the synthesis of one glucose molecule is:

a. 30
b. 38
c. 40
d. 48

Ans. (d) 48

98. The light and dark reaction of photosynthesis are linked by:

a. NADP and ATP
b. $NADPH_2$
c. $NADPH_2$ and ATP
d. None of these

Ans. (c) $NADPH_2$ and ATP

99. C_4 cycle is considered as recently evolved pathway as an adaptation to:

a. Hot and dry climate
b. Dry and cold climate
c. Temperate climate
d. Dry and humid climate

Ans. (a) Hot and dry climate

100. Anoxygenic photosynthesis is a characterstic to:

a. Bacteria
b. Fungi
c. Algae
d. Higher plant

Ans. (a) Bacteria

101. One of the following is not a limiting factor in photosynthesis:

a. Co_2
b. Water
c. Light
d. O_2

Ans. (c) Light

102. Which of the following algae are used to study calvin cycle?

a. Scenedesmus and chlorococcus
b. Scenedesmus and chlorella
c. Chlorella only
d. None of these

Ans. (b) Scenedesmus and chlorella

103. Photorespiration process found in plant:

a. Injurious to plant
b. Is a defense mechanism
c. Increase photosynthetic yield
d. All of these

Ans. (b) Is a defense mechanism

104. The source of energy for CO_2 fixation is:

a. O_2
b. Temp
c. Light
d. Water

Ans. (c) Light

105. Who received the Nobel prize for working on green plant?

a. Hill
b. Khorana
c. Calvin
d. Beadle

Ans. (c) Calvin

106. Which one of the following pigments is characteristically not found in the chloroplast?

a. Chlorophyll
b. Carotene
c. Xanthophylls
d. Anthocyanin

Ans. (d) Anthocyanin

107. An example of photosynthetic inhibitor is:

a. DCPIP
b. DCMU
c. DPCIP
d. DCPIP

Ans. (b) DCMU

108. Besides water, light and CO_2, photosynthesis requires

a. NADP
b. ATP
c. RuBP
d. ADP

Ans. (c) RuBP

109. During photosynthesis, when PGA is changed in to phosphoglyceraldehyde, the following process occurs:

a. Reduction
b. Oxidation
c. Hydrolysis
d. Electrolysis

Ans. (a) Reduction

110. Cyclic photo-phosphorylation result in the formation of:

a. ADP
b. ATP
c. NADH
d. $NADPH_2$

Ans. (b) ATP

111. In the phosphorylation process, energy is derived from:

a. Glucose
b. Maltose
c. Electron
d. Cytochromes

Ans. (c) Electron

112. Which elements are required for the synthesis of chlorophyll molecule?

a. Iron and chlorine
b. Iron and calcium
c. Iron and magnesium
d. Iron and potassium

Ans. (c) Iron and magnesium

113. A water soluble pigment is:

a. Carotene   b. Anthocyanin

c. Chlorophyll   d. PEP Carboxylate

Ans. (b) Anthocyanin

114. The chloroplast contains the highest quantity of:

a. RuBP carboxylase   b. Rubp oxygenase

c. PEP carboxylase   d. PEP oxygenase

Ans. (a) RuBP carboxylase

115. An essential raw material for food manufacturing in green plant is:

a. CO_2 b. Mineral salt

c. NADPH   d. FAD

Ans. (a) CO_2

116. Rate of photosynthetic process is independent of:

a. Quality of light

b. Duration of light

c. Duration of temperature

d. Quantity of light

Ans. (b) Duration of light

117. The magnesium in a chlorophyll molecule is located in the:

a. Center of chlorophyll   b. Center of porpyrin

c. Phytol tail   d. None of these

Ans. (b) Center of porpyrin

118. The correct chemical formula for chlorophyll b is:

a. $C_{55}H_{72}O_5N_4Mg$ b. $C_{55}H_{77}O_6N_4Mg$

c. $C_{55}H_{70}O_6N_4Mg$ d. $C_{55}H_{72}O_5N_4Mg$

Ans. (c) $C_{55}H_{70}O_6N_4Mg$

119. Scientists who received the Noble prize for physiology and medicine for their work on green plant are

a. Calving and hill

b. Calvin and Borlaug

c. Bateson and purnnet

d. Beadle and tatum

Ans. (b) Calvin and Borlaug

120. Moll's malf leaf experiment shows relationship between:

a. Photosynthesis and respiration

b. Photosynthesis and light

c. Photosynthesis and CO_2

d. Photosynthesis and temp.

Ans. (c) Photosynthesis and CO_2

121. In plants, the radiant energy is stored in the form of chemical energy isn:

a. ATP   b. ADP

c. $NADPH_2$ d. Glucose

Ans. (d) Glucose

122. Starch containing plastids are called:

a. Alyloplast   b. Amyloplast

c. Aleuroplasts   d. Chloroplast

Ans. (b) Amyloplast

123. Thylakoids in grana have enzymes for:

a. C3 cycle   b. C4 cycle

c. Photophosphorylation   d. None of these

Ans. (c) Photophosphorylation

124. Which one of the following is a correct statement in reference to photosynthesis?

a. ATP molecules are formed

b. NAD molecules are formed

c. ATP molecule are not formed

d. Reduced NAD is generated

Ans. (a) ATP molecules are formed

125. Kranz type of leaf anatomy is found in plants having:

a. C_3 and C_4 cycle   b. C_2 and C_4 cycle

c. C_2 and C_3 cycle   d. None of these

Ans. (a) C_3 and C_4 cycle

126. The first stable product of carbon assimilation is:

a. Acetyl CoA   b. Pyruvic acid

c. Phosphoglyceric acid   d. RuBP

Ans. (c) Phosphoglyceric acid

127. PEPCO enzymes are found in:

a. C_3 plant   b. C_2 plant

c. C_4 plant   d. None of these

Ans. (c) C_4 plant

128. Cyclic photophosphorylation involves:

a. PSI

b. PSI and mesophyll cell

c. PSII

d. PSII and thylakoid

Ans. (a) PSI

129. The primary electron acceptor of PSI is:

a. Ferredoxin   b. Plastoquinone

c. Plastocyanin   d. Cytochrome

Ans. (a) Ferredoxin

130. The term assimilatory powers in photosynthesis refers to:

a. Reduction of CO_2
b. Oxidation of CO_2
c. Photolysis of water
d. Formation of ATP and $NADPH_2$

Ans. (d) Formation of ATP and $NADPH_2$

131. Manufacturing of fructose in C_4 path way is found in:

a. Subsidiary cell
b. Guard cell
c. Bundle sheath
d. Mesophyll cells

Ans. (c) Bundle sheath

132. Which of the following are C_4 plants?

a. Maize and wheat
b. Wheat and rice
c. Maize and ananas
d. All of these

Ans. (c) Maize and ananas

133. In C_4 cycle, in the first step:

a. CO_2 combined with PGA
b. CO_2 combined with PEP
c. CO_2 combined with RuBP
d. None of these

Ans. (b) CO_2 combined with PEP

134. During ATP synthesis, electrons pass through:

a. O_2
b. CO_2
c. Cytochrome
d. Water

Ans. (c) Cytochrome

135. During primary photochemical acts, the first active chlorophyll is located in:

a. P_{700}
b. P_{685}
c. P_{680}
d. P_{785}

Ans. (c) P_{680} .

136. C4 plnts usually lack:

a. Photorespiration
b. Transpiration
c. Calvin cycle
d. Photosynthesis

Ans. (a) Photorespiration

137. In zea mays, calvin cycle:

a. Occurs in the stroma of bundle sheath chloroplast
b. Occurs in the stroma of mesophyll cell
c. Occurs in the grana of bundle sheath chloroplast
d. None of these

Ans. (a) Occurs in the stroma of bundle sheath chloroplast

138. The initial enzyme of calvin cycle is:

a. PEP
b. PEPCO
c. CoA
d. RUBISCO

Ans. (d) RUBISCO

139. The number of ATP and NADPH2 molecules required for the synthesis of one glucose molecule is:

a. 12 and 16
b. 12 and 18
c. 18 and 12
d. 18 and 30

Ans. (c) 18 and 12

140. The CO_2 acceptor in C4 cycle is:

a. Phosphoenol pyruvate
b. Ribulose 1,5 biphoshpate
c. Oxaloacetic acid
d. Phosphoglycolic acid

Ans. (a) Phosphoenol pyruvate

141. In dark reaction:

$6CO_2 + A + 12\ NADPH + H^+ \rightarrow C_6H_{12}O_6 + 6H_2O + B + 18H_3PO_4 + 12NADP$, A and B are respectively:

a. 6 ATP and 6 ADP
b. 12 ATP and 12 ADP
c. 18 ATP and 18 ADP
d. none of these

Ans. (c) 18 ATP and 18 ADP

142. Hatch and Slack cycle is not found in:

a. Zea mays
b. Triticum aestivum
c. Oryza sataiva
d. Saccharum officinarum

Ans. (b) Triticum aestivum

143. Chemiosmotic phosphorylation depends upon:

a. ATP breaking in to ADP and Pi
b. An electrochemical gradience
c. ADP breaking in to ATP and Pi
d. None of these

Ans. (b) An electrochemical gradience

144. Quantum yield of photosynthesis declines in red light but becomes normal when it is followed by blue light. This phenomenon is called:

a. Red drop effect
b. Emerson effect
c. Englemans effect
d. Blackmans effect

Ans. (b) Emerson effect

145. Electrons excited from photosystem II pass directly to:

a. Plastoquinone
b. Plastocyanin
c. Ferredoxin
d. None of these

Ans. (a) Plastoquinone

146. Which of the following technique was used by calvin for tracing the pathway of photosynthesis?

a. Electrophoresis   b. Spectrophotometry

c. Chromatography   d. All of these

Ans. (c) Chromatography

147. Solarisation of chlorophyll is:

a. Photo-oxidation   b. Photo-reduction

c. Oxido-reduction   d. Oxido-oxidation

Ans. (a) Photo-oxidation

148. What is the common between photosynthesis and respiration?

a. Light   b. Temperature

c. Cytochromes   d. ADP formation

Ans. (c) Cytochromes

149. CO_2 fixation in C_4 pathway takes place in:

a. Subsidiary cell   b. Guard cell

c. Bundle sheath   d. Mesophyll cell

Ans. (d) Mesophyll cell

150. Who for the first time experimentally demonstrated that oxygen released during photosynthesis comes from water?

a. Ruben and kamen

b. Calvin

c. Hill and neil

d. Fleming

Ans. (a) Ruben and kamen

151. First law of thermodynamics deals with.

a. Conservation of mass

b. Conservation of both mass and energy

c. Conservation of energy

d. All of these

Ans. (c) Conservation of energy

152. First law of thermodynamics may be stated as:

a. $Q = \Delta E - W$ b. $\Delta E = Q + W$

c. $\Delta E = Q - W$ d. $W = \Delta E + Q$

Ans. (c) $\Delta E = Q - W$

153. The heat of formation of carbon dioxide is –90.4 kcal. This shows that:

a. CO_2 is isothermal compound

b. CO_2 is exothermic compound

c. CO_2 is endothermic compound

d. All of the above

Ans. (b) CO_2 is exothermic compound

154. The sign of enthalpy change "H for an endothermic reaction reaction is:

a. Positive

b. Negative

c. May be positive or negative

d. None of the above

Ans. (a) Positive

155. Heat evolved is given:

a. –ve sign   b. +ve sing

c. No sign   d. None of the above

Ans. (a) –ve sign

156. If total enthalpy of reactants and products are Hr and Hp respectively, then for an exothermic reaction:

a. $H_R > H_P$ b. $H_R < H_P$

c. $H_R = H_P$ d. None of the above

Ans. (a) $H_R > H_P$

157. Select the correct relation:

a. $Q_V = \Delta E$ b. $Q_P = -\Delta H$

c. $Q_P = QV$ d. $Q_P = \Delta E$

Ans. (a) $Q_V = \Delta E$

158. The relation between heat of a reaction of constant pressure and at constant volume is:

a. $Q_P = Q_V + \Delta n \times RT$ b. $Q_P = Q_V - \Delta n \times RT$

c. $Q_V = Q_P + \Delta n \times RT$ d. $Q_V = Q_P - \Delta n \times RT$

Ans. (a) $Q_P = Q_V + \Delta n \times RT$

159. ΔH is related to ΔE by the equation:

a. $\Delta H = \Delta E + \Delta n \times RT$

b. $\Delta H = \Delta E - \Delta n \times RT$

c. $\Delta H = \Delta E \times PV$

d. None the above

Ans. (a) $\Delta H = \Delta E + \Delta n \times RT$

160. Enthalpy H is defined as:

a. $H = E \times PV$

b. $H = E + PV$

c. $H = E - PV$

d. None of the above

Ans. (b) $H = E + PV$

161. By convention the enthalpy of an element in standard state is assumed to be:

a. 5   b. 10

c. 0   d. 100

Ans. (c) 0

162. Condition of standard state are:

   a. 2°C and 1 atm   b. 25°C and 1 atm
   c. 15°C and 1 atm   d. 5°C and 1 atm

Ans. (b) 25°C and 1 atm

163. The heat of formation of compounds:

   a. May be positive or negative
   b. Is always negative
   c. Is always positive
   d. Is zero in standard state

Ans. (a) May be positive or negative

164. Select the correct order:

   a. 1 erg > 1 joule > 1 cal
   b. 1 joule > 1 erg > 1 cal
   c. 1 erg > 1 cal > 1 joule
   d. 1 cal > 1 joule > 1 erg

Ans. (d) 1 cal > 1 joule > 1 erg

165. The heat of neutralization of a strong acid with a strong base:

   a. Depends upon the nature of acid
   b. Is a constant value
   c. Depends upon the nature of base
   d. None of the above

Ans. (b) Is a constant value

166. Heat of neutralization of acetic acid with sodium hydroxide is expected to be about:

   a. –13.7 kcal   b. –14.7 kcal
   c. –13.4 kcal   d. –15.5 kcal

Ans. (c) –13.4 kcal

167. The quantity of heat which must be supplied to decompose a compound into its elements is equal to the heat evolved during the formation of that compound from the elements." This statement is called:

   a. Le Chatelier's principle
   b. Joule's principle
   c. Hess's law
   d. Lavoisier and Laplace Law

Ans. (d) Lavoisier and Laplace Law

168. The resultant heat change in a chemical reaction is the same whether it takes place in one or several stage". This statement is called

   a. Hess's law
   b. Le Chatelier's Principle
   c. Joule Thomson principle
   d. None of the above

Ans. (a) Hess's law

169. Heat of combustion, "H, of methane, ethane, ethylene and acetylene gases are –212.8, –373.0, –337.0 and -310.5 kcal respectively at the same temperature. The best fuel among these gases is:

   a. Ethylene   b. Ethane
   c. Methane   d. Acetylene

Ans. (c) Methane

170. The equation,

$$c(s) + \frac{1}{2}O_2(g) = CO(g);\ \Delta H = -26.4\ kcal$$ **shows that:**

   a. Carbon monoxide is endothermic compound
   b. Carbon monoxide is exothermic compound
   c. Reaction is endothermic
   d. Above reaction is not possible

Ans. (b) Carbon monoxide is exothermic compound

171. If no heat is transferred to and from the system during a process, the process is called:

   a. Adiabatic   b. Isothermal
   c. Isobaric   d. Cyclic

Ans. (a) Adiabatic

172. If temperature is kept constant throughout a process, the process is called:

   a. Isobestic   b. Isobaric
   c. Isothermal   d. Adiabatic

Ans. (c) Isothermal

173. The heat of combustion, ΔH, of hydrogen gas at 25°C is –68.4 kcal. The heat of formation of water liquid at 25°C

   a. – 68.4 kcal   b. – 38.4 kcal
   c. – 92.4 kcal   d. None of the above

Ans. (a) – 68.4 kcal

174. The apparatus used from measuring the heat of reactions at constant volume is called:

   a. Colorimeter   b. Pyrometer
   c. Calorimeter   d. Pyknometer

Ans. (c) Calorimeter

175. The bond energy of C–H bond in CH_4 from thermo-chemical equation, $C(g) + 4H(g) \rightarrow CH_4(g)$; ΔH= –397.8 kcal is expected to be about:

   a. +99.45 kcal
   b. +379.8 kcal
   c. +100 kcal
   d. +95.0 kcal

Ans. (a) +99.45 kcal

176. The heat of reaction does not depend upon:

a. Physical state of reactants and products

b. The method by which final products are obtained from reactants

c. Temperature of the reaction

d. Whether the reactions is carried out at constant pressure or at constant volume

Ans. (b) The method by which final products are obtained from reactants

177. The reaction, $N_2(g) + O_2(g) = 2NO(g)$; "H = +21.6 is:

a. Isothermic   b. Endothermic

c. Explosive   d. Exothermic

Ans. (b) Endothermic

178. In the reaction, $H_2(g) + Cl_2(g) = 2HCl(g) + 44.0$ kcal:

a. Enthalpy of products is equal to the enthalpy of reactant

b. Enthalpy of products is twice the enthalpy of reactant

c. Enthalpy of products is greater than the enthalpy of reactant

d. None of these

Ans. (c) Enthalpy of products is greater than the enthalpy of reactant

179. Heat of formation of CO(g) and CO2(g) are –26.4 and –94.0 kcal respectively. The heat of combustion of carbon monoxide is:

a. +120.0 kcal   b. – 67.6 kcal

c. + 35.4 kcal   d. – 68.0 kcal

And. (b) – 67.6 kcal

180. An endothermic reaction is one in which?

a. Heat is converted into electricity

b. Heat is absorbed

c. Heat is given out

d. Heat is converted into mechanical work

Ans. (b) Heat is absorbed

181. Which wavelength of light is absorbed maximum by chlorophyll a?

a. 400 nm   b. 690 nm

c. 695 nm   d. 680 nm

Ans. (d) 680 nm

182. What is the by product of bacterial photosynthesis?

a. H_2S b. S

c. K   d. O_2

Ans. (b) S

183. Photosynthetic bacteria do not contain:

a. PS I   b. Plastocynin

c. PS II   d. Both a and b

Ans. (c) PS II

184. Bacterial photosynthesis involves:

a. PS I only   b. PS II only

c. Both PS I and PS II   d. None of these

Ans. (a) PS I only

185. Following are chemosynthetic bacteria:

a. Sulphur bacteria   b. Nitrifying bacteria

c. Methane becteria   d. All of these

Ans. (d) All of these

186. Which process was first discovered in Rhodospirillum rubrum?

a. Phosphorylation

b. Cyclic photophosphorylation

c. Non-cyclic photophosphorylation

d. Photolysis of water

Ans. (b) Cyclic photophosphorylation

187. Substrate for photorespiration is:

a. Malic acid   b. Formic acid

c. Glycolate   d. Glucornic acid

Ans. (c) Glycolate

188. Photorespiration involves:

a. Glyoxylate cycle   b. Glycolate cycle

c. Cori cycle   d. None of these

Ans. (b) Glycolate cycle

189. RUBISCO behaves like an axygenase when:

a. Temperature is increase

b. Co_2 is reduce

c. O_2/CO_2 ratio is increased

d. All of these

Ans. (d) All of these

190. Which of the following is produced as a by-product during photorespiration?

a. O_2 b. H_2O

c. CO_2 d. H_2O_2

Ans. (d) H_2O_2

191. Transamination reaction occurs during:

a. Respiration   b. Transpiration

c. Photosynthesis   d. Photorespiration

Ans. (d) Photorespiration

192. NAD is reduced to NADH2 in:

a. Transpiration
b. Respiration
c. Photorespiration
d. None of these

Ans. (c) Photorespiration

193. In C3 plants like paddy, the photosynthetic yield is reduced due to:

a. Transpiration
b. Respiratioin
c. Photosynthesis
d. None of these

Ans. (b) Respiratioin

194. Which of the following processes protect oxidation of chlorophyll?

a. Photorespiration
b. Transpiration
c. Photosynthesis
d. Respiration

Ans. (a) Photorespiration

195. Banana fruits are rich in starch, but how does it reach in the fruit is correctly explained is:

a. Starch grains are transported through xylem
b. Sucrose is transported to fruit where it polymerises in to starch
c. Starch grains are transported through phloem
d. None of these

Ans. (b) Sucrose is transported to fruit where it polymerises in to starch

196. The photosynthetic products are translocated to various parts of plant in the form of

a. Maltose
b. Sucrose
c. Glucose
d. Starch

Ans. (b) Sucrose

197. In a ringed plant:

a. Shoot die first
b. Root die first
c. Both die simultaneously
d. None of these

Ans. (b) Root die first

198. Cucurbitaceous plants are least affected by ringing because of:

a. Large cambium cells
b. External phloem
c. Internal phloem
d. Regeneration of phloem

Ans. (c) Internal phloem

199. Photorespiration of favoured by:

a. Low O_2 and low CO_2
b. High CO_2 and low O_2
c. High O_2 and low CO_2
d. None of these

Ans. (c) High O_2 and low CO_2

200. A cell organelle associated with photorespiration is:

a. Lysosome
b. Peroxisome
c. Mitochondria
d. Ribosome

Ans. (b) Lysosome

201. Plants are considered purifiers of air due to process of:

a. Respiration
b. Transpiration
c. Photosynthesis
d. Transcription

Ans. (c) Photosynthesis

202. In respiration there is a conversion of :

a. Kinetic in to potential energy
b. Potential in to kinetic energy
c. Radiant in to kinetic energy
d. All of these

Ans. (b) Potential in to kinetic energy

203. When fatty seeds are maturing, the R.Q. will be

a. More than unity
b. Unity
c. Less than unity
d. Equal to unity

Ans. (a) More than unity

204. The connecting link between glycolysis and krebs cycle is:

a. Acetyl CoA
b. Pyruvic acid
c. Cytochromes
d. None of these

Ans. (a) Acetyl CoA

205. Krebs cycle takes place in mitochondria in its:

a. Matrix
b. F1 partical
c. Inner membrane
d. Outermembrane

Ans. (a) Matrix

206. Krebs cycle starts with the formation of a six carbon compound from a reaction in between:

a. Pyruvic acid and Acetyl CoA
b. Oxaloacetic acid and Acetyl CoA
c. Oxaloacetic acid and Acetyl CoA
d. None of these

Ans. (c) Oxaloacetic acid and Acetyl CoA

207. During the conversion of pyruvic acid in to acetyl CoA, following are formed:

a. CO_2 and water
b. O_2 and water
c. CO_2 and NADH2
d. CO_2 and ATP

Ans. (c) CO_2 and NADH2

208. In chlorella, when one molecule of glucose is aerobically and completely oxidised, the number of ATP molecules formed are:

    a. 6   b. 12
    c. 24   d. 36

Ans. (d) 36

209. Guanosine triphosphate is formed during conversion of:

    a. Succinyl CoA in to succinic acid
    b. Succinic acid in to fumaric acid
    c. Fumaric acid in to malic acid
    d. None of these

Ans. (a) Succinyl CoA in to succinic acid

210. The universal hydrogen acceptor is:

    a. FAD   b. NADPH
    c. ATP   d. NAD

Ans. (d) NAD

211. The efficiency of aerobic respiration is

    a. 45%   b. 50%
    c. 60%   d. 75%

Ans. (b) 50%

212. In krebs cycle, the mineral activator required for enzyme aconitase is :

    a. Mg   b. Fe
    c. Ca   d. Zn

Ans. (b) Fe

213. During aerobic respirations, the substrate which enters the mitochondria is:

    a. Glucose   b. Sucrose
    c. Pryuvic acid   d. Acetyl CoA

Ans. (c) Pryuvic acid

214. In prokaryotes, the complete oxidation of a molecule of glucose results in net gain of

    a. 2 molecules of ATP
    b. 36 molecules of ATP
    c. 18 molecules of ATP
    d. 4 molecules of ATP

Ans. (b) 36 molecules of ATP

215. Stearic acid is oxidised in:

    a. Ribosome
    b. Peroxisome
    c. Cytoplasm
    d. Mitochondria

Ans. (c and d) Cytoplasm and Mitochondria

216. Cut apple fruits when kept dipped in ascorbic acid do not turn brown because ascorbic acid

    a. Inhibits activity of polyphenol oxidase
    b. Prevents drying of cut surface
    c. Repairs all injury caused by cutting
    d. All of these

Ans. (a) Inhibits activity of polyphenol oxidase

217. Which one of the following has an inbibitory effect on respiration?

    a. CO_2 b. O_2
    c. N   d. B

Ans. (a) CO_2

218. The oxidation of ethyl alcohol takes place in :

    a. Ribosome   b. Peroxisome
    c. Mitochondria   d. Cytosol

Ans. (c) Mitochondria

219. Which one of the following has higher amount of energy?

    a. FAD   b. NAD
    c. FADH2   d. NADH2

Ans. (a) FAD

220. What will be the value of RQ in Bryophyllum leaves during day time?

    a. Less than unity   b. More than unity
    c. Equal to unity   d. Zero

Ans. (d) Zero

221. Cut surfaces of fruits and vegetables often become dark because:

    a. Dirty knife makes it dark
    b. Dust of air makes it dark
    c. Tannins are formed
    d. Oxidation of tannic acid due to presence of iron in traces from knife

Ans. (d) Oxidation of tannic acid due to presence of iron in traces from knife

222. Which one of the following is a polluting organelle?

    a. Mitochondria   b. Ribosome
    c. Lysosome   d. Peroxisome

Ans. (a) Mitochondria

223. The enzyme carboxylase requires amineral activator. It is

    a. Mg   b. K
    c. Ca   d. Fe

Ans. (a) Mg

224. How many ATP molecules are formed on complete oxidation of a glucose molecule through hexose monophosphate shunt cycle?

a. 2　　　　　　　　b. 4
c. 36　　　　　　　d. 38

Ans. (c) 36

225. The correct sequence of Krebs cycle is:

a. Isocitric acid → oxalosuccinic acid → citric acid
b. Isocitric acid → citric acid → alpha keto glutaric acid
c. Isocitric acid → oxalosuccinic acid → alpha ketoglutaric acid
d. None of these

Ans. (c) Isocitric acid → oxalosuccinic acid → alpha ketoglutaric acid

226. How many ATP molecules are formed from complete oxidation of acetyl CoA:

a. 6 ATP　　　　　b. 12 ATP
c. 18 ATP　　　　d. 24 ATP

Ans. (b) 12 ATP

227. The increased rate of respiration during fruit ripening is called:

a. Climacteric　　b. Pasteur effect
c. Photosynthesis　d. Fermentation

Ans. (a) Climacteric

228. Which of the following causes loss of two protons and two electron:

a. Fermentation
b. Dehydrogenation
c. Dehydration
d. Carboxylation

Ans. (b) Dehydrogenation

229. Where does formation of Acetyl CoA from pyruvic acid take place?

a. Ribosome
b. Mitochondria
c. Glyoxysome
d. Cytosol

Ans. (b) Mitochondria

230. An organelle involved with the break down of fats before final oxidation is:

a. Mitochondria
b. Ribosome
c. Glyoxysome
d. Cytosol

Ans. (c) Glyoxysome

231. Potato tubers are larger in plants grown at Darjeeling than grown in Andhra Pradesh. It is because there the rate of:

a. Respiration is high
b. Photosynthesis is high
c. Respiration is low
d. None of these

Ans. (c) Respiration is low

232. An indispensable role in energy metabolism is played by:

a. Phosphorus　　b. Potassium
c. Iron　　　　　d. Calcium

Ans. (a) Phosphorus

233. In glycolysis, there is a net gain of 2 ATP molecules and two molecules of:

a. FADH2　　　　b. NADH2
c. NADPH2　　　d. NAD

Ans. (b) NADH2

234. In TCA cycle, the hydrogen atoms removed at succinate level are accepted by:

a. ATP　　　　　b. NAD
c. FAD　　　　　d. CoA

Ans. (c) FAD

235. R.Q. is higher when respiratory substrate is:

a. Glucose　　　　b. Sucrose
c. Formic acid　　d. Malic acid

Ans. (d) Malic acid

236. In hexose monophosphate shunt, the hydrogen acceptor is:

a. FAD　　　　　b. NAD
c. NADP　　　　d. FADH

Ans. (c) NADP

237. R.Q. of C39H74O6 is:

a. 0.55　　　　　b. 1.12
c. 0.7　　　　　d. 1.3

Ans. (c) 0.7

238. The factors required to link glycolysis with organic acid cycle are:

a. NAD and CoA
b. Lipic acid
c. TPP and Mg
d. All of these

Ans. (d) All of these

239. The ratio os energy released between anaerobic and aerobic respiration:

a. 1:2 b. 1:3
c. 1:15 d. 1:18

Ans. (d) 1:18

240. The number of CO_2 molecule released between anaerobic and aerobic respiration is:

a. 0 b. 1
c. 2 d. 3

Ans. (a) 0

241. How many NADH2 are produced during the aerobic oxidation of alpha ketogutarate:

a. 1 b. 2
c. 3 d. 4

Ans. (b) 2

242. The connecting link between β-oxidation and Krebs cycle is:

a. Malic acid b. Citric acid
c. Acetyl CoA d. None of these

Ans. (d) None of these

243. In photosynthesis and respiration, the energy is derived form:

a. Electron flow across cytochromes
b. Oxygen
c. CO_2
d. All of the above

244. Plants can convert fatty acids to sugars by a process called:

a. Calvin cycle
b. Krebs cycle
c. Glycolysis
d. Glyoxylate cycle

Ans. (d) Glyoxylate cycle

245. R.Q. of germinating caster seed is:

a. 1 b. >1
c. <1 d. 2

Ans. (c) <1

246. The glycolate metabolism occurs in:

a. Mitochondria
b. Lysosomes
c. Peroxisomes
d. Ribosome

Ans. (c) Peroxisomes

247. Oxidative phosphorylation involves simultaneous oxidation and phosphorylation to finally produce:

a. ATP b. NAD
c. FAD d. FADH

Ans. (b) NAD

248. The activity of enzyme hexokinase, which catalyse glucose to glucose 6-posphate. Is inhibited by glucose 6-phosphate, it is an example of:

a. Competitive inhibition
b. Non competitive inhibition
c. Feedback allosteric inhibition
d. None of these

Ans. (c) Feedback allosteric inhibition

249. An example of polycistronic enzyme is:

a. Pepsin b. Rennin
c. Papin d. RNA polymerase

Ans. (d) RNA polymerase

250. Enzyme ligase is used for:

a. Joining the pieces of DNA
b. Denaturation of DNA
c. Digestion of fat
d. Splitting of DNA

Ans. (a) Joining the pieces of DNA

251. A bacterium having radioactive thymidine is allowed to multiply in an medium containing non-radioactive thymidine for two generation. What percentage of bacteria should contain radioactive DNA?

a. 20 b. 30
c. 40 d. 50

Ans. (d) 50

252. Replication of DNA takes place in the presence of:

a. DNA polymerase and DNA ligase
b. DNA polymerase, ligase and RNA polymerase
c. Topoisomrase, ligase, nuclease
d. DNA polymerase only

Ans. (b) DNA polymerase, ligase and RNA polymerase

253. DNA replication is:

a. Semi-continuous and conservative
b. Discontinuous and semi conservative
c. Conservative and semi discontinuous
d. None of these

Ans. (b) Discontinuous and semi conservative

254. **One of the following statement is incorrect with regards to β-DNA:**
    a. A + G = C + T
    b. A + T = C + G
    c. A + C = G + T
    d. None of these

Ans. (b) A + T = C + G

255. **Which of the following plays important role in breaking and reassembling one strand of DNA?**
    a. Topoisomerase
    b. Ligase
    c. Helicase
    d. Single strand binding protein

Ans. (a) Topoisomerase

256. **The direction of DNA replication is:**
    a. 5′ → 3′
    b. 3′ → 5′
    c. 2′ → 3′
    d. All of the above

Ans. (a) 5′ → 3′

257. **The okazaki fragments consist of :**
    a. DNA + RNA
    b. DNA + PRIMER
    c. DNA ONLY
    d. RNA ONLY

Ans. (c) DNA ONLY

258. **The amino acid is attached to t-RNA in its.**
    a. 5′ end
    b. 3′ end
    c. Varies from place to place
    d. Anticodon end

Ans. (b) 3′ end

259. **Which one is the most stable kind of RNA found in a cell?**
    a. r RNA
    b. t RNA
    c. m RNA
    d. hn RNA

Ans. (d) hn RNA

260. **The enzyme primase is infact:**
    a. DNA polymerase I
    b. RNA polymerase
    c. Helicase
    d. Topoisomerase

Ans. (a) DNA polymerase I

261. **The role of sigma factor in transcription is:**
    a. Initiation
    b. Elongation
    c. Termination
    d. Translocation

Ans. (a) Initiation

262. **The initiator codon is:**
    a. UUU
    b. AUG
    c. UGA
    d. GGG

Ans. (b) AUG

263. **In eukaryotes, m RNA is formed by:**
    a. DNA
    b. RNA
    c. hn RNA
    d. All of these

Ans. (c) hn RNA

264. **In an operon, the RNA polymerase binds to:**
    a. Repressor
    b. Promoter
    c. Operator
    d. Regulator

Ans. (b) Promoter

265. **How many sense codons are found in a eukaryotic cell?**
    a. 46
    b. 64
    c. 61
    d. 62

Ans. (c) 61

266. **In mitochondria, how many t RNA can read codons for twenty amino acid?**
    a. 22
    b. 23
    c. 24
    d. 25

Ans. (a) 22

267. **The discovery of replication of DNA has been made on:**
    a. Neurospora crassa
    b. Drosophila
    c. *E. coli*
    d. None of these

Ans. (c) *E. coli*

268. **The popular name Kornberg enzyme refer to:**
    a. DNA polymerase
    b. RNA polymerase
    c. Transcriptase
    d. Endonuclease

Ans. (a) DNA polymerase

269. **Which one of the following does not code for any protein?**
    a. Introns
    b. Exons
    c. Overlapping gene
    d. None of these

Ans. (a) Introns

270. **When a single anticodon can recognise more than one codon of m-RNA, it refers to:**
    a. Gene flow hypothesis
    b. Wobble hypothesis
    c. Template hypothesis
    d. None of these

Ans. (b) Wobble hypothesis

271. The translation termination triplet is:

a. UGG   b. AAU

c. AUG   d. UAA

Ans. (d) UAA

272. DNA is transcribed by some viral RAN using the enzyme:

a. Endonuclease   b. RNA polymerase

c. Reverse transcriptase   d. Helicase

Ans. (c) Reverse transcriptase

273. Constitutive genes are those genes which are active:

a. During differentiation stages

b. During developmental stage

c. Throughout life time

d. At any stage of life

Ans. (c) Throughout life time

274. Enzymes synthesised in lac operon are:

a. Lactase, permease and glactosidase

b. Permease, glactase and lactase

c. Permease, galactosidse and transacetylase

d. None of these

Ans. (c) Permease, galactosidse and transacetylase

275. In lac operon model, an operon consists of:

a. One operator gene and one structural gene

b. One promoter gene and one structural gene

c. Regulator gene, promoter gene and operator gene

d. None of these

Ans. (b) One promoter gene and one structural gene

276. In tryptophan operon, a repressor consists of co-repressor and apo-repressor. These two are made up of:

a. Tryptophan and protein

b. RNA and tryptophan

c. DNA and tryptophan

d. RNA and protein

Ans. (a) Tryptophan and protein

277. The colinearity hypothesis indicates that:

a. The sequence of nucleotides in gene correlates with the sequence of amino acids in protein

b. Genes are arranged linearly in both strands of DNA

c. Genes afe arranged linearly in both strands of RNA

d. None of these

Ans. (a) The sequence of nucleotides in gene correlates with the sequence of amino acids in protein

278. Which is the most short lived RNA?

a. r RNA   b. m RNA

c. t RNA   d. None of these

Ans. (b

279. Mark the incorrect match:

a. HIV – AIDS

b. TMV – dsDNA

c. TMV – ssDNA

d. Capsid protein coat of virus

Ans. (c) TMV – ssDNA

280. Enzyme important in genetic engineering are:

a. Helicase

b. Ligase

c. Topoisomerase

d. Restriction enzymes

e. Both a and d

Ans. (e) Both a and d

281. Which of the following is general formula of monosaccharides?

a. $Cn(H_2O)_{2n}$ b. $C_2n(H_2O)$

c. $Cn(H_2O)_n$ d. $Cn(HO)_n$

Ans. (c) $Cn(H_2O)_n$

282. Reducing sugar having:

a. A free keto group

b. A free aldehyde group

c. OH group at one end

d. Free aldenyde or keto group

Ans. (d) Free aldenyde or keto group

283. Which of the following is a imino acid?

a. Asparagines   b. Proline

c. Glycine   d. Threonine

Ans. (b) Proline

284. Which amino acid have longest side chain?

a. Lysine and leucine   b. Arginine

c. Arginine and lysine   d. Asparagine

Ans. (c) Arginine and lysine

285. Polysaccharides are polymers of simple sugars which are covalently linked by :

a. Phosphodiester bonds

b. Glycosidic bonds

c. Peptide bonds

d. Hydrogen bonds

Ans. (b) Glycosidic bonds

286. Cellulose and starch are glucose polymers but differ in which of the following:

i. Starch is soluble whereas cellulose is insoluble

ii. Glucose polymers in cellulose linked by b(1–4) whereas in starch by a(1–4) linkage

iii. Cellulose is linear whereas starch is branched polymer

iv. a(1–4) linkage present in starch but absent in cellulose

Choose the correct answer:

a. i, ii, iv
b. i, ii, iii, iv
c. i, ii, iii
d. i, ii only

Ans. (b) i, ii, iii, iv

287. Chitin is found in fungal cell walls and in exoskeleton of insects and crustaceans. The monomer unit of chitin is :

a. Galactose
b. Fructose
c. Glucose
d. N-acetyl glucosamine

Ans. (d) N-acetyl glucosamine

288. Glycogen is a :

a. Polymer of fructose
b. Linear polymer
c. Branched polymer
d. Polymer of galactose

Ans. (c) Branched polymer

289. Which of the following amino acid have aromatic side chains?

a. Tryptophane
b. Tyrosine
c. Phenylalanine
d. All of these

Ans. (b) Tyrosine

290. None-polar aliphatic side chains are present in :

a. Glutamine
b. Asparagine
c. Alanine
d. Cystine

Ans. (c) Alanine

291. A-carboxyl group of one amino acid is covalently linked to the α-amino group of next amino acid by

a. Sulphide bond
b. Amide bond
c. Hydrogen bond
d. Phosphodiester bond

Ans. (b) Amide bond

292. α-helix is a sencondary structure of protein. α-right-handed helix contain:

a. 2.6 amino acid residues per turn
b. 4.6 amino acid residues per turn
c. 3.6 amino acid residues per turn
d. 5.6 amino acid residues per turn

Ans. (c) 3.6 amino acid residues per turn

293. β-pleated sheet present in:

a. Primary proteins
b. Fibroin
c. Globular protein
d. None of these

Ans. (b) Fibroin

294. The correct folding of tertiary proteins *in vivo* is assisted by proteins called :

a. Domains
b. Motifs
c. Chaperones
d. Families

Ans. (c) Chaperones

295. Cholesterol and other lipids are transported to specific targets by lipoproteins. In blood cholesterol is carried out by :

a. VLDL
b. LDL
c. IDL
d. DDT

Ans. (b) LDL

296. Gangliosides are carbohydrate rich sphingolipids that contain acidic sugars. These acidic sugars are called :

a. α-ketoglutaric acid
b. Aspartic acid
c. Sialic acid
d. Amino acids

Ans. (c) Sialic acid

297. which of the following is fatty acid containing compound ?

a. Sugarcane juice
b. Waxes
c. Triacylglycerol
d. Both 'a' 'b'

Ans. (d) Both 'a' 'b'

298. The double bonds of all naturally occurring unsaturated fatty acids are in the:

a. d-configuration
b. Trans-configuration
c. Cis-configuration
d. L-configuration

Ans. (c) Cis-configuration

299. The melting point of fatty acids is influenced by:

a. Length and degree of unstauration of hydrocarbon chain
b. Only degree of unsaturation
c. Only length of hydrocarbon chain
d. None of the above

Ans. (a) Length and degree of unstauration of hydrocarbon chain

300. The number of t-RNA molecules in every cell is at least :

a. 15
b. 10
c. 20
d. 25

Ans. (c) 20

301. The C_4, C_5 and N_3 of pyrimidine base are derived from:

   a. Aspartic acid   b. Serine
   c. Glutamic acid   d. Glycine

Ans. (a) Aspartic acid

302. A portion of uric acid is converted to urea and ammonia by intestinal:

   a. Urogenolysis   b. Ureotolysis
   c. Uricolysis   d. Ureolysis

Ans. (c) Uricolysis

303. The end product of purine catabolism in other mammals except man is:

   a. Ammonia   b. Allantonin
   c. Uric acid   d. Creatinine

Ans. (b)

304. The number of nucleotide pairs present in one turn of DNA is:

   a. 10   b. 6
   c. 4   d. 8

Ans. (a) 10

305. The N_3 and N_9 of purine are derived from the amide nitrogen of:

   a. Glutamate   b. Asparagines
   c. Glutamine   d. Aspartic acid

Ans. (c) Glutamine

306. The net excretion of total uric acid in 24 hours in a normal man is:

   a. 300–500 mg
   b. 200–400 mg
   c. 100–300 mg
   d. 400–600 mg

Ans. (d) 400–600 mg

307. The three important units of DNA are:

   a. Bases, 3-deoxyribose and phosphoric acid
   b. Bases, ribose and phosphoric acid
   c. Bases, 2-deoxyribose and phosphoric acid
   d. All of these above

Ans. (c) Bases, 2-deoxyribose and phosphoric acid

308. DNA is denatured by:

   a. Acid
   b. Alkali
   c. Heat
   d. All of these

Ans. (d) All of these

309. Synthesis of RNA molecule is terminated by a signal by a signal which is recognized by:

   a. δ factor   b. p-(Rho) factor
   c. α-factor   d. σ factor

Ans. (b) p-(Rho) factor

310. The carbon atoms at positions 4 and 5 and the N atom at position 7 of purine base are supplied from:

   a. Valine   b. Glycine
   c. Alanine   d. Serine

Ans. (b) Glycine

311. All α-amino acids are optically active *except*:

   a. Glycine   b. Alanine
   c. Serine   d. Phenylalanine

Ans. (c) Serine

312. In many proteins, the hydrogen bonding produces a regular coiled arrangement called :

   a. γ-helix   b. β-helix
   c. α-helix   d. δ-helix

Ans. (c) α-helix

313. α-helix is stabilized by:

   a. Disulphide bond   b. Covalent bond
   c. Ionic bond   d. Hydrogen bond

Ans. (d) Hydrogen bond

314. The distance travelled per turn of α-helix is:

   a. 0.54 nm   b. 0.44 nm
   c. 0.34 nm   d. 0.64 nm

Ans. (a) 0.54 nm

315. The space covered by each amino acid residue of α-helix is:

   a. 0.25 nm   b. 0.18 nm
   c. 0.15 nm   d. 0.35 nm

Ans. (c) 0.15 nm

316. Glutamate dehydrogenase is a:

   a. Dimer   b. Monomer
   c. Tetramer   d. All of these

Ans. (c) Tetramer

317. When egg albumin is coagulated (by heating)

   a. Only tertiary structure is changed
   b. Only primary structure is changed
   c. Secondary and tertiary structures are changed
   d. Only secondary structure is changed

Ans. (c) Secondary and tertiary structures are changed

318. Oxidative conversion of many amino acids to their corresponding a-keto acids occurs in mammalian:

 a. Adipose tissue
 b. Pancreae
 c. Intestine
 d. Liver and kidney

Ans. (d) Liver and kidney

319. Synthesis of glutamine is accompanied by the hydrolysis of:

 a. ATP
 b. ADP
 c. TPP
 d. Creatine phosphate

Ans. (a) ATP

320. In brain, the major mechanism for removal of ammonia is the formation of :

 a. Asparagines
 b. Aspartate
 c. Glutamine
 d. Glutamic acid

Ans. (c) Glutamine

321. The metabolism of protein is integrated with that of carbohydrate and fat through:

 a. Malate
 b. Oxaloacetate
 c. Isocitrate
 d. Citrate

Ans. (b) Oxaloacetate

322. Sulphur of sulphur containing amino acid is removed as:

 a. SO_2
 b. $BaSO_4$
 c. H_2SO_4
 d. SO_3

Ans. (c) H_2SO_4

323. Transamination is a:

 a. Physical process
 b. Irreversible process
 c. Reversible process
 d. None of these

Ans. (c) Reversible process

324. Which of the following can not undergo transamination?

 a. Threonine
 b. Alanine
 c. Serine
 d. Valine

Ans. (a) Threonine

325. The process of transamination requires:

 a. FAD
 b. ATP
 c. NAD^+
 d. PLP

Ans. (d) PLP

326. In small intestine trypsin hydrolyses peptide linkage containing:

 a. Aspartate
 b. Serine
 c. Arginine
 d. Histidine

Ans. (c) Arginine

327. The unwanted amino acids abstracted from the tissues are either used up by the tissue or in the liver converted into:

 a. Ammonia
 b. Urea
 c. Uric acid
 d. Ammonium salt

Ans. (b) Urea

328. In humans, nitrogen of amino acid is removed as:

 a. Uric acid
 b. Ammonia
 c. Urea
 d. All of these

Ans. (c) Urea

329. The building up and broken down of protoplasm are noncerned with the metabolism of:

 a. Minerals
 b. Proteins
 c. Urea
 d. All of these

Ans. (b) Proteins

330. The most important sugar concerned with human biochemistry is:

 a. Lactose
 b. Sucrose
 c. Glucose
 d. Fructose

Ans. (c) Glucose

331. Which of the following is not a monosaccharide?

 a. Glucose
 b. Fructose
 c. Lactose
 d. Galactose

Ans. (c) Lactose

332. Possible number of isomers of glucose is:

 a. 12
 b. 4
 c. 8
 d. 16

Ans. (d) 16

333. Which of the following is not a disaccharide?

 a. Sucrose
 b. Maltose
 c. Starch
 d. Lactose

Ans. (c) Starch

334. Which of the following is epimer of glucose?

 a. Cellulose
 b. Fructose
 c. Ribose
 d. Galactose

Ans. (d) Galactose

335. Cellulose is made up of the molecules of:

a. γ-glucose   b. β-glucose
c. α-glucose   d. δ-glucose

Ans. (b) β-glucose

336. Iodine solution gives no colour with?

a. Cellulose   b. Starch
c. Glycogen   d. Dextrin

Ans. (a) Cellulose

337. Which of the following monosaccharide has maximum rate of absorption in the intestine?

a. Mannose   b. Fructose
c. Glucose   d. Galactose

Ans. (d) Galactose

338. Which of the following sugar does not reduce Fehling's solution?

a. Sucrose   b. Lactose
c. Fructose   d. Glucose

Ans. (c) Fructose

339. Barfoed's solution is not reduced by:

a. Sucrose   b. Glucose
c. Ribose   d. Mannose

Ans. (a) Sucrose

340. Each branch of amylopectin is at an interval of glucose units:

a. 24–30   b. 34–40
c. 44–50   d. 14–20

Ans. (a) 24–30

341. Human heart muscles contain:

a. D-arabinose   b. D-ribose
c. D-xylose   d. D-lyxose

Ans. (d) D-lyxose

342. The absorption of glucose is interfered by the deficiency of:

a. Thiamine   b. Fe^{++}
c. Mg^{++} d. Vitamin A

Ans. (a) Thiamine

343. Glycogen synthetase activity is depressed by:

a. Cyclic-AMP
b. Insulin
c. Fructokinase
d. Glucose

Ans. (a) Cyclic-AMP

344. The branching enzyme acts on the glycogen when the main chain is lengthened by :

a. 50–100 glucose units
b 1–6 glucose units
c. 6–11 glucose units
d. 200–500 glucose units

Ans. (c) 6–11 glucose units

345. The two triose phosphate molecules involved in one of the important steps of glycolysis are :

a. Dihydroxyacetone phosphate and glyceraldehydes-1 phosphate
b. Dihydroxyacetone phosphate and glycol phosphate
c. Dihydroxyacetone phosphate and glyceraldehydes-3 phosphate
d. Dihydroxyacetone phosphate and glyceraldehydes-2 phosphate

Ans. (c) Dihydroxyacetone phosphate and glyceraldehydes-3 phosphate

346. Activation of the inactive phosphorylase is stimulated by:

a. Cyclic-AMP   b. ATP
c. NAD^+ d. None of these

Ans. (a) Cyclic-AMP

347. The main product of glycolysis (i.e. anaerobic condition) in skeletal muscles is:

a. A-ketoglutarate   b. Pyruvate
c. Lactate   d. succinate

Ans. (a) A-ketoglutarate

348. Cyclic AMP is formed from ATP by the enzyme adenylate cyclase which is activated by the hormone:

a. Epinephrine   b. Insulin
c. Testosterone   d. Progesterone

Ans. (a) Epinephrine

349. Pyruvate is accumulated by the dieartry deficiency of :

a. Vitamin B_6 b. Vitamin B_2
c. Vitamin B_1 d. Vitamin B_{12}

Ans. (c) Vitamin B_1

350. The synthesis of adenylate cyclase is increased by:

a. GH
b. FSH
c. ACTH
d. TH

Ans. (d) TH

351. Hexokinase has a high affinity for glucose than:

a. Galactokinase
b. Fructokinase
c. Glucokinase
d. All of these

Ans. (a) Galactokinase

352. Conversion of fructose 1, 6 diphosphate to fructose-6 phosphate is stimulated by:

a. Glucagon
b. ACTH
c. Insulin
d. None of these

Ans. (a) Glucagon

353. Fructokinase is present in:

a. Brain
b. Intestine
c. Heart
d. Adipose tissue

Ans. (b) Intestine

354. The carrier of the citric acid cycle is:

a. Oxaloacetate
b. Malate
c. Fumarate
d. Succinate

Ans. (a) Oxaloacetate

355. Glucose-6-PO$_4$ is absent in:

a. Heart
b. Adipose tissue
c. Kidney
d. Brain

Ans. (b) Adipose tissue

356. The conversion of citrate to isocitrate is catalysed by:

a. Isocitrase
b. Citrase
c. Aconitase
d. Decarboxylase

Ans. (c) Aconitase

357. Dihydroxyacetone phosphate and glyceraldehydes-3-phosphate are interconverted by:

a. Diphosphotriose isomerase
b. Phosphotriose isomerase
c. Triose isomerase
d. Dihydroxyacetone phosphorylase

Ans. (b) Phosphotriose isomerase

358. Insulin is given in the form of:

a. Insulin in alcohol
b. Insulin in water
c. Protamine zinc insulin
d. Insulin in tissue fluid

Ans. (c) Protamine zinc insulin

359. diabetes mellitus is characterised by:

a. Glycosuria
b. Polyurea
c. Polydispia
d. All of these

Ans. (d) All of these

360. The amount of sugar in urine of a normal individual is:

a. 0.5%
b. 0.05%
c. 1%
d. 71%

Ans. (b) 0.05%

361. The heptose ketose formed in HMP shunt is:

a. Mannoheptose
b. Glucoheptose
c. Galactoheptose
d. Sedoheptulosea

Ans. (d) Sedoheptulosea

362. Hexose monophosphate pathway of oxidation of glucose is active only in:

a. Liver
b. Lactating mammary gland
c. Adipose tissue
d. All of these

Ans. (d) All of these

363. In human being, galactose is most easily available by conversion of:

a. Maltase
b. Fructose
c. Glucose
d. Milk

Ans. (d) Milk

364. Lactose is formed in mammary gland under the influence of lactose synthetase by the reaction of:

a. Glucose and galactose
b. UDP galactose and glucose
c. UDP glucose and UDP galactose
d. UDP glucose and galactose

Ans. (b) UDP galactose and glucose

365. Which of the following is not a mucopolysaccharide?

a. Chondriotin
b. Inulin
c. Sialic acid
d. Heparin

Ans. (b) Inulin

366. Mucopolysaccharides consist of repeating units of disaccharide molecule consisting of:

a. Three monosaccharides
b. Two monosaccharides
c. Uronic acid + acylated amino sugar
d. Glucose + amino sugar

Ans. (c) Uronic acid + acylated amino sugar

367. Function of brain is disturbed when the blood glucose level falls from the normal fasting value 80 mg /100 ml to:

a. 40 mg/100 ml   b. 10 mg/100 ml
c. 20 mg/100 ml   d. 60 mg /100 ml

Ans. (c) 20 mg/100 ml

368. The renal threshold value for glucose is:

a. 80 mg/100 ml   b. 120 mg/100 ml
c. 200 mg/100 ml   d. 180 mg/100 ml

Ans. (d) 180 mg/100 ml

369. Which is not glucogenic substance in human being?

a. Glycerol   b. Lactate
c. Amino acid   d. Propionate

Ans. (d) Propionate

370. In one HMP shunt, one molecule of glucose is oxidized with the net generation of:

a. 35 moles of ATP   b. 36 moles of ATP
c. 38 moles of ATP   d. 39 moles of ATP

Ans. (a) 35 moles of ATP

371. The hydrogen acceptor used in HMP shunt is:

a. ADP   b. NAD^+
c. $NADP^+$ d. ATP

Ans. (c) $NADP^+$

372. In liver, the enzyme fructokinase converts fructose to:

a. Fructose-6-PO_4
b. Fructose-1-PO^4
c. Glucose-1-PO^4
d. Fructose 1, 6 diphosphate

Ans. (b) Fructose-1-PO^4

373. The enzyme hexokinase can phosphorylate fructose as well as glucose. The affinity than or enzyme is:

a. Equal for glucose and fructose
b. Great for fructose than glucose
c. Great for glucose than for fructose
d. Small for glucose than fructose

Ans. (c) Great for glucose than for fructose

374. One complete Kreb-s cycle starting from oxaloacetate produces:

a. 12 ATP   b. 6 ATP
c. 3 ATP   d. 24 ATP

Ans. (a) 12 ATP

375. The net number of moles of ATP produced when one glucosyl unit of glycogen undergoes glycolysis under anaerobic conditions is:

a. 2   b. 3
c. 4   d. 1

Ans. (b) 3

376. The net number of moles of ATP produced when one free glucose molecule undergoes glycolysis under aerobic conditions is:

a. 3   b. 8
c. 9   d. 2

Ans. (b) 8

377. DNA finger printing has proved useful in forensic science. It involves the use of:

a. c-DNA
b. r-RNA
c. Ministellites
d. bacterial DNA

Ans. (c) Ministellites

378. The purpose of cloning is to:

a. Lost genotype
b. Preserve genotype
c. Replace original genotype
d. None of these

Ans. (b) Preserve genotype

379. Which is a genetic vector:

a. Cosmid   b. Phage
c. Plasmid   d. All of these

Ans. (d) All of these

380. Lipids are:

a. Soluble in both water and organic solvents
b. Soluble in water
c. Soluble in organic solvents
d. Insoluble in both water and organic sovents

Ans. (c) Soluble in organic solvents

381. Δ^8 indicates a double bond between carbon atoms:

a. 8 and 9   b. 7 and 8
c. 6 and 8   d. 9 and 10

Ans. (a) 8 and 9

382. Esters of long chain fatty acids with long chain monohydric alcohols are called:

a. Protein   b. Waxes
c. Fats   d. Carbohydrate

Ans. (b) Waxes

383. Essential fatty acids contain:

a. One double bond   b. Three double bond
c. Two double bond   d. All of these

Ans. (d) All of these

384. Naturally occurring fatty acids usually contains:

a. Carbon atoms remain absent
b. Odd number of carbon atoms
c. Even number of carbon atoms
d. None of these

Ans. (c) Even number of carbon atoms

385. Animal fats mainly contain:

a. Serine and linolenic amino acids
b. Linoleic and linolenic acids
c. Stearic and palmitic acids
d. Citric and oxalic acids

Ans. (c) Stearic and palmitic acids

386. Side chain of archidonic acid contains the number of double bonds:

a. 4   b. 3
c. 2   d. 5

Ans. (a) 4

387. Hydrolysis of fat alkali is called:

a. Transduction
b. Saponification number
c. Saponification
d. Recombination

Ans. (c) Saponification

388. Lecithin contains a nitrogenous base called:

a Choline   b. Ethanolamine
c. Insitol   d. Lecine

Ans. (a) Choline

389. Cephalin are compound lipids which contain:

a. Asparagines
b. Myoinositol
c. Ethanolamine
d. Both 'a' and 'b'

Ans. (d) Both 'a' and 'b'

390. Lecithins are soluble in ordinary fat solvents *except:*

a. Ethanol   b. Benzene
c. Methanol   d. Acetone

Ans. (d) Benzene

391. Lecithins combine with protein to form:

a. Phosphoprotein
b. Lipoprotein
c. Mucoprotein
d. Glycoprotein

Ans. (b) Lipoprotein

392. The protein moiety of lipoprotein is known as:

a. Preprotein   b. Apoprotein
c. Pseudoprotein   d. Post protein

Ans. (b) Apoprotein

393. Which of the following is steroid hormone?

a. Androgens   b. Estrogens
c. Corticoids   d. All of these

Ans. (d) All of these

394. In sphingomyelins, the alcoholic moiety is:

a. Glycerol   b. Glycol
c. Sphingosine   d. Acetyl alcohol

Ans. (c) Sphingosine

395. Gangiliosides are the glycolipids occurring in:

a. Brain   b. Kidney
c. Liver   d. Muscle

Ans. (a) Brain

396. Very low density lipoproteins also known as:

a. β-lipoprotein   b. α-lipoprotein
c. Pre-β-liprotein   d. γ-lipoprotein

Ans. (c) Pre-β-liprotein

397. In gangliosides, the sugar protein may be:

a. Amino acid
b. Sialic acid
c. Acetylated amino sugar
d. α-ketoglutaric acid

Ans. (b) Sialic acid

398. The main source of cholesterol is:

a. Animal fats   b. Vegetables
c. Egg yolk   d. All of these

Ans. (c) Egg yolk

399. Digestion of fat starts in:

a. Stomach
b. Mouth
c. Small intestine
d. Large intestine

Ans. (c) Small intestine

400. Lipids are emulsified by the action of:
- a. Ergosterol
- b. Lipoprotein
- c. Cholesterol
- d. Bile salts

Ans. (d) Bile salts

401. The majority of the absorbed fat appears in the form of :
- a. HDL
- b. LDL
- c. VLDL
- d. Chylomicrons

Ans. (d) Chylomicrons

402. Lipase present in the stomach can not hydrolyze fats due to:
- a. Acidity
- b. Neutrality
- c. High acidity
- d. Alkalinity

Ans. (c) High acidity

403. Fatty acids are mainly oxidized by:
- a. γ-oxidation
- b β-oxidation
- c. α-oxidation
- d. None of these

Ans. (b) β-oxidation

404. During oxidation, long chain fatty acids are first converted to acyl-Co-A in the:
- a. Cytosol
- b. Lysosome
- c. Microsome
- d. Mitochondria

Ans. (a) Cytosol

405. Activation of lower fatty acids occurs within the:
- a. Mitochondria
- b. Microsome
- c. Lysosome
- d. Cytosol

Ans. (a) Mitochondria

406. The enzyme thiokinase catalyzing the activation of fatty acids requires the cofactor:
- a. Mg^{++}
- b. Ca^{++}
- c. Mn^{++}
- d. K^+

Ans. (a) Mg^{++}

407. Long chain fatty acids are activated with in the cytosol while the further steps of oxidation take place in mitochondria. Thus the long chain acyl-Co-A peneterates mitochondria in the presence of:
- a. Palmitate
- b. Sorbitol
- c. Carnitine
- d. Na^+

Ans. (c) Carnitine

408. During one set of β-oxidation of a fatty acid, the number of carbon atoms removed in/are:
- a. 1
- b. 2
- c. 3
- d. Not definite

Ans. (b) 2

409. Acyl-Co-A is converted to α, β-unsaturated acyl Co-A by the enyme acyl-Co-A dehydrogenase in the presence of coenzyme :
- a. $NADP^+$
- b. NAD^+
- c. FAD^+
- d. ATP

Ans. (c) FAD^+

410. The final product of β-oxidation of an odd numbered carboxylic acid is :
- a. α-ketoglutaric acid
- b. Acetyl-Co-A
- c. Propionyl Co-A
- d. Oxalic acid

Ans. (c) Propionyl Co-A

411. Prostaglandins are used for:
- a. The prevention of conception
- b. The induction of menstruation
- c. The termination of pregnancy
- d. All of these

Ans. (d) All of these

412. Synthesis of prostaglandins is inhibited by:
- a. Fluoride ion
- b. Asprin
- c. Cyanide ion
- d. Arsenate ion

Ans. (b) Asprin

413. All active prostaglandins have a common double bond which lies:
- a. Between C_{17} and C_{18} and has *cis* configuration
- b. Between C_{13} and C_{14} and has *cis* configuration
- c. Between C_{13} and C_{14} and has *trans* configuration
- d. Between C_{17} and C_{18} and has *trans* configuration

Ans. (c) Between C_{13} and C_{14} and has *trans* configuration

414. In human blood, the Mg per cent of cholesterol is:
- a. 50–100
- b. 20–80
- c. 140–250
- d. 300–600

Ans. (c) 140–250

415. Cholesterol contains 27 carbon molecules which are derived from:
- a. Higher fatty acid molecule
- b. Acetate molecule
- c. Co-A molecule
- d. Carbon dioxide and glucose molecule

Ans. (b) Acetate molecule

416. Of the 27 carbon atoms of cholesterol, how many derived are from the CH_3 group of the acetate (CH_3COO^-) molecule:

a. 15   b. 14

c. 13   d. 27

Ans. (a) 15

417. Biosynthesis of cholesterol in the liver is suppressed by:

a. Talking   b. Fasting

c. Dietary cholesterol   d. Both (a) and (b)

Ans. (d) Both (a) and (b)

418. Fatty liver results in the deficiency of:

a. Stearic acid   b. Pantothenic acid

c. Vitamin A   d. Caproic acid

Ans. (b) Pantothenic acid

419. The number of ATP moles liberated during the oxidation of one mole of palmitic acid to CO_2 and H_2O is:

a. 130   b. 128

c. 131   d. 129

Ans. (d) 129

420. Under normal conditions the fate of acetyl-Co-A is:

a. Conversion to acetoacetate

b. Conversion to acetone

c. Entry to citric acid cycle

d. None of the above

Ans. (c) Entry to citric acid cycle

421. When concentration of ketone bodies in human blood increases, the condition is known as:

a. Ketonemia   b. Ketonuria

c. Ketosis   d. Ketogenesis

Ans. (a) Ketonemia

422. Enzymes responsible for ketone body formation are found mainly in:

a. Chromosomes   b. Nucleus

c. Mitochondria   d. Extrahepatic tissue

Ans. (c) Mitochondria

423. Ketone bodies are utilized in:

a. Chromosomes

b. Nucleus

c. Mitochondria

d. Extrahepatic tissue

Ans. (d) Extrahepatic tissue

424. Under prolonged starvation brain takes energy from:

a. Carbohydrates   b. Acetoacetate

c. Fats   d. Proteins

Ans. (b) Acetoacetate

425. Fatty acid synthesis takes place in:

a. Mitochondria   b. Cytosol

c. Microsomes   d. Chloroplast

Ans. (b) Cytosol

426. Fatty acid oxidation takes place in:

a. Cytosol   b. Mitochondria

c. Chloroplast   d. Microsomes

Ans. (b) Mitochondria

427. Acetyl Co-A carboxylase, involved in the carboxylation of acetyl Co-A contain :

a. Cyanocobalmine   b. Biotin

c. Pyridoxal   d. None of these

Ans. (b) Biotin

428. The dehydrogenating steps in the β-oxidation of fatty acid utilize:

a. $NADP^+$ b. NAD^+

c. NADH   d. NADPH

Ans. (b) NAD^+

429. Lengthening of fatty acid in mitochondria and microsomes takes place by the addition of:

a. Leucine and arginine respectively

b. Citric acid and oxalic acid respectively

c. Aetyle Co-A and propionyl Co-A respectively

d. Alanine and lysine respectively

Ans. (c) Aetyle Co-A and propionyl Co-A respectively

CHECK YOU GRASP

1. **Which vitamin is a constituent of FMN?**
   - a. Tocoferol
   - b. Nicotinic acid
   - c. Riboflavin
   - d. Nicotinamide

2. **Which of the following is general formula of monosaccharides?**
   - a. $Cn(H_2O)_{2n}$
   - b. $C_2n(H_2O)$
   - c. $Cn(H_2O)_n$
   - d. $Cn(HO)_n$

3. **Which of the following is epimer of glucose?**
   - a. Cellulose
   - b. Fructose
   - c. Ribose
   - d. Galactose

4. **The connecting link between glycolysis and krebs cycle is:**
   - a. Acetyl CoA
   - b. Pyruvic acid
   - c. Cytochromes
   - d. None of these

5. **Which elements play important role in photolysis of water?**
   - a. Mg and Cl
   - b. Mg and Mo
   - c. Mn and Cl
   - d. Fe and Mg

6. **One of the following is not a limiting factor in photosynthesis:**
   - a. CO_2
   - b. Water
   - c. Light
   - d. O_2

7. **An ayurvedic medicine isabgol is obtained from:**
   - a. Root
   - b. Leaves
   - c. Seeds
   - d. Stem

8. **The term assimilatory powers in photosynthesis refers to:**
   - a. Reduction of CO_2
   - b. Oxidation of CO_2
   - c. Photolysis of water
   - d. Formation of ATP and $NADPH_2$

9. **In gangliosides, the sugar protein may be:**
   - a. Amino acid
   - b. Sialic acid
   - c. Acetylated amino sugar
   - d. α-ketoglutaric acid

10. **One complete Kreb-s cycle starting from oxaloacetate produces:**
    - a. 12 ATP
    - b. 6 ATP
    - c. 3 ATP
    - d. 24 ATP

11. **Biosynthesis of cholesterol in the liver is suppressed by:**
    - a. Talking
    - b. Fasting
    - c. Dietary cholesterol
    - d. Both (a) and (b)

12. **One of the following statement is incorrect with regards to β-DNA:**
    - a. $A + G = C + T$
    - b. $A + T = C + G$
    - c. $A + C = G + T$
    - d. None of these

13. **How many ATP molecules are formed on complete oxidation of a glucose molecule through hexose monophosphate shunt cycle?**
    - a. 2
    - b. 4
    - c. 36
    - d. 38

14. **the coenzyme FMN and FAD incorporate a vitamin in its structure which is:**
    - a. Vit. C
    - b. Vit. A
    - c. Vit.B_2
    - d. Vit. K

15. **Cholesterol and other lipids are transported to specific targets by lipoproteins. In blood cholesterol is carried out by:**
    - a. VLDL
    - b. LDL
    - c. IDL
    - d. DDT

In case of less than 80% score, go through brief Review and Glance one again from chapter

Key: 1-c 2-c 3-d 4-a 5-c 6-c 7-c 8-d 9-b 10-a 11-d 12-b 13-c 14-c 15-b

8

Enzyme Engineering

1. **In plants, enzymes are present**
   a. Only in leaves
   b. Only in storage organs
   c. Only in flowers
   d. In all the living cells of the plant body

   Ans. (d) In all the living cells of the plant body

2. **Enzymes are useful because they**
   a. Catalyse biochemical reactions in the plant body
   b. Supply energy
   c. Enhance the absorption of water
   d. Are important structural components

   Ans. (a) Catalyse biochemical reactions in the plant body

3. **The enzymes which act normally within cells are called**
   a. Endoenzymes
   b. Exoenzymes
   c. Apoenzymes
   d. Ferment

   Ans. (a) Endoenzymes

4. **The scientists associated with the study of enzymes include**
   a. Buchner   b. Went
   c. Sumner   d. Both a and c

   Ans. (d) Both a and c

5. **'Enzymes are proteins', was suggested by**
   a. Pasteur
   b. Leeuwenhoek
   c. Miller
   d. Sumner

   Ans. (d) Sumner

6. **Noble Prize for discovering enzyme was given to**
   a. Fischer   b. Altmann
   c. Fleming   d. Buchner

   Ans. (d) Buchner

7. **Which of the following enzymes was first isolated and purified in the form of crystal**
   a. Amylase   b. Ribonuclease
   c. Urease   d. Pepsin

   Ans. (c) Urease

8. **Urease, the first enzyme crystallized, was crystallized by**
   a. J. Northrop   b. E. Buchner
   c. Louis Pasteur   d. J.B. Sumner

   Ans. (d) J.B. Sumner

9. **Number of enzymes known now-a-days is approximately**
   a. 1,000   b. 2,000
   c. 3,000   d. 4,000

   Ans. (b) 2,000

10. **Enzymes are basically made up of**
    a. Proteins   b. Vitamins
    c. Carbon   d. Fats

    Ans. (a) Proteins

11. **Enzymes are made up of**
    a. Carbohydrates   b. Fats
    c. Proteins   d. DNA

    Ans. (c) Proteins

12. **An enzyme can be synthesized by chemically bonding together the molecules of**
    a. Carbohydrates   b. Amino acids
    c. Lipase   d. CO_2

    Ans. (b) Amino acids

13. **Enzymes are polymers of**
    a. Amino acids
    b. Hexose carbon
    c. Fatty acids
    d. Inorganic phosphate

    Ans. (a) Amino acids

14. **Which one of the following statement if true for the enzyme**
    a. All enzymes are proteins
    b. All proteins are enzymes
    c. All enzymes are not proteins
    d. All enzymes are vitamins

Ans. (c) All enzymes are not proteins

15. **Which enzyme is not proteinaceous**
    a. Isozyme
    b. Ribozyme
    c. Holozyme
    d. Trypsin

Ans. (b) Ribozyme

16. **Ribozyme is**
    a. RNA without sugar
    b. RNA without phosphate
    c RNA having enzyme activity
    d. RNA with extra phosphate

Ans. (c) RNA having enzyme activity

17. **The non-protein part of an enzyme is called**
    a. Holoenzyme
    b. Prosthetic group
    c. Apoenzyme
    d. None of the above

Ans. (b) Prosthetic group

18. **The protein part of an enzyme is called**
    a. Holoenzyme
    b. Prosthetic group
    c. Apoenzyme
    d. All of the above

Ans. (c) Apoenzyme

19. **When coenzyme combines with apoenzymes, it is called**
    a. Holoenzyme
    b. Cofactor
    c. Isoenzyme
    d. Prosthetic group

Ans. (a) Holoenzyme

20. **Coenzyme is**
    a. Always a protein
    b. Often a vitamin
    c. Always an inorganic compound
    d. Often a metal

Ans. (b) Often a vitamin

21. **Cytochrome oxidase contains**
    a. Iron
    b. Magnesium
    c. Cobalt
    d. Mercury

Ans. (a) Iron

22. **Some metal known as cofactors of enzymes are**
    a. Ca^{++}, Zn^{++}, Mn^{++}
    b. Zn^{++}, Ca^{++}
    c. K^+, Co^{++}
    d. All of the above

Ans. (d) All of the above

23. **What will happen to an enzyme when apoenzyme is separated from its metal component**
    a. Activity will be increased
    b. Activity will be lost
    c. Activity will be decreased
    d. There will be no change in the activity

Ans. (b) Activity will be lost

24. **NADP is**
    a. An enzyme
    b. A part of soluble RNA
    c. A part of transfer RNA
    d. A coenzyme

Ans. (d) A coenzyme

25. **FAD or FMN is a coenzyme; which vitamin is incorporated in its structure**
    a. Vitamin B_1
    b. Vitamin B_2
    c. Vitamin B_6
    d. Vitamin C

Ans. (b) Vitamin B_2

26. **The nature of coenzyme is**
    a. Non proteinaceous
    b. Proteinaceous
    c. Both a and b
    d. None of the above

Ans. (a) Non proteinaceous

27. **During enzyme activity, the coenzyme**
    a. Acts as a donor or acceptor of atoms which are added to or removed from the substrates
    b. Are important in oxidation-reduction reactions
    c. Both a and b
    d. None of the above

Ans. (c) Both a and b

28. **Which of the following are coenzymes**
    a. NAD, NADP, FAD, FMN
    b. Vitamin, Fe, Cu
    c. $NADPH_2$, Ca, Co
    d. NAD, K, CoA

Ans. (a) NAD, NADP, FAD, FMN

29. **Out of total enzymes present in the cell, mitochondrion alone has**
    a. 95%
    b. 20%
    c. 64%
    d. 70%

Ans. (d) 70%

30. Which of the following is iron porphyrin coenzyme or cofactor

a. Coenzyme A
b. Cytochrome
c. NAD
d. FAD

Ans. (b) Cytochrome

31. The ratio of enzyme: substrate molecules can be as high as

a. 1:1000
b. 1:10,000
c. 1:50,000
d. 1:100,000

Ans. (d) 1:100,000

32. The turnover number of the fastest enzyme is

a. 10^5
b. 10^4
c. 18×10^4
d. 4×10^6

Ans. (d) 4×10^6

33. Which among the following has highest turnover number

a. Urease
b. Carbonic anhydrase
c. Catalase
d. Pepsin

Ans. (c) Catalase

34. Which among the following has highest catalytic efficiency

a. Catalse
b. Urease
c. Carbonic anhydrase
d. Pepsin

Ans. (c) Carbonic anhydrase

35. The number of enzyme units per mg of protein is known as

a. Molecular activity
b. Specific activity
c. Turnover number
d. Molar activity

Ans. (b) Specific activity

36. Amount of enzyme transforming 1 μmole of substrate per minute at 25°C under optimal conditions of measurement is called

a. Specific activity
b. Unit of enzyme (activity)
c. Catalytic centre activity
d. Enzyme purity

Ans. (b) Unit of enzyme (activity)

37. Which of the following statements is incorrect

a. At optimum pH, the activity of enzyme is maximum
b. Enzymes are not affected by hydrogen ion concentration

c. The optimum pH for pepsin is 2.0
d. The optimum pH for trypsin is 8.8

Ans. (b) Enzymes are not affected by hydrogen ion concentration

38. At temperature below the freezing point, an enzyme is

a. Slightly activated
b. Killed
c. Inactivated
d. Unaffected

Ans. (c) Inactivated

39. How is the rate of enzyme-catalyzed reactions affected by every 10°C rise of temperature

a. Halves
b. Doubles
c. Becomes four times
d. Remains unchanged

Ans. (b) Doubles

40. At which temperature, the enzyme activity would be maximum

a. 35°C
b. 45°C
c. 55°C
d. 60°C

Ans. (a) 35°C

41. Most of the enzymes are inactivated at temperature above

a. 25°C
b. 45°C
c. 55°C
d. 80°C

Ans. (b) 45°C

42. At boiling temperature, an enzyme is

a. Killed
b. Denatured
c. Inactivated
d. Unaffected

Ans. (b) Denatured

43. On boiling/treating with strong acid or alkali/treating with pepsin, an enzyme loses its catalytic activity because

a. It is a protein
b. It burns
c. It is a functional substances
d. It is a lipoprotein

Ans. (a) It is a protein

44. Which part of an active enzyme is denatured by heat

a. Apoenzyme
b. Holoenzyme
c. Coenzyme
d. Activator

Ans. (a) Apoenzyme

45. Enzymes catalyses a reaction in _____

   a. Forward direction
   b. Backward direction
   c. Both ways
   d. Either ways

Ans. (d) Either ways

46. Enzymes differ from inorganic catalysts in

   a. Having a high diffusion rate
   b. Working at high temperature
   c. Not being used up in reactions
   d. Being proteinaceous in nature

Ans. (d) Being proteinaceous in nature

47. What is true about enzymes

   a. All act best at pH 7.0
   b. All are amino acids
   c. All are proteins
   d. All act best at 0°C

Ans. (c) All are proteins

48. Which of the following is not an attribute of enzymes

   a. These are proteinaceous in nature
   b. These speed up the rate of biochemical reaction
   c. These are specific in nature
   d. These are used up in reaction

Ans. (d) These are used up in reaction

49. Enzymes are sensitive to

   a. Light
   b. Wind velocity
   c. Change in pH
   d. Rainfall

Ans. (c) Change in pH

50. Dry seeds can endure higher temperature than the germinating seeds because

   a. Dry seeds are hard
   b. Seedlings are tender
   c. Dry seeds have more reserve food
   d. Hydration makes the enzyme more sensitive to temperature

Ans. (d) Hydration makes the enzyme more sensitive to temperature

51. Zymogens are

   a. Enzyme acting upon starch
   b. Groups of zymase enzymes
   c. Inactive enzyme precursors
   d. None of the above

Ans. (c) Inactive enzyme precursors

52. Enzymes which are slightly different in molecular structure, but can perform identical activities are called

   a. Isoenzymes
   b. Homoenzymes
   c. Apoenzymes
   d. Coenzymes

Ans. (a) Isoenzymes

53. Lactic dehydrogenase (LDH) which catalyses pyruvate to lactate is an example of

   a. Apoenzyme
   b. Antienzyme
   c. Isoenzyme
   d. Coenzyme

Ans. (c) Isoenzyme

54. An enzyme which catalyses the rearrangement of molecular structure and forms a compound of same molecular weight is called

   a. Ligase
   b. Oxidoreductase
   c. Isomerase
   d. Hydrolase

Ans. (c) Isomerase

55. The transfer of a group from a donor molecule to an acceptor molecule is catalysed by

   a. Transferase
   b. Isomerase
   c. Protease
   d. Hydrolytic enzymes

Ans. (a) Transferase

56. Transferases are involved in the transfer of

   a. Methyl group
   b. Amino group
   c. Phosphate group
   d. All of these

Ans. (d) All of these

57. Oxidative enzymes occur in

   a. Lysosomes
   b. Golgi bodies
   c. Mitochondria
   d. Ribosomes

Ans. (c) Mitochondria

58. Hydrolases are involved in the hydrolysis of

   a. Esters
   b. Lipids
   c. Proteins
   d. All of these

Ans. (d) All of these

59. Ligases are involved in the synthesis of

   a. C-C bonds
   b. C-N bonds
   c. C-O bonds
   d. All of these

Ans. (d) All of these

60. Esterase belongs to

a. Oxidoreductases   b. Carboxylases

c. Hydrolases   d. Transferases

Ans. (c) Hydrolases

61. Which of the following is a hydrolytic enzyme

a. Esterase   b. Carbohydrase

c. Protease   d. All of these

Ans. (d) All of these

62. The enzyme converting starch into maltose is

a. Invertase   b. Hydrogenase

c. Maltase   d. Diastase

Ans. (d) Diastase

63. Diastase enzyme helps in the digestion of

a. Starch   b. Proteins

c. Fats   d. Amino acids

Ans. (a) Starch

64. Which of the following enzymes acts upon fatty acids

a. Amylase   b. Ligase

c. Trypsin   d. Peptidase

Ans. (b) Ligase

65. Lipase enzyme acts upon

a. Water   b. Protein

c. Fat   d. Sugar

Ans. (c) Fat

66. Which enzyme is required to digest the reserve food material (lipid) in castor seeds

a. Lipase   b. Diastase

c. Amylase   d. Protease

Ans. (a) Lipase

67. In seeds, digestion is made possible at relatively low temperature by

a. Auxins

b. Proteins

c. Enzymes

d. Nitrogenous complex substances

Ans. (c) Enzymes

68. In the cell, digestive enzymes are mostly located in

a. Lysosomes

b. Cell wall

c. Chromosomes

d. Ribosome

Ans. (a) Lysosomes

69. An enzyme acts by

a. Reducing activation energy

b. Increasing activation energy

c. Increasing reaction time

d. Decreasing reaction time

Ans. (a) Reducing activation energy

70. Which of the following is correct in an enzyme-controlled reaction (E = enzyme; S = Substrate, P = Product)

a. $E + S \leftrightarrow E + P$ b. $E + S \leftrightarrow ES \leftrightarrow E + P$

c. $E + S \leftrightarrow ES \leftrightarrow E$ d. $E + S \leftrightarrow P \leftrightarrow E + P$

Ans. (b) $E + S \leftrightarrow ES \leftrightarrow E + P$

71. Turnover number of enzyme depends upon

a. Molecular weight of enzyme

b. Size of enzyme molecule

c. Active sites of enzyme molecule

d. Concentration of substrate molecule

Ans. (c) Active sites of enzyme molecule

72. Which of the following is the best evidence for template theory of enzyme action

a. Compounds similar in structure to the substrate inhibit the reaction

b. Enzymes speed up reaction by definite amount

c. Enzymes determine the direction of a reaction

d. Enzymes are found in living organisms and increase the rate

Ans. (a) Compounds similar in structure to the substrate inhibit the reaction

73. The enzyme is said to be working at maximum efficiency

a. When substrate concentration is increased to point of saturation

b. When substrate concentration is low

c. When substrate coming in contact with active site are negligible

d. None of the above is true

Ans. (a) When substrate concentration is increased to point of saturation

74. When the action of the enzyme is inhibited in the presence of a substance which closely resembles the substrate molecule, then the inhibition is known as

a. Feedback inhibition

b. Non-competitive inhibition

c. Allosteric inhibition

d. Competitive inhibition

Ans. (d) Competitive inhibition

75. In competitive inhibition, which of the following is true

a. $E + I \leftrightarrow EI$
b. $E + I \leftrightarrow EI + S \leftrightarrow ESI$
c. $S + I \leftrightarrow SI$
d. $ES + I \leftrightarrow ESI$

Ans. (a) $E + I \leftrightarrow EI$

76. Non-competitive inhibitors are those which

a. Alter the structure or protein molecule
b. Get attached on the active site
c. Activate the enzyme
d. Break the bonds which are responsible for the formation of active sites

Ans. (a) Alter the structure or protein molecule

77. The product of an enzyme-catalyzed reaction can act as inhibitor of the reaction. This mechanism of control is known as

a. Feedback inhibition
b. Competitive inhibition
c. Metabolic antagonism
d. Repression

Ans. (a) Feedback inhibition

78. In feedback inhibition, a metabolic pathway is switched off by

a. Competitive inhibition
b. Denaturation
c. Accumulation of end product
d. Allosteric inhibition

Ans. (d) Allosteric inhibition

79. Which of the following statements is incorrect

a. Enzymes hasten the completion of a reaction
b. The two terms 'substrate' and 'product' signify the starting and ending materials of a reaction
c. Enzymes are affected by the reactions they catalyse
d. Enzyme exhibit specificity for the reactions there catalyse

Ans. (c) Enzymes are affected by the reactions they catalyse

80. Enzymes, vitamins and hormones can be classified in a single category of biological chemicals because all of them

a. Are proteins
b. Are synthesized in organisms
c. Enhance the oxidative metabolism
d. Aid in regulating metabolism

Ans. (d) Aid in regulating metabolism

81. Which enzymes can digest plant protein?

a. Pepsin
b. Erepsin
c. Rennin
d. All the above

Ans. (a) Pepsin

82. Enzymes as they exist inside the cell are

a. In solid form
b. In crystalline form
c. In solution form
d. In colloidal form

Ans. (d) In colloidal form

83. Feedback inhibition is affected by

a. End product
b. First product
c. Enzymes
d. External factor

Ans. (a) End product

84. K_m value refers to

a. Maximum reaction velocity
b. Near maximum reaction velocity
c. One half of the maximum reaction velocity
d. Threshold value

Ans. (c) One half of the maximum reaction velocity

85. The substrate concentration at which an enone half of the maximum reaction velocityzyme attains half its maximum velocity is called

a. Threshold value
b. Half life
c. Michaelis Menton constant
d. Concentration coefficient

Ans. (c) Michaelis Menton constant

86. For the enzyme action

a. Value of K_m is low
b. Value of K_i is low·
c. Value of K_m is high
d. Value of K_i is high

Ans. (b) Value of K_i is low

87. The function of an enzyme is

a. To cause chemical reactions which would not occur otherwise
b. To change the rates of chemical reactions
c. To control the equilibrium points of reactions
d. To change the direction of reactions

Ans. (b) To change the rates of chemical reactions

88. The organic compounds which have transient association with apoenzymes are called

a. Holoenzyme
b. Coenzyme
c. Prosthetic group
d. None of these

Ans. (b) Coenzyme

89. Iron is a cofactor responsible for the catalytic action of

a. Sucrose　　　　　b. Lipase

c. Catalase　　　　　d. Cellulose

Ans. (c) Catalase

90. The fastest acting enzyme is

a. Peroxidase

b. Amylase

c. Carbonic anhydrase

d. Phosphoglyceromutase

Ans. (c) Carbonic anhydrase

91. The enzyme bromelain is obtained from

a. Papaya　　　　　b. Pineapple

c. Saliva　　　　　d. Witches broom

Ans (b) Pineapple

92. The evolution of oxygen from H_2O_2 in a living tissue is catalysed by

a. MnO_2　　　　　b. Peroxidase

c. SnO_2　　　　　d. Invertase

Ans. (b) Peroxidase

93. The enzyme sucrose acts on

a. Sucrose only　　　　b. Any disaccharide

c. Starch and sucrose　　d. Any organic molecule

Ans. (a) Sucrose only

94. The active site of an enzyme is formed by some of its

a. R groups on the amino acids

b. Amino groups of amino acids

c. Carboxyl groups of the amino acids

d. Exposed sulphur bonds

Ans. (a) R groups on the amino acids

95. Upon binding the substrate at one site, other sites on an enzyme become more reactive. This is called

a. Allosteric inhibition　　b. Specificity

c. Co-operativity　　　　d. Activation

Ans. (c) Co-operativity

96. Which of these inactivates an enzyme by changing enzyme shape

a. Allosteric inhibitor

b. Competitive inhibitor

c. Irreversible inhibitor

d. Multienzyme complex

Ans. (a) Allosteric inhibitor

97. Which of these inactivates an enzyme by denaturing it

a. Allosteric inhibitor

b. Competitive inhibitor

c. Irreversible inhibitor

d. Multienzyme complex

Ans. (c) Irreversible inhibitor

98. The specificity of an enzyme is governed by the tertiary structure. In forming a tertiary structure, bonds develop between certain amino acids. The resulting shape provides for the substrate

a. Spatial fit

b. Bonding fit

c. Spatial and bonding fit both

d. Neither spatial nor bonding fit

Ans. (c) Spatial and bonding fit both

99. Only a substrate with a particular shape is help by the enzyme. It is due to

a. Spatial fit of the active site

b. Bonding fit of the active site

c. Both spatial and bonding fit of the active site

d. Neither spatial nor bonding fit of the active site

Ans. (a) Spatial fit of the active site

100. Bonding fit of an enzyme is the presence of certain active sites

a. Within the grooves in the surface of tertiary structure

b. Outside the grooves on the surface of tertiary surface

c. Both within and outside the grooves in the surface of tertiary structure

d. Formed as a result of quaternary structure

Ans. (a) Within the grooves in the surface of tertiary structure

101. Specificity of the bonding fit for a particular reaction is the result of

a. R groups on the amino acids

b. Amino groups of amino acids

c. Carboxyl groups of the amino acids

d. Exposed sulphur bonds

Ans. (a) R groups on the amino acids

102. Which of the following statements is correct?

a. Enzymes can substitute one another

b. No other enzyme can substitute for a missing enzyme

c. A few enzymes can substitute a given enzyme

d. While some enzymes can be substituted by other enzymes, there is no substitute for most of the enzymes

Ans. (b) No other enzyme can substitute for a missing enzyme

103. All the enzymes of a multienzyme complex are arranged together in

a. Solution of ATP
b. Membrane
c. Quaternary protein
d. Coenzyme

Ans. (b) Membrane

104. During feedback inhibition, the high concentrations of the end product of a metabolic pathway

a. Slow down the enzymes which control earlier steps in the pathway
b. Switch off the enzymes which control earlier steps in the pathway
c. Slow down or switch off the enzymes which control earlier steps in the pathway
d. Denature the enzymes which control earlier steps in the pathway

Ans. (c) Slow down or switch off the enzymes which control earlier steps in the pathway

105. Feedback inhibition quite often involves

a. Competitive inhibition
b. Irreversible inhibition
c. Allosteric inhibition
d. All the above

Ans. (c) Allosteric inhibition

106. Glutamate pyruvate transaminase enzyme is an example of

a. Qxidoreductases
b. Transferases
c. Lyases
d. Ligases

Ans. (b) Transferases

107. Most of the digestive enzymes belongs to the category

a. Qxidoreductases
b. Transferases
c. Hydrolases
d. Lyases

Ans. (c) Hydrolases

108. Histidine decarboxylase enzyme belongs to the category

a. Qxidoreductases
b. Isomerases
c. Lyases
d. Ligases

Ans. (c) Lyases

109. Which enzyme require energy for their action and obtain it from the hydrolysis of ATP

a. Qxidoreductases
b. Transferases
c. Ligases
d. Lyases

Ans. (c) Ligases

110. The enzyme pyruvate carboxylase combines pyruvic acid and CO_2 to form oxaloacetic acid at the expense of ATP. The enzyme is

a. An isomerase
b. A ligase
c. A lyase
d. A transferase

Ans. (b) A ligase

111. The activity of an enzyme declines

a. Above the optimum temperature
b. Below the optimum temperature
c. Both above and below the optimum temperature
d. Below the minimum and above the maximum temperature

Ans. (c) Both above and below the optimum temperature

112. Pepsinogen (inactive form of enzyme pepsin) is converted into its active form by

a. Isomerism
b. Hydrolysis
c. Oxidation
d. Reduction

Ans. (b) Hydrolysis

113. Most intracellular enzymes function best

a. At neutral pH
b. In acidic conditions
c. In basic conditions
d. Either neutral or acidic conditions

Ans. (a) At neutral pH

114. The protein-digesting enzyme trypsin functions best is

a. pH 7.0
b. pH 6.5
c. pH 7.5
d. pH 8.5

Ans. (d) pH 8.5

115. On reaching the stomach, the enzyme salivary amylase is inactivated by

a. Pepsinogen
b. Pepsin
c. Hydrochloric acid
d. Mucous

Ans. (c) Hydrochloric acid

116. The inhibition of succinic acid dehydrogenase by malonic acid is an example of

a. Competitive inhibition
b. Allosteric inhibition
c. Feedback inhibition
d. Irreversible inhibition

Ans. (a) Competitive inhibition

117. Sulpha drugs are used for the control of bacterial pathogens because they cause

a. Competitive inhibition of folic acid synthesis
b. Allosteric inhibition of folic acid synthesis
c. Feedback inhibition of folic acid synthesis
d. Irreversible inhibition of folic acid synthesis

Ans. (a) Competitive inhibition of folic acid synthesis

118. Cyanide kills an organism by inhibiting

a. Hexokinase
b. Cytochrome oxidase
c. Succinate dehydrogenase
d. Histidine decarboxylase

Ans. (b) Cytochrome oxidase

119. How many categories of enzymes have been recognized by IUB

a. 5   b. 6
c. 7   d. 8

Ans. (b) 6

120. Which ions are toxic for enzyme activity

a. Mn^{++} b. K^+
c. Na^{++} d. Hg^{++}

Ans. (d) Hg^{++}

121. The enzyme Hexokinase which catalyses glucose to Glucose-6-phosphate in glycolysis is inhibited by Glucose-6-phosphate. This is an example of

a. Feedback allosteric inhibition
b. Positive feedback
c. Competitive inhibition
d. Non-competitive inhibition

Ans. (a) Feedback allosteric inhibition

122. If temperature is increased from 3°C to 45°C, the rate enzyme activity will

a. Only increase
b. Only decrease
c. Initially increase then decrease
d. Initially decrease then increase

Ans. (c) Initially increase then decrease

123. The name enzyme was coined by

a. Kuhne
b. Buchner
c. Berzelius
d. Dubrunfaut

Ans. (a) Kuhne

124. Nobel Prize for discovering emzymes was given to

a. Kuhne   b. Duclaux
c. Buchner   d. Dubrunfaut

Ans. (c) Buchner

125. Who confirmed protein nature of enzymes

a. Monod et al.   b. Arber et al
c. Berzelius   d. Northrop

Ans. (d) Northrop

126. Number of known enzymes is

a. 500   b. 5400
c. 1500   d. Over 2000

Ans. (d) Over 2000

127. Molecular weight of the smallest enzyme (bacterial ferredoxin) is

a. 6000   b. 5400
c. 4500   d. 3500

Ans. (a) 6000

128. A nonproteinaceous enzyme is

a. Lysozyme   b. Ribozyme
c. Ribonuclease-P   d. Both b and c

Ans. (d) Both b and c

129. Many enzymes are produced in inactive state called

a. Allosteric enzyme
b. Enzyme precursor
c. Proenzyme or zymogen
d. Both b and c

Ans. (d) Both b and c

130. An autocatalytic enzyme is

a. Pepsin   b. Trypsin
c. Chymotrypsin   d. All the above

Ans. (d) All the above

131. Pepsin is

a. Simple enzyme   b. Exoenzyme
c. Endoenzyme   d. Both a and b

Ans. (d) Both a and b

132. Which one is a conjugate enzyme

a. Succinate dehydrogenase
b. Urease
c. Trypsin
d. Both a and b

Ans. (a) Succinate dehydrogenase

133. An enzyme made of both protein and nonprotein parts is together called

a. Coenzyme
b. Endoenzyme
c. Exoenzyme
d. Holoenzyme

Ans. (d) Holoenzyme

134. An apoenzyme is a

a. Vitamin
b. Amino acid
c. Carbohydrate
d. Protein

Ans. (d) Protein

135. Nonprotein part of holoenzyme is

a. Vitamin
b. Cofactor
c. Fatty acid
d. Zymogen

Ans. (b) Cofactor

136. Vitamins are generally involved in forming component of enzyme called

a. Apoenzyme
b. Holoenzyme
c. Prosthetic group
d. Coenzyme and prosthetic group

Ans. (d) Coenzyme and prosthetic group

137. Loosely attached organic cofactor of holoenzyme is called

a. Modular
b. Prosthetic group
c. Coenzyme
d. Ligase

Ans. (c) Coenzyme

138. Firmly attached organic cofactor of holoenzyme is

a. Transferase
b. Activator
c. Modulator
d. Prosthetic group

Ans. (d) Prosthetic group

139. Coenzyme is often a

a. Carbohydrate
b. Protein
c. Vitamin
d. Fatty acid

Ans. (c) Vitamin

140. Part of enzyme where substrate is changed into product is called

a. Allosteric site
b. Active site
c. Cofactor
d. Prosthetic group

Ans. (b) Active site

141. Which one gives rise to coenzyme

a. B_2
b. B_1
c. Nicotinamide
d. All the above

Ans. (d) All the above

142. Each step of a metabolic pathway has its

a. Own cofactor
b. Enzyme
c. Coenzyme
d. One to several enzymes

Ans. (b) Enzyme

143. In certain metabolic pathways, a number of enzymes are required. These multienzyme complexes occur enclosed in

a. Membrane
b. Area with ATP
c. Microbodies
d. Endoplasmic reticulum

Ans. (a) Membrane

144. Inorganic cofactor is often called

a. Coenzyme
b. Prosthetic group
c. Modulator
d. Activator

Ans. (d) Activator

145. Active site of an enzyme is formed of

a. Amino groups of some amino acids
b. Carboxyl groups of some amino acids
c. –HS bonds of amino acids
d. R-groups of selected amino acids

Ans. (d) R-groups of selected amino acids

146. Different molecular forms of an enzyme having the same substrate specificity are

a. Zymogens
b. Coenzymes
c. Isoenzymes
d. Allosteric enzymes

Ans. (c) Isoenzymes

147. An allosteric enzyme has

a. One active site
b. One active site and one allosteric site
c. Active site and two types of allosteric sites
d. Two types of active sites

Ans. (c) Active site and two types of allosteric sites

148. Allosteric enzymes have allosteric sites for

a. Both activation and inhibition
b. Inhibition only
c. Activation only
d. Reduction in activation energy

Ans. (a) Both activation and inhibition

149. Turn-over number of the fastest enzyme is

a. 18×10^4 b. 10^4
c. 36×10^6 d. 10^5

Ans. (c) 36×10^6

150. The fastest enzyme is

a. Urease   b. Carbonic anhydrase
c. Trypsin   d. Pepsin

Ans. (b) Carbonic anhydrase

151. Substrate concentration at which an enzyme attains half its maximum velocity is

a. Threshold value
b. Half life
c. Michaelis-Menten constant
d. Concentration coefficient

Ans. (c) Michaelis-Menten constant

152. Enzyme that does not follow K_m values is

a. Exoenzyme   b. Allosteric enzyme
c. Isoenzyme   d. Pepsin

Ans. (b) Allosteric enzyme

153. K_m value is

a. Maximum reaction velocity
b. Near maximum reaction velocity
c. One half of maximum reaction velocity
d. Threshold value

Ans. (c) One half of maximum reaction velocity

154. The word appended at the end of enzyme name is

a. –ose   b. –ase
c. –in   d. –sin

Ans. (b) –ase

155. The word –ase added to enzyme is

a. Suffix   b. Prefix
c. Interpolation   d. Conjugation

Ans. (a) Suffix

156. The suffix -ase to enzyme names was proposed by

a. Duclaux   b. Buchner
c. Northrop   d. Pasteur

Ans. (a) Duclaux

157. The enzymes catalysting breakdown without addition of water are called

a. Lyases   b. Hydrolases
c. Ligases   d. Oxidoreductases

Ans. (a) Lyases

158. The enzymes that act on starch are

a. Esterases   b. Amylases
c. Proteases   d. Lipases

Ans. (b) Amylases

159. Enzyme aldolase which helps in combining dihydroxy acetone phosphate with glyceraldehydes phosphate belongs to the category of

a. Ligases   b. Hydrolases
c. Transferases   d. Lyases

Ans. (d) Lyases

160. Enzyme taking part in converting dihydroxyacetone phosphate to glyceraldehydes phosphate belongs to the class of

a. Isomerases   b. Hydrolases
c. Ligases   d. Transferases

Ans. (a) Isomerases

161. Enzyme lipase is capable of hydrolyzing

a. Starch   b. Fat
c. Protein   d. Cellulose

Ans. (b) Fat

162. Substrate for enzyme sucrase is

a. Any disaccharide
b. Starch and cane sugar
c. Cane sugar
d. Milk sugar

Ans. (c) Cane sugar

163. Enzyme required for hydrolyzing the food reserve in castor seed is

a. Amylase   b. Lipase
c. Protease   d. Diastase

Ans. (b) Lipase

164. Epimerase belongs to the class of enzymes

a. Hydrolases
b. Ligases
c. Isomerases
d. Oxidoreductases

Ans. (c) Isomerases

165. Enzymes catalyzing bonding of two components with the help of ATP are

a. Transferases
b. Ligases
c. Lyases
d. Phosphorylases

Ans. (b) Ligases

166. Enzymes used in breaking DNA at specific sites are

a. DNA-ases
b. Endonucleases
c. Restriction endonucleases
d. Exonucleases

Ans. (c) Restriction endonucleases

167. Restriction endonucleases were discovered by

a. Arber et al
b. Monod et al
c. Cech et al
d. Altman et al

Ans. (a) Arber et al

168. IUB has divided enzymes into classes

a. 4
b. 5
c. 6
d. 7

Ans. (c) 6

169. Most of the digestive enzymes belong to the class of

a. Lyases
b. Hydrolases
c. Oxidoreductases
d. Transferases

Ans. (b) Hydrolases

170. Constitutive enzymes are

a. Operational all the time
b. House keeping enzymes
c. Alloenzymes
d. Both a and b

Ans. (d) Both a and b

171. Repressible enzyme is

a. Present all the time
b. Functional almost all the time
c. Repressed in presence of a specific chemical
d. All the above

Ans. (d) All the above

172. Gaucher's disease is due to the deficiency of the enzyme

a. α -Fucosidase
b. β -Galactosidase
c. β -Glucosidase
d. Sphingomyelinase

Ans. (c) β -Glucosidase

173. An example of ligases is

a. Succinate thiokinase
b. Alanine racemase
c. Fumarase
d. Aldolase

Ans. (a) Succinate thiokinase

174. An example of lyases is

a. Glutamine synthetase
b. Fumarase
c. Cholinesterase
d. Amylase

Ans. (b) Fumarase

175. Activation or inactivation of certain key regulatory enzymes is accomplished by covalent modification of the amino acid

a. Tyrosine
b. Phenylalanine
c. Lysine
d. Serine

Ans. (d) Serine

176. The enzyme which can add water to a carbon-carbon double bond or remove water to create a double bond without breaking the bond is

a. Hydratase
b. Hydroxylase
c. Hydrolase
d. Esterase

Ans. (a) Hydratase

177. Fischer's 'lock and key' model of the enzyme action implies that

a. The active site is complementary in shape to that of substance only after interaction.
b. The active site is complementary in shape to that of substance
c. Substrates change conformation prior to active site interaction
d. The active site is flexible and adjusts to substrate

Ans. (b) The active site is complementary in shape to that of substance

178. From the Lineweaver-Burk plot of Michaelis-Menten equation, Km and Vmax can be determined when V is the reaction velocity at substrate concentration S, the X-axis experimental data are expressed as

a. 1/V
b. (B) V
c. 1/S
d. (D) S

Ans. (c) 1/S

179. A sigmoidal plot of substrate concentration ([S]) verses reaction velocity (V) may indicate

a. Michaelis-Menten kinetics
b. Co-operative binding
c. Competitive inhibition
d. Non-competitive inhibition

Ans. (b) Co-operative binding

180. The K_m of the enzyme giving the kinetic data as below is

a. –0.50   b. –0.25

c. +0.25   d. +0.33

Ans. (d) +0.33

181. The kinetic effect of purely competitive inhibitor of an enzyme

a. Increases K_m without affecting V_{max}

b. Decreases K_m without affecting V_{max}

c. Increases V_{max} without affecting K_m

d. Decreases V_{max} without affecting K_m

Ans. (a) Increases K_m without affecting V_{max}

182. If curve X in the graph (below) represents no inhibition for the reaction of the enzyme with its substrates, the curve representing the competitive inhibition, of the same reaction is

a. A   b. B

c. C   d. D

Ans. (a) A

183. An inducer is absent in the type of enzyme:

a. Allosteric enzyme

b. Constitutive enzyme

c. Co-operative enzyme

d. Isoenzymic enzyme

Ans. (b) Constitutive enzyme

184. In reversible non-competitive enzyme activity inhibition

a. V_{max} is increased

b. K_m is increased

c. K_m is decreased

d. Concentration of active enzyme is reduced

Ans. (d) Concentration of active enzyme is reduced

185. In reversible non-competitive enzyme activity inhibition

a. Inhibitor bears structural resemblance to substrate

b. Inhibitor lowers the maximum velocity attainable with a given amount of enzyme

c. K_m is increased

d. K_m is decreased

Ans. (b) Inhibitor lowers the maximum velocity attainable with a given amount of enzyme

186. In competitive enzyme activity inhibition

a. The structure of inhibitor generally resembles that of the substrate

b. Inhibitor decreases apparent K_m

c. K_m remains ineffective

d. Inhibitor decreases V_{max} without affecting K_m

Ans. (a) The structure of inhibitor generally resembles that of the substrate

187. In enzyme kinetics V_{max} reflects

a. The amount of an active enzyme

b. Substrate concentration

c. Half the substrate concentration

d. Enzyme substrate complex

Ans. (a) The amount of an active enzyme

188. In enzyme kinetics K_m implies

a. The substrate concentration that gives one half V_{max}

b. The dissocation constant for the enzyme substrate comples

c. Concentration of enzyme

d. Half of the substrate concentration required to achieve V_{max}

Ans. (b) The dissocation constant for the enzyme substrate comples

189. In competitive enzyme activity inhibition

a. Apparent K_m is decreased

b. Apparent K_m is increased

c. V_{max} is increased

d. V_{max} is decreased

Ans. (b) Apparent K_m is increased

190. In non competitive enzyme activity inhibition, inhibitor

a. Increases K_m b. Decreases K_m

c. Does not effect K_m d. Increases K_m

Ans. (c) Does not effect K_m

191. An enzyme catalyzing oxidoreduction, using oxygen as hydrogen acceptor is

a. Cytochrome oxidase

b. Lactate dehydrogenase

c. Malate dehydrogenase

d. Succinate dehydrogenase

Ans. (a) Cytochrome oxidase

192. The enzyme using some other substance, not oxygen as hydrogen acceptor is

a. Tyrosinase

b. Succinate dehydrogenase

c. Uricase

d. Cytochrome oxidase

Ans. (b) Succinate dehydrogenase

193. **An enzyme which uses hydrogen acceptor as substrate is**

    a. Xanthine oxidase
    b. Aldehyde oxidase
    c. Catalase
    d. Tryptophan oxygenase

Ans. (c) Catalase

194. **Enzyme involved in joining together two substrates is**

    a. Glutamine synthetase
    b. Aldolase
    c. Gunaine deaminase
    d. Arginase

Ans. (a) Glutamine synthetase

195. **The pH optima of most of the enzymes is**

    a. Between 2 and 4   b. Between 5 and 9
    c. Between 8 and 12   d. Above 12

Ans. (b) Between 5 and 9

196. **Coenzymes are**

    a. Heat stable, dialyzable, non protein organic molecules
    b. Soluble, colloidal, protein molecules
    c. Structural analogue of enzymes
    d. Different forms of enzymes

Ans. (a) Heat stable, dialyzable, non protein organic molecules

197. **An example of hydrogen transferring coenzyme is**

    a. CoA   b. NAD$^+$
    c. Biotin   d. TPP

Ans. (b) NAD$^+$

198. **An example of group transferring coenzyme is**

    a. NAD$^+$ b. NADP$^+$
    c. FAD   d. CoA

Ans. (d) CoA

199. **Cocarboxylase is**

    a. Thiamine pyrophosphate
    b. Pyridoxal phosphate
    c. Biotin
    d. CoA

Ans. (c) Biotin

200. **A coenzyme containing non aromatic hetero ring is**

    a. ATP   b. NAD
    c. FMN   d. Biotin

Ans. (d) Biotin

201. **A coenzyme containing aromatic hetero ring is**

    a. TPP   b. Lipoic acid
    c. Coenzyme Q   d. Biotin

Ans. (a) TPP

202. **Isoenzymes are**

    a. Chemically, immunologically and electrophoretically different forms of an enzyme
    b. Different forms of an enzyme similar in all properties
    c. Catalysing different reactions
    d. Having the same quaternary structures like the enzymes

Ans. (a) Chemically, immunologically and electrophoretically different forms of an enzyme

203. **Isoenzymes can be characterized by**

    a. Proteins lacking enzymatic activity that are necessary for the activation of enzymes
    b. Proteolytic enzymes activated by hydrolysis
    c. Enzymes with identical primary structure
    d. Similar enzymes that catalyse different Reaction

Ans. (b) Proteolytic enzymes activated by hydrolysis

204. **The isoenzymes of LDH**

    a. Differ only in a single amino acid
    b. Differ in catalytic activity
    c. Exist in 5 forms depending on M and H monomer contents
    d. Occur as monomers

Ans. (c) Exist in 5 forms depending on M and H monomer contents

205. **The normal value of CPK in serum varies between**

    a. 4–60 IU/L   b. 60–250 IU/L
    c. 4–17 IU/L   d. > 350 IU/L

Ans. (a) 4–60 IU/L

206. **Factors affecting enzyme activity**

    a. Concentration   b. pH
    c. Temperature   d. All of these

Ans. (d) All of these

207. **Which of the following is a substrate specific enzyme?**

    a. Hexokinase
    b. Thiokinase
    c. Lactase
    d. Aminopeptidase

Ans. (c) Lactase

209. Coenzymes combine with

a. Proenzymes
b. Apoenzymes
c. Holoenzymes
d. Antienzymes

Ans. (b) Apoenzymes

210. Coenzymes are required in which of the following reactions?

a. Oxidation-reduction
b. Transamination
c. Phosphorylation
d. All of these

Ans. (d) All of these

211. Which of the following coenzyme takes part in hydrogen transfer reactions?

a. Tetrahydrofolate
b. Coenzyme A
c. Coenzyme Q
d. Biotin

Ans. (c) Coenzyme Q

212. Which of the following coenzyme takes part in oxidation-reduction reactions?

a. Pyridoxal phosphate
b. Lipoic acid
c. Thiamin diphosphate
d. None of these

Ans. (b) Lipoic acid

213. In conversion of glucose to glucose-6-phsophate, the coenzyme is

a. Mg^{++}
b. ATP
c. Both (A) and (B)
d. None of these

Ans. (b) ATP

214. A coenzyme required in transamination reactions is

a. Coenzyme A
b. Coenzyme Q
c. Biotin
d. Pyridoxal phosphate

Ans. (d) Pyridoxal phosphate

215. Coenzyme A contains a vitamin which is

a. Thiamin
b. Ascorbic acid
c. Pantothenic acid
d. Niacinamide

Ans. (c) Pantothenic acid

216. Cobamides contain a vitamin which is

a. Folic acid
b. Ascorbic acid
c. Pantothenic acid
d. Vitamin B_{12}

Ans. (d) Vitamin B_{12}

217. A coenzyme required in carboxylation reactions is

a. Lipoic acid
b. Coenzyme A
c. Biotin
d. All of these

Ans. (c) Biotin

218. Which of the following coenzyme takes part in tissue respiration?

a. Coenzyme Q
b. Coenzyme A
c. NADP
d. Cobamide

Ans. (a) Coenzyme Q

219. The enzyme hexokinase is a

a. Hydrolase
b. Oxidoreductase
c. Transferase
d. Ligase

Ans. (c) Transferase

220. Which of the following is a proteolytic enzyme?

a. Pepsin
b. Trypsin
c. Chymotrypsin
d. All of these

Ans. (d) All of these

221. Enzymes which catalyse binding of two substrates by covalent bonds are known as

a. Lyases
b. Hydrolases
c. Ligases
d. Oxidoreductases

Ans. (c) Ligases

222. The induced fit model of enzyme action was proposed by

a. Fischer
b. Koshland
c. Mitchell
d. Markert

Ans. (b) Koshland

223. Allosteric inhibition is also known as

a. Competitive inhibition
b. Non-competitive inhibition
c. Feedback inhibition
d. None of these

Ans. (c) Feedback inhibition

224. An allosteric enzyme is generally inhibited by

a. Initial substrate of the pathway
b. Substrate analogues
c. Product of the reaction catalysed by allosteric enzyme
d. Product of the pathway

Ans. (d) Product of the pathway

225. **When the velocity of an enzymatic reaction equals** V_{max}, **substrate concentration is**

   a. Half of K_m
   b. Equal to K_m
   c. Twice the K_m
   d. Far above the K_m

   Ans. (d) Far above the K_m

226. **In Lineweaver-Burk plot, the y-intercept represents**

   a. V_{max}
   b. K_m
   c. K_m
   d. $1/K_m$

   Ans. (b) K_m

227. **In competitive inhibition, the inhibitor**

   a. Competes with the enzyme
   b. Irreversibly binds with the enzyme
   c. Binds with the substrate
   d. Competes with the substrate

   Ans. (d) Competes with the substrate

228. **Competitive inhibitors**

   a. Decrease the Km
   b. Decrease the Vmax
   c. Increase the Km
   d. Increase the Vmax

   Ans. (c) Increase the Km

229. **Competitive inhibition can be relieved by raising the**

   a. Enzyme concentration
   b. Substrate concentration
   c. Inhibitor concentration
   d. None of these

   Ans. (b) Substrate concentration

230. **Physostigmine is a competitive inhibitor of**

   a. Xanthine oxidase
   b. Cholinesterase
   c. Carbonic anhydrase
   d. Monoamine oxidase

   Ans. (b) Cholinesterase

231. **Carbonic anhydrase is competitively inhibited by**

   a. Allopurinol
   b. Acetazolamide
   c. Aminopterin
   d. Neostigmine

   Ans. (b) Acetazolamide

232. **Serum lactate dehydrogenase rises in**

   a. Viral hepatitis
   b. Myocardial infarction
   c. Carcinomatosis
   d. All of these

   Ans. (d) All of these

233. **Which of the following serum enzyme rises in myocardial infarction?**

   a. Creatine kinase
   b. GOT
   c. LDH
   d. All of these

   Ans. (d) All of these

234. **From the following myocardial infarction, the earliest serum enzyme to rise is**

   a. Creatine Kinase
   b. GOT
   b. GPT
   d. LDH

   Ans. (a) Creatine Kinase (b) GOT

235. **Proenzymes**

   a. Chymotrysinogen
   b. Pepsinogen
   c. Both (A) and (B)
   d. None of these

   Ans. (b) Pepsinogen

236. **Alkaline phosphatase is present in**

   a. Liver
   b. Bones
   c. Placenta
   d. All of these

   Ans. (d) All of these

237. **Which of the following isoenzyme of lactate dehydrogenase is raised in serum in myocardial infarction?**

   a. LD_1
   b. LD_2
   c. LD_1 and LD_2
   d. LD_5

   Ans. (c) LD_1 and LD_2

238. **Enzymes which are always present in an organism are known as**

   a. Inducible enzymes
   b. Constitutive enzymes
   c. Functional enzymes
   d. Apoenzymes

   Ans. (b) Constitutive enzymes

239. **Inactive precursors of enzymes are known as**

   a. Apoenzymes
   b. Coenzymes
   c. Proenzymes
   d. Holoenzymes

   Ans. (c) Proenzymes

240. **Whcih of the following is a proenzyme?**

   a. Carboxypeptidase
   b. Aminopeptidase
   c. Chymotrypsin
   d. Pepsinogen

   Ans. (d) Pepsinogen

241. Allosteric enzymes regulate the formation of products by

a. Feedback inhibition
b. Non-competitive inhibition
c. Competitive inhibition
d. Repression-derepression

Ans. (a) Feedback inhibition

242. Regulation of some enzymes by covalent modification involves addition or removal of

a. Acetate   b. Sulphate
c. Phosphate   d. Coenzyme

Ans. (c) Phosphate

243. Covalent modification of an enzyme generally requires a

a. Hormone   b. cAMP
c. Protein kinase d. All of these

Ans. (d) All of these

244. An inorganic ion required for the activity of an enzyme is known as

a. Activator   b. Cofactor
c. Coenzyme   d. None of these

Ans. (b) Cofactor

245. The first enzyme found to have isoenzymes was

a. Alkaline Phosphatase
b. Lactate dehydrogenase
c. Acid Phosphatase
d. Creatine kinase

Ans. (b) Lactate dehydrogenase

246. Lactate dehydrogenase is located in

a. Lysosomes   b. Mitochondria
c. Cytosol   d. Microsomes

Ans. (c) Cytosol

247. Lactate dehydrogenase is a

a. Monomer   b. Dimer
c. Tetramer   d. Hexamer

Ans. (c) Tetramer

248. Ceruloplasmin is absent in

a. Cirrhosis of liver
b. Wilson's disease
c. Menke's disease
d. Copper deficiency

Ans. (b) Wilson's disease

249. Ceruloplasmin oxidizes

a. Copper   b. Iron
c. Both (A) and (B) d. None of these

Ans. (b) Iron

250. Creatine kinase is present in all of the following except:

a. Liver   b. Myocardium
c. Muscles   d. Brain

Ans. (a) Liver

251. Alkaline phosphatase is present in

a. Liver   b. Bones
c. Intestinal mucosa d. All of these

Ans. (d) All of these

252. All of the following are zinc-containing enzymes except:

a. Acid phosphatase
b. Alkaline phosphatase
c. Carbonic anhydrase
d. RNA polymerase

Ans. (a) Acid phosphatase

253. All of the following are iron-containing enzymes except:

a. Carbonic anhydrase b. Catalase
c. Peroxidase   d. Cytochrome oxidase

Ans. (a) Carbonic anhydrase

254. Biotin is a coenzyme for

a. Pyruvate dehydrogenase
b. Pyruvate carboxylase
c. PEP carboxykinase
d. Glutamate pyruvate transminase

Ans. (b) Pyruvate carboxylase

255. Enzymes accelerate the rate of reactions by

a. Increasing the equilibrium constant of reactions
b. Increasing the energy of activation
c. Decreasing the energy of activation
d. Decreasing the free energy change of the reaction

Ans. (c) Decreasing the energy of activation

256. Kinetics of an allosteric enzyme are explained by

a. Michaelis-Menten equation
b. Lineweaver-Burk plot
c. Hill plot
d. All of these

Ans. (c) Hill plot

257. Covalent modification of an enzyme usually involves phosphorylation /dephosphorylation of

a. Serine residue
b. Proline residue
c. Hydroxylysine residue
d. Hydroxyproline residue

Ans. (a) Serine residue

258. V_{max} of an enzyme may be affected by

a. pH
b. Temperature
c. Non-competitive inhibitors
d. All of these

Ans. (d) All of these

259. In enzyme assays, all the following are kept constant *except*:

a. Substrate concentration
b. Enzyme concentration
c. pH
d. Temperature

Ans. (b) Enzyme concentration

260. If the substrate concentration is much below the k_m of the enzyme, the velocity of the reaction is

a. Directly proportional to substrate concentration
b. Not affected by enzyme concentration
c. Nearly equal to V_{max}
d. Inversely proportional to substrate concentration

Ans. (a) Directly proportional to substrate concentration

261. Enzymes requiring NAD as co-substrate can be assayed by measuring change in absorbance at

a. 210 nm
b. 290 nm
c. 340 nm
d. 365 nm

Ans. (c) 340 nm

262. Different isoenzymes of an enzyme have the same

a. Amino acid sequence
b. Michaelis constant
c. Catalytic activity
d. All of these

Ans. (c) Catalytic activity

263. The Michaehis-menten hypothesis:

a. Postulates the formation of an enzyme substrate complex
b. Enables us to calculate the isoelectric point of an enzyme

c. States that the rate of a chemical reaction may be independent of substrate concentration
d. States that the reaction rate is proportional to substrate concentration

Ans. (a) Postulates the formation of an enzyme substrate complex

264. Schardinger's enzyme is

a. Lactate dehydrogenase
b. Xanthine dehydrogenase
c. Uric oxidase
d. L amino acid dehydrogenase

Ans. (b) Xanthine dehydrogenase

265. Tryptophan pyrolase is currently known as

a. Tryptophan deaminase
b. Tryptophan dioxygenase
c. Tryptophan mono oxygenase
d. Tryptophan decarboxylase

Ans. (b) Tryptophan dioxygenase

266. An enzyme which brings about lysis of bacterial cell wall is

a. Amylase   b. Lysozyme
c. Trypsin   d. Lipase

Ans. (b) Lysozyme

267. Trypsin has no action on

a. Hemoglobin   b. Albumin
c. Histone   d. DNA

Ans. (d) DNA

268. Multiple forms of the same enzymes are known as

a. Zymogens   b. Isoenzymes
c. Proenzymes   d. Pre-enzymes

Ans. (b) Isoenzymes

269. In non-competitive enzyme action

a. V_{max} is increased
b. Apparent k_m is increased
c. Apparent k_m is decreased
d. Concentration of active enzyme molecule is reduced

Ans. (c) Apparent k_m is decreased

270. An allosteric enzyme influences the enzyme activity by

a. Competing for the catalytic site with the substrate
b. Changing the specificity of the enzyme for the substrate

c. Changing the conformation of the enzyme by binding to a site other than catalytic site

d. Changing the nature of the products formed

Ans. (c) Changing the conformation of the enzyme by binding to a site other than catalytic site

271. Which of the following regulatory reactions involves a reversible covalent modification of an enzyme?

a. Phosphorylation of serine OH on the enzyme

b. Allosteric modulation

c. Competitive inhibition

d. Non-competitive inhibition

Ans. (a) Phosphorylation of serine OH on the enzyme

272. A competitive inhibitor of an enzyme has which of the following properties?

a. It is frequently a feedback inhibitor

b. It becomes covalently attached to an enzyme

c. It decreases the V_{max}

d. It interferes with substrate binding to the enzyme

Ans. (d) It interferes with substrate binding to the enzyme

273. When [s] is equal to Km, which of the following conditions exist?

a. Half the enzyme molecules are bound to substrate

b. The velocity of the reaction is equal to V_{max}

c. The velocity of the reaction is independent of substrate concentration

d. Enzyme is completely saturated with substrate

Ans. (a) Half the enzyme molecules are bound to substrate

274. Which of the following statements about an enzyme exhibiting allosteric kinetics with cooperative interaction is false?

a. A plot of V-Vk [s] has a sigmoidal shape

b. An inhibitor may increase the apparent K_m

c. Line weaver Berk plot is useful for determining Km and V_{max}

d. Removal of allosteric inhibitor may result in hyperbolic V-S [s] plot

Ans. (d) Removal of allosteric inhibitor may result in hyperbolic V-S [s] plot

275. Pantothenic acid acts on

a. NADP

b. NADPH

c. FAD

d. CoA

Ans. (b) NADPH

276. Vitamin deficiency that causes fatty liver includes all *except*:

a. Vitamin E

b. Pyridoxine

c. Retionic acid

d. Pantothenic acid

Ans. (c) Retionic acid

277. In which of the following types of enzymes an inducer is not required?

a. Inhibited enzyme

b. Cooperative enzyme

c. Allosteric enzyme

d. Constitutive enzyme

Ans. (d) Constitutive enzyme

278. In which of the following types of enzyme water may be added to a C—C double bond without breaking the bond?

a. Hydrolase

b. Hydratase

c. Hydroxylase

d. Esterase

Ans. (b) Hydratase

279. 'Lock' and 'Key' model of enzyme action proposed by Fisher implies that

a. The active site is flexible and adjusts to substrate

b. The active site requires removal of PO_4 group

c. The active site is complementary in shape to that of the substrate

d. Substrates change conformation prior to active site interaction

Ans. (c) The active site is complementary in shape to that of the substrate

280. In competitive inhibition of enzyme action

a. The apparent K_m is decreased

b. The apparent K_m is increased

c. V_{max} is decreased

d. Apparent concentration of enzyme molecules decreased

Ans. (b) The apparent K_m is increased

281. In competitive inhibition which of the following kinetic effect is true?

a. Decreases both K_m and V_{max}

b. Increases both K_m and V_{max}

c. Decreases K_m without affecting V_{max}

d. Increases K_m without affecting V_{max}

Ans. (d) Increases K_m without affecting V_{max}

282. Enzymes are required in traces because they

    a. Have high turnover number

    b. Remain unused at the end of reaction and are re used

    c. Show cascade effect

    d. All are correct

Ans. (d) All are correct

283. An organic substance bound to an enzyme and essential for the activity of enzyme is called

    a. Holoenzyme   b. Apoenzyme

    c. Coenzyme   d. Isoenzyme

Ans. (c) Coenzyme

284. Enzyme catalysed reactions occur in

    a. Pico seconds   b. Micro seconds

    c. Milli seconds   d. None of these

Ans. (c) Milli seconds

285. An enzyme can accelerate a reaction up to

    a. 1010 times   b. 101 times

    c. 10100 times   d. 10 times

Ans. (a) 1010 times

286. In plants, enzymes occur in

    a. Flowers only

    b. Leaves only

    c. All living cells

    d. Storage organs only

Ans. (c) All living cells

287. Zymogen is a

    a. Vitamin   b. Enzyme precursor

    c. Modulator   d. Hormone

Ans. (b) Enzyme precursor

288. Cofactor (Prosthetic group) is a part of holoenzyme, it is

    a. Inorganic part loosely attached

    b. Accessory non-protein substance attached firmly

    c. Organic part attached loosely

    d. None of these

Ans. (b) Accessory non-protein substance attached firmly

289. A protein having both structural and enzymatic traits is

    a. Myosin   b. Collagen

    c. Trypsin   d. Actin

Ans. (a) Myosin

290. Enzymes are different from catalysts in

    a. Being proteinaceous

    b. Not used up in reaction

    c. Functional at high temperature

    d. Having high rate of diffusion

Ans. (a) Being proteinaceous

291. Enzymes, vitamins and hormones are common in

    a. Being proteinaceous

    b. Being synthesized in the body of organisms

    c. Enhancing oxidative metabolism

    d. Regulating metabolism

Ans. (d) Regulating metabolism

292. Dry seeds endure higher temperature than germinating seeds as

    a. Hydration is essential for making enzymes sensitive to temperature

    b. Dry seeds have a hard covering

    c. Dry seeds have more reserve food

    d. Seedlings are tender

Ans. (a) Hydration is essential for making enzymes sensitive to temperature

293. Coenzymes FMN and FAD are derived from vitamin

    a. C

    b. B_6

    c. B_1

    d. B_2

Ans. (d) B_2

294. Template/lock and key theory of enzyme action is supported by

    a. Enzymes speed up reaction

    b. Enzymes occur in living beings and speed up certain reactions

    c. Enzymes determine the direction of reaction

    d. Compounds similar to substrate inhibit enzyme activity

Ans. (d) Compounds similar to substrate inhibit enzyme activity

295. Combination of apoenzyme and coenzyme produces

    a. Prosthetic group

    b. Holoenzyme

    c. Enzyme substrate complex

    d. Enzyme product complex

Ans. (b) Holoenzyme

296. Enzyme inhibition caused by a substance resembling substrate molecule is

a. Competitive inhibition
b. Non-competitive inhibition
c. Feedback inhibition
d. Allosteric inhibition

Ans. (a) Competitive inhibition

297. An enzyme brings about

a. Decrease in reaction time
b. Increase in reaction time
c. Increase in activation energy
d. Reduction in activation energy

Ans. (d) Reduction in activation energy

298. Feedback inhibition of enzyme is influenced by

a. Enzyme
b. External factors
c. End product
d. Substrate

Ans. (c) End product

299. Coenzyme is

a. Often a vitamin
b. Always an inorganic compound
c. Always a protein
d. Often a metal

Ans. (a) Often a vitamin

300. Genetic engineering requires enzyme:

a. DNA ase
b. Amylase
c. Lipase
d. Restriction endonuclease

Ans. (d) Restriction endonuclease

301. Which is not true about inorganic catalysts and enzymes?

a. They are specific
b. Inorganic catalysts require specific not needed by enzymes
c. They are sensitive to pH
d. They speed up the rate of chemical reaction

Ans. (b) Inorganic catalysts require specific not needed by enzymes

302. Key and lock hypothesis of enzyme action was given by

a. Fischer
b. Koshland
c. Buchner
d. Kuhne

Ans. (a) Fischer

303. An example of feedback inhibition is

a. Allosteric inhibition of hexokinase by glucose-6-phosphate
b. Cyanide action on cytochrome
c. Sulpha drug on folic acid synthesizer bacteria
d. Reaction between succinic dehydrogenase and succinic acid

Ans. (a) Allosteric inhibition of hexokinase by glucose-6-phosphate

304. Feedback term refers to

a. Effect of substrate on rate of enzymatic reaction
b. Effect of end product on rate reaction
c. Effect of enzyme concentration on rate of reaction
d. Effect of external compound on rate of reaction

Ans. (b) Effect of end product on rate reaction

305. Allosteric inhibition

a. Makes active site unifit for substrate
b. Controls excess formation and end product
c. Both (A) and (B)
d. None of these

Ans. (c) Both (A) and (B)

306. The ratio of enzyme to substrate molecules can be as low as

a. 1 : 100,000
b. 1 : 500,000
c. 1 : 10,000
d. 1 : 1,000

Ans. (a) 1 : 100,000

307. Vitamin B_2 is component of coenzyme:

a. Pyridoxal phosphate
b. TPP
c. NAD
d. FMN/FAD

Ans. (d) FMN/FAD

308. K_m value of enzyme is substrate concentration at

a. $\frac{1}{2} V_{max}$
b. $2 V_{max}$
c. $\frac{1}{2} V_{max}$
d. $4 V_{max}$

Ans. (d) $4 V_{max}$

309. Part of enzyme which combines with nonprotein part to form functional enzyme is

a. Apoenzyme
b. Coenzyme
c. Prosthetic group
d. None of these

Ans. (c) Prosthetic group

310. Who got Nobel Prize in 1978 for working on enzymes?

a. Koshland   b. Arber and Nathans

c. Nass and Nass   d. H.G. Khorana

Ans. (a) Koshland

311. Site of enzyme synthesis in a cell is

a. Ribosomes   b. RER

c. Golgi bodies   d. All of these

Ans. (b) RER

312. The fruit when kept is open, tastes bitter after 2 hours because of

a. Loss of water from juice

b. Decreased concentration of fructose in juice

c. Fermentation by yeast

d. Contamination by bacterial enzymes

Ans. (d) Contamination by bacterial enzymes

313. Hexokinase (Glucose + ATP → Glucose-6–P + ADP) belongs to the category:

a. Transferases   b. Lysases

c. Oxidoreductases   d. Isomerases

Ans. (c) Oxidoreductases

314. Which enzyme is concerned with transfer of electrons?

a. Desmolase   b. Hydrolase

c. Dehydrogenase   d. Transaminase

Ans. (a) Desmolase

315. The best example of extracellular enzymesm (exoenzyme) is

a. Nucleases

b. Digestive enzymes

c. Succinic dehydrogenase

d. None of these

Ans. (c) Succinic dehydrogenase

316. Which mineral element controls the activity of Nitrate reductase?

a. Fe   b. Mo

c. Zn   d. Ca

Ans. (a) Fe

317. Name the enzyme that acts both as carboxylase at one time and oxygenase at another time.

a. PEP carboxylase

b. RuBP carboxylase

c. Carbonic anyhdrase

d. None of these

Ans. (b) RuBP carboxylase

318. A metabolic pathways is a

a. Route taken by chemicals

b. Sequence of enzyme facilitated chemical reactions

c. Route taken by an enzyme from one reaction to another

d. Sequence of origin of organic molecules

Ans. (b) Sequence of enzyme facilitated chemical reactions

319. The energy required to start an enzymatic reaction is called

a. Chemical energy   b. Metabolic energy

c. Activation energy   d. Potential energy

Ans. (c) Activation energy

320. Out of the total enzymes present in a cell, a mitochondrion alone has

a. 4%   b. 70%

c. 95%   d. 50%

Ans. (b) 70%

321. Creatine phosphokinase isoenzyme is a marker for

a. Kidney disease   b. Liver disease

c. Myocardial infarction   d. None of these

Ans. (c) Myocardial infarction

322. Which inactivates an enzyme by occupying its active site?

a. Competitive inhibitor

b. Allosteric inhibitor

c. Non-competitive inhibitor

d. All of these

Ans. (a) Competitive inhibitor

323. Which one is coenzyme?

a. ATP   b. Vitamin B and C

c. CoQ and CoA   d. All of these

Ans. (d) All of these

324. The active site of an enzyme is formed by

a. R group of amino acids

b. NH_2 group of amino acids

c. CO group of amino acids

d. Sulphur bonds which are exposed

Ans. (a) R group of amino acids

325. Carbonic anhydrase enzyme has maximum turn over number (36 million). Minimum turn over number for an enzyme

a. DNA polymerase

b. Lysozyme

c. Penicillase

d. Lactase dehydrogenase

Ans. (b) Lysozyme

326. In cell, digestive enzymes are found mainly in

a. Vacuoles   b. Lysosomes

c. Ribosomes   d. Lomasomes

Ans. (b) Lysosomes

327. Substrate concentration at which an enzyme attains half its maximum velocity is

a. Threshold value

b. Michaelis-Menton constant

c. Concentration level

d. None of these

Ans. (b) Michaelis-Menton constant

328. Which enzyme hydrolyses starch?

a. Invertase   b. Maltase

c. Sucrase   d. Diastase

Ans. (b) Maltase

329. Enzymes functional in cell or mitochondria are

a. Endoenzymes

b. Exoenzymes

c. Apoenzymes

d. Holoenzymes

Ans. (c) Apoenzymes

330. The enzymes present in the membrane of mitochondria are

a. Flavoproteins and cytochromes

b. Fumarase and lipase

c. Enolase and catalase

d. Hexokinase and zymase

Ans. (a) Flavoproteins and cytochromes

331. A mitochondrial marker enzyme is

a. Aldolase

b. Amylase

c. Succinic dehydrogenase

d. Pyruvate dehydrogenase

Ans. (c) Succinic dehydrogenase

332. The enzyme used in polymerase chain reaction (PCR) is

a. Taq polymerase

b. RNA polymerase

c. Ribonuclease

d. Endonuclease

Ans. (d) Endonuclease

333. Which of the following is a microsomal enzyme inducer?

a. Indomethacin   b. Clofibrate

c. Tolbutamide   d. Glutethamide

Ans. (d) Glutethamide

334. Identify the correct molecule which controls the biosynthesis of proteins in living organisms.

a. DNA   b. RNA

c. Purines   d. Pyrimidines

Ans. (a) DNA

335. The tear secretion contains an antibacterial enzyme known as

a. Zymase   b. Diastase

c. Lysozyme   d. Lipase

Ans. (c) Lysozyme

336. Identify one of the canbonic anhydrase inhibitor that inhibit only luminal carbonic anhydrase enzyme

a. Methazolamide

b. Acetazolamide

c. Dichlorphenamide

d. Benzolamide

Ans. (b) Acetazolamide

337. Group transferring Co-enzyme is

a. CoA   b. NAD^+

c. $NADP^+$ d. FAD^+

Ans. (a) CoA

338. The co-enzyme containing an automatic hetero ring in the structure is

a. Biotin

b. TPP

c. Sugar phosphate

d. Co-enzyme

Ans. (c) Sugar phosphate

339. The example of hydrogen transferring co-enzyme is

a. $B_6–PO_4$ b. $NADP^+$

c. TPP   d. ATP

Ans. (d) ATP

340. Enzyme catalyzed hydrolysis of proteins produces amino acid of the form

a. D   b. DL

c. L   d. Racemic

Ans. (c) L

341. Transaminase activity needs the Coenzyme:

a. ATP

b. B_6–PO_4

c. FADT

d. NAD^+

Ans. (b) B_6–PO_4

342. The biosynthesis of urea occurs mainly in the liver

a. Cytosol

b. Mitochondria

c. Microsomes

d. Nuclei

Ans. (b) Mitochondria

343. Bile salts make emulsification with fat for the action of

a. Amylose

b. Lipase

c. Pepsin

d. Trypsin

Ans. (b) Lipase

344. All of the following compounds are intermediates of TCA cycle *except*:

a. Maleate

b. Pyruvate

c. Oxaloacetate

d. Fumarate

Ans. (b) Pyruvate

345. In conversion of lactic acid to glucose, three reactions of glycolytic pathway are circumvented, which of the following enzymes do not participate?

a. Pyruvate carboxylase

b. Phosphoenol pyruvate carboxy kinase

c. Pyruvate kinase

d. Glucose-6-phosphatase

Ans. (b) Phosphoenol pyruvate carboxy kinase

346. In the normal resting state of human most of the blood glucose burnt as fuel is consumed by

a. Liver

b. Brain

c. Adipose tissue

d. Muscles

Ans. (b) Brain

347. A regulator of the enzyme glucogen synthase is

a. Citric acid

b. Pyruvate

c. Glucose-6-PO_4

d. GTP

Ans. (c) Glucose-6-PO_4

348. A specific inhibitor for succinate dehydrogenase is

a. Arsenite

b. Malonate

c. Citrate

d. Fluoride

Ans. (b) Malonate

349. During the functioning of biosensor, which of the following sequences of event occurs?

a. Enzymatic/cellular reaction $\rightarrow$ detector $\rightarrow$ transducer

b. Enzymatic/cellular reaction $\rightarrow$ transducer $\rightarrow$ detector

c. Enzymatic/cellular reaction $\rightarrow$ pressure gauge $\rightarrow$ time

d. Enzymatic/cellular reaction $\rightarrow$ vibrator $\rightarrow$ mechanical signal

Ans. (b) Enzymatic/cellular reaction $\rightarrow$ transducer $\rightarrow$ detector

350. An immobilized enzyme being used in continuous plug flow reactor exhibits an effectiveness factor (η) of 1.2. The value of η being greater than one could be apparently due to one of the following reasons. Identify the correct reasons.

a. The enzyme follows substrate inhibited kinetics with intern pore diffusion initiation

b. The enzyme experiences external film diffusion limitation

c. The enzyme follows sigmoid kinetic

d. The immobilized enzyme is operationally unstable

Ans. (c) The enzyme follows sigmoid kinetic

351. The degree of inhibition for non-competitive inhibition of an enzyme catalyzed reaction

a. Increase with increase substrate concentration

b. Reaches a maxima with increase in substrate concentration and then decreases

c. Is independent of substrate concentration

d. Decreases with increase in substrate concentration

Ans. (b) Reaches a maxima with increase in substrate concentration and then decreases

352. An enzyme following Michaelis-Menten kinetics with $V_m = 2.5$ mmol m^{-3}s^{-1} and km = 5.0 mM was used to carry out the reaction in a batch stirred reactor. Starting with an initial substrate concentration of 0.1 M, the time required for 50% conversion of the substrate will be about

a. 01 hr

b. 06 hr

c. 02 hr

d. 12 hr

Ans. (b) 06 hr

353. The maximum reaction velocity (V_m) for an enzyme catalyzed reaction was experimentally measured at two different temperatures of following results were obtained

Temperature, °C	–27	37
V_m mmolm^{-3}s^{-1}	2.25	4.50

The energy of activation for the reaction is

a. 12834 cal mol^{-1} b. 25668 cal mol^{-1}

c. 6417 cal mol^{-1} d. 19251 cal mol^{-1}

Ans. (a) 12834 cal mol^{-1}

354. Inversion of sucrose by immobilized invertase follows substrate inhibited kinetics. The reaction rate (V) in mol mhr^{-1} can be expressed as

$$V = 800 \frac{(S)}{\left\{ 400 + 50(S) + (S)^2 \right\}}$$

Where, (S) is sucrose concentration
The immobilized invertase preparation is used in a CSTR with 100 mol m^{-3} sucrose concentration in the feed stream. If the reaction velocity passes through a maxima at (S) = 20 mol m^{-3} the feed flow rate for a reactor volume of 1 m^3 to get the maximum productivity from reactor should be

a. 0.11 m^{-3}hr^{-1}

b. 1.10 m^{-3}hr^{-1}

c. 5.05 m^{-3}hr^{-1}

d. None of these

Ans. (a) 0.11 m^{-3}hr^{-1}

355. Enzyme papin is used with success to

a. Increase meat production

b. Leaven bread

c. Ripen papaya fruit

d. Tenderize meat

Ans. (d) Tenderize meat

356. Which one of the following reactions used for the purpose of recycling enzymes in bioprocesses?

a. Isomerization

b. Immobilization

c. Phosphorylation

d. Polymerization

Ans. (b) Immobilization

357. Match the industrial application of the following enzymes:

A Penicillinase	1. Pharmaceutical
B Pectinase	2. Leather
C Trypsin	3. Wine
D Rennin	4. Dairy

Codes

	A	B	C	D
a.	4	3	1	2
b.	1	3	2	4
c.	1	2	3	4
d.	4	2	3	1

Ans. (b) 1 3 2 4

358. Which one of the following techniques is NOT ideal for immobilized cell-free enzyme?

a. Physical entrapment by encapsulation

b. Covalent surface bonding to surface carriers

c. Physical bonding by flocculation

d. Covalent chemical bonding by cross-linking the precipitate

Ans. (c) Physical bonding by flocculation

359. The enzyme where catalysis involves transfer of electrons are named as

a. Isomerase   b. Transferases

c. Oxidoreductase   d. Lyases

Ans. (c) Oxidoreductase

360. The graph shows a Lineweaver-Burke plot for an enzyme catalyzed reaction

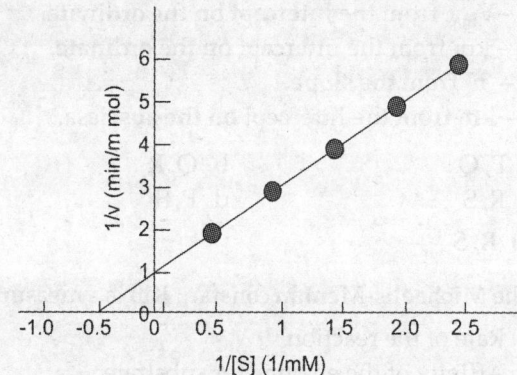

Which of the following statements is correct?

a. V_{max} is 5 M mol/min and with competitive inhibition V_{max} remains unchanged

b. K_m is 2M mol/min and with competitive inhibition both K_m and V_{max} both decreases

c. K_m is 0.5 mM and with competitive inhibition V_{max} increases but K_m remain

d. K_m is 2.0 mM and with competitive inhibition K_m increases but V_{max} remains unchanged

Ans. (d) K_m is 2.0 mM and with competitive inhibition K_m increases but V_{max} remains unchanged

361. Data for Questions 13 and 14 The kinetic data for an enzymatic in the presence and absence of inhibitors are plotted in the following figure

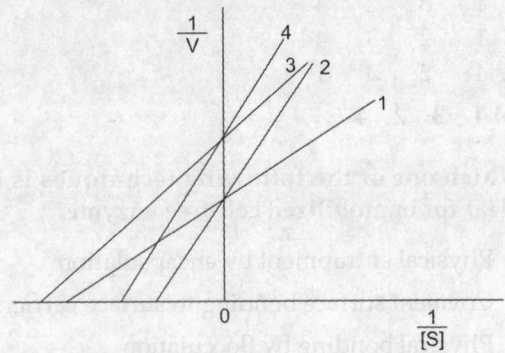

Which line represents kinetics without inhibitors?
a. Line 1
b. Line 2
c. Line 3
d. Line 4

Ans. (b) Line 2

362. Which line represents kinetics of non competitive inhibition?

a. Line 1
b. Line 2
c. Line 3
d. Line 4

Ans. (d) Line 4

363. Using Hill equation for an enzyme $[s]_0 = (v_0 km/ V_{max} - v_0)^{1/n}$ and the plot of $\log_{10} (v_0/V_{max} - v_0)$ vs $\log_{10} [s]_0$ one can find out

P – V_{max} from the intercept on the ordinate.
Q – km from the intercept on the ordinate.
R – 'n' from the slope.
S – km from the intercept on the abscissa.

a. P, Q
b. Q, R
c. R, S
d. P, S

Ans. (c) R, S

364. The Michaelis-Menton constant Km is a measure of

a. Rate of the reaction
b. Affinity of the enzyme for substrate
c. Concentration of enzyme-substrate [ES] intermediate
d. None of these

Ans. (b) Affinity of the enzyme for substrate

365. The Michaelis – Menton constant, Km is

a. Numerically equal to ½ V_{max}
b. Dependent on enzyme concentration
c. Independent of pH
d. Numerically equal to the substrate concentration that gives half-maximal velocity

Ans. (d) Numerically equal to the substrate concentration that gives half-maximal velocity

366. Most industrial enzymes are obtained from

a. Plants
b. Animal tissues
c. Microbes
d. Insects

Ans. (c) Microbes

367. The turnover number of chymotrypsin is 100 s^{-1} and for DNA polymerase it is 15 S^1. This means that

a. Chymotrypsin binds to its substrates with higher affinity than does DNA polymerase
b. The velocity of chymotrypsin reaction is always greater than that of DNA polymerase
c. The velocities of reaction catalysed by both enzymes of saturatic substrate levels could be equal if 6.7 times more DNA polymerase than chymotrypsin where used
d. The velocities of chymotrypsin reactions at particular enzyme concentration and saturating substrate levels is lower than that of DNA polymerase reaction under the same condition

Ans. (c) The velocities of reaction catalysed by both enzymes of saturatic substrate levels could be equal if 6.7 times more DNA polymerase than chymotrypsin where used

368. Enzyme catalysis of chemical reaction

a. Increases the forward and reverse reaction rates
b. Decreases "Gˆ" so that the reaction can proceed spontaneously
c. Increases the energy of transition state
d. Decreases the entropy of reactions

Ans. (a) Increases the forward and reverse reaction rates

369. The factor likely to increase the rate of reaction catalyzed by a surface immobilized enzyme is/are

a. Increase agitation of the bulk liquid containing the substrate
b. Continued replacement of the bulk liquid containing the substrate
c. Increased concentration of the substrate in the bulk liquid
d. All of the above

Ans. (d) All of the above

370. Which of the following cases are likely to lead to faster rates of catalyzing by an enzyme immobilized on a negatively charged support?

a. A positively charged substrate and negatively charged product
b. A negatively charged substrate and positively charged product

c. A positively charged substrate and positively charged product

d. None of these

Ans. (a) A positively charged substrate and negatively charged product

371. On doubling the enzyme concentration, the kinetic parameters that changes are

a. K_m b. V_{max}

c. K_{cat} d. Both V_{max} and K_{cat}

Ans. (d) Both V_{max} and K_{cat}

372. An enzyme does the following in catalyzing a reaction

a. Stabilizes the substrate

b. Decreases the equilibrium constant

c. Increases the forward reaction rate

d. Hasten the approach of rate equilibrium

Ans. (b) Decreases the equilibrium constant

373. Ki indicates

a. Competitive inhibition

b. Denaturation of enzyme

c. Reaction velocity

d. All the above

Ans. (a) Competitive inhibition

374. Km value of enzyme is substrate concentration at

a. $\frac{1}{4} V_{max}$ b. $2 V_{max}$

c. $\frac{1}{2} V_{max}$ d. $4 V_{max}$

Ans. (c) $\frac{1}{2} V_{max}$

375. The ratio of enzyme to substrate molecules can be

a. 1 : 100,000   b. 1 : 500,000

c. 1 : 10,000   d. 1 : 1,000

Ans. (a) 1 : 100,000

376. Which one value is required for enzyme action?

a. Low k_m

b. High k_m

c. Low k_i

d. High k_i

Ans. (c) Low k_i

377. Turn-over number of an enzyme is dependent upon

a. Size of enzyme

b. Active site

c. Molecular weight of enzyme

d. Concentration of substrate

Ans. (c) Molecular weight of enzyme

378. Competitive inhibition is due to

a. Protein poison

b. Substrate analogue

c. Non-availability of activation energy

d. Short wave radiation

Ans. (b) Substrate analogue

379. End product inhibition is called

a. Substrate regulation

b. Feed back regulation

c. Irreversible inhibition

d. Non competitive inhibition

Ans. (b) Feed back regulation

380. Non competitive inhibition often results in

a. Changing in enzyme structure

b. Blocking of active site

c. Non synthesis of enzyme

d. Non availability of cofactor

Ans. (a) Changing in enzyme structure

381. Template theory of enzyme action was given by

a. Fischer

b. Koshland

c. Moned et al

d. Michaelis and Menton

Ans. (a) Fischer

382. Enzyme our immobilized through

a. Covalently attaching to solid support

b. Cross-linking

c. Entrapping in gel

d. All of the above

Ans. (d) All of the above

383. Enzyme used in detergents are

a. Amylases

b. Lipases

c. Proteases

d. Glucoisomerase

Ans. (c) Proteases

384. Enzyme TPA or tissue Plasminogen activator is used for

a. Dissolving blood clots

b. Maintaining plasma contents

c. Clearing turbidity of juices

d. Stimulating thromboplastin production

Ans. (a) Dissolving blood clots

385. **Enzyme immobilization is**
    a. Conversion of active enzyme into inactive enzyme form
    b. Provide enzyme with protective covering
    c. Changing soluble enzyme into insoluble state
    d. None of the above

Ans. (b) Provide enzyme with protective covering

386. **Which of the following is the molecular weight of mRNA?**
    a. 15,000 to 30,000
    b. 20,000 to 35,000
    c. 25,000 to 40,000
    d. 30,000 to 50,000

Ans. (d) 30,000 to 50,000

387. **α-helix in protein can be labeled**
    a. 3.6_{13} helix
    b. 4.4_{16} helix
    c. 2.6_{12} helix
    d. None of these

Ans. (c) 2.6_{12} helix

388. **When a protein is denatured the freedom of rotation about bonds in both the polypeptide backbone and the side chain is**
    a. Increased
    b. Decreased
    c. Increased in the backbone only
    d. Increased in the side chain only

Ans. (a) Increased

389. **The term milimol is written as**
    a. M.M
    b. V.M
    c. uuM
    d. mM

Ans. (d) mM

390. **The phenomenon by which the synthesis of a set of enzyme leading to a product from outside is known as**
    a. Repression
    b. Depression
    c. Suppression
    d. None of these

Ans. (a) Repression

391. **Autolytic function is shown by**
    a. Enzymes
    b. DNA
    c. Hormones
    d. RNA

Ans. (a) Enzymes

392. **K_m is**
    a. The dissociation constant for the enzyme substrate complex
    b. Equal to half the substrate concentration required to achieve V_{max}

    c. Identical for all isozymes of an enzyme
    d. The substrate concentration that gives one-half V_{max}

Ans. (d) The substrate concentration that gives one-half V_{max}

393. **Di-isopropyl fluorophosphates (DEF) reacts with serine proteases stoichiometrically and irreversibly and therefore is a**
    a. Competitive inhibitor
    b. Non-competitive inhibitor
    c. Uncompetitive inhibitor
    d. Repressor

Ans. (b) Non-competitive inhibitor

394. **In non-competitive inhibition**
    a. The concentration of active enzyme molecules is reduced
    b. V_{max} is increased
    c. The concentration of active enzyme molecules is unchanged
    d. The apparent K_m is increased

Ans. (a) The concentration of active enzyme molecules is reduced

395. **In an enzyme assay in which substrate concentration is much lower then K_m, the rate**
    a. Approaches V_{max}
    b. Shows zero-order kinetics
    c. It proportional to substrate concentration
    d. Is independent of enzyme concentration

Ans. (c) It proportional to substrate concentration

396. **Isoenzymes**
    a. Are enzymes that exist in more than one amino acid sequence in the same species
    b. Cannot ne distinguished in a geiven species except immunologically
    c. By definition must have the same amino aicd composition
    d. Are single polypeptide chains that differ by an amino acid replacement

Ans. (a) Are enzymes that exist in more than one amino acid sequence in the same species

397. **Which of the following is not a component of coenzyme A?**
    a. Adenylic acid
    b. Pantothenic acid
    c. Cysteamine
    d. Acetic acid

Ans. (d) Acetic acid

398. As a coenzyme, pyruvate decarboxylase requires

a. Coenzyme A
b. NAD$^+$
c. FMN
d. Thiamine pyrophosphate

Ans. (d) Thiamine pyrophosphate

399. Dehydrogenases use as coenzymes all of the following *except:*

a. NAD$^+$
b. NADP
c. FAD
d. Ferriprotoporphyrin

Ans. (d) Ferriprotoporphyrin

400. Which of the following is an essential cofactor in carboxylation reactions?

a. Coenzyme A   b. Biotin
c. CTP   d. Lipoic acid

Ans. (b) Biotin

401. The enzyme that catalyses the reaction $2H_2O \rightarrow 2H_2O + O_2$ is a

a. Dehydrogenase   b. Peroxidase
c. Catalase   d. Hydrolase

Ans. (c) Catalase

402. Which enzyme will cleave leucyl-glycyl-proline to leucine and glycyl-proline?

a. Carboxypeptidase
b. Glycylglycyl peptidase
c. Aminopeptidase
d. Chymotrypsin

Ans. (c) Aminopeptidase

403. An enzyme of saliva that hydrolyzes starch is

a. Pepsin
b. β-Amylase
c. Lysozyme
d. α-Amylase

Ans. (d) α-Amylase

404. The isoenzymes of lactate dehydrogenase

a. Demonstrate the evolutionary development of this enzyme
b. Range from monomers to tetramers
c. Differ only in a single amino acid
d. Exist in 5 forms depending upon the content of M and H monomers

Ans. (d) Exist in 5 forms depending upon the content of M and H monomers

405. The nerve gas, DFP, has been a useful reagent in enzyme chemistry. At the active site of many hydrolytic enzymes of DFP combines with

a. Histidine   b. Serine
c. Lysine   d. Aspartate

Ans. (b) Serine

406. The isocitrate dehydrogenase reaction is analogous to (performs the same type of chemical reaction)

a. Pyruvate dehydrogenase
b. α-ketoglutarate dehydrogenase
c. β-hydroxyacyl-CoA dehydrogenase
d. 6-phosphogluconate dehydrogenase

Ans. (d) 6-phosphogluconate dehydrogenase

407. Antimetabolites act by

a. Competitive inhibition when they combine irreversibly with an enzyme
b. Competitive inhibition when they combine reversibly with an enzyme
c. Non-competitive inhibition if there is no relation between degree of inhibition and substrate concentration
d. Lactate dehydrogenase

Ans. (b) Competitive inhibition when they combine reversibly with an enzyme

408. K_m and V_{max} can be determined from the Lineweaver – Burk plot of the Michaelis – Menton equation shoen below. Where V is the reaction velocity at substrate concentrations S, the X-axis experimental data are expressed as

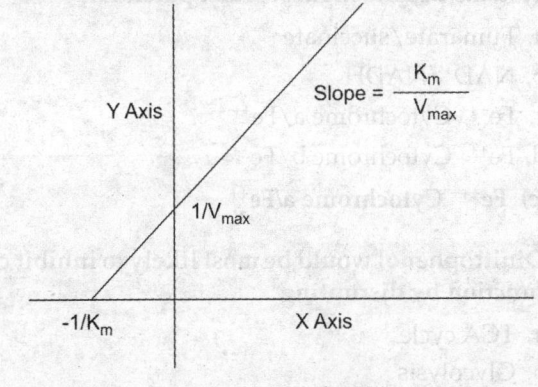

a. 1/V   b. V
c. 1/S   d. S

Ans. (c) 1/S

409. All the following gastrointestinal enzymes are secreted as inactive zymogens (proenzymes) *except:*

a. Ribonuclease   b. Pepsin
c. Trypsin   d. Chymotrypsin

Ans. (a) Ribonuclease

410. Which enzyme has the greatest specificity for peptide bonds on the carboxyl side of a cationic amino acid side chain?

a. Carboxypeptidase   b. Trypsin

c. Rennin   d. Pepsin

Ans. (b) Trypsin

411. Which of the following statements about myosin is true?

a. It is a spherically symmetric molecule

b. It is low in α-helix content

c. It is a zinc-requiring enzyme

d. It is an actin-binding protein

Ans. (d) It is an actin-binding protein

412. If an enzyme behaves according to classic Michaelis-Menton kinetics, from a double reciprocal plot of velocity versus substrate concentration, the value for the Michaelis constant (K_m) of the substrate can be determined graphically as the

a. Slope of curve

b. Point of infection of the curve

c. Absolute value of the intercept of the curve with the X-axis

d. Reciprocal of the absolute value of the intercept of the curve with the Y-axis

Ans. (d) Reciprocal of the absolute value of the intercept of the curve with the Y-axis

413. Which of the following oxidation-reduction systems has the highest redox potential?

a. Fumarate/succinate

b. $NAD^+/NADH$

c. Fe^{+++} Cytochrome a/Fe^{++}

d. Fe^{+++} Cytochrome b/Fe^{++}

Ans. (c) Fe^{+++} Cytochrome a/Fe^{++}

414. Dinitrophenol would be most likely to inhibit cell function by disrupting

a. TCA cycle

b. Glycolysis

c. Hepatic gluconeogenesis

d. Oxidative phosphorylation

Ans. (d) Oxidative phosphorylation

415. Polymyxin is unique among chemotherapeutic agents because it is bactericidal in the absence of cell growth. it exerts its effect by

a. Detergent-like disruption of membranes

b. Binding of DNA polymerase

c. Binding to DNA as an insertion its effect by

d. Binding to polysome-bound mRNA

Ans. (a) Detergent-like disruption of membranes

416. Cycloserine inhibits transpeptidation in the formation of the peptidoglycan cell wall network of gram positive organisms. This action of cycloserine is competitively inhibited by

a. L-lysine   b. D-alanine

c. D-glutamine   d. D-serine

Ans. (b) D-alanine

417. Some antibiotics act as ionophores, which means that they

a. Increase cell membrane permeability to specific ions

b. Inhibit both translation and transcription

c. Inhibit only translation

d. Interfere directly with bacterial cell-wall synthesis

Ans. (a) Increase cell membrane permeability to specific ions

418. De novo synthesis of an enzyme, promoted by the substrate on which it acts, is characterized by the term

a. Induction

b. Gratuity

c. Activation

d. Derepression

Ans. (a) Induction

419. Control of metabolic pathway may be exerted by enzyme repression or induction. In vertebrates, this form of enzyme control α curs primarily in the

a. Heart

b. Brain

c. Liverd

d. Skeletal muscle

Ans. (c) Liverd

420. A hypothetical biosynthetic pathway is shown in the diagram below. A microbial organism defective in one enzyme of this path is grown in a medium containing X. Large amounts of M and L are found in the organism but none of Z. in which enzyme is the mutation expressed?

a. Enzyme A

b. Enzyme B

c. Enzyme C

d. Enzyme D

Ans. (c) Enzyme C

421. The activity of most single polypeptide enzymes can be represented by the hyperbolic curve A shown below. However, the activity of homotropic regulatory enzymes shows a sigmoid dependence on substrate concentration, curve B. this sigmoid relationship between substrate concentration and reaction velocity indicates that

a. Homotropic enzymes are polymers

b. Homotropic enzymes catalyzes reactions more slowly than single polypeptide enzymes

c. The reaction rate is independent of substrate concentration

d. The binding of one substrate molecule enhances subsequent substrate binding and activity

Ans. (d) The binding of one substrate molecule enhances subsequent substrate binding and activity

422. Which of the following statements concerning trypsinogen and chymotrypsinogen are false?

a. They have considerable homologies in primary sequence

b. They are secreted by exocrine cells in the pancreas

c. They are exopeptidases

d. They can be converted into active enzymes by limited digestion with trypsin

Ans. (c) They are exopeptidases

423. It is true of most enzymes that they

a. Increase the rapidity of the reaction they catalyze

b. Are specific for the substrate as well as the substrate as well as the reaction catalyzed

c. Are large polypeptides with a molecular weight greater than 5,000 daltons

d. All of the above

Ans. (d) All of the above

424. Proteins that contain a porphyrin ring include

a. Catalase
b. Cytochrome
c. Haemoglobin
d. All the above

Ans. (d) All the above

425. Which of the following proteins contain iron?

a. Haemoglobin
b. Cytochrome C
c. Peroxidase
d. All of the above

Ans. (d) All of the above

426. Which of the following statements about sickle cell anaemia are true?

a. It is widely distributed in areas of high malaria fatality

b. It results from a single amino acid change in haemoglobin

c. It is seen in homozygous individuals only

d. All of these

Ans. (d) All of these

427. Which of the following statements about isozymes of a given enzyme are true?

a. They have different substrate specificities

b. They may exhibit different K_m values for substances or cofactors

c. They are composed of distinct multimeric complexes

d. They usually exhibit identical electrophoretic mobility

Ans. (b) They may exhibit different K_m values for substances or cofactors

(c) They are composed of distinct multimeric complexes

428. Heavy chains of I_gG antibody may be separated from light chains with

a. Ethanolamine
b. Pepsin
c. Papain
d. Mercaptoethanol

Ans. (d) Mercaptoethanol

429. Which of the following enzymes was first isolated and purified in the form of crystals

a. Urease
b. Pepsin
c. Amylase
d. Ribonuclease

Ans. (a) Urease

430. FAD and FMN is a coenzyme which vitamin is incorporated into its structure

a. Vitamin B_2
b. Vitamin B_1
c. Vitamin B_6
d. Vitamin C

Ans. (a) Vitamin B_2

431. Zymogens are

a. Enzymes acting upon starch

b. Group of zymase enzymes

c. Inactive enzymes precursors

d. None of the above

Ans. (c) Inactive enzymes precursors

432. Which of the following is iron porphyrin coenzymes or cofactor

a. CoA

b. Cytochrome

c. NAD

d. FAD

Ans. (b) Cytochrome

433. The non protein part of enzyme called

 a. Holoenzymes　　　b. Prosthetic group
 c. Apoenzymes　　　d. None of these

Ans. (b) Prosthetic group

434. Enzymes are sensitive to

 a. pH　　　　　　b. Rain fall
 c. Wing velocity　　d. Light

Ans. (a) pH

435. The protein part of an enzymes known as

 a. Holoenzymes
 b. Apoenzymes
 c. Prosthetic group
 d. None of the above

Ans. (b) Apoenzymes

436. NADP is

 a. Enzymes activator
 b. Electron acceptors
 c. Ion carrier
 d. All living cells of plant body

Ans. (b) Electron acceptors

437. In plants enzymes are present in

 a. Only in leaves
 b. Only in flowers
 c. Only in storage organs
 d. Hydrogen acceptor

Ans. (d) Hydrogen acceptor

438. Cytochrome oxidase contains

 a. Magnesium　　　b. Cobalt
 c. Mercury　　　　d. Iron

Ans. (d) Iron

439. NADP is

 a. An enzyme
 b. A part of s-RNA
 c. A coenzyme (coenzyme II)
 d. A part of t-RNA

Ans. (c) A coenzyme (coenzyme II)

440. In seeds digestion is made possible at relatively low temperature by

 a. Auxins
 b. Nitrogenous substance
 c. Proteins
 d. Enzymes

Ans. (d) Enzymes

441. The first enzyme that reduces nitrates to nitrites and ammonia in plant is

 a. Glutamine synthetase
 b. Glutamate dehydrogenase
 c. Nitrite reductase
 d. Nitrate reductase

Ans. (d) Nitrate reductase

442. Out of total enzymes present in the cell mitochondria alone has

 a. 4%　　　　　　b. 95%
 c. 70%　　　　　d. No enzymes

Ans. (c) 70%

443. Which of the following is the best evidence for template theory of enzymes action

 a. Compounds similar in structure to the substrate inhibit the reaction
 b. Enzymes speed up the reaction by definite amount
 c. Enzymes determine the direction of a reaction
 d. Enzymes are found in living organism and increase the rate of certain reaction

Ans. (a) Compounds similar in structure to the substrate inhibit the reaction

444. Enzymes are basically made up of

 a. Fats　　　　　b. Carbon
 c. Vitamins　　　d. Proteins

Ans. (d) Proteins

445. Enzymes are proteins it was suggested by

 a. Summer
 b. Pasteur
 c. Miller
 d. Leeuwenhoek

Ans. (a) Summer

446. Esterase belongs to

 a. Oxidation reduction enzymes
 b. Carboxylase
 c. Hydrolytic enzymes
 d. Transferase

Ans. (c) Hydrolytic enzymes

447. Enzymes are different from inorganic, catalysts in

 a. Being proteinaceous in nature
 b. Not being used up in reaction
 c. Working at high temperature
 d. Having a high diffusion rate

Ans. (a) Being proteinaceous in nature

448. Which of the following is not an attribute of enzymes

a. They are proteinaceous in nature
b. They speed up the rate of biochemical
c. They are specific in nature
d. They are used in reaction

Ans. (d) They are used in reaction

449. When coenzyme is combined with apoenzyme it is called

a. Co-factor
b. Holoenzyme
c. Substrate enzyme complex
d. Vitamin A

Ans. (b) Holoenzyme

450. LDH (Lactic dehydrogenase) which catalyzed pyruvate to lactate is an example of

a. Apoenzyme
b. Antienzyme
c. Isoenzyme
d. Co-enzyme

Ans. (c) Isoenzyme

451. Enzymes which convert starch into maltase is

a. Maltase
b. Diastase
c. Invertase
d. Hydrogenase

Ans. (b) Diastase

452. At temperature below the freezing point enzyme is

a. Slightly activated
b. Killed
c. Inactivated
d. Unaffected

Ans. (c) Inactivated

453. Enzymes, vitamins and hormones can be classified into a single category of biological chemicals because all of them

a. Aid in regulating metabolism
b. Are proteins
c. Are synthesized in organism
d. Enhance the oxidation metabolism

Ans. (a) Aid in regulating metabolism

454. Diastase enzymes digest or enzymes diastase helps in the digestion of

a. Proteins
b. Fats
c. Amino acid
d. Starch (polysaccharides)

Ans. (d) Starch (polysaccharides)

455. The product of an enzymes catalysed reaction can act as inhibitors of the reaction. This mechanism of control is known as

a. Repressor
b. Competitive inhibition
c. Feedback inhibition
d. Metabolic antagonism

Ans. (c) Feedback inhibition

456. Dry seeds can endure higher temperature than the germinating deeds because

a. Dry seeds have more reserve food
b. Dry seeds are hard
c. The seedlings are tender
d. Hydration makes the enzymes more sensitive to temperature

Ans. (d) Hydration makes the enzymes more sensitive to temperature

457. At boiling temperature an enzyme is

a. Unaffected
b. Killed
c. Inactivated
d. Denaturated

Ans. (d) Denaturated

458. A huge amount of starch is stored in potatoes which are underground. This is made possible by

a. Synthesis of sugar in the potatoes
b. Activity of enzymes which convert starch into sugar and sugar back into starch after it has of starch the potato
c. Migration of starch from aerial parts
d. Migration of starch from the soil

Ans. (b) Activity of enzymes which convert starch into sugar and sugar back into starch after it has of starch the potato

459. An enzyme that catalyses the rearrangement of molecular structure and forms a compound of same molecular weight is called

a. Hydrolase
b. Isomerase
c. Oxido reductase
d. Ligase

Ans. (b) Isomerase

460. Blocking of active site of an enzyme is a kind of

a. Feedback inhibition
b. Non competitive inhibition
c. Allosteric inhibition
d. Competitive inhibition

Ans. (d) Competitive inhibition

461. Enzymes which act normally within cells are called

a. Apoenzymes   b. Exoenzymes
c. Endoenzymes   d. Ferments

Ans. (c) Endoenzymes

462. Enzymes which are solitary different in molecular structure but can perform identical activities are called

a. Apoenzymes   b. Isoenzymes
c. Coenzymes   d. Homoenzymes

Ans. (b) Isoenzymes

463. The plant proteinases or endopeptidases enzyme is

a. Trypsin   b. Papain
c. Pepsin   d. Urease

Ans. (b) Papain

464. Which of the following statement is not correct

a. All enzymes are thermostable
b. All enzymes are biocatalysts
c. All enzymes are proteins
d. All proteins are enzymes

Ans. (d) All proteins are enzymes

465. The activity of succinic dehydrogenase is inhibited by

a. Glycolate   b. Pyruvate
c. Phosphoglycerate   d. Malonate

Ans. (d) Malonate

466. In feedback inhibition a metabolic pathway is switched off by

a. Lack of a substrate
b. By a rise in temperature
c. Competitive inhibition
d. Accumulation of end product

Ans. (d) Accumulation of end product

467. An enzyme acts by

a. Increasing the pH
b. Decreasing the pH
c. Reducing the energy of activation
d. Increasing the energy of activation

Ans. (c) Reducing the energy of activation

468. T. Cech and S. Altman got noble prize in 1989 for

a. Viral infection
b. Mechanism of DNA synthesis
c. Catalytic role of RNA (ribozyme)
d. All the above

Ans. (c) Catalytic role of RNA (ribozyme)

469. The enzyme is said to be working at maximum efficiency

a. When substrate coming in contact with active site are negligible
b. When substrate concentration is increased to point of saturation
c. When substrate concentration is low
d. None of these

Ans. (b) When substrate concentration is increased to point of saturation

470. Which enzyme is required to digest the reserve food material (liquid) in castor seeds

a. Amylase   b. Protease
c. Diastase   d. Lipase

Ans. (d) Lipase

471. Hydrolases are involved in the hydrolysis of

a. Proteins   b. Esters
c. Lipids   d. All the above

Ans. (d) All the above

472. Which of the following statement is incorrect

a. The two terms substrate and product signify the starting and ending materials of a reaction
b. Enzymes hasten the completion of a reaction
c. Enzymes exhibit specificity for the reaction they catalyze
d. Enzymes are affected by the reactions they catalyze

Ans. (d) Enzymes are affected by the reactions they catalyze

473. Some metals known as cofactors of enzymes are

a. K^+, Co^{++} b. $Ca^{++}, Zn^{++}, Mn^{++}$
c. Zn^{++}, Ca^{++} d. All the above

Ans. (d) All the above

474. During enzyme activity the coenzyme acts as

a. Activator of oxidation reduction reactions
b. A donor or acceptor of atoms which are added to or removed from the substrates
c. Both a and b
d. None of these

Ans. (c) Both a and b

475. Amount of enzyme transforming one mole, of substrate per minute at 25°C under optimal conditions of measurement is called

a. Enzyme purity   b. Specific activity
c. Unit of enzyme activity   d. Catalytic centre activity

Ans. (c) Unit of enzyme activity

476. What will happen to an enzyme when apoenzyme is separated from it metal component

    a. Activity will be lost

    b. Activity will be increased

    c. Activity will be decreased

    d. There will be no change in the activity

Ans. (a) Activity will be lost

477. Which of the following are coenzymes

    a. NAD, K, CoA

    b. Vitamin, Fe, Cu

    c. NAD, NADP, FAD, FMN

    d. $NADPH_2$, Ca, Co

Ans. (c) NAD, NADP, FAD, FMN

478. Turn over number of enzyme depends upon

    a. Size of enzyme molecule

    b. Molecular weight of enzyme

    c. Active sites of enzyme molecule

    d. Concentration of substrate molecule

Ans. (c) Active sites of enzyme molecule

479. Which of the following is correct in an enzyme controlled reaction (E = enzyme, S = substrate, P = product)

    a. E + S = ES = E

    b. E + S = ES = E + P

    c. E + S = E + P

    d. E + S = P = E + P

Ans. (b) E + S = ES = E + P

480. Non competitive inhibition can result in

    a. Blocking of active site

    b. Non availability of cofactor

    c. Change in enzyme structure

    d. Non synthesis of enzymes

Ans. (c) Change in enzyme structure

481. Induced fit theory of enzyme action was given be

    a. Buchner   b. Kuhne

    c. Koshland   d. Fischer

Ans. (c) Koshland

482. Enzyme taking part in converting dihydroxy acetone phosphate to glyceraldehydes phosphate belongs to the type of

    a. Ligases   b. Transferases

    c. Isomerases   d. Hydrolases

Ans. (c) Isomerases

483. The fastest enzyme is

    a. Trypsin   b. Pepsin

    c. Carbonic anhydrase   d. Urease

Ans. (c) Carbonic anhydrase

484. The enzyme used for alcohol formation by fermentation is

    a. Invertase   b. Lipase

    c. Amylase   d. Zymase

Ans. (d) Zymase

485. Feedback inhibition is caused by blocking of enzymes by

    a. Chemicals produced by hormones

    b. Hormones

    c. Competitive inhibition

    d. Accumulated end products

Ans. (d) Accumulated end products

486. A substance unrelated to substrate reversibly changes the activity of an enzyme. It is

    a. Allosteric subunit

    b. Competitive inhibitor

    c. Allosteric modulator

    d. Non competitive inhibitor

Ans. (b) Competitive inhibitor

487. Feedback inhibition is induced by

    a. Enzyme   b. Catalyst

    c. End product   d. Substrate

Ans. (c) End product

488. Enzymes as they exist inside the cell are

    a. In solid form   b. In crystalline form

    c. In colloidal form   d. In solution form

Ans. (c) In colloidal form

489. In genetic engineering some important enzymes are used, one of them is

    a. Topoisomerase

    b. Helicase

    c. Restriction endonuclease

    d. Translocase

Ans. (c) Restriction endonuclease

490. Enzymes are useful because they

    a. Are important structural components

    b. Supply energy

    c. Enhance the absorption of water

    d. Catalyse biochemical reactions in the plant body

Ans. (d) Catalyse biochemical reactions in the plant body

491. Urease, the first enzyme crystallized by

a. Louis pasteur   b. J.B. Summer
c. E. Buchner   d. J. Northrop

Ans. (b) J.B. Summer

492. Which enzyme is not proteinaceous

a. Holozyme   b. Trypsin
c. Ribozyme   d. Isozyme

Ans. (c) Ribozyme

493. Which one of the following statements is true for the enzymes

a. All enzymes are proteins
b. All proteins are enzyme
c. All enzymes are not proteins
d. All enzymes are vitamins

Ans. (a) All enzymes are proteins

494. The scientists associated with the study of enzyme include

a. Went   b. Buchner
c. Summer   d. Both b and c

Ans. (d) Both b and c

495. The nature of coenzyme is

a. Proteinaceous   b. Non proteinaceous
c. Both a and b   d. None of these

Ans. (d) None of these

496. Which of the following statements is incorrect

a. The optimum pH for trypsin is 8.8
b. At optimum pH, the activity of enzyme is maximum
c. Enzymes are not affected by hydrogen ion concentration
d. The optimum pH for pepsin is 2.0

Ans. (c) Enzymes are not affected by hydrogen ion concentration

497. Which part of an active enzyme is denatured by heat

a. Coenzyme   b. Apoenzyme
c. Holoenzyme   d. Activator

Ans. (b) Apoenzyme

498. How is the rate of enzyme catalysed reactions affected by every 10°C rise of temperature

a. Halves
b. Becomes four times
c. Doubles
d. Remains unchanged

Ans. (c) Doubles

499. On boiling or treating with strong acid or alkali an enzymes loses its catalytic activity because

a. It is a lipoprotein
b. It burns
c. It is a protein
d. It is functional substance

Ans. (c) It is a protein

500. At which temperature the enzyme activity would be maximum

a. 60°C   b. 55°C
c. 45°C   d. 35°C

Ans. (d) 35 °C

501. Which of the following is not an attribute of enzymes

a. The speed up the rate of biochemical reaction
b. These are specific in nature
c. They are used up in reaction
d. These are proteinaceous in nature

Ans. (c) They are used up in reaction

502. Transferases are involved in the transfer of

a. Phosphate group   b. Amino group
c. Methyl group   d. All of the above

Ans. (d) All of the above

503. The transfer of a group from a donor molecule to an acceptor molecule is catalyzed by

a. Protease   b. Isomerase
c. Transferase   d. Hydrolytic enzymes

Ans. (c) Transferase

504. Activation energy is required by

a. Non catalyzed reactions
b. Catalyzed reaction
c. Both a and b
d. None of the above

Ans. (c) Both a and b

505. Which of the following is a hydrolytic enzyme

a. Protease   b. Esterase
c. Carbohydrase   d. All of the above

Ans. (d) All of the above

506. Ligases are involved in the synthesis of

a. C-O bonds
b. C-N bonds
c. C-C bonds
d. All of the above

Ans. (d) All of the above

507. In competitive inhibition which of the following is true

a. ES + I = ESI   b. S + I = SI

c. E + I = EI   d. E + I = EI + S = ESI

Ans. (c) E + I = EI

508. Many vitamins are necessary to the cell

a. To increase immunity

b. To act as coenzymes

c. To provide energy

d. To help in digestion

Ans. (b) To act as coenzymes

509. Coenzyme is often a

a. Fatty acid   b. Vitamin

c. Protein   d. Carbohydrate

Ans. (b) Vitamin

510. Coenzyme functions in association with a

a. Apoenzyme   b. Protein

c. Holoenzyme   d. Vitamin

Ans. (a) Apoenzyme

511. The enzymes catalyzing breakdown without addition of water are called

a. Ligases   b. Lysases

c. Hydrolases   d. Oxidoreductases

Ans. (b) Lysases

512. Amylopectin acts upon

a. Polysaccharide in any medium

b. Polysaccharide in acidic medium

c. Polysaccharide in alkaline medium

d. Polysaccharide in neutral medium

Ans. (c) Polysaccharide in alkaline medium

513. Coenzyme is

a. Always a protein

b. Often a vitamin

c. Always an inorganic compound

d. Often a metal

Ans. (b) Often a vitamin

514. An enzyme can be synthesized by chemically bonding together molecules of

a. Carbohydrates

b. Amino acids

c. Lipases

d. CO_2

Ans. (b) Amino acids

515. A coenzyme is

a. Same enzyme that occurs in different tissues such as heart and muscle

b. One that shares the function of other enzyme

c. Organic or inorganic in nature and helps activate metabolic enzymes

d. Organic non protein in nature and helps to activate metabolic enzymes

Ans. (d) Organic non protein in nature and helps to activate metabolic enzymes

516. Enzymes are the polymers of

a. Hexose carbon   b. Fatty acids

c. Amino acids   d. Inorganic phosphate

Ans. (c) Amino acids

517. The enzyme which hydrolyse starch is

a. Sucrase   b. Cellulase

c. Amylase   d. Invertase

Ans. (c) Amylase

518. Ribozyme is

a. RNA without sugar

b. RNA without phosphate

c. RNA having enzyme activity

d. RNA with extra phosphate

Ans. (c) RNA having enzyme activity

519. The release of adenyl cyclase from the cell membrane changes

a. ATP into ADP

b. ADP into ATP

c. cAMP into ATP

d. ATP into cAMP

Ans. (d) ATP into cAMP

520. Proteinaceous nature of the enzyme was established by obtaining crystalline form of urease from Jack beans in 1926 by

a. Buchner   b. Summer

c. Pouling   d. Northrop

Ans. (b) Summer

521. Which of the following enzyme is not proteinaceous in nature

a. Coenzyme

b. Ribozyme

c. Succinic dehydrogenase

d. Catalase

Ans. (b) Ribozyme

522. Turn over number of an enzyme depends on its

a. Concentration of enzyme

b. Size of enzyme

c. Number of active sites

d. Molecular weight

Ans. (c) Number of active sites

523. Which has coenzyme activity

a. Purine   b. Pyrimidine

c. Urease   d. Both a and b

Ans. (c) Urease

524. Which one is not a simple enzyme

a. Amylase   b. Pepsin

c. Urease   d. Dehydrogenase

Ans. (d) Dehydrogenase

525. UbQ (ubiquinone) is

a. Activator

b. Protein cofactor

c. Non protein coenzyme

d. Protein coenzyme

Ans. (c) Non protein coenzyme

526. The enzyme used to dissolve blood clot in coronary artery is

a. Thrombokinase   b. Rennin

c. Streptokinase   d. Tyrosinase

Ans. (c) Streptokinase

527. The metallic ion acting as activator of ATPase in cell membrane

a. Fe^{++} b. K^+

c. Na^+ d. Mg^{++}

Ans. (c) Na^+

528. Enzyme responsible for RNA directed DNA synthesis is

a. DNA polymerase

b. Helicase

c. Reverse transcriptase

d. Topoisomerase

Ans. (c) Reverse transcriptase

529. Which of the following enzyme is functional in maize grain during germination

a. Maltase   b. Diastase

c. Urease   d. Zymase

Ans. (b) Diastase

530. Cytochrome oxidase is a marker enzyme for

a. Circular DNA of mitochondria

b. Outer membrane of mitochondria

c. Inner membrane of mitochondria

d. Matrix of mitochondria

Ans. (c) Inner membrane of mitochondria

531. The enzymes are highly specific in their action. This specificity of an enzyme if due to

a. RNA

b. Specific coenzymes

c. Arrangement of amino acids

d. Active site

Ans. (c) Arrangement of amino acids

532. The stoppage of an enzymatic (biological) reaction by the end product of reaction is called

a. End product inhibition

b. Feed back inhibition

c. Negative inhibition

d. All of the above

Ans. (d) All of the above

533. Coenzyme is a part of enzyme

a. Vitamin A

b. Inorganic metal activator

c. Non protein organic part attached firmly

d. Non protein organic part attached loosely

Ans. (d) Non protein organic part attached loosely

534. In competitive inhibition

a. Inhibitor block site

b. Inhibitor resembles the substrate in molecular structure

c. Inhibitor has no effect on allosteric site

d. All are correct

Ans. (d) All are correct

535. If the prosthetic group or non protein part of an conjugation enzyme (Holoenzyme) is removed then

a. Enzyme becomes inactive

b. K_m constant increases

c. Activity of enzyme decreases

d. Enzyme starts inhibiting the reaction

Ans. (a) Enzyme becomes inactive

536. Where does reaction occur between enzyme and substrate

a. Allosteric site   b. Prosthetic group

c. Active site   d. None of the above

Ans. (c) Active site

537. Induced fit theory of Koshland states that

a. Active sites are inactive and do not participate

b. Active sites are static like a key

c. Active sites undergo geometrical conformational changes

d. None of these

Ans. (c) Active sites undergo geometrical conformational changes

538. Cyanide kill an animal by inhibiting cytochrome oxidase (enzyme of respiratory chain). Is does not bind with active site this is an examples of

a. Feedback inhibition

b. Noncompetitive inhibition

c. Competitive inhibition

d. Allosteric inhibition

Ans. (b) Noncompetitive inhibition

539. The spoilage of food can be prevented by keeping it in cold storage. It is due to

a. More availability of pure oxygen in cold storage

b. Reduced respiration

c. Reduced enzyme activity of bacteria

d. Reduced enzyme activity in substrate molecules

Ans. (c) Reduced enzyme activity of bacteria

540. Which inactivates an enzyme by occupying its active sites

a. Noncompetitive inhibition

b. Competitive inhibition

c. Allosteric inhibition

d. All of the above

Ans. (b) Competitive inhibition

541. Which is not an attribute of enzymes

a. Regulator

b. Specificity

c. Procaine

d. Used in reaction

Ans. (d) Used in reaction

542. Sometimes enzymes are named according to the source from which they are obtained such as papain from papaya. Name of the enzymes obtained from pineapple

a. Maltose   b. Bromelain

c. Sucrose   d. Pineollelase

Ans. (b) Bromelain

543. The Q_{10} for enzyme activity is

a. 3–4   b. 2–3

c. 1–2   d. 1–3

Ans. (b) 2–3

544. According to IUB system, isomerases belong to which class

a. IV   b. V

c. III   d. I

Ans. (b) V

545. As temperature changes from 30 to 45°C the rate of enzyme activity will

a. Increase

b. Decrease

c. First decrease and then increase

d. First increase and then decrease

Ans. (d) First increase and then decrease

546. IUB has divided enzymes with how many classes?

a. 6   b. 5

c. 4   d. 8

Ans. (a) 6

547. Why is heat used to sterilized non living object in tissue culture

a. Proteins lose their tertiary structure due to break down of bonds

b. Proteins are denatured at temperature above 55°C

c. Both correct

d. Only a is correct

Ans. (c) Both correct

CHECK YOU GRASP

1. The scientists associated with the study of enzymes include

a. Buchner   b. Went

c. Sumner   d. Both a and c

2. Which enzyme is not proteinaceous

a. Isozyme   b. Ribozyme

c. Holozyme   d. Trypsin

3. Ribozyme is

a. RNA without sugar

b. RNA without phosphate

c. RNA having enzyme activity

d. RNA with extra phosphate

4. The non-protein part of an enzyme is called

a. Holoenzyme

b. Prosthetic group

c. Apoenzyme

d. None of the above

5. In Lineweaver-Burk plot, the y-intercept represents

a. V_{max} b. K_m

c. K_m d. $1/K_m$

6. In competitive inhibition, the inhibitor

a. Competes with the enzyme

b. Irreversibly binds with the enzyme

c. Binds with the substrate

d. Competes with the substrate

7. Competitive inhibitors

a. Decrease the Km

b. Decrease the Vmax

c. Increase the Km

d. Increase the Vmax

8. In enzyme kinetics V_{max} reflects

a. The amount of an active enzyme

b. Substrate concentration

c. Half the substrate concentration

d. Enzyme substrate complex

9. A demonstrable inducer is absent in

a. Allosteric enzyme

b. Constitutive enzyme

c. Inhibited enzyme

d. Co-operative enzyme

10. Whcih of the following is a proenzyme?

a. Carboxypeptidase   b. Aminopeptidase

c. Chymotrypsin   d. Pepsinogen

11. What is true about enzymes

a. All act best at pH 7.0

b. All are amino acids

c. All are proteins

d. All act best at 0°C

12. Zymogens are

a. Enzyme acting upon starch

b. Groups of zymase enzymes

c. Inactive enzyme precursors

d. None of the above

13. Which one is coenzyme?

a. ATP   b. Vitamin B and C

c. CoQ and CoA   d. All of these

14. The active site of an enzyme is formed by

a. R group of amino acids

b. NH_2 group of amino acids

c. CO group of amino acids

d. Sulphur bonds which are exposed

In case of less than 80% score, go through brief Review and Glance one again from chapter

Key: 1-d   2-b   3-c   4-b   5-b   6-d   7-c   8-a   9-b   10-d   11- c   12-c   13-d   14-a

9

Plant and Animal Physiology

1. **'Plant Physiology' book was written by**
   - a. Singh and Purohit
   - b. Salisburry and Ross
   - c. Wiebe
   - d. Albert

   Ans. (b) Salisburry and Ross

2. **Enzyme for conversion of ammonia to amino acid is**
   - a. Nitrate reductase
   - b. Nitrite reductase
   - c. Alanine transferase
   - d. Glutamine synthetase

   Ans. (d) Glutamine synthetase

3. **Important function of leghaemoglobin in root nodules is**
   - a. O_2 regulation
   - b. N_2 fixation
   - c. Water regulation
   - d. All

   Ans. (a) O_2 regulation

4. **The externally thin strands of cytoplasm is termed as**
   - a. Primary cell wall
   - b. Secondary cell wall
   - c. Middle lamella
   - d. Plasmodesmata

   Ans. (d) Plasmodesmata

5. **In plants, genetic material is present in**
   - a. Nucleus and mitochondria
   - b. Nucleus only
   - c. Mitochondria and chloroplast
   - d. Nucleus, chloroplast and mitochondria

   Ans. (d) Nucleus, chloroplast and mitochondria

6. **The main function of endoplasmic reticulum is**
   - a. Fat synthesis
   - b. Protein synthesis
   - c. Disease resistance
   - d. Chlorophyll synthesis

   Ans. (b) Protein synthesis

7. **An enzyme associated with decarboxylation reaction in photosynthetic reaction of C_4 plants is**
   - a. Pyruvate dikinase
   - b. Malic acid dehydrogenase
   - c. PEP carboxylase
   - d. Malic enzymes

   Ans. (d) Malic enzymes

8. **Golgi bodies was discovered in 1898 by**
   - a. Camillio Golgi
   - b. Stanley
   - c. Farmer and Moori
   - d. Flemming

   Ans. (a) Camillio Golgi

9. **RNA synthesis in nucleus participate in protein synthesis in**
   - a. Nucleus
   - b. Cytosol
   - c. Chloroplast
   - d. Spherosome

   Ans. (b) Cytosol

10. **Which cell organelle is the site of chemical activity in cells, perhaps over half of the cell's metabolism**
    - a. Chloroplast
    - b. Nucleus
    - c. Mitochondria
    - d. ER

    Ans. (c) Mitochondria

11. **Photorespiration is high in**
    - a. Maize
    - b. Sugarcane
    - c. Pineapple
    - d. Rice

    Ans. (d) Rice

12. **Tick out which is not correctly matched**
    - a. Chloroplast – chlorophyll
    - b. Chromoplast – red pigments
    - c. Leucoplast – storage proteins
    - d. Nucleolus – fat

    Ans. (d) Nucleolus – fat

13. **Spherosomes are related with**
    - a. Chlorophyll
    - b. Red pigments
    - c. Power
    - d. Fat

    Ans. (d) Fat

253

14. Theoretically possible quantum yield in photosynthesis is

a. 0.12
b. 0.9
c. 0.8
d. 0.4

Ans. (a) 0.12

15. Ribosomes are produced in

a. ER(rough)
b. Nucleolus
c. Mitochondria
d. Chloroplast

Ans. (b) Nucleolus

16. The pigments which produce the colour of many flowers or the red of red maple leaves are generally stored in

a. Vacuole
b. Chromoplast
c. Lysosome
d. Dictyosome

Ans. (a) Vacuole

17. Ultimate electron donor in mitochondrial e^- transport chain is

a. Cytochrome A
b. Cytochrome B
c. Ubiquinone
d. Plastoquinone

Ans. (c) Ubiquinone

18. The hydrogen atoms on the surface of the oxygen atom are distributed apart at a right angle of

a. 90°
b. 105°
c. 120°
d. 180°

Ans. (b) 105°

19. The strongest bond is

a. Ionic bond
b. Covalent bond
c. Hydrogen bond
d. Van der Waals

Ans. (a) Ionic bond

20. The weakest bond is

a. Covalent bond
b. Van der waals
c. Ionic bond
d. Hydrogen bond

Ans. (b) Van der waals

21. Latent heat of vaporization (water to vapour) is

a. 80 cal
b. 540 cal
c. 586 cal
d. 620 cal

Ans. (c) 586 cal

22. Latent heat of fusion (ice to water) is

a. 540 cal
b. 620 cal
c. 80 cal
d. 40 cal

Ans. (c) 80 cal

23. Important radiant generated in pentose phosphate pathway of glucose degradation is

a. NADH
b. ATP
c. Ferridoxin
d. NADPH

Ans. (d) NADPH

24. Glyoxysomes functions in breakdown of

a. Acetyl CoA
b. Amino acids
c. Sugars
d. Fatty acids

Ans. (d)

25. The Brownian movement was discovered in 1827 by the Scottish botanist

a. Tyndall
b. Robert brown
c. Murrfy
d. Stayler

Ans. (b) Robert brown

26. Calcium is an imp. Constituent of

a. Protein
b. Cell wall
c. Chloroplast
d. Nucleic acid

Ans. (b) Cell wall

27. Maximum free radicals production is takes place in

a. Germination
b. Flowering
c. Fruiting
d. Senescence

Ans. (d) Senescence

28. Precursor for ethylene biosynthesis is

a. Methionine
b. Alanine
c. Ornithine
d. Tryptophan

Ans. (a) Methionine

29. In a rapidly transpiring plant the water column in xylem will be

a. Positive pressure
b. Negative presssure
c. High root presssure
d. No pressure

Ans. (b) Methionine

30. Transpiration is measured by

a. Lysimeter
b. Photometer
c. Tensiometer
d. Auxanometer

Ans. (b) Photometer

31. Stomata are regulated by

a. N
b. P
c. K
d. Ca

Ans. (c) K

32. Plant lost water in transpiration upto the extent of

a. 80%
b. 90%
c. 95%
d. 99%

Ans. (d) 99%

33. The world tallest tree is

a. Sequoia sempervirens
b. Eucalyptus regans
c. Psendotsuga menziesii
d. Ailanthus excelsa

Ans. (a) Sequoia sempervirens

34. Proteins that bind to TATA box in promoters region are

a. Coactivators
b. Coregulators
c. Enhancers
d. Transcriptional factors

Ans. (d) Transcriptional factors

35. The chemical nature of GA_3 is

a. Phenolic
b. Terpene
c. Purine
d. Indole

Ans. (b) Terpene

36. Site of oxidative electron transport in cell is

a. Mitochondria
b. Chloroplast
c. Nucleus
d. Cytoplasm

Ans. (a) Mitochondria

37. Guttation is not favoured under

a. Low humidity
b. High humidity
c. Low root pressure
d. High humidity and low root pressure

Ans. (c) Low root pressure

38. The basic elements of the cohesion theory for the ascent of sap are

a. Driving force
b. Hydration
c. Cohesion of water
d. All

Ans. (d) All

39. The xylem and phloem elements in the plant are surrounded by a layer of living cells called

a. Casparian strips
b. Pericycle
c. Stele
d. Endodermis

Ans. (b) Pericycle

40. Which part of root absorb water and minerals

a. Root cap
b. Root hairs
c. Epidermis
d. Endodermis

Ans. (b) Root hairs

41. Fluid mosaic model of cell membrane is given by

a. Daniel and Davson
b. Robertson
c. Robercook
d. Singer and Nicholson

Ans. (d) Singer and Nicholson

42. The stage of seeds showing no germination because of internal conditions of seed is termed as

a. Dormancy
b. Quinscence
c. Recalciterant
d. Longetivity

Ans. (a) Dormancy

43. A plant hormone, which is primary regulator of abscission process is

a. Ethylene
b. Auxin
c. ABA
d. Gibberellins

Ans. (c) ABA

44. Growing of plant in soilless nutrient solution is referred as

a. Aeroponics
b. Hydroponics
c. Xeroponics
d. None

Ans. (b) Hydroponics

45. Most of the wheat cultivars are

a. Day neutral
b. Short day plants
c. Qualitative long day plants
d. Quantitative long day plants

Ans. (c) Qualitative long day plants

46. The critical conc. of micronutrients needed in tissue is equal to or less than

a. 1 ppm
b. 10 ppm
c. 100 ppm
d. 1000 ppm

Ans. (c) 100 ppm

47. Rice grain is deficient in

a. Lysine
b. Glysine
c. Isoleucine
d. Alanine

Ans. (a) Lysine

48. Storage of elements in vacuoles occurs under

a. Deficient zone
b. Critical zone
c. Luxury consumption
d. Toxic zone

Ans. (c) Luxury consumption

49. Chelates are

a. Organic in nature   b. Inorganic in nature
c. Both a and b   d. None

Ans. (a) Organic in nature

50. Siderophores produced by fungi and bacteria in soil are the source of

a. Zn   b. Fe
c. Cu   d. Mn

Ans. (b) Fe

51. The young leaves of terminal bud at first typically hooked, finally dying back at tips and margins are the deficiency symptoms of

a. K   b. Fe
c. Ca   d. Cu

Ans. (c) Ca

52. The young leaves chlorotic, principal veins remain typically green, stalks slender and short are the deficiency symptoms of

a. Fe   b. Cu
c. Mn   d. B

Ans. (a) Fe

53. Iron stored in chloroplast as an iron protein complex is called

a. Calmodulin   b. Phytoferritin
c. Chloroferritin   d. Chromoferritin

Ans. (b) Phytoferritin

54. Initiation of protein synthesis in eukaryotic mRNA requires

a. 3' poly A tail   b. 5' poly A tail
c. 5' cap   d. 3' cap

Ans. (c) 5' cap

55. The first sign of switch over from vegetative stage to reproductive stage in wheat is

a. Ear emergence stage
b. Double ridge stage
c. Terminal spikelet stage
d. Anthesis stage

Ans. (b) Double ridge stage

56. Abundant P in plants related with

a. Early maturity
b. Delay maturity
c. Accumulation of anthocyanin pigments
d. Both b and c

Ans. (d) Both b and c

57. Increase in temp. at anthesis stage in wheat results in

a. Increased grain size
b. Decreased grain size
c. Increased duration of grain growth
d. No effect

Ans. (b) Decreased grain size

58. An ideal type of rice with small, thick and erect leaf was proposed by

a. Tsunoda
b. Tanaka
c. Yoshida
d. Murata

Ans. (c) Yoshida

59. Increase in wheat yield potential so far results from

a. Increase in HI
b. Increase in dry matter production
c. Increase in stem weight
d. Increase in leaf weight

Ans. (a) Increase in HI

60. Most commonly grown crop plants are included in

a. Halophytes
b. Glycophytes
c. Sciophytes
d. Xerophytes

Ans. (b) Glycophytes

61. Acytelene reduction to ethylene is measured as

a. Nitrate reduction
b. Glutamate synthase activity
c. Nitrite reduction
d. N_2 fixation

Ans. (d) N_2 fixation

62. The gray speck of oats, 'marsh spot of peas', and speckled yellows of sugar beets are the deficiency symptoms of

a. Cu   b. Mn
c. Fe   d. Zn

Ans. (b) Mn

63. The 'heart rot' of beets, 'stem crack' of celery, 'water core' of turnip and 'drought spot' of apples are the deficiency symptoms of

a. B   b. Ca
c. Zn   d. Cu

Ans. (a) B

64. Optimum temp. for maximum crop development in wheat is

a. 10 –15°C
b. 20–25°C
c. 25–30°C
d. 30–35°C

Ans. (b) 20–25°C

65. 'little leaf' and 'rosette' of apple, 'white bud' of maize are the deficiency symptoms of

a. Fe
b. Zn
c. Cl
d. Mo

Ans. (b) Zn

66. Under an excessive light level the synthesis of which of the following is found increased

a. Antheraxanthin
b. Violaxanthin
c. Zeaxanthin
d. All

Ans. (c) Zeaxanthin

67. In citrus plant, die back disease is the result of deficiency

a. N
b. P
c. B
d. Cu

Ans. (d) Cu

68. Which micronutrient is essential for the synthesis of 'auxin'

a. Cu
b. Mn
c. Zn
d. Si

Ans. (c) Zn

69. 'Whiptail' disease of cauliflower is due to deficiency of

a. Cu
b. Cl
c. Ca
d. Mo

Ans. (d) Mo

70. Direct reduction of O_2 by photosystem-I leads to the formation of

a. H_2O_2
b. Superoxide anion radical
c. Singlet oxygen
d. Singlet exited state of O_2

Ans. (a) H_2O_2

71. Which of the following is not a colligative property

a. Depression of freezing point
b. Refractive index
c. Lowering of vapour pressure
d. Elevation of boiling point

Ans. (b) Refractive index

72. The optimum pH of nutrient solution in nutrient solution culture is

a. 4
b. 6
c. 8
d. 9

Ans. (b) 6

73. Acid rains are due to following gases are

a. CO_2 and CO
b. Ozone and CO_2
c. NO_2 and SO_2
d. NH_3 and CO_2

Ans. (c) NO_2 and SO_2

74. Tumor inducing principle in Agrobacterium is in

a. T-DNA
b. Ti-plasmid
c. t-RNA
d. none

Ans. (a) T-DNA

75. Mycorrhiza (association of fungi with roots of higher plants) increased the availability of

a. Fe
b. N
c. P
d. B

Ans. (c) P

76. VAM is mostly used in

a. Perennial trees
b. Annual crops
c. Biennial crops
d. All

Ans. (a) Perennial trees

77. If the accumulation ratio in absorption of nutrients is greater than one then it is known as

a. Active absorption
b. Passive absorption
c. Adsorption
d. None

Ans. (a) Active absorption

78. Which one of the following is a most harmful pollutant by automobiles

a. SO_2
b. CO
c. N_2O
d. SO_2

Ans. (b) CO

79. ^{14}C has a half life of

a. 14 days
b. 100 years
c. 5730 years
d. 6000 years

Ans. (c) 5730 years

80. Mass flow mechanism was proposed by

a. Darwin
b. Munch
c. Hugo de Vries
d. Banda

Ans. (b) Munch

81. **hn RNA strands for**

a. Homogeneous nuclear RNA
b. Heterogeneous nuclear RNA
c. Heterocyclic nuclear RNA
d. All

Ans. (b) Heterogeneous nuclear RNA

82. **Isotopes differs in**

a. Electrons and protons
b. Protons and neutrons
c. Neutrons only
d. Electrons and neutrons

Ans. (c) Neutrons only

83. **The process in which sugars are raised to high conc. in phloem cells close to a source is known as**

a. Xylem loading
b. Phloem loading
c. Phloem conc
d. Phloem deloading

Ans. (b) Phloem loading

84. **The breakdown of large molecules to small molecules and this process often releases energy is called as**

a. Anabolism
b. Catabolism
c. Both a and b
d. None

Ans. (b) Catabolism

85. **One curie of activity is equivalent to**

a. 3.7×10^4 disintegration per sec.
b. 3.7×10^1 disintegration per sec.
c. 3.7×10^{10} disintegration per sec.
d. 3.7×10^7 disintegration per sec.

Ans. (c) 3.7×10^{10} disintegration per sec.

86. **Climatric rise in respiration is observed in**

a. Mango
b. Citrus
c. Grapes
d. Cherries

Ans. (a) Mango

87. **Callus is induced to form roots in the medium of**

a. Auxin only
b. Cytokinins only
c. More Cytokinins than Auxin
d. More Auxin than Cytokinins

Ans. (d) More Auxin than Cytokinins

88. **S containing amino acids is /are**

a. Cysteine
b. Methionine
c. Lysine
d. Both a and b

Ans. (d) Both a and b

89. **Which group of enzymes form double bonds by elimination of a chemical groups**

a. Kinases
b. Lyases
c. Polymerases
d. Ligases

Ans. (b) Lyases

90. **Electrophoresis was developed to separate**

a. Fats
b. carbohydrates
c. Vitamins
d. Proteins

Ans. (d) Proteins

91. **Ripening is delayed by synthesis of antisense ACC synthetase RNA in which fruit**

a. Tomato
b. Grapes
c. Citrus
d. Cherries

Ans. (a) Tomato

92. **Blue light is always less efficient in photosynthesis than**

a. White
b. Red
c. Orange
d. Violet

Ans. (b) Red

93. **Recognition site of t- RNA is**

a. Anticodon
b. Loop I
c. Loop IV
d. 3' OH end

Ans. (a) Anticodon

94. **Chlorophyll are green because they**

a. Reflect green light
b. Absorb green light
c. Transmit green light
d. None

Ans. (b) Absorb green light

95. **RNA – DNA hybridization to quantify gene expression at mRNA level is called as**

a. Southern blotting
b. Slot-blot technique
c. Western blotting
d. Northern blotting

Ans. (d) Northern blotting

96. **Wavelength of visible light is**

a. 260–350 nm
b. 360–760 nm
c. 390–760 nm
d. 400–700 nm

Ans. (c) 390–760 nm

97. **Plastocyanin protein contain**

a. Fe
b. Cu
c. P
d. Mo

Ans. (b) Cu

98. Z –scheme of electron transport first proposed by

    a. Hill and Bendall
    b. Hatch and Boardman
    c. Haliwell
    d. Calwin

Ans. (a) Hill and Bendall

99. How many photons are required to produce one molecule of oxygen

    a. 4   b. 8
    c. 12   d. 16

Ans. (b) 8

100. Brassino steroid is present in

    a. Mustard   b. Cotton
    c. Wheat   d. Sunflower

Ans. (a) Mustard

101. In C_3 plant, which enzyme first react with CO_2 to form PGA

    a. Invertases   b. Rubisco
    c. Oxaloacetate   d. PEP

Ans. (b) Rubisco

102. Hormone associated with 'acid growth theory' is

    a. GA_3 b. Cytokinin
    c. Auxin   d. Ethylene

Ans. (c) Auxin

103. Protein content in pulses ranges from

    a. 10 –15%   b. 20 –25%
    c. 25 –30%   d. 40 –45%

Ans. (b) 20 –25%

104. Protein content of cereals ranges from

    a. 8–12%   b. 12–15%
    c. 15–20%   d. 20–25%

Ans. (a) 8–12%

105. Nitrate reductase is found in

    a. Chloroplast   b. Golgibodies
    c. Mitochondria   d. Cytoplasm

Ans. (d) Cytoplasm

106. Natural inhibitor of IAA oxidases is

    a. Caffeic acid
    b. Coumaric acid
    c. ABA
    d. Lactic acid

Ans. (b) Coumaric acid

107. In C_4 plants, the first stable product of photo-synthesis is

    a. PGA   b. Malic acid
    c. Oxalic acid   d. Tartaric acid

Ans. (c) Oxalic acid

108. Close association of chloroplast, peroxisomes and mitochondria in a leaf cell are related with

    a. Photosynthesis   b. Respiration
    c. Photorespiration   d. None

Ans. (c) Photorespiration

109. How many ATP are required to produce 1 mole of hexose in photosynthesis

    a. 8   b. 18
    c. 28   d. 38

Ans. (b) 18

110. Instrument used for measuring 'stomatal pressure' is

    a. Porometer   b. Callipers
    c. Photometer   d. Micronare

Ans. (a) Porometer

111. Who coined the term 'biological clock'

    a. Went   b. Borthwick
    c. Salisburry   d. Bunning

Ans. (d) Bunning

112. Most dangerous gas for depletion of ozone layer is

    a. Chlorine   b. CFC
    c. Benzene   d. CO_2

Ans. (b) CFC

113. Which process is also known as glycolate pathway

    a. Photosynthesis   b. Respiration
    c. β-oxidation   d. Photorespiration

Ans. (d) Photorespiration

114. The present level of CO_2 in atmosphere is

    a. 210–250 ppm   b. 295–300 ppm
    c. 360–370 ppm   d. 420–460 ppm

Ans. (c) 360–370 ppm

115. In C_4 plants, enzyme responsible for the synthesis of malic acid is

    a. PEP carboxylase   b. Rubisco
    c. Isomerise   d. Kinase

Ans. (a) PEP carboxylase

116. Element for most of dehydrogenase is

　　a. Ca　　　　　　b. Mo
　　c. Mg　　　　　　d. Zn

Ans. (d) Zn

117. Lysimeter is used in measurement of

　　a. Light
　　b. Transpiration
　　c. Lysine content
　　d. Water potential

Ans. (b) Transpiration

118. Agave americana is a

　　a. C_3 plant　　　　b. C_4 plant
　　c. CAM plant　　　　d. None

Ans. (c) CAM plant

119. The most striking feature of CAM plants is formation of malic acid at

　　a. Morning　　　　b. Afternoon
　　c. Evening　　　　d. Night

Ans. (d) Night

120. Select the families to which CAM plants belong

　　a. Bromeliaceae　　b. Cactaceae
　　c. Orchidaceae　　　d. All

Ans. (d) All

121. Photosynthetic inhibition by O_2 is called as

　　a. Hill reaction
　　b. Warburg's effect
　　c. Feed back inhibition
　　d. Competitive effect

Ans. (b) Warburg's effect

122. Among the following statements which one is not correct about photosynthesis

　　a. Light captured by PS-I and electron passed to PS-II
　　b. O_2 is released from photolysis of water
　　c. ATP from electron transport chain with PS-I, PS-II
　　d. Light independent reactions uses energy rich molecules to reduce CO_2

Ans. (a) Light captured by PS-I and electron passed to PS-II

123. Among following which is antioxidant

　　a. Quinines
　　b. Tocopherols
　　c. Phenols
　　d. Sorbitols

Ans. (b) Tocopherols

124. Which ecosystem has highest net primary productivity per unit area

　　a. Tropical seasonal forest
　　b. Tropical rain forest
　　c. Cultivated lands
　　d. Savanna

Ans. (b) Tropical rain forest

125. The irradiance at which photosynthesis is equal to respiration rate (net CO_2 exchange is zero) is called

　　a. Light compensation point
　　b. Light saturation point
　　c. Solar constant
　　d. PAR

Ans. (a) Light compensation point

126. The CO_2 conc. at which photosynthetic fixation just balances respiratory loss is known as

　　a. O_2 compensation point
　　b. O_2 saturation point
　　c. CO_2 compensation point
　　d. CO_2 saturation point

Ans. (c) CO_2 compensation point

127. The transpiration ratio is highest for

　　a. C_3 plants　　　　b. C_4 plants
　　c. CAM plants　　　　d. None

Ans. (a) C_3 plants

128. Photosynthesis inhibited by 21% O_2 in

　　a. C_3 plants　　　　b. C_4 plants
　　c. CAM plants　　　　d. None

Ans. (b) C_4 plants

129. For C_3 plants, the optimum temperature for photosynthesis is

　　a. 15–25°C　　　　b. 25–30°C
　　c. 30–47°C　　　　d. 35°C

Ans. (a) 15–25°C

130. Respiratory quotient for carbohydrates is approximately

　　a. 0.5　　　　　　b. 1.0
　　c. 1.33　　　　　　d. 0.7

Ans. (b) 1.0

131. Respiratory quotient for fatty acid is

　　a. 0.7　　　　　　b. 0.5
　　c. 1.33　　　　　　d. 2.0

Ans. (a) 0.7

132. Respiratory quotient for organic acid is

a. 0.7 b. 1.0
c. 1.33 d. >1.0

Ans. (c) 1.33

133. The end product of glycolysis is

a. Glucose b. Sucrose
c. Pyruvic acid d. NADH

Ans. (c) Pyruvic acid

134. Glycolysis takes place in

a. Mitochondria b. Chloroplast
c. Cytoplasm d. Nucleus

Ans. (c) Cytoplasm

135. Electron transport system take place in which part of mitochondria

a. Matrix
b. Cristae
c. Outer membrane
d. Inner membrane

Ans. (b) Cristae

136. Krebs cycle produces

a. 18 ATP b. 30 ATP
c. 32 ATP d. 36 ATP

Ans. (b) 30 ATP

137. First time IAA from human urine was isolated by

a. Kogl b. Went
c. Adns d. Miller

Ans. (a) Kogl

138. The term 'skototropism' is associated with whom

a. Jumper and Jones
b. Mayber and Mayer
c. Strong and Ray
d. Hans and Knot

Ans. (c) Strong and Ray

139. Pollen germination requires the following element

a. B b. K
c. Ca d. Si

Ans. (a) B

140. Who first isolated 'zeatin' from corn seed

a. Wiesner b. Miller
c. Zeigler d. Letham

Ans. (d) Letham

141. Storage protein in beans is

a. Insulin b. Globulins
c. Phaseoline d. Tripsin

Ans. (c) Phaseoline

142. Main organic acid in pineapple is

a. Citric acid
b. Pyruvic acid
c. Malic acid
d. Acetic acid

Ans. (c) Malic acid

143. Sulphate reduction in leaves take place in

a. Mitochondria
b. Chloroplast
c. Glyoxisomes
d. Peroxisomes

Ans. (b) Chloroplast

144. Polymer of cellulose is

a. β-D glucose b. α-D glucose
c. Fructose d. Glucose

Ans. (a) β-D glucose

145. In which cell organelle, PEP carboxylation is taking place in C_4 plants

a. Epidermal cells
b. Mesophyll cells
c. Xylem cells
d. Bundle sheath cells

Ans. (b) Mesophyll cells

146. Cyanide resistant respiration follow

a. Pentose phosphate pathway
b. Krebs cycle
c. Glycolysis
d. None

Ans. (a) Pentose phosphate pathway

147. Green house gas for global warming is

a. O_2 b. CH_4
c. SO_2 d. CO_2

Ans. (d) CO_2

148. Amino acid produced in photorespiration

a. Serine
b. Arginine
c. Tryptophan
d. Methionine

Ans. (a) Serine

149. In monocots and dicots accumulation of which hormone causes collapse and lysis of mature cortical cells in the root, leading to a tissue with large air spaces

a. Auxin   b. Gibberellins
c. Ethylene   d. ABA

Ans. (c) Ethylene

150. Aerenchyma is related with

a. ABA   b. Ethylene
c. Cytokinin   d. Auxin

Ans. (b) Ethylene

151. When starch reacts with iodine produces colour

a. Yellow   b. Blue
c. Green   d. Red

Ans. (b) Blue

152. Under aerobic conditions microbes grow slower but uses more sugar and produces more CO_2 and ethanol, this phenomenon known as

a. Warburg's effect   b. Pasteur effect
c. Both a and b   d. None

Ans. (b) Pasteur effect

153. Enzyme used to cut double stranded RNA is

a. DNAase
b. Reverse transcriptase
c. Restriction endonuclease
d. Lipase

Ans. (c) Restriction endonuclease

154. Which one can not pass across membrane by diffusion

a. CO_2 b. O_2
c. H_2O d. H^+

Ans. (d) H^+

155. In many species, the gradual decrease in respiration is reversed by a sharp increase, known as

a. Non climacteric   b. Climacteric
c. Both   d. None

Ans. (b) Climacteric

156. Conversion of organic nitrogen to NH_4 by soil microbes is called

a. Amminization
b. Ammonification
c. Nitrification
d. Mineralization

Ans. (b) Ammonification

157. Denitrification occurs in

a. Water logged soil   b. Well aerated soils
c. Alkali soils   d. Acidic soils

Ans. (a) Water logged soil

158. C_3 cycle of carbon fixation takes place in

a. Nucleus
b. Thylakoid of chloroplast
c. Stroma of chloroplast
d. Cytosol

Ans. (c) Stroma of chloroplast

159. The process by which N_2 is reduced to ammonium is called

a. Nitrification
b. N_2 fixation
c. Denitrification
d. Ammonia volatilization

Ans. (b) N_2 fixation

160. How many electrons are required for conversion of NO_2^- to NH_4^+

a. 4   b. 6
c. 8   d. 10

Ans. (b) 6

161. Mature root nodule made largely of

a. Diploid cells   b. Tetraploid cells
c. Hexaploid cells d. None

Ans. (b) Tetraploid cells

162. The main function of leghaemoglobin is

a. Fe supply   b. Water supply
c. O_2 supply   d. All

Ans. (c) O_2 supply

163. N_2 fixation is carried out by enzyme

a. Nitrate reductase   b. Nitrite reductase
c. Nitrogenase   d. Rubisco

Ans. (c) Nitrogenase

164. Nitrogenase consists of

a. Fe protein   b. Mo protein
c. Fe–Mo protein   d. none

Ans. (c) Fe –Mo protein

165. Which one of the following is P mobilize

a. VAM   b. Rhizobium
c. BGA   d. Clostridium

Ans. (a) VAM

166. 'Dormin' is coined by

a. Skoog

b. Wareig

c. Addicot

d. Wilkins

Ans. (b) Wareig

167. Kranz type of anatomy is found in

a. Sunflower

b. Soybean

c. Sorghum

d. Spinach

Ans. (c) Sorghum

168. How many Calvin cycles are needed to produce one molecule of glucose

a. 1

b. 3

c. 6

d. 9

Ans. (c) 6

169. The ureides is the major nitrogen compound transported from root nodules to other parts of plant in

a. Soybean

b. Wheat

c. Sugarcane

d. Sugarbet

Ans. (a) Soybean

170. How many quanta are there in 1 μ Einstein

a. 5.074×10^{23}

b. 6.02×10^{17}

c. 6.02×10^{-23}

d. 6.02×10^{23}

Ans. (b) 6.02×10^{17}

171. Unit of pressure in SI system

a. Atmosphere

b. Dynes per square cm

c. Pascal

d. mm of mercury

Ans. (c) Pascal

172. One millimole of $CaCO_3$ weight is

a. 100g

b. 1g

c. 1.0g

d. 0.1g

Ans. (d) 0.1g

173. In process of nitrate reduction, the oxidation no. of nitrogen changes from

a. +3 to +5

b. +5 to –3

c. +6 to –3

d. –2 to +5

Ans. (b) +5 to –3

174. Reduction of nitrite to ammonium ions is catalysed by nitrite reductase in

a. Chloroplast

b. Proplastids of roots

c. Both a and b

d. Cytoplasm

Ans. (c) Both a and b

175. Flowering stimulus is perceived by

a. Shoot apex

b. Leaves

c. Buds

d. Flowers

Ans. (b) Leaves

176. 1- amino-cyclopropane-1-carboxylic acid (ACC) is a close precursor of

a. ABA

b. Ethylene

c. Salicylic acid

d. GA

Ans. (b) Ethylene

177. The first step of assimilation of sulphate is catalyzed by

a. ATP sulfurylase

b. APS sulfotransferase

c. Pyrophosphatase

d. Cysteine synthetase

Ans. (a) ATP sulfurylase

178. Coconut fat is a rich source of

a. Palmitic acid

b. Stearic acid

c. Lauric acid

d. Ricinoleic acid

Ans. (c) Lauric acid

179. Phytoalexins includes

a. Pisatin

b. Phaseolin

c. Isocoumarin

d. All

Ans. (d) All

80. Antimicrobial compounds synthesized by plants when infected with microbes are

a. Betalin

b. Phytoalexins

c. Flavones

d. Flavonols

Ans. (b) Phytoalexins

181. Flavonoides includes

a. Anthocyanins

b. Flavonols

c. Flavones

d. All

Ans. (d) All

182. Betalains have role in

a. Germination

b. Pollination

c. Fruit setting

d. Ripening

Ans. (b) Pollination

183. The first alkaloid to be isolated and crystallized was the

a. Nicotine

b. Cocaine

c. Morphine

d. Caffeine

Ans. (c) Morphine

184. Nicotine is produced only in

a. Roots   b. Leaves
c. Stem   d. Seed

Ans. (a) Roots

185. A cell lacking cell wall is also lack in

a. Biomembrane   b. Chloroplast
c. ER   d. Mitochondria

Ans. (b) Chloroplast

186. cDNA stands for

a. Copy DNA
b. Cyclic DNA
c. Complementary DNA
d. Both a and b

Ans. (c) Complementary DNA

187. Dry weight is commonly obtained by drying the freshly harvested plant material at

a. 60–70°C   b. 70–80°C
c. 90–100°C   d. 100–105°C

Ans. (b) 70–80°C

188. In bamboos, which live more than half century, flowering occurs only

a. Once   b. Twice
c. Thrice   d. Not countable

Ans. (a) Once

189. Fluorescence which is sensitive to the conditions of photothermal traps are said to be

a. Constant Fluorescence
b. Dead Fluorescence
c. Background Fluorescence
d. Variable Fluorescence

Ans. (d) Variable Fluorescence

190. The century plant exist for a decade or more than before flowering ...... and dying

a. Once   b. Twice
c. Thrice   d. Not countable

Ans. (a) Once

191. Grana stacks of thylakoid membranes are high in

a. PS-I
b. PS-II
c. Cyt b or f
d. Chloroplast a or b

Ans. (b) PS-II

192. In the great majority of plant species, seed germination begins with

a. Radical   b. Epicotyl
c. Both a and b   d. None

Ans. (a) Radical

193. Phyllotaxis is related with arrangement of

a. Roots   b. Branches
c. Leaves   d. Flowers

Ans. (c) Leaves

194. Oxygenase function of Rubisco was first shown by

a. Andrews and Lorimer
b. Ogren and Bowes
c. Guttendge
d. Went

Ans. (b) Ogren and Bowes

195. Major form of carbon transfer in plants is by

a. Sucrose   b. Glucose
c. Fructose   d. Maltose

Ans. (a) Sucrose

196. The term auxin was first used in 1926 by

a. Frits went   b. Jacobs
c. Goldsmith   d. Yabuta

Ans. (a) Frits went

197. Photorespiration increases at warm temperature due to

a. Ratio of dissolved chloroplast O_2 to CO_2 is lower
b. Ratio of dissolved chloroplast O_2 to CO_2 is higher
c. Ratio of dissolved chloroplast O_2 to CO_2 is not affected
d. Ratio of dissolved chloroplast O_2 to CO_2 is equal

Ans. (b) Ratio of dissolved chloroplast O_2 to CO_2 is higher

198. IAA is chemically similar to the amino acid

a. Methionine
b. Tryptophan
c. Serine
d. Proline

Ans. (b) Tryptophan

199. Apical dominance is the result of

a. Auxins
b. Cytokinins
c. Ethylene
d. GA

Ans. (a) Auxins

200. The bakane (foolish seedling) disease of rice is caused by

a. Gibberella fujikuroi

b. Claviceps fuziformis

c. Xanthomonas oryzae

d. None

Ans. (a) Gibberella fujikuroi

201. The compound, gibberellins was isolated from fungus in 1930s by

a. Went

b. Yabuta and Hayashi

c. Anthony Trewavas

d. Crozier

Ans. (b) Yabuta and Hayashi

202. Which nutrient is related with water oxidizing enzyme complex

a. P

b. Mn

c. Cu

d. Fe

Ans. (b) Mn

203. Activator of carbonic anhydrase

a. Mn

b. P

c. Cu

d. Zn

Ans. (d) Zn

204. Which element is related with cytochrome

a. P

b. Zn

c. Cu

d. Fe

Ans. (d) Fe

205. The precursor of gibberellic acid is

a. Mevalonic acid

b. Kaurene

c. Violaxanthene

d. None

Ans. (b) Kaurene

206. Which plant hormone promote germination of dormant seed and growth of dormant buds

a. Auxin

b. GA

c. Cytokinins

d. ABA

Ans. (b) GA

207. During germination, embryo normally provides which hormone to the aleurone layer for the manufacturing of hydrolytic enzymes

a. IAA

b. ABA

c. Cytokinins

d. GA_3

Ans. (d) GA_3

208. Zeatin had first been identified by

a. Letham

b. Gottlieb Haberlandt

c. Steward

d. Skoog

Ans. (a) Letham

209. Natural occurring cytokinin is /are

a. Zeatin

b. Kinetin

c. Both a and b

d. Benzyl adenine

Ans. (c) Both a and b

210. The precursor of cytokinins is

a. Violaxanthene

b. Isopentenyl adenine

c. Campastrall

d. Kaurene

Ans. (b) Isopentenyl adenine

211. Which one of the following delay senescence and increase nutrient sink activity

a. Auxin

b. GA

c. ABA

d. Cytokinins

Ans. (d) Cytokinins

212. Which plant hormone is a volatile hormone

a. ABA

b. Ethylene

c. Cytokinins

d. Auxin

Ans. (b) Ethylene

213. Which gas is considered as antagonist to ethylene action

a. O_2

b. N_2

c. CO_2

d. CH_4

Ans. (c) CO_2

214. Precursor of abscisic acid (ABA)

a. Violaxanthene

b. Xanthoxin

c. Isopentenyl adenine

d. Methionine

Ans. (a) Violaxanthene

215. The hormone ABA was first identified and characterized chemically in 1963 by

a. Frederick T. Addicott

b. Milborrow

c. Bradford

d. None

Ans. (a) Frederick T. Addicott

216. The major functions of ABA is / are

a. Inhibition of RNA synthesis

b. Inhibition of translation

c. Effect on plasma membrane

d. All

Ans. (d) All

217. Precursor of brassinosteroides is

a. Adenine   b. Campastrall
c. Violaxanthine   d. Kaurene

Ans. (b) Campastrall

218. Growth movement toward (positive) or away (negative) from the earth's gravitational pull is known as

a. Photoperiodism   b. Phototropism
c. Gravitropism   d. Plagiotropism

Ans. (c) Gravitropism

219. Aminoethoxyvinylglycine (AVG) inhibits

a. Alternate bearing in mango
b. Photosynthetic e⁻ transport
c. Ethylene biosynthesis
d. Cyanide resistant respiration

Ans. (c) Ethylene biosynthesis

220. Which one of the following is not correctly matched

a. TIBA–inhibit polar transport of IAA
b. SHAM–inhibit cyanide resistant respiration
c. Atrazine–inhibit Photosynthetic e⁻ transport
d. None

Ans. (d) None

221. Law of inhibitory factor is given by

a. VH Blackman   b. RF Blackman
c. RD Asana   d. CM Donald

Ans. (b) RF Blackman

222. Which scientist worked on drought tolerance

a. R D Asana   b. C M Donald
c. HA Borthwick   d. VH Blackman

Ans. (a) R D Asana

223. Select the pair which is not correctly matched

a. LAR-leaf area per unit plant dry weight
b. SLA-leaf area per unit leaf dry weight
c. SLW-leaf dry weight per unit leaf area
d. None

Ans. (d) None

224. The main function of jasmic acid is

a. Promote leaf senescence
b. Steroid growth promoter
c. Control nastic movements
d. Decrease senescence

Ans. (a) Promote leaf senescence

225. The main function of salicylic acid is

a. Control nastic movements
b. Promote leaf senescence
c. Increase resistance to plant pathogen's infection
d. Reduces water stress

Ans. (c) Increase resistance to plant pathogen's infection

226. Select the pair which is not correctly matched

a. Transamination – Brassin and Kriman
b. Photoperiodism – Garner and Allard
c. Ascorbic acid – Chinoy
d. None

Ans. (d) None

227. The main function of turgorins is

a. Control nastic movements
b. Promote leaf senescence
c. Increase resistance to plant pathogen's infection
d. Steroid growth promoter

Ans. (a) Control nastic movements

228. The term vernalization relates

a. To low temperature promotion of flowering
b. To low temperature promotion of early germination
c. To high temperature for early ripening
d. None

Ans. (a) To low temperature promotion of flowering

229. Which of the following is/are day neutral plants

a. Cotton   b. Buckwheat
c. Sunflower   d. All

Ans. (d) All

230. Who named the florigen

a. Skoog   b. Knott
c. Chailakhayan   d. Salisbury

Ans. (c) Chailakhayan

231. In vernalization the seeds are allowed to germinate for some time and then are given cold temperature treatments by keeping them at

a. 0 to 5°C   b. 0 to 20°C
c. 10–20°C   d. 20–25°C

Ans. (a) 0 to 5°C

232. He movement of secondary branches of roots and stem growing at right angle is known as

a. Plagiogeotropic   b. Apogeotropic
c. Diageotropic   d. none

Ans. (c) Diageotropic

233. Parthenocarpy means formation of fruits without seed is found in

a. Bananas   b. Pineapple

c. Melons   d. All

Ans. (d) All

234. The example of non-climacteric fruits is /are

a. Oranges   b. Lemons

c. Pepper   d. All

Ans. (d) All

235. When dormancy occurs due to unfavourable environmental conditions is known as

a. Innate dormancy

b. Imposed dormancy

c. Induced dormancy

d. All

Ans. (b) Imposed dormancy

236. The phenomenon in which germination of seeds is affected by light, such seeds are known as

a. Photoperiodic   b. Thermoperiodic

c. Photoblastic   d. Vernalized

Ans. (c) Photoblastic

237. Positive photoblastic plants includes

a. Nicotiana tabacum   b. Nigella damascena

c. Silene armeria   d. Nemophila insignis

Ans. (a) Nicotiana tabacum

238. Off season flowering in plants is positive by giving treatment of

a. Photoperiodism   b. Vernalization

c. Both a and b   d. Thermoperiodism

Ans. (c) Both a and b

239. Maleic hydrazide is used to

a. Suppress flowering and emergence of suckers

b. Induce seed germination

c. Enhance ripening

d. All

Ans. (a) Suppress flowering and emergence of suckers

240. Pomato (a hybrid of potato and tomato) produced by

a. Cytoplasmic fusion

b. Protoplasmic fusion

c. Nuclear fusion

d. None

Ans. (b) Protoplasmic fusion

241. The principle of electrophoresis were first made in 1807 by

a. Alexander Reuss   b. Michael Faraday

c. EH Du Bosi Raymond   d. Lambert

Ans. (a) Alexander Reuss

242. In year 1906, who initiated the idea of chromatography

a. Michael Faraday   b. AJP Martin

c. Michael Tswett   d. RLM Synge

Ans. (c) Michael Tswett

243. The term protoplasm was introduced by

a. Purkinje (1840)   b. Purkinje (1860)

c. Von Mohl (1846)   d. Virchow (1855)

Ans. (a) Purkinje (1840)

244. Who first time reported the presence of ribosomes in cell

a. Palade   b. Haguenau

c. Robinson and Brown   d. Benda

Ans. (a) Palade

245. Intracellular digestion, autophagy, aging and autolysis are the functions of

a. Mitochondria   b. Lysosomes

c. Peroxisomes   d. Spherosomes

Ans. (b) Lysosomes

246. Vacuoles are surrounded by

a. Plasma membrane   b. Cell wall

c. Tonoplast   d. Lipid bilayer

Ans. (c) Tonoplast

247. Which cell organelle concerned with glyoxylate metabolism

a. Spherosomes   b. Lysosomes

c. Ribosomes   d. Glyoxysomes

Ans. (d) Glyoxysomes

248. Diffusion of liquid into gas results in the formation of

a. Foam   b. Precious stones

c. Clouds   d. Smoke

Ans. (c) Clouds

249. The adsorption of water by hydrophilic colloids is called

a. Diffusion   b. Imbibition

c. Plasmolysis   d. Mass flow

Ans. (b) Imbibition

250. The total amount of water present in soil is called as

    a. Holard   b. Chesard

    c. Echard   d. Water table

Ans. (a) Holard

251. Who gave the transpiration pull or cohesion tension theory of ascent of sap

    a. Unger   b. Dixon and Jolly

    c. Milburn and Johnson   d. Stephan Hales

Ans. (b) Dixon and Jolly

252. Guttation is take place through

    a. Stomata   b. Hydathode

    c. Leaf veins   d. Guard cells

Ans. (b) Hydathode

253. Which instrument used to measure stomatal opening

    a. Porometer   b. Photometer

    c. IRGA   d. Manometer

Ans. (a) Porometer

254. 'Tea yellow' disease is caused by deficiency of

    a. N   b. P

    c. S   d. B

Ans. (c) S

255. General starvation is the deficiency symptom of

    a. N   b. P

    c. K   d. Ca

Ans. (a) N

256. Blossom end rot is the deficiency symptom of

    a. Ca   b. Mg

    c. B   d. Mo

Ans. (a) Ca

257. In tobacco, 'sand drown' disease is found due to deficiency of

    a. Ca   b. Mg

    c. Fe   d. Cu

Ans. (b) Mg

258. Copper deficiency in cereals, oats, beet and pulses causes

    a. Exanthema or die back

    b. White tip disease

    c. Rosette

    d. Frenching

Ans. (b) White tip disease

259. Which of the following statements is correct about diffusion?

    a. It is very rapid over long distances

    b. It requires an expenditure of energy by the cell

    c. It is a passive process

    d. It occurs when molecules move from a region of lower concentration to one of higher concentration

Ans. (c) It is a passive process

260. Osmosis is a form of diffusion in which

    a. The solute moves freely from a region of higher concentration to one of higher concentration through a semi permeable membrane

    b. The solvent moves through a semi permeable membrane from region, where a solute is in higher concentration to region of lower concentration

    c. The solvent moves through a semi permeable membrane from higher solvent concentration to lower solvent concentration

    d. Solute as well as solvent moves freely from a region of higher concentration to one of higher concentration through a semi permeable membrane

Ans. (c) The solvent moves through a semi permeable membrane from higher solvent concentration to lower solvent concentration

261. I place a cell in a solution .Over a period of time, I notice that the cell shrinks ,as if it is losing water which of the following seems likely?

    a. The solution is a strong buffer

    b. The solution is an acid

    c. The solution has more dissolved solutes than the cell does

    d. The solution has more dissolved solutes than the cell does

Ans. (c) The solution has more dissolved solutes than the cell does

262. Water potential

    a. Of a solution is always greater than for pure water

    b. Is the potential energy of water in a system

    c. Is a measure of the level of the active movement of water a system

    d. Is never zero

Ans. (b) Is the potential energy of water in a system

263. If a plant cell is placed in deionised water the potential of that cell becomes

    a. More positive because the pressure potential becomes more positive

    b. More positive because the osmotic potential becomes more negative

c. More positive because the pressure potential becomes more negative

d. Less negative because the pressure potential becomes more positive

Ans. (d) Less negative because the pressure potential becomes more positive

264. The sap of a plant cell has an osmotic potential of -10 bars and there is a wall pressure of 2 bars . When this cell is placed in a solution with an osmotic potential of -3 bars the force causing water to enter the cell is

    a. −8 bar   b. −7 bar

    c. −5 bar   d. −3 bar

Ans. (c) −5 bar

265. A root cortex cell has a solute potential of −0.5 MPa. The water potential of the soil is −0.3 MPa. At what turgor pressure would the root cortex cell no longer take up water?

    a. 0 MPa   b. −0.15 MPa

    c. +0.15 MPa   d. +0.2 MPa

Ans. (d) +0.2 MPa

266. A limp lettuce leaf has an osmotic potential = −4 MPa. The lettuce leaf is placed into a beaker of pure water. When the cells of the lettuce leaf are fully turgid the water potential of the leaf cells will be

    a. +4 MPa   b. +8 MPa

    c. −4 MPa   d. 0.0 MPa

Ans. (d) 0.0 MPa

267. Space between cell wall and plasma membrane in a plasmolysed cell is occupied by

    a. Pure water   b. Air

    c. Cell sap   d. Plasmolysing solution

Ans. (d) Plasmolysing solution

268. In a flaccid cell

    a. DPD = OP   b. DPD = TP

    c. DPD = OP−TP   d. None

Ans. (a) DPD = OP

269. A cell at incipient plasmolysis, with a solute potential of −2000 KPa, is placed in a solution of water potential −1200KPa. The direction of flow of water will be

    a. From cell to solution

    b. From solution to cell

    c. Data incomplete

    d. No flow of water

Ans. (b) From solution to cell

270. If both leaf water potential and leaf osmotic potential in mid afternoon on a hot summer day equals − 15 bars

    a. The leaf is probably wilted

    b. The whole plant is at the permanent point

    c. Leaf cells have highest wall pressure

    d. The soil is at the plant's permanent wilted point

Ans. (a) The leaf is probably wilted

271. Which of the following plays no role in the movement of water through the xylem of plants?

    a. Capillarity

    b. Root pressure

    c. H^+/ATPase pump at the xylem element membrane

    d. Transpirational pull

Ans. (c) H^+/ATPase pump at the xylem element membrane

272. Water cohesion

    a. Creates the pulling force which pulls water upward in the xylem

    b. Causes water to move from the xylem into the phloem in response to differences in water concentration

    c. Is an energy requiring process

    d. Is responsible for making the column of water

Ans. (d) Is responsible for making the column of water

273. The class of water in the soil, that provides most of the water of plants and is thus the most important, is

    a. Gravitational   b. Field capacity

    c. Capillary   d. Hygroscopic

Ans. (c) Capillary

274. Halophytes such as mangroves meet high osmotic pressures in the soil. They overcome the problem of water uptake by

    a. Increase in the root to shoot ratio

    b. Reduction in the number of stomata to reduce transpiration

    c. Accumulation of electrolytes in the vacuoles

    d. Growth at relatively high humidity to reduce transpiration

Ans. (c) Accumulation of electrolytes in the vacuoles

275. Root pressure is a /an

    a. Non-osmotic phenomenon

    b. Osmotic phenomenon

    c. Positive hydrostatic pressure

    d. More than one correct

Ans. (d) More than one correct

276. Which of the following statement is correct?

a. Members of gymnosperm show high root pressure
b. Actively transpiring plants show high root pressure
c. Root pressure is mainly responsible for ascent of sap
d. None

Ans. (d) None

277. Transpiration pull depends on

a. Adhesion of water molecules to the walls of phloem cells
b. Capillarity
c. The very negative water potential of the atmosphere
d. Cohesion of water molecules to each other

Ans. (c) The very negative water potential of the atmosphere

278. The source of energy driving the transport of water through the xylem is

a. ATP produced by photosynthesis
b. ATP generated by respiration
c. The sun
d. Transpiration

Ans. (c) The sun

279. The water within xylem vessels moves toward the top of a tree (long distances) as a result of

a. Atmospheric pressure on roots
b. Active transport of ions into the vascular bundle
c. Evaporation of water through stoma
d. The force of root pressure

Ans. (c) Evaporation of water through stoma

280. Which combination of characteristic of a vessel element is most important foe water movement in the xylem?

a. Rigid cell wall, cell death at maturity, end walls absent
b. Rigid cell wall, reduction in size of plastids and mitochondria, end walls present
c. Rigid cell wall, living cell membrane, and walls absent
d. Flexible cell wall, nucleus anchored to the cell membrane, end walls present

Ans. (c) Rigid cell wall, living cell membrane, and walls absent

281. Which of the following properties of water is most directly related to its ability to rise in the capillary spaces of plants?

a. Neutral Ph
b. High density
c. Low compressibility
d. High surface tension

Ans. (d) High surface tension

282. Which of the following observations shows that ion uptake in plants is energy dependent?

a. Ion uptake shows saturation kinetics
b. Ion uptake rates are different for different ions
c. Some ions accumulate against a concentration gradient
d. Some ions enter the symplast before reaching the endodermis

Ans. (c) Some ions accumulate against a concentration gradient

283. How does a plant accumulate ions from the soil, which has a lower concentration than that in the plant?

a. Applies pressure to push ions into the cell
b. Applies tension to pull the ions into the cell
c. Expends energy to transport ions against concentration gradient
d. Roots grow around soil particles trapping the ions in a cell

Ans. (c) Expends energy to transport ions against concentration gradient

284. Which statement about the function of the casparian strip is correct?

a. It prevents excess transpiration from leaves
b. It regulates ions movement into root vascular cylinder
c. It prevent disease causing organisms from invading the plant
d. It is the pathway for nutrient transfer from xylem to phloem

Ans. (b) It regulates ions movement into root vascular cylinder

285. Mark the correct statements

a. Resistance to water flow in root cortex will be higher for symplastic pathway
b. Major pathway followed by ions from the epidermis to tracheary element of root is symplastic
c. The casparian strip prohibits H_2O from passing through the apoplast
d. Absorption of ions in plants is controlled by carriers and pumps
e. All

Ans. (e) All

286. Ion absorption by plant roots

a. Can be explained by the nutrient-carrier hypothesis
b. Is basically ions passively soaking in root cells along with soil water

c. Explains the movement of ions from a dilute soil solution into a more concertrated solution

d. More than one correct

Ans. (d) More than one correct

287. When a cell membrane moves substances from a region of lower concentration to a region og higher concentration, and expends energy in the process, this type of movement is called

a. Osmosis
b. Diffusion
c. Active transport
d. Facilitate diffusion

Ans. (c) Active transport

288. Ion absorption by symplast occurs

a. Passively by facilitated diffusion
b. Actively by primary and secondary active transport
c. Passively by free diffusion
d. Both a and b

Ans. (d) Both a and b

289. In plant roots, the casparian strip is correctly described by which of the following?

a. It is located in the walls between endodermal cells and cortex cells
b. It provides energy for the active transport of minerals into the vascular bundle from the cortex
c. It ensures that all minerals are absorbed from the soil in equal amounts
d. It ensures that all water and dissolved substances must pass through a cell before entering the vascular bundle

Ans. (d) It ensures that all water and dissolved substances must pass through a cell before entering the vascular bundle

290. Ion transport in root occurs

a. Passively through channels
b. Actively through channels
c. Actively through carriers
d. Through both symplast and apoplast

Ans. a, c, and d.

291. Ion channels

a. Always require ATP in order to function
b. Are always open
c. Are integral membrane proteins
d. Are responsible for the selective permeability of a membrane

Ans. (c) Are integral membrane proteins, (d) Are responsible for the selective permeability of a membrane

292. The casparian strip

a. Limits the pathway available to water and solutes, forcing them to enter the symplast
b. Surrounds the root vascular tissue
c. Allows water to move down a water potential gradient
d. Is made of suberin

Ans. All

ANIMAL PHYSIOLOGY

1. Which is true for the autonomic nervous system?

a. The sympathetic nervous system always stimulates the organ system
b. The parasympathetic nervous system always stimulates the organ system
c. It depends on the organ system whether the division stimulates or inhibits it
d. None of these

Ans. (c) It depends on the organ system whether the division stimulates or inhibits it

2. Which of the following statement is true?

a. Nodes of Ranvier are most easily seen in cross-section of peripheral nerve
b. Most nerves contain afferent and efferent fiber and thus carry both motor and sensory signals
c. Peripheral nerve is similar to smooth muscle in terms of the connective tissue investment
d. None of these

Ans. (b) Most nerves contain afferent and efferent fiber and thus carry both motor and sensory signals

3. Which of the following cells is responsible for myelin formation in the peripheral nervous system?

a. Schwann cell
b. Microglial cell
c. Astrocyte
d. All of these

Ans. (a) Schwann cell

4. Which of the following is not done by glial cells?

a. Producing insulating sheaths around axons
b. Giving metabolic support to neurons
c. Receiving and conducing electrochemical signals
d. Removing debris after the death of a neuron

Ans. (c) Receiving and conducing electrochemical signals

5. The perineurium is the connective tissue layer

a. Surrounding an entire nerve
b. Surrounding individual axons in the CNS

c. Surrounding individual axons in the PNS

d. Surrounding fascicles of axons in the PNS

Ans. (d) Surrounding fascicles of axons in the PNS

6. The system that controls smooth muscle, cardiac muscle, and gland activity is the

a. Autonomic nervous system

b. Somatic nervous system

c. Skeletal division

d. None of these

Ans. (a) Autonomic nervous system

7. Neurotransmitters are removed from the synaptic deft by

a. Diffusion   b. Cellular uptake

c. Enzymatic breakdown   d. Axonal transport

Ans. a, b, c.

8. Which of the following is true of the sympathetic nervous system?

a. It's voluntarily controlled via the forebrain

b. It's voluntarily controlled via the reticular formation

c. It uses different neurotransmitters at the ganglion and at the synaptic cleft

d. It's a subdivision of the somatic nervous system

Ans. (c) It uses different neurotransmitters at the ganglion and at the synaptic cleft

9. The effect of parasympathetic nervous stimulation on the heart is

a. Increased activity of the SA node

b. Increased activity of the AV node

c. Increased force of contraction

d. Slowing of the heart

Ans. (d) Slowing of the heart

10. The action potential of a neuron

a. Is terminated by efflux of Na^+

b. Is terminated by efflux of K^+

c. Declines in amplitude as it moves along the axon

d. None of these

Ans. (b) Is terminated by efflux of K^+

11. Action potentials are conducted more rapidly in

a. Larger diameter axons than small diameter axons

b. Small diameter axons than large diameter axons

c. Unmyelinated than myelinated axons

d. Axons that lack a warpping of Schwann cell

Ans. (a) Larger diameter axons than small diameter axons

12. An inhibitory neuron could affect the neuron with which it synapses by

a. Producing an IPSP within the neuron

b. Increasing K+ efflux from the neuron

c. Hyperpolarizing the neuron

d. All of the above

Ans. (d) All of the above

13. Which of the following comparisons are true?

a. Nerve impulses produce their effects quickly, whereas hormonal responses generally are slower.

b. Nervous system effects are brief, whereas endocrine system effects are longer lasting

c. The nervous system can stimulate or inhibit the release of hormones by the endocrine system

d. All of the above

Ans. (d) All of the above

14. Long term reflex action such as cycling and swimming are controlled by

a. Cerebellum   b. Spinal cord

c. Cerebrum   d. Hypothalamus

Ans. (a) Cerebellum

15. Which of the following sequence describes the passage of an action potential in the neuron?

a. Dendrite, cell body, axon, synaptic cleft

b. Dendrite, synaptic cleft, cell body, axon

c. Axon, cell body, dendrite, synaptic cleft

d. None of these

Ans. (a) Dendrite, cell body, axon, synaptic cleft

16. Which of the following statements are true?

a. The frequency of impulses and the number of activated sensory neurons encodes differences in stimuli intensity

b. Larger-diameter axons conduct nerve impulses faster than smaller-diameter ones

c. The diameter of an axon and the presence or absence of a myelin sheath are the most important factors that determine the speed of nerve impulse propagation

d. All of the above

Ans. (d) All of the above

17. Which of the following statements are true?

a. Two of more neurotransmitters nay be present in many neurons

b. An excitatory neurotransmitter can never be inhibitory regardless of the neuron that produces it

c. The catecholamine neurotransmitter acetylcholine is synthesized from the amino acid tyrosine

d. Both a and b

Ans. (d) Both a and b

18. The most sensitive vertebrate chemoreceptor known are the

a. Organs of corti of humans

b. Olfactory receptors of mammals

c. Taste receptors of fishes

d. Rod and cone cells of mammals

Ans. (c) Taste receptors of fishes

19. Which of the following statement is correct?

a. The function of the crystalline lens is t bend light rays and focus them on the optic nerve

b. Near sightedness is a condition resulting from loss of lens elasticity

c. The space anterior to the lens is filled with the vitreous humor

d. None of these

Ans. (b) Near sightedness is a condition resulting from loss of lens elasticity

20. The fovea of the eye

a. Is the region of highest visual acuity

b. Contain only rods

c. Contain only cones

d. Contain only red and green cones

Ans. (a) Is the region of highest visual acuity

21. The fluid that fills the posterior chamber of the eye is the

a. Choroid humor

b. Vitreous humor

c. Aqueous humor

d. None of these

Ans. (b) Vitreous humor

22. Some diseases damage the hair cells in the ear. When the damage to the outer hair cells is greater than the damage to the inner hair cells

a. The K^+ concentration in perilymph is decreased

b. The K^+ concentrations in endolymph is decreased

c. The affected hair cells fail the shorten when exposed to sound

d. The perception of vertical acceleration is disrupted

Ans. (c) The affected hair cells fail the shorten when exposed to sound

23. The basilar membrane of the cochlea

a. Vibrates in a pattern determined by the form of the travelling wave in the fluids in the cochlea

b. Vibrates when the body is subjected to linear acceleration

c. Covers the oval window and the round window

d. All of these

Ans. (a) Vibrates in a pattern determined by the form of the travelling wave in the fluids in the cochlea

24. Most of the CO_2 transported in the blood

a. Dissolved in plasma

b. In carbamino compounds formed from plasma protein

c. Bound to Cl^-

d. In the form of HCO_3^-

Ans. (d) In the form of HCO_3^-

25. Which of the following has the greatest effect on the ability of blood to transport oxygen?

a. pH of plasma

b. Temperature of the blood

c. Amount of haemoglobin in the blood

d. None of these

Ans. (c) Amount of haemoglobin in the blood

26. Variations in which of the following components of blood or cerebrospinal fluid do not affect respiration

a. Arterial H+ concentration

b. Arterial HCO3- concentration

c. Arterial Na+ concentration

d. cerebrospinal fluid CO_2 concentration

Ans. (c) Arterial Na+ concentration

27. The most important factor in determining the percent oxygen saturation of haemoglobin is

a. Acidity

b. The temperature

c. The partial pressure of carbon dioxide

d. The partial pressure of oxygen

Ans. (d) The partial pressure of oxygen

28. The most abundant protein in human blood is

a. Albumin   b. Globulin

c. Haemoglobin   d. Transferring

Ans. (c) Haemoglobin

29. Leukopenia is a term used to described

a. High RBC count   b. High WBC count

c. Low WBC count   d. Low RBC count

Ans. (c) Low WBC count

30. Which of the following contains oxygenated blood in an adult human?

a. Right atrium   b. Pulmonary vein

c. Pulmonary artery   d. All of these

Ans. (b) Pulmonary vein

31. Which of the following is the most muscular chamber in a bird's heart of a mammal's heart?

a. The left atrium   b. The left ventricle

c. The right atrium   d. The right ventricle

Ans. (b) The left ventricle

32. Which of the following statement about circulatory systems is true?

a. Hormones are transported in the blood

b. All invertebrates have an open circulatory system

c. Capillaries have thicker walls than veins

d. The systemic circulation carries blood to and from the lungs

Ans. (a) Hormones are transported in the blood

33. Which one of the following series represents the correct path of blood circulation?

a. Right atrium, left ventricle, lungs left atrium, left ventricle, body

b. Left atrium, left ventricle, right atrium, right ventricle, lungs, body

c. Right atrium, right ventricle, lungs, left atrium, left ventricle, body

d. None of these

Ans. (c) Right atrium, right ventricle, lungs, left atrium, left ventricle, body

34. Which of the following statement about the heart is false?

a. Contraction is initiated by a nerve impulse

b. The heart contains a number of cells with an unstable membrane potential

c. The heart contains a number of cells with a stable membrane potential

d. None of these

Ans. (a) Contraction is initiated by a nerve impulse

35. The *lub* of the *lub-dub* sound the heart makes is caused by the

a. Closing of the mitral and tricuspid valves

b. Closing of the pulmonary and aortic valves

c. Sound of blood rushing in to the atria

d. Sound of blood rushing in to the ventricle

Ans. (a) Closing of the mitral and tricuspid valves

36. If communication between the SA node and the AV node became blocked, which will most likely occur?

a. The rate of atrial contraction will decrease

b. The rate of ventricular contraction will decrease

c. Stroke volume will increase to 5L/beat

d. Afterload will increase

Ans. (b) The rate of ventricular contraction will decrease

37. When compared to arteries, veins generally

a. Have more muscle in the tunica media

b. Are thinner walled

c. Carry faster moving blood

d. Have thicker endothelium

Ans. (b) Are thinner walled

38. Which of the following is the primary factor regulation normal coronary blood flow?

a. Systolic wall tension

b. Mycocardial oxygen consumption

c. Aortic diastolic pressure

d. Coronary perfusion pressure

Ans. (c) Aortic diastolic pressure

39. Administration of a local anaesthetic with epinephrine will most likely produce which of the following cardiovascular effect?

a. Increased diastolic blood pressure

b. Increased heart beat

c. Decreased heart rate

d. Decreased systolic blood pressure

Ans. (b) Increased heart beat

40. The lymphatic system

a. Is an open circulatory system

b. Contains one-way valves

c. Returns fluids to the bloodstream

d. All of the above

Ans. (d) All of the above

41. Fluid is driven through the lymphatic system by

a. Squeezing of the lymphatic vessels by the body's muscles

b. Contractions of the lymph nodes

c. Pressure created by the pumping of the heart

d. Contraction of the walls of the lymphatic vessels

Ans. (a) Squeezing of the lymphatic vessels by the body's muscles

42. Which of the following statements are correct?

a. Passive exhalation results from elastic recoil of the chest wall and lungs
b. Air flow during breathing is due to a pressure gradient between the lungs and the atmospheric air
c. During normal breathing the pressure between the two pleural layers is always sub-atmospheric
d. All of the above

Ans. (d) All of the above

43. Which of the following factors affect the rate of external respiration?

a. Partial pressure differences of the gases
b. Surface area for gas exchange
c. Diffusion distance
d. Solubility and molecular weight of the gases
e. All of the above

Ans. (e) All of the above

44. Which gas law that states that each gas in a mixture exerts its own pressure as if all the other gases were not present?

a. Henry's law
b. Dalton's law
c. Boyle's law
d. Haldane's law

Ans. (b) Dalton's law

45. Which of the following statements are true?

a. It is impossible for people to kill themselves by holding their breath
b. Emotional stimuli can alter respiration
c. Certain chemical stimulation alter the rate and depth of breathing
d. All of the above

Ans. (d) All of the above

46. On the summit of Mt. Everest, where the barometric pressure is about 250 mm Hg, the partial pressure of O_2 is about

a. 0.1 mm Hg
b. 0.5 mm Hg
c. 5.0 mm Hg
d. 50 mm Hg

Ans. (d) 50 mm Hg

47. The tidal volume in a normal man at rest is about

a. 0.5 L
b. 1.2 L
c. 2.5 L
d. 3.5 L

Ans. (a) 0.5 L

48. Which of the following is responsible for the movement of O_2 from the alveoli in to the blood in the pulmonary capillaries?

a. Passive diffusion
b. Secondary active transport
c. Filtration
d. Active transport

Ans. (a) Passive diffusion

49. Concerning the functional histology of the kidney

a. The superficial nephrons have short loops of henle; thus, they have a low capacity to reabsorb salt
b. In dehydration, the blood flow to deep nephrons tends to increase
c. The deep nephrons have long loops of henle; thus have a high capacity to reabsorb salt and water
d. All of these

Ans. (d) All of these

50. Which of the following is a function of the kidneys?

a. Release of hormones
b. Maintenance of plasma pH
c. Maintenance of plasma
d. All of these

Ans. (d) All of these

51. In the distal convoluted tubule of the nephrons

a. Sodium reabsorption requires energy
b. Secretion of potassium does not require energy
c. Water reabsorption requires energy
d. Ammonia is secreted

52. Reabsorption of chloride ions from the glomerular filtrate in the kidney tubule is carried out by

a. Active transport
b. Passive transport
c. Diffusion
d. Osmosis

Ans. (c) Diffusion

53. Drinking which of the following would lead to the highest rate of ADH secretion and release?

a. Two liters of distilled water
b. Two liters of sea water
c. Two liters of iso-osmotic saline
d. Two liters of human blood plasma

Ans. (b) Two liters of human blood plasma

54. An increase secretion of rennin would be expected to have what effect on sodium excretion and potassium excretion in urine?

a. Increase in Na+ excretion and increase K+ excretion
b. Increase in Na+ excretion and decrease K+ excretion

c. Decrease in Na+ excretion and increase K+ excretion

d. Decrease in Na+ excretion and decrease K+ excretion

Ans. (c) Decrease in Na+ excretion and increase K+ excretion

55. Which of the following is not a function of atrial natriuretic peptide?

a. It acts to decrease aldosterone release from the adrenal cortex

b. It acts to increase urine output

c. It acts to increase blood pressure

d. It acts to decrease ADH release

Ans. (c) It acts to increase blood pressure

56. Which of the following is incorrect?

a. Aldosterone is mad in the hypothalamus and released from the anterior pituitary

b. Aldosterone affects water reabsorption

c. Aldosterone stimulates the secretion of K+

d. None of these

Ans. (a) Aldosterone is mad in the hypothalamus and released from the anterior pituitary

57. The majority of reabsorption occurs in the

a. Renal capsule

b. Collecting duct

c. Proximal convoluted tubule

d. Ascending limb of the loop of Henle

Ans. (c) Proximal convoluted tubule

58. Concerning water reabsorption by the proximal tubule

a. Main driving forces for water reabsorption in the proximal tubule are solute uptake and oncotic pressure in peritubular capillaries

b. A significant amount of water uptake in the proximal tubule is dependent on sodium uptake by the Na+/H+ antiports present in their luminal membrane

c. Bothe a and b

d. None of these

Ans. (c) Bothe a and b

59. Concerning arterial blood pressure regulation

a. Main driving forces for water reabsorption in the proximal tubule are solute uptake and oncotic pressure in peritubular capillaries

b. Prostaglandins and dopamine and bradykinin are vasodilators

c. ADH, angiotensin II and epinephrine are vasoconstrictors

d. None of these

Ans. (d) None of these

60. The following is/are correct for the countercurrent multiplier system

a. The ascending limb of the loop of Henle transports Nacl by active transport

b. The descending limb is quite permeable to water

c. The fluid of the ascending limb becomes relatively dilute

d. All of the above are correct

Ans. (d) All of the above are correct

61. The site of production of cholecystokinin and secretin is the

a. Small intestine   b. Large intestine

c. Stomach   d. Pancreas

Ans. (a) Small intestine

62. Which of the following is not a function of the liver?

a. Storage of glucose   b. Production of bile

c. Storage of vitamin C   d. None of these

Ans. (c) Storage of vitamin C

63. The gall ballbladder

a. Produces bile

b. Is attached to the pancreas

c. Stores and concentrates bile

d. Produces cholecystokinin

Ans. (c) Stores and concentrates bile

64. Which structure thickens in certain regions of the alimentary canal in order to act as a sphincter?

a. Circular layer of the muscularis externa

b. Longitudinal layer of the muscularis mucosae

c. Circular layer of the muscularis mucosae

d. None of these

Ans. (a) Circular layer of the muscularis externa

65. The 3 pairs of extrinsic salivary glands are the

a. Parotid, submandibular, and sublingual

b. Parotid, submandibular, and buccal

c. Parotid, sublingual, and ethmodial

d. Parotid, buccal, and submaxillary

Ans. (c) Parotid, sublingual, and ethmodial

66. The gastric gland cell whose absence could lead to pernicious anemia is the

a. Parietal cell

b. Goblet cell

c. Chief cell

d. Mucous neck cell

Ans. (a) Parietal cell

67. A major function of the large intestine is to

a. Remove waste materials

b. Secrete digestive enzymes

c. Secrete water in order to regulate blood volume

d. All of the above

Ans. (a) Remove waste materials

68. Which of the following statements are correct

a. Mechanical digestion occurs in the stomach

b. Cholecystokinin, gastrin and secretin are produced by an enteroendocrine cells

c. Pancreas, small intestine and salivary glands produce digestive enzyme

d. Mucous neck cell, chief cells, parietal cells present in the stomach

e. All of the above

Ans. (e) All of the above

69. Each of the following statement about Brunner's glands is correct *except*:

a. They produce a serous secretion rich in digestive enzyme

b. They are characteristic component of the duodenal wall

c. They lie in the submucosal layer

d. All of the above

Ans. (a) They produce a serous secretion rich in digestive enzyme

70. Which of the following statement is/are correct?

a. Pepsinogen is synthesized and released by chief cells

b. Hormones mainly involved in controlling pancreatic exocrine secretions are cholecystokinin and secretin

c. Chief cells in children secrete an enzyme rennin

d. All of the above are correct

Ans. (d) All of the above are correct

71. The function of the hepatic portal circulation is to

a. Collect absorbed nutrients for metabolic processing or storage

b. Carry toxins to the venous system for disposal thru the urinary trac

c. Hormone distribution

d. Transfer bile to the liver from the pancreas

Ans. (a) Collect absorbed nutrients for metabolic processing or storage

72. Which of the following is false of the small intestine?

a. Most rapid absorption of galactose

b. First site of protein hydrolysis

c. Site of the majority of water absorption in the GI tract

d. Site of carbohydrate, protein and fat digestion

Ans. (b) First site of protein hydrolysis

73. Digestive processes in the large intestine include

a. Mass peristalsis

b. Absorption of some vitamins and electrolytes

c. Elimination of cellulose-base material

d. All of the above

Ans. (d) All of the above

74. Hormones

a. Generally utilize negative feedback mechanisms to regulate their secretion

b. Will only cause an effect on cells with receptors for the hormone

c. Can regulate the responsiveness of the target tissue by controlling the number of receptors for the hormone

d. All of the above

Ans. (d) All of the above

75. The pituitary gland's posterior lobe produces two hormones, i.e.

a. Progesterone and estradiol

b. Cortisone and corticosterone

c. Vasopressin and oxytocin

d. None of the above

Ans. (c) Vasopressin and oxytocin

76. In which of the following combinations is the name of the hormone, its chemical type and its tissue of origin correctly matched ?

a. Aldosterone → peptide → pancreas

b. ACTH → polypeptide → adrenal cortex

c. Glucagons → peptide → adrenal cortex

d. Vasopression → peptide → posterior pituitary

Ans. (d) Vasopression → peptide → posterior pituitary

77. Which of the following hormones does not act by a second messenger system

a. Glucagon

b. Epinephrine

c. Testosterone

d. Follicle stimulating hormone

Ans. (c) Testosterone

78. Which hormone binds to intracellular receptors

a. Growth hormone

b. Insulin

c. Triiodothyronine

d. Thyroid stimulating hormone

Ans. (c) Triiodothyronine

79. Which of the following hormones does not act by a second messenger system

a. Aldosterone

b. Glucagon

c. Luteinizing hormone

d. None of these

Ans. (c) Luteinizing hormone

80. Which one of the following statements with respect to testosterone is not true?

a. Testosterone receptor mutant is embryonic lethal

b. Testosterone receptor is essential for male reproduction

c. Testosterone is produce in female rats

d. Testosterone is not essential for fetal growth

Ans. (a) Testosterone receptor mutant is embryonic lethal

81. Administration of estrogen to adult male rats results in

a. Decreased testosterone production

b. Decrease luteinizing hormone and testo-sterone production

c. Increased estrogen secretion in the testis

d. None of the above

Ans. (d) None of the above

82. Radioactive iodine can be incorporated in to

a. Threonine

b. Tyrosine

c. Serine

d. Leucine

Ans. (b) Tyrosine

83. The receptor for which of the following hormones is a transcription factor?

a. Estradiol

b. Glucagon

c. Insulin

d. Adrenalin

Ans. (a) Estradiol

84. The development of adult characteristics in a molting insect is promoted by

a. Ecdysone   b. Thyroxine

c. Juvenile hormone d. Pheromone

Ans. (a) Ecdysone

85. The fight-or-flight response is developed by hormones of the

a. Adrenal medulla   b. Hypothalamus

c. Adrenal cortex   d. None of these

Ans. (a) Adrenal medulla

86. Epinephrine and nor-epinephrine functions as both hormones and

a. Neurotransmitters

b. Ions to promote action potentials

c. Fuel for cellular respiration

d. Solutes to promote osmotic flow

Ans. (a) Neurotransmitters

87. All the hormones of the adrenal cortex are synthesized from

a. Cholesterol   b. Tyrosine

c. Fats   d. Glycoproteins

Ans. (a) Cholesterol

88. Thyroxine and triidothyronine, produce by the thyroid gland, are synthesized from iodine and

a. Glycoprotein   b. Cholesterol

c. Tyrosine   d. Phenylalanine

Ans. (c) Tyrosine

89. The parathyroid glands are located adjacent to the

a. Parathyroid gland b. Thyroid gland

c. Pancreas   d. Adenoids

Ans. (b) Thyroid gland

90. A person with diabetes mellitus does not secrete enough

a. Sugar   b. Glucagons

c. Epinephrine   d. Insulin

Ans. (d) Insulin

91. The nerouns of a person with diabetes mellitus do not produce sufficient

a. Fatty acid   b. Enzymes

c. Vitamins   d. ATP

Ans. (d) ATP

92. Which of the following are true concerning androgens?

a. They stimulate the male pattern of development

b. They contribute to sex drive in males and females

c. They stimulate protein synthesis

d. All of the above

Ans. (d) All of the above

93. Which of the following hormones is a modified amino acid?

a. Epinephrine　　　　b. Progesterone

c. Estrogen　　　　　 d. Prostaglandin

Ans. (a) Epinephrine

94. Thyroxin is important in the control of

a. Diabetes mellitus

b. Calcium uptake

c. Cellular metabolic rates

d. Mitochondrial respiration

Ans. (c) Cellular metabolic rates

95. The primary target organ of aldosterone action is

a. Liver

b. Kidney

c. Heart

d. Pancreas

Ans. (b) Kidney

10

Microbiology and Pathology

1. Who is credited with discovery of bacteria?

  a. Louis pasteur   b. Leewenhoek

  c. Needham   d. Tyndall

Ans. (b) Leewenhoek

2. Founder of modern bacteriology is

  a. Leewenhoek   b. Pasteur

  c. Robert Koch   d. None

Ans. (b) Pasteur

3. Founder of bacteriological techniques is

  a. Pasteur   b. Koch

  c. Gram   d. Buchner

Ans. (b) Koch

4. Gram staining was discovered by gram in year

  a. 1762   b. 1932

  c. 1884   d. 1890

Ans. (c) 1884

5. Gram stain used is an example of

  a. Simple stain   b. Differential stain

  c. Acid fast stain   d. None

Ans. (b) Differential stain

6. Acid fast staining used for such bacteria

  a. Mycobacterium   b. Rhizobium

  c. Bacillus sp.   d. Clostridium

Ans. (a) Mycobacterium

7. Counter stain used in gram staining

  a. Ethyl alcohol   b. Iodine solution

  c. Crystal violet   d. Safranin

Ans. (d) Safranin

8. Agar-Agar was developed by

  a. Joseph lister   b. Koch

  c. Hesse   d. Pasteur

Ans. (c) Hesse

9. Facultative free living 'N' fixing bacterium

  a. Rhizobium   b. Azotobacter

  c. Klebsiella   d. None

Ans. (c) Klebsiella

10. Cubical packets of 8 cells is called in bacteria

  a. Staphylococcus   b. Diplococcus

  c. Bacillus   d. Sarcina

Ans. (d) Sarcina

11. Braun's lipoprotein is present in

  a. Gram +ve bacteria   b. Gram -ve bacteria

  c. Bacteriophage   d. Yeast

Ans. (b) Gram -ve bacteria

12. In endospore staining which one is used

  a. Malachite green   b. Basic fuschin

  c. Indian ink   d. Methylene blue

Ans. (a) Malachite green

13. Pseudomorein is present in which organism

  a. Archaebacteria   b. Eubacteria

  c. Eukaryote   d. Fungi

Ans. (a) Archaebacteria

14. Mesosomes are well developed in

  a. Gram +ve bacteria   b. Yeast

  c. *E.coli*   d. Mycoplasma

Ans. (a) Gram +ve bacteria

15. Energy parasite

  a. Spirilla   b. Mycoplasma

  c. Chlaymidia   d. Archaebacteria

Ans. (c) Chlaymidia

16. Example of pleomorphic bacteria

  a. Acetobacter   b. Azotobacter

  c. Achromobacter   d. Arthrobacter

Ans. (d) Arthrobacter

17. N–reserve materials in cyanobacteria

a. Volutin granular
b. PHB
c. Polysaccharidesd.
d. Cyanophycin granules

Ans. (d) Cyanophycin granules

18. Cyst formation is characteristic feature of

a. Acetobacter   b. Arthrobacter
c. Azotobacter   d. None

Ans. (c) Azotobacter

19. Lysozyme treated cells of gram +ve bacteria are called

a. Protoplast   b. Sphaeroplast
c. Cytoplasm   d. None

Ans. (a) Protoplast

20. Bacteria having especially high rate of respiration

a. Rhizobium   b. Azotobacter
c. E.coli   d. Acetobacter

Ans. (b) Azotobacter

21. Lysozyme treated cells of gram -ve bacteria are called

a. Protoplast   b. Sphaeroplast
c. Cytoplasm   d. Mesosomes

Ans. (b) Sphaeroplast

22. Species of mycoplasma are inhibited by

a. Penicillin   b. Tetramycin
c. Both   d. None

Ans. (b) Tetramycin

23. Xanthomonas is an example of

a. Monotrichous   b. Peritrichous
c. Lophotrichous   d. Cephalotrichous

Ans. (a) Monotrichous

24. Test organism for pasteurization is

a. Coxicella burnetti
b. Clostridium pasteurizanum
c. Bacillus subtilis
d. Bacillus steareothermophillus

Ans. (a) Coxicella burnetti

25. Ray fungi is the name given to

a. Rhizopus   b. Yeast
c. Actinomycetes   d. Mycoplasma

Ans. (c) Actinomycetes

26. Actinomycetes are

a. Gram +ve, aerobic   b. Gram +ve, anaerobic
c. Gram -ve, aerobic   d. Gram -ve, anaerobic

Ans. (a) Gram +ve, aerobic

27. Example for microaerophilic N_2 fixer

a. Rhizobium   b. Azotobacter
c. E.coli   d. Frankia

Ans. (d) Frankia

28. Citric acid is produced by

a. Aspergillus niger   b. Acetobacter
c. Acetobutylicum   d. none

Ans. (a) Aspergillus niger

29. Vitamin B_2 is produced by

a. Ashbya gossypii   b. Pseudomonas
c. Brevibacterium   d. None

Ans. (a) Ashbya gossypii

30. Bacitracin is produced by

a. Bacillus subtilis   b. Aspergillus niger
c. E. coli   d. Yeast

Ans. (a) Bacillus subtilis

31. Production of vinegar is by

a. Bacillus subtilis   b. Azotobacter
c. Glucanobacter   d. none

Ans. (c) Glucanobacter

32. First antifungal antibiotic

a. Cycloheximide   b. Aureofungin
c. Neomycin   d. Nystatin

Ans. (d) Nystatin

33. Neomycin is produced by

a. S. Nouesii   b. S. fradiae
c. S. Erthyreus   d. S. Venezuelea

Ans. (b) S. fradiae

34. Inhibitory action of penicillin is

a. Cell wall synthesis b. Protein synthesis
c. Both   d. None

Ans. (a) Cell wall synthesis

35. Organism involved in swiss cheese ripening

a. Penicillium sp.   b. Propionibacterium
c. Streptococcus sp.   d. None

Ans. (a) Penicillium sp.

36. Phosphorus solubilising microorganism

a. VAM b. Mucor
c. Rhizopus d. *E.coli*

Ans. (a) VAM

37. The term mycorrhiza is coined by

a. Frank b. Hartig
c. De bary d. Winogradasky

Ans. (a) Frank

38. Name the scientists involved in commercial production of Penicillin

a. Alexander Flemming b. Florey and Chain
c. Tulsane Brothers d. Louis Pasteur

Ans. (b) Florey and Chain

39. Development of plants due to increase in number of cells is called

a. Hypertrophy b. Hypotrophy
c. Hyperplasia d. Hypoplasia

Ans. (c) Hyperplasia

40. Name the bacterium producing endospore is

a. Bacillus b. Agrobacterium
c. Xanthomonas d. *E.coli*

Ans. (a) Bacillus

41. The most resistant form of microbial life in the bacteria is

a. Cyst b. Endospore
c. Vegetative stage d. None

Ans. (b) Endospore

42. UV light is most germicidal at the wavelength of

a. 245 nm b. 255 nm
c. 265 nm d. None

Ans. (c) 265 nm

43. UV light are microcidal due to the formation of

a. Pyrine dimers
b. Pyrimidene dimmers
c. DNA damage
d. RNA damage

Ans. (b) Pyrimidene dimmers

44. Low pH of media inhibits the growth of

a. Bacteria b. Molds
c. Both d. None

Ans. (a) Bacteria

45. Canning is a food preservation technique first derived by

a. Appert b. Pasteur
c. Buchner d. Menton

Ans. (a) Appert

46. Which of the following is/are bioinsecticides

a. Bacillus thuringiensis b. Bacillus popilliae
c. Both d. None

Ans. (c) Both

47. Fumaric acid produced by

a. Aspergillus niger b. Aspergillus terrus
c. Aspergillus fumigates d. Rhizopus nigricans

Ans. (d) Rhizopus nigricans

48. Ionizing radiation to sterilize materials is called

a. Ionization b. Pasteurization
c. Cold sterilization d. Tyndallisation

Ans. (c) Cold sterilization

49. Rhizosphere was coined by

a. Hiltner b. Beijernick
c. Winogradasky d. None

Ans. (a) Hiltner

50. ATP needed for N_2 fixation

a. 12 b. 16
c. 28 d. 32

Ans. (b) 16

51. Factor which does not affect legume root nodulation

a. Temperature b. Light
c. Combined N_2 d. H^+ ion conc.

Ans. (b) Light

52. Microaerophillic N_2 fixing bacteria

a. Azotobacter b. Azospirillum
c. Clostridium d. Enterobacter

Ans. (b) Azospirillum

53. Bacteria which can ferment sugar faster than yeast

a. Clostridium b. Bacillus
c. Thiobacillus d. Zygomonas

Ans. (d) Zygomonas

54. Father of soil microbiology is

a. Winogradasky b. Beijernick
c. Hiltner d. Spermi

Ans. (a) Winogradasky

55. Glycolysis inhibition in the presence of oxygen is called

a. Warburg effect
b. Hypoglycolytic effect
c. Pasteur effect
d. None

Ans. (c) Pasteur effect

56. Wood sugar is

a. Glucose
b. Mannose
c. Xylose
d. Arabinose

Ans. (c) Xylose

57. A mat of organism formed at the surface of a liquid culture is called

a. Biofilm
b. Pellicle
c. Scum
d. Foam

Ans. (c) Scum

58. Alginates are isolated from

a. Rhodophyta
b. Bryophyta
c. Chlorophyta
d. Phaeophyta

Ans. (d) Phaeophyta

59. The first antiseptic agent used was

a. Mercuric chloride
b. Carbolic acid
c. Alcohol
d. Hyposolution

Ans. (b) Carbolic acid

60. All bacteria having a conjugative plasmid will have

a. Drug resistance
b. Sex pili
c. Flagella
d. All of the above

Ans. (b) Sex pili

61. A fluorescent dye used in fluorescent microscopy is

a. Acridine orange
b. Phosphotungstic acid
c. Ethium bromide
d. Luciferin

Ans. (c) Ethium bromide

62. A mutation with multiple effect on the phenotype is called

a. Multiple mutation
b. Frame shift mutation
c. Pleotropic mutation
d. None

Ans. (d) None

63. Which among the following is used for insertion of foreign DNA into cells?

a. Agrobacterium
b. Vaccinia virus
c. Hela cells
d. All of these

Ans. (a) Agrobacterium

64. Starting material for wine making is

a. Molasses
b. Barley malt
c. Grape juice
d. Beet root mash

Ans. (c) Grape juice

65. Virus quantification in a given sample is done by

a. End point efflux
b. End point dilution
c. End point titration
d. All of these

Ans. (b) End point dilution

66. Which among the following is a flagellated cyanobacteria?

a. Chroococcum
b. Nostoc
c. Both a and b
d. None

Ans. (d) None

67. Which among the following is a restriction modification in DNA?

a. Capping
b. Tailing
c. Methylation
d. Phosphorylation

Ans. (c) Methylation

68. First antifungal antibiotic is

a. Nystatin
b. Cycloheximide
c. Aureofungin
d. None

Ans. (a) Nystatin

69. A medium in which different types of micro-organisms exhibit different growth forms so that they could be distinguished is called

a. Selective medium
b. Synthetic medium
c. Differential medium
d. Preferential medium

Ans. (c) Differential medium

70. Cell–cell interaction and differentiation is mostly studied on

a. Arabidopsis thaliana
b. Cenorabditis elegens
c. *E.coli*
d. Dictyostlium discodeum

Ans. (d) Dictyostlium discodeum

71. Milky disease is caused by

a. Bacillus thuringiensis
b. Lactobacillus lactis
c. Bacillus papillae
d. None

Ans. (c) Bacillus papillae

72. A bacterial cell which lacks a chromosome but contains all the components for transcription and translation

    a. Maxi cell   b. Empty cell

    c. Mini cell   d. Ghost cell

Ans. (c) Mini cell

73. Fractional sterilization is

    a. Appertization   b. Pasteurization

    c. Tyndalization   d. Cold sterilization

Ans. (c) Tyndalization

74. In gram staining the alcohol acts on

    a. Teichoic acid   b. Peptidoglycan

    c. Periplasm   d. Membrane lipids

Ans. (d) Membrane lipids

75. Partial diploid in bacteria is called

    a. Merozygote   b. Heterokaryon

    c. False zygote   d. None

Ans. (a) Merozygote

76. Specialized N fixing cells in filamentous cyanobacteria are

    a. Akinites   b. Endospores

    c. Cysts   d. Heterocysts

Ans. (d) Heterocysts

77. Cell to cell communication in legume rhizobium symbiosis is carried out by

    a. Lectins

    b. Flavanoids

    c. Isoflavons

    d. Haemoglobin

Ans. (a) Lectins

78. Bacterial endospores are characterized by the presence of

    a. Diaminopimelic acid

    b. Polybetahydroxy butyrate

    c. Dipicolinic caid

    d. All

Ans. (c) All

79. In leghaemoglobin the heme portion is specified by

    a. Plantgenes

    b. Bacterial genes

    c. Both

    d. None

Ans. (b) Bacterial genes

80. Giemsa stain are used as particularly applicable for staining

    a. Rickettsias   b. Spores

    c. Protozoa   d. Both a and c

Ans. (d) Both a and c

81. Name the organism which are predatory on bacteria

    a. Virus   b. Viroid

    c. Bdellovibrios   d. Prion

Ans. (c) Bdellovibrios

82. In cocoa fermentation the microbial inoclumn used is of

    a. Aspergillus niger   b. Candida krusei

    c. Rhizopus oryzae   d. None

Ans. (b) Candida krusei

83. Riboflavin can be obtained by microbial fermentation using fungi

    a. Ashbya gossypii   b. Rhizopus oryzae

    c. Sacchromycetes   d. None

Ans. (a) Ashbya gossypii

84. Tetracycline is effective against

    a. Gram +ve bacteria   b. Gram -ve bacteria

    c. Fungi   d. Broad spectrum

Ans. (d) Broad spectrum

85. Bacitracin is effective against

    a. Gram +ve bacteria   b. Gram -ve bacteria

    c. Fungi   d. Broad spectrum

Ans. (a) Gram +ve bacteria

86. Pili are filamentous hair like structures on the surface of only

    a. Gram +ve bacteria   b. Gram -ve bacteria

    c. Both   d. None

Ans. (b) Gram -ve bacteria

87. The phenomenon of inhibiting the growth of bacteria without killing them

    a. Bactericidal   b. Bacteriostatic

    c. Both   d. None

Ans. (b) Bacteriostatic

88. A cell wall component which anchors the outer membrane of enteric gram negative bacteria to the peptidoglycan layer

    a. Teichoic acid   b. Lignic acid

    c. Braun lipoprotein   d. None

Ans. (c) Braun lipoprotein

89. Protein coat of a virus

a. Capsule   b. Capsid

c. Envelope   d. Coat

Ans. (b) Capsid

90. An antiviral substance produced by animal tissue

a. Virion   b. Interferon

c. Antibody   d. Antigen

Ans. (b) Interferon

91. Nitrogenous enzyme first isolated from

a. Clostridium pasteurianum

b. Bacillus sp.

c. Azotobacter

d. Penicillium

Ans. (a) Clostridium pasteurianum

92. Fungi used for bioassay of biotin

a. Neurospora   b. Yeast

c. Aspergillus   d. Penicillium

Ans. (a) Neurospora

93. Which is a plant pathogen bacteria

a. Shigella   b. *E. coli*

c. Salmonella   d. Erwinia

Ans. (d) Erwinia

94. Anaerobic free living N fixing bacterium

a. Azotobacter   b. Acetobacter

c. Kelbsiella   d. Clostridium

Ans. (d) Clostridium

95. Virus – "Contangium vivum fluidum" was given by

a. A. Mayer   b. Beijernick

c. Iwanoski   d. None

Ans. (b) Beijernick

96. Itaconic acid produced by

a. Aspergillus terrus

b. Aspergillus itaconicus

c. Both

d. None

Ans. (c) Both

97. Phagocytosis is discovered by

a. Robert Koch   b. Elie Metchnikoff

c. Joseph Lister   d. Fanny Hesse

Ans. (b) Elie Metchnikoff

98. Lipopolysaccharide is found in cell wall of

a. Gram +ve bacteria

b. Gram –ve bacteria

c. Both

d. Fungi

Ans. (b) Gram –ve bacteria

99. In autoclave which form of heat is used?

a. Dry heat   b. Moist heat

c. Vaccum heat   d. None

Ans. (a) Dry heat

100. Who developed cell free fermentation of modern science?

a. Koch   b. Pasteur

c. Buchner   d. None

Ans. (c) Buchner

101. Nitrogenase enzyme has how many components?

a. 1   b. 2

c. 3   d. 4

Ans. (c) 3

102. Antiseptic surgery is given by

a. Joseph lister   b. Koch

c. Schrcedes   d. Jenner

Ans. (a) Joseph lister

103. Number of chromosome in bacteria

a. 0   b. 2

c. 1   d. Many

Ans. (c) 1

104. Murein is present in

a. Cyanobacteria

b. Halobacterium

c. Methanobacterium

d. None

Ans. (a) Cyanobacteria

105. Sterols are present in

a. Eubacteria   b. Fungi

c. Mycoplasma   d. None

Ans. (c) Mycoplasma

106. Father of bacteriology

a. Eichels   b. Woose

c. Haeckenl   d. Chester

Ans. (a) Eichels

107. Microorganism which are associated with non legumes
a. Anabaena   b. Klebsiella
c. Both   d. None

Ans. (c) Both

108. In archaebacteria which one is present in cell wall?
a. Murein   b. Pseudomurein
c. Both   d. None

Ans. (b) Pseudomurein

109. Mesosomes are well developed in
a. E. coli
b. Proteus vulgaris
c. Bacillus
d. None

Ans. (c) Bacillus

110. Smallest self replicating prokaryotes capable of generating their own energy
a. Mycoplasma   b. Virus
c. Chlamydia   d. Rickettias

Ans. (a) Mycoplasma

111. Species of mycoplasma are inhibited by
a. Penicillin   b. Tetracycline
c. Both   d. None

Ans. (b) Tetracycline

112. Principal sites for CO_2 fixation in autotrophic prokaryotes
a. Chromosomes
b. Carboxysomes
c. Both
d. None

Ans. (b) Carboxysomes

113. Which one is not correct about mesosomes?
a. Prominemty in gram + ve bacteria
b. Prominemty in gram -ve bacteria
c. Helps in cell division
d. Helps in DNA replication

Ans. (b) Prominemty in gram -ve bacteria

114. In gram + ve bacteria flagella
a. Only M ring is present
b. Only S ring is present
c. Only S and M rings are present
d. All rings L, P, S and M are present

Ans. (c) Only S and M rings are present

115. Bacteria are commonly seen in soils such as
a. Acidic   b. Neutral
c. Alkaline   d. Saline

Ans. (b) Neutral

116. In archaebacteria, first aminoacid to initiate a new polypeptide chain
a. Methionine   b. Cysteine
c. Lysine   d. None

Ans. (a) Methionine

117. Amylases produced by
a. Aspergillus sp.   b. Bacillus sp.
c. Both   d. None

Ans. (c) Both

118. Lipase produced by
a. Bacillus subtilis   b. Rhizopus sp.
c. Aspergillus sp.   d. None

Ans. (b) Rhizopus sp.

119. Red pigment produced by
a. Serratia   b. Micrococcus
c. Both   d. None

Ans. (a) Serratia

120. Bacillus is a
a. Psychrophillic   b. Thermophillic
c. Osmophillic   d. Gas former

Ans. (b) Thermophillic

121. Commercial (now a days) production of penicillin is
a. Penicillium notatum
b. Penicillium chrysogenium
c. Aspergillus sp.
d. None

Ans. (b) Penicillium chrysogenium

122. Antibiotic streptomycin was isolated by
a. Buiknokles
b. Flemming
c. Walksman
d. Duggar

Ans. (c) Walksman

123. An aminoglycoside antibiotic
a. Penicillin   b. Streptomycin
c. Tetracycline d. None

Ans. (b) Streptomycin

124. Mesophiles have temperature range of

a. 25–45°C   b. 15–30°C

c. 20–45°C   d. 15–45°C

Ans. (d) 15–45°C

125. Root surface that can be colonized by the microbes

a. Rhizosphere   b. Rhizoplane

c. Both   d. None

Ans. (b) Rhizoplane

126. Numbers of layers surrounding the heterocyst

a. 1   b. 2

c. 3   d. 4

Ans. (c) 3

127. Heterocyst lack

a. PS I   b. PS II

c. Both   d. None

Ans. (a) PS I

128. Fungi used for bioassay of pantothenic acid

a. Yeast   b. Neurospora

c. Mucor   d. Aspergillus

Ans. (a) Yeast

129. Fermenting organism involved in yoghurt

a. Streptococcus   b. Aspergillus

c. Podiococcus   d. None

Ans. (a) Streptococcus

130. Microbe used for sarurkraut preparation

a. A. Niger   b. Streptococcus sp.

c. Leuconostoc sp.   d. None

Ans. (c) Leuconostoc sp.

131. Ropiness of unpacked bread is due to growth of

a. Bacillus subtilis   b. A. Niger

c. Streptococcus sp.   d. Clostridium sp.

Ans. (a) Bacillus subtilis

132. Example of chemolithotroph

a. *E.coli*   b. Bacillus

c. Azotobacter   d. Nitrosomonas

Ans. (d) Nitrosomonas

133. Iron bacteria which oxidises ferrous into ferric compound

a. Leptothrix   b. Beggiotoa

c. Both   d. None

Ans. (a) Leptothrix

134. Nitrate reductase enzyme present in

a. Cytoplasm   b. Chloroplast

c. Mitochondria   d. Nucleus

Ans. (a) Cytoplasm

135. Test organism for phenol coefficient

a. Salmonella typhii

b. Staphylococcus aureus

c. Both

d. None

Ans. (c) Both

136. Microbe involved in fibre retting

a. Micrococcus sp.

b. Bacillus subtilis

c. Clostridium butrycium

d. Lactobacillus sp.

Ans. (c) Clostridium butrycium

137. Microbe involved in tobacco curing

a. Micrococcus sp.   b. Bacillus subtilis

c. A. Niger   d. Lactobacillus sp.

Ans. (a) Micrococcus sp.

138. Urea degrading bacteria

a. Bacillus pasturi

b. Clostridium pasteurianum

c. A. Niger

d. Micrococcus sp.

Ans. (a) Bacillus pasturi

139. 'P' solubilizing bacteria

a. Bacillus megatherium

b. Clostridium pasteurianum

c. A. Niger

d. Micrococcus sp.

Ans. (a) Bacillus megatherium

140. Example of eukaryotic inhibitor antibiotic

a. Cycloheximide   b. Penicillium

c. Tetracycline   d. Streptomycin

Ans. (a) Cycloheximide

141. Lactose sugar of milk is converted into lactic acid by

a. Streptococcus lactis

b. Lactobacillus sp.

c. Clostridium sp.

d. None

Ans. (b) Lactobacillus sp.

142. Which of the following is used to detect the presence of HIV?

a. ELISA test
b. Benedict's test
c. Widal test
d. Biuret's test

Ans. (a) ELISA test

143. Which of the following does not produce any enzyme?

a. Amoeba
b. Virus
c. Bacteria
d. Fungi

Ans. (b) Virus

144. A virus that may not destroy the host

a. Virulent phage
b. Temperate phage
c. Cyano phage
d. Lytic cycle

Ans. (b) Temperate phage

145. Prions are

a. Organism containing only nucleic acid
b. Proteins which are capable of replications in certain mammalian cells
c. Small cells which are infectious
d. Fungal toxins

Ans. (b) Proteins which are capable of replications in certain mammalian cells

146. A virions is a

a. Infectious nucleic acid
b. Infectious virus particle
c. A virus parasite on bacteria
d. None

Ans. (b) Infectious virus particle

147. Which bacterium solublizes tricalcium phosphate in soluble rock phosphates in soils

a. Bacillus polymyxa
b. Pseudomonas striata
c. Spirillum lipoferum
d. Both a and b

Ans. (b) Pseudomonas striata

148. Number of flagella in cyanobacteria are

a. 0
b. 1
c. 2
d. 3

Ans. (a) 0

149. Type of relationship between Acetobacter diazotrophicus and sugarcane is

a. Symbiotic
b. Associative
c. Endophytic
d. Free living

Ans. (c) Endophytic

150. Example of VAM fungi

a. Pisoletecis
b. Sclerotenia
c. Glomus
d. Trichoderma

Ans. (c) Glomus

151. Chemolithotrophs are those bacteria which can utilize

a. Inorganic material as the energy source
b. Light as the energy source
c. Organic compound as the electron source
d. Crude oil as carbon source

Ans. (a) Inorganic material as the energy source

152. The spirochete responsible for syphilis is

a. Borellia
b. Spirocheta
c. Leptospira
d. Treponema

Ans. (d) Treponema

153. A lysogen of *E. coli* becomes resistant to further infection by bacteriophage lambda because

a. *E. coli* no longer contains receptors on its cell surface
b. One copy of phage is already present inside the cell
c. Presence of repressor in cell
d. *E. coli* is dead

Ans. (b) One copy of phage is already present inside the cell

154. All the members of genus Bacillus are known as

a. Their ability to break down sulphur containing compounds
b. Their ability to form spores
c. Their ability to live in the absence of oxygen
d. The capsules they possess

Ans. (b) Their ability to form spores

155. Autoclaves are routinely used in labs for sterilization. It acts by

a. Disrupting crll membranes
b. Denaturing proteins
c. Changing physically membrane lipids
d. All

Ans. (d) All

156. Mycoplasmas are different from other prokaryotes by

a. Presence of chitin in cell walls
b. Presence of murein in cell walls
c. Presence of protein in cell walls
d. Absence of cell wall itself

Ans. (d) Absence of cell wall itself

157. During conjugation

a. Cell to cell contact required
b. Naked DNA transferred
c. Bacteriophage mediates DNA transfer
d. Only plasmid is transferred from donar to recipient

Ans. (a) Cell to cell contact required

158. Archaeal cells usually do not contain peptidoglycan, rather contain pseudopeptidoglycan which is mainly composed of

a. N-acetylmuramic acid and L- aminoacid
b. N-acetyltalosaminuronic acid and D- aminoacid
c. N-acetylmuramic acid D- aminoacid
d. N-acetyltalosaminuronic acid L- aminoacid

Ans. (d) N-acetyltalosaminuronic acid L- aminoacid

159. Chalamydiae are distinguished by all the following characteristics *except*:

a. They are tiny bacteria
b. Their developmental cycle includes an elementary body and a reticulate body
c. They cause rocky mountain spotted fever and typhus
d. They multiply only in living cells

Ans. (c) They cause rocky mountain spotted fever and typhus

160. Pasteurization of milk is done by

a. Boiling the milk for 20 minutes
b. Heating the milk at 72°C for 30 minutes
c. Heating the milk at 72°C for 20 minutes
d. Heating the milk at 62°C for 30 minutes

Ans. (d) Heating the milk at 62°C for 30 minutes

161. The group of organism which uses light as energy source and CO_2 as the principal carbon source

a. Photoheterotrophs
b. Chemoautotrophs
c. Chemoheterotrophs
d. Photoautotrophs

Ans. (d) Photoautotrophs

162. Which one of the following sequences has helped in identifying eukaryotes. Eubacteria and archaebacterial cell types?

a. Signature sequence
b. Signal sequence
c. Shine-dalgarno sequence
d. Aminoacid sequence

Ans. (a) Signature sequence

163. Media containing spores and thermolabile constituents are sterilized by

a. Pasteurization
b. UV irradiation
c. Dry heat
d. Tyndallisation

Ans. (b) UV irradiation

164. A highly aerobic and metabolically versatile organism used in oil spill clearing is

a. Mycobacterium smegmatis
b. Azotobacter vinelandii
c. Pseudomonas cepacia
d. Leuconostoc mesenteroides

Ans. (c) Pseudomonas cepacia

165. Penicillin and lysozyme prevent synthesis and cause lysis, respectively, of cell walls of

a. Micrococcus lysodeikticus
b. *E. coli*
c. S. Cerevisiae
d. Methanobacterium barkeri

Ans. (a) Micrococcus lysodeikticus

166. In an $F^+ \times F^-$ cross

a. F^+ cell becomes an hfr cell
b. F^- cell becomes an hfr cell
c. F^+ cell becomes an F^- cell
d. F^- cell becomes an F^+ cell

Ans. (d) F^- cell becomes an F^+ cell

167. A bacterial cell that is mostly haploid, but is diploid for some regions of the genome is called

a. Heterodiploid
b. Pseudodiploid
c. Half diploid
d. Mero diploid

Ans. (d) Mero diploid

168. Interferon

a. Is species specific
b. Reacts directly with virus particles to inactivate them
c. Reacts with cells, and the affected cells then become resistant to a no. of different values
d. Is constitutively produced at high levels in cells but require an inducer for activity

Ans. (c) Reacts with cells, and the affected cells then become resistant to a no. of different values

169. Bacteria which directly convert atmospheric nitrogen into NH_4^+ are called

a. Denitrifying bacteria
b. Nitrifying bacteria
c. Nitrogen fixing bacteria
d. b and c

Ans. (c) Nitrogen fixing bacteria

170. Pili represent

    a. Extra chromosomal genetic elements

    b. Protoplasmic outgrowths of donor cells

    c. Small flagella

    d. Special bacterial cells

Ans. (b) Protoplasmic outgrowths of donor cells

171. Streaming of protoplasm is absent in

    a. Parenchyma and collenchymas cells

    b. Bacterial cells and vessels

    c. Cells of higher plants

    d. Cells of hydrilla

Ans. (b) Bacterial cells and vessels

172. Which of the following is essential for living cells?

    a. Flagella

    b. Capsule

    c. Cell wall

    d. Cytoplasmic membrane

Ans. (d) Cytoplasmic membrane

173. Bacterial flagella impart motility to the cell by

    a. Undulating membrane

    b. Rotatory membrane

    c. Gliding

    d. Both a and b

Ans. (b) Rotatory membrane

174. Bacteria broth cultures eventually stop growing and enter stationary phase because they

    a. Deplete essential nutrients

    b. Accumulate toxic products

    c. Become too crowded

    d. Both a and b

Ans. (d) Both a and b

175. Genome of organism includes genes from

    a. Chromosome

    b. Mitochondria

    c. Plasmids

    d. All

Ans. (d) All

176. A virion is a

    a. Naked, infectious piece of DNA

    b. Complete, infectious virus particle

    c. Nucleic acid without a capsid

    d. Naked, infectious piece of RNA

Ans. (b) Complete, infectious virus particle

177. Animal viruses usually penetrate a host cell by

    a. Injection   b. Exocytosis

    c. Endocytosis   d. A vector

Ans. (c) Endocytosis

178. An envelope is acquired during which of the following steps?

    a. Penetration   b. Release

    c. Lysis   d. Assembly

Ans. (b) Release

179. A virus with RNA–dependent RNA polymerase

    a. Synthesizes DNA from RNA template

    b. Synthesizes dsRNA from RNA template

    c. Synthesizes dsRNA from DNA template

    d. Transcribes mRNA from DNA

Ans. (b) Synthesizes dsRNA from RNA template

180. Ability of a virus to infect an organism is regulated by

    a. Host species

    b. Type of cells

    c. Availability of an attachment site

    d. All

Ans. (d) All

181. Which of the following statement is incorrect?

    a. Bacteria divide by binary fission

    b. No. of bacteria increases exponentially

    c. Bacterial growth is defined in terms of population size

    d. None

Ans. (d) None

182. HIV, a retrovirus contains

    a. Two copies of negative sense ssRNA

    b. One ssRNA

    c. Two copies of dsRNA

    d. Two copies of positive sense ssRNA

Ans. (d) Two copies of positive sense ssRNA

183. Bacteria that must have organic molecules both for energy and as a source of carbon are called

    a. Photoautotrophs   b. Photoheterotrophs

    c. Chemoheterotrophs   d. Chemoautotrophs

Ans. (c) Chemoheterotrophs

184. Bacteria that get their energy by fermentation and for whom oxygen is lethal are called

    a. Obligate anaerobes   b. Obligate aerobes

    c. Facultative aerobes   d. Facultative anaerobes

Ans. (a) Obligate anaerobes

185. Bacteria (Treponema pallidium) that cause the venereal disease syphilis are

a. Pseudomonads   b. Purple nonsulfur

c. Rickettsias   d. Spirochetes

Ans. (d) Spirochetes

186. Heterocyst of cyanobacteria

a. Specialized for oxygenic photosynthesis

b. Forms spores

c. Specialized for gamete formation

d. Specialized for N_2 fixation

Ans. (d) Specialized for N_2 fixation

187. What is true about *E. coli*?

a. It is a parasite in the liver of man

b. It shows syngamy and meiosis

c. It exhibits alternation of generation

d. It lives symbiotically in the colon of humans

Ans. (d) It lives symbiotically in the colon of humans

188. Periplasm is

a. Found in both gram –ve and gram + ve bacteria

b. Found to contain specific bacterial lipids

c. Space between two plasma membrane

d. Artifact from microscopic aberrations

Ans. (a) Found in both gram –ve and gram + ve bacteria

189. Which is true for bacteria?

a. Bacteria lack DNA

b. Mitochondria and nuclear membrane is present

c. Nuceoid is the region which contains DNA

d. RNA acts as genetic material

Ans. (c) Nuceoid is the region which contains DNA

190. Plasmids do which of the following?

a. Direct synthesis of conjugation pili

b. Provide resistance to certain antibiotics

c. Induce the formation of tumors in plants

d. All

Ans. (d) All

191. Retrovirus RNA encodes for all of the following genes, *except:*

a. gag   b. pol

c. env   d. ela

Ans. (d) ela

192. Which of the following statement is false?

a. Most bacteria in nature are lysogens

b. Lysogenic phage contains ds DNA

c. Biosynthesis of DNA containing animal virus occur in nucleus

d. TMV is minus ssRNA virus

Ans. (d) TMV is minus ssRNA virus

193. Retroviruses have RNA genome, however they replicaye through ds DNA formation. This process involves

a. Polymerase coded by virus itself

b. Polymerase coded by host

c. Host DNA polymerase

d. Unknown mechanism

Ans. (a) Polymerase coded by virus itself

194. Bacteriophage MS2

a. Contains ds DNA as genetic material

b. Contains ss RNA and infect only F⁺ *E. coli*

c. Contains minus (–) stranded RNA

d. Does not require pili for infection to E. coli

Ans. (b) Contains ss RNA and infect only F⁺ E. Coli

195. RNA as genetic material found in which of the following organism?

a. Plasmodium

b. Staphylococcus aureus

c. Schizosaccharomyces cerevisiae

d. Polio virus

Ans. (d) Polio virus

196. Which one of the following viruses replicate in the cytoplasm?

a. SV40   b. Adenovirus

c. Vaccinia virus   d. Herpex simplex virus

Ans. (c) Vaccinia virus

197. Oncoprotein Ras is a

a. Kinase   b. ATPase

c. GTPase   d. Phosphotase

Ans. (c) GTPase

198. Bacteriophage M13 contains as its genetic material

a. ssRNA   b. dsRNA

c. ss DNA   d. ds DNA

Ans. (c) ss DNA

199. Genome of cauliflower mosaic virus is

a. +ve stranded RNA

b. ss DNA

c. ds DNA

d. dsRNA

Ans. (c) ds DNA

200. Infectious ssRNAs in plants that are not associated with any protein are called

a. Viruses
b. Viroids
c. Prions
d. Satellite viruses

Ans. (b) Viroids

PATHOLOGY

201. In 1845, the late blight of potato destroyed the potato crop of Ireland was caused by

a. Phytophthora infestans
b. Alternaria solani
c. Pythium aphanidermatum
d. Pseudomonas solanacearum

Ans. (a) Phytophthora infestans

202. In 1943, Bengal had faced a serious famine which cause a great loss in rice yield was caused by

a. Helminthosporium oryzae
b. Colletotrichum falcatum
c. Pyricularia oryzae
d. Fusarium udum

Ans. (a) Helminthosporium oryzae

203. Who is the father of plant pathology?

a. TJ Burill
b. Needham
c. Anton de Bary
d. EJ Butler

Ans. (c) Anton de Bary

204. Who advanced the gene for gene concept of disease resistance and susceptibility in 1946

a. Flor
b. Vanderplank
c. Gaumann
d. Muller

Ans. (a) Flor

205. Who describes the first plant nematode disease, the seed gall caused by A nguina tritici in1743 AD

a. Berkeley
b. Kuhn
c. Needham
d. NA Cobb

Ans. (c) Needham

206. Who is the father of American Nematology?

a. Kuhn
b. H Schacht
c. NA Cobb
d. TJ Burill

Ans. (c) NA Cobb

207. Who is considered founder of virology?

a. Beijernick
b. AE Mayer
c. WM Stanley
d. TO Diener

Ans. (a) Beijernick

208. The first Indian scientist who collected and identified fungi in India?

a. EJ Butler
b. KR Kirtikar
c. JF Dastur
d. KC Mehta

Ans. (b) KR Kirtikar

209. 'Fungi and disease in plants' was written in 1918 by

a. J F Dastur
b. BB Mundakur
c. EJ Butler
d. R. Prasad

Ans. (c) EJ Butler

210. 'Fungi and plant diseases' was written by

a. BB Mundakur
b. J F Dastur
c. G Rangaswami
d. KC Mehta

Ans. (a) BB Mundakur

211. In bacteria, variability is caused by

a. Conjugation
b. Transformation
c. Transduction
d. All

Ans. (d) All

212. Who done most of his work on rust diseases in India

a. R Prasad
b. KC Mehta
c. BB Mundakur
d. EJ Butler

Ans. (b) KC Mehta

213. Citrus canker, which originated from China is caused by pathogen

a. Xanthomonas campestris pv. Citri
b. Albugo candida
c. Erwinia amylovora
d. Claviceps fusiformis

Ans. (a) Xanthomonas campestris pv. Citri

214. Citrus greening disease mainly confined to

a. North India
b. South India
c. East India
d. West India

Ans. (a) North India

215. Select the disease caused by mycoplasma like organisms

a. Brinjal little leaf
b. Rice yellow dwarf
c. Sugarcane grassy shoot
d. Sesamum phyllody
e. All

Ans. (e) All

216. **Select the organism which cannot synthesize protein by own enzymes**
    a. Bacteria
    b. Mycoplasma
    c. RLO
    d. Virus

Ans. (d) Virus

217. **Sandak spike disease of sandal is caused by**
    a. Bacteria
    b. Virus
    c. Fungi
    d. MLO

Ans. (d) MLO

218. **Tick out the sexual spores of fungi**
    a. Chlamydospores
    b. Sporangiospores
    c. Zoospores
    d. Zygospores

Ans. (d) Zygospores

219. **'white blisters of crucifers' is caused by pathogen**
    a. Pythium debarynam
    b. Albugo candida
    c. Sclerospora sorghi
    d. Plasmopora viticola

Ans. (b) Albugo candida

220. **Who is the father of plant pathology in India?**
    a. E J Butler
    b. KC Mehta
    c. BB Mundakur
    d. R Prasad

Ans. (a) E J Butler

221. **Downey mildew of bajra is caused by**
    a. Sclerospora sorghi
    b. Sclerospora sacchari
    c. S. graminicola
    d. Pernospora parasitica

Ans. (c) S. graminicola

222. **Rust fungi completing their life cycle on one host are called**
    a. Polymorphic
    b. Autoecious
    c. Heteroecious
    d. None

Ans. (b) Autoecious

223. **Promycelium in Rust fungi bears**
    a. Basidiospores
    b. Aeciospores
    c. Uredia
    d. Telia

Ans. (a) Basidiospores

224. **Effective control of late blight of potato is possible by use of**
    a. Sanitation measures
    b. Spray of metalaxl
    c. Bordeaux mixture
    d. All

Ans. (d) All

225. **Bacterial colony known is**
    a. Spore
    b. Mycelium
    c. Ooze
    d. Hypha

Ans. (c) Ooze

226. **Albugo candida causes white blisters or white rust of crucifers is**
    a. Obligate parasite
    b. Obligate saprophite
    c. Facultative parasite
    d. Facultative saprophyte

Ans. (a) Obligate parasite

227. **Albugo candida produces**
    a. Basidiospores
    b. Ascospores
    c. Zoospores
    d. Oospores

Ans. (d) Oospores

228. **Green ear or downey mildew of pearlmillet was first time reported in India by**
    a. K C Mehta
    b. E J Butler
    c. BB Mundakur
    d. R Prasad

Ans. (b) E J Butler

229. **Downey mildew disease of pearlmillet is primarilya**
    a. Seed borne
    b. Air borne
    c. Soil borne
    d. Water borne

Ans. (c) Soil borne

230. **Stem gall of coriander is caused by**
    a. Protomyces macrosporus
    b. Plasmopara viticola
    c. Peronospora pisi
    d. None

Ans. (a) Protomyces macrosporus

231. **Symptoms of powdery mildew of pea first appears on**
    a. Stem
    b. Roots
    c. Leaves
    d. Flowers

Ans. (c) Leaves

232. **Disease caused by Leptosphaeria sacchari in sugarcane is**
    a. Red rot
    b. Black rot
    c. Ring spot
    d. None

Ans. (c) Ring spot

233. Disease ergot of rye produces sclerotia is caused by

a. Claviceps purpurea   b. C. fusiformis
c. C. sativae   d. All

Ans. (a) Claviceps purpurea

234. Loose smut of wheat is

a. Internally seed borne   b. Externally seed borne
c. Both a and b   d. None

Ans. (a) Internally seed borne

235. Covered smut of barley is

a. Internally seed borne
b. Externally seed borne
c. Both a and b
d. None

Ans. (b) Externally seed borne

236. Which fungicide give effective control of covered smut of barley

a. Vitavax   b. Ceresan
c. Agrosan 5W   d. Sulphur dust

Ans. (a) Vitavax

237. Loose smut of barley is

a. Internally seed borne
b. Externally seed borne
c. Soil borne
d. All

Ans. (a) Internally seed borne

238. False smut of sugarcane can be controlled by adopting

a. Avoid the practice of ratooning
b. Disinfection of setts before planting
c. Removal of smutted whips from the field
d. All

Ans. (d) All

239. Infection of smut of maize occurs during

a. Vegetative stage   b. Reproductive stage
c. After flowering   d. Before sowing

Ans. (a) Vegetative stage

240. Grain smut of sorghum is externally seed borne disease caused by pathogen

a. Sphacelotheca reiliana
b. Sphacelotheca cruenta
c. Sphacelotheca sorghi
d. Tolyposporium enrenbergii

Ans. (c) Sphacelotheca sorghi

241. Smut of pearlmillet is a

a. Internally seed borne   b. Externally seed borne
c. Soil borne   d. All

Ans. (c) Soil borne

242. Karnal bunt of wheat first time reported in Karnal by Mitra in

a. 1929   b. 1931
c. 1941   d. 1951

Ans. (b) 1931

243. Karnal bunt of wheat is caused by

a. Neovossia indica   b. Tilletia horrida
c. Urocystis tritici   d. Ustilago tritici

Ans. (a) Neovossia indica

244. Karnal bunt of wheat gives foul smell in the field due to the presence of volatile compound

a. Tetramethyl amine
b. Trimethyl amine
c. Diallyl propyl sulphide
d. Allyl propyl disulphide

Ans. (b) Trimethyl amine

245. The causal organism Neovossia indica produces

a. Urediospores   b. Zoospores
c. Oospores   d. Teliospores

Ans. (d) Teliospores

246. The causal organism of bunt of rice is

a. Urocystis tritici
b. Tilletia foetida
c. Neovossia horrid
d. None

Ans. (c) Neovossia horrid

247. Effective control of flag smut of wheat can be done by adopting of

a. Use of resistant varieties
b. Seed treatment
c. Crop rotation
d. All

Ans. (d) All

248. Black rust or stem rust of wheat is caused by

a. Puccinia graminis tritici
b. Puccinia striformis
c. Puccinia recondita
d. Melampsora lini

Ans. (a) Puccinia graminis tritici

249. Which type of spores of Puccinia graminis tritici infect the barberry plant

a. Teliospores

b. Urediospores

c. Basidiospores

d. Aeciospores

Ans. (c) Basidiospores

250. In rust cycle the cereal host is infected by

a. Urediospores

b. Aeciospores

c. Teliospores

d. Basidiospores

Ans. (b) Aeciospores

251. Yellow rust of wheat is caused by

a. Puccinia striformis

b. Puccinia recondita

c. Puccinia graminis tritici

d. Puccinia hordei

Ans. (a) Puccinia striformis

252. In India the leaf rust of coffee was first time recorded in

a. 1856

b. 1870

c. 1880

d. 1943

Ans. (b) 1870

253. Rust of linseed and flax is caused by

a. Puccinia recondite

b. Puccinia striformis

c. Puccinia graminis tritici

d. Melampsora lini

Ans. (d) Melampsora lini

254. Rust of linseed and flax can be controlled by spray of

a. Borax

b. Dithane M-45

c. Vitavax

d. Agrosan GN

Ans. (a) Borax

255. Early blight of potato produces

a. Conidia

b. Telia

c. Uredia

d. Acecia

Ans. (a) Conidia

256. Early blight of potato is

a. Soil borne disease

b. Air borne

c. Seed borne

d. All

Ans. (a) Soil borne disease

257. Effective control of early blight of potato, which fungicide is most suitable

a. Zineb

b. Dithane M-45

c. Blitox

d. Difolatan

Ans. (b) Dithane M-45

258. Leaf spot or tikka disease of groundnut is caused by

a. Cercospora arachidicola

b. Cercosporidium personatum

c. Both a and b

d. Drechslera graminea

Ans. (c) Both a and b

259. Brown Leaf spot disease of rice is caused by

a. Drechslera graminea

b. Cercospora arachidicola

c. Xanthomonas oryzae

d. Pyricularia oryzae

Ans. (a) Drechslera graminea

260. Fungus of Drechslera oryzae produces toxins which are highly toxic to rice seedling, name of such toxin is

a. ABA

b. Trimethyl amine

c. Isobutylene

d. Cochliobolin

Ans. (d) Cochliobolin

261. Pathogen of rice blast or rotten neck is

a. Ustilago tritici

b. Pyricularia oryzae

c. Alternaria alternate

d. None

Ans. (b) Pyricularia oryzae

262. Tea rust is caused by

a. MLO

b. Virus

c. Bacteria

d. Algae

Ans. (d) Algae

263. Colletotrichum falcatum produces

a. Zygospores

b. Oospores

c. Ascospores

d. Conidiospores

Ans. (d) Conidiospores

264. Wilt of pigeonpea is caused by

a. Fusarium udum

b. Gibbrella indica

c. Rhizopus nigricans

d. Aspergillus flavus

Ans. (a) Fusarium udum

265. For the effective control of wilt, pigeonpea should be intercropped with

a. Maize
b. Pearlmillet
c. Sorghum
d. Mung

Ans. (c) Sorghum

266. The most important symptom of wilt of cotton is

a. Necrosis
b. Yellowing of tissues
c. Discolouration of tissues and plugging of vessels by hyphae
d. All

Ans. (c) Discolouration of tissues and plugging of vessels by hyphae

267. Wilt disease of sugarcane was first time reported in India from

a. Punjab
b. Tamilnadu
c. Bihar
d. U.P.

Ans. (c) Bihar

268. Pathogen responsible for charcoal rot of soyabean is

a. Ascochyta rabiei
b. Macrophomina phaseolina
c. Rhizoctonia solani
d. Penicillium

Ans. (b) Macrophomina phaseolina

269. Incidence of black scurf of potato is more in

a. Sandy soil
b. Clay soil
c. Alluvial soil
d. Loam soil

Ans. (a) Sandy soil

270. Attack of sheath blight of rice is more during

a. Germination
b. Active tillering stage
c. Flowering
d. All

Ans. (b) Active tillering stage

271. The nematodes are

a. Monoblastic
b. Duoblastic
c. Triploblastic
d. all

Ans. (c) Triploblastic

272. The nematodes lack organs for

a. Circulation
b. Respiration
c. Both a and b
d. Excretory

Ans. (c) Both a and b

273. Citrus greening caused by

a. Fastidious bacteria
b. Fungi
c. Virus
d. MLO

Ans. (a) Fastidious bacteria

274. Uredospores of puccinia graminis are disseminated by

a. Wind
b. Animals
c. Insects
d. Birds

Ans. (a) Wind

275. G + C content of prokaryotes is

a. 20%
b. 30%
c. 50%
d. 70%

Ans. (a) 20%

276. MLO first discovered by

a. Louis pasteur
b. Leuvenhoeck
c. Kuch
d. Mendal

Ans. (a) Louis pasteur

277. Plant pathology written by

a. RS Singh
b. Agrios
c. VS Singh
d. AP Sinha

Ans. (b) Agrios

278. In north India and central India, the black rust inoculums cause from

a. South
b. Hilly area
c. From USA
d. From Nepal

Ans. (a) South

279. Plant disease written by

a. BB Mundakur
b. RS Singh
c. Agrios
d. KC Mehta

Ans. (b) RS Singh

280. MLO disease transmitted by

a. Leaf hopper
b. Aphid
c. Whitefly
d. Animals

Ans. (a) Leaf hopper

281. Teliospores of rust have germpores in number

a. 1
b. 2
c. 3
d. 4

Ans. (b) 2

282. Alternate host of black rust

a. Barberi
b. Bajra
c. Jowar
d. wheat

Ans. (a) Barberi

283. Hot water treatment of seed is useful for control of

a. Loose smut
b. Covered smut
c. Rust
d. Powdery mildew

Ans. (a) Loose smut

284. Smut of maize caused by

a. Ustilago tritici
b. Ustilago maydis
c. Ustilago hordei
d. None

Ans. (b) Ustilago maydis

285. Sterility mosaic disease of pigeonpea spread by

a. Virus
b. Aphid
c. Whitefly
d. Mites

Ans. (d) Mites

286. Phyllody disease of sesamum spread by

a. Leaf hopper
b. Jassid
c. Aphid
d. Whitefly

Ans. (a) Leaf hopper

287. Fungi imperfecti includes in

a. Deuteromycotina
b. Basidiomycotina
c. Ascomycotina
d. Oomycetes

Ans. (a) Deuteromycotina

288. Rust includes in

a. Deuteromycotina
b. Basidiomycotina
c. Ascomycotina
d. Oomycetes

Ans. (b) Basidiomycotina

289. Smut includes in

a. Deuteromycotina
b. Basidiomycotina
c. Ascomycotina
d. Oomycetes

Ans. (b) Basidiomycotina

290. Powdery mildew includes in

a. Deuteromycotina
b. Basidiomycotina
c. Ascomycotina
d. Oomycetes

Ans. (c) Ascomycotina

291. Downy mildew includes in

a. Oomycetes
b. Chytridiomycetes
c. Zygomycetes
d. Hypochytridiomycetes

Ans. (a) Oomycetes

292. Downy mildew of pea caused by

a. Pernospora pisi
b. Albugo candida
c. Erysiphae polygoni
d. None

Ans. (a) Pernospora pisi

293. Father of Indian Mycology

a. EJ Butler
b. KC Mehta
c. Mundakur
d. RS Singh

Ans. (a) EJ Butler

294. In 2005 which pathological scientist got Borlaug award

a. Rattan Lal
b. VL Chopra
c. CD Mayee
d. S Nagrajan

Ans. (d) S Nagrajan

295. Micrografting is used to produce plants free from

a. Virus
b. RLO's
c. MLO's
d. Bacteria

Ans. (a) Virus

296. Black heart is a physiological disorder of

a. Tomato
b. Chilli
c. Potato
d. Cabbage

Ans. (c) Potato

297. Tungro disease of rice is spread by

a. Nephotettix virescens
b. Sogatella furcifera
c. Nilaparvata lugens
d. Thrips tabaci

Ans. (a) Nephotettix virescens

298. Panama wilt is a disease of

a. Bamboo
b. Mango
c. Pineapple
d. Banana

Ans. (d) Banana

299. VAM is

a. Bacteria
b. Fungi
c. Virus
d. Algae

Ans. (b) Fungi

300. 'Buck eye rot' is a disease of which crop

a. Water chestnut
b. Sweet potato
c. Pods of garden pea
d. Tomato fruits

Ans. (a) Water chestnut

301. The major storage fungi that effects the food grain is

a. Rhizobium   b. Mucor

c. Cercospora   d. Aspergillus

Ans. (d) Aspergillus

302. Loose smut is controlled by

a. Soil treatment   b. Seed treatment

c. Chemical spray   d. None

Ans. (b) Seed treatment

303. Yellow leaf mosaic of bhindi crop spreads by

a. Jassids   b. Borers

c. Jassids and Borers   d. None

Ans. (c) Jassids and Borers

304. Yellow mosaic virus disease of moong is spread by

a. Bemisia tabaci   b. Aphir crassivora

c. Nephotettix viruscens   d. Amrasca bigulitula

Ans. (b) Aphir crassivora

305. Heterodera avenne is

a. Root knot nematode   b. Cyst nematode

c. Lesion nematode   d. Lance nematode

Ans. (b) Cyst nematode

306. Panama disease of banana is prevented by

a. Spraying zinc carrier

b. Spraying copper fungicide

c. Application of lime to soil

d. Providing adequate irrigation

Ans. (c) Application of lime to soil

307. Which one of the following fungicide is not systemic in nature

a. Vitavax   b. Thiram

c. Benlate   d. Topsin

Ans. (b) Thiram

308. Little leaf of brinjal is caused by a

a. Fungus   b. Bacteria

c. Virus   d. Mycoplasma

Ans. (d) Mycoplasma

309. Bacterial diseases are controlled by use of chemicals

a. Kelthane

b. Fungicide

c. Antibiotics

d. Viricides

Ans. (c) Antibiotics

310. Application of potash increases

a. Resistance to water logging

b. Frost resistance in plants

c. Disease resistance in plants

d. None

Ans. (c) Disease resistance in plants

311. Decomposition of organic matter in submerged soil is carried out by

a. Bacteria   b. Actinomycetes

c. Fungi   d. Earthworm

Ans. (a) Bacteria

312. Margosa is a highly effective product in reducing root knot population belongs to

a. Acacia arabica   b. Azadirachta indica

c. Citrullus colosynthes   d. Pongamia glabra

Ans. (b) Azadirachta indica

313. In plant buckling, puckering and blistering symptoms are produced by

a. Bacteria   b. Fungi

c. Viruses   d. Mycoplasma

Ans. (c) Viruses

314. The fungi which transmit plant viruses belong to class

a. Basidiomycetes

b. Ooomycetes

c. Zygoomycetes

d. Plasmodiophoromycetes

Ans. (d) Plasmodiophoromycetes

315. For quick and accurate detection of viruses can be done by

a. ELISA   b. HADAS

c. IEM   d. All

Ans. (d) All

316. Potato virus diseases are spread by

a. Aphids   b. Jassids

c. Nematodes   d. Tuber moth

Ans. (a) Aphids

317. Leaf curl of tomato is spread by

a. Jassids

b. White fly

c. Aphids

d. Nematodes

Ans. (b) White fly

318. Bunchy top of banana is caused by

a. Nematodes   b. Fungi

c. White fly   d. Leaf hoppers

Ans. (d) Leaf hoppers

319. Yellow mosaic of legumes was first reported in India from

a. Shimla   b. Solan

c. Delhi   d. Kanpur

Ans. (c) Delhi

320. Potato spindle tuber disease is transmitted

a. Mechanically   b. Biologically

c. Water   d. All

Ans. (a) Mechanically

321. Suicidal germination take place in

a. Dodder

b. Striga

c. Loranthus

d. Dendrophthoe falcate

Ans. (b) Striga

322. Ozone is toxic to expanding leaves of almost all types of plant at the conc. of equal or more than

a. 0.1 ppm   b. 0.2 ppm

c. 0.3 ppm   d. 0.5 ppm

Ans. (a) 0.1 ppm

323. SO_2 is toxic to plants at or above

a. 0.1–0.3 ppm   b. 0.3–0.5 ppm

c. 0.5–0.7 ppm   d. 1 ppm

Ans. (b) 0.3–0.5 ppm

324. Black heart of potato is the result of

a. High temp. during transit

b. Poor ventilation in the store

c. High temp. of soil during growth and maturation of tubers in the crop field

d. All

Ans. (d) All

325. Bordeaux mixture was first time used for the control of

a. Downey mildew of grape vines

b. Powdery mildew of pea

c. Root rot of beet

d. Damping off of pea

Ans. (a) Downey mildew of grape vines

326. Damping off and leaf blight are very effectively checked by

a. Bordeaux mixture   b. Burgundy mixture

c. Thiram   d. Copper oxychloride

Ans. (d) Copper oxychloride

327. Dinocap is sold in market as

a. Bravo   b. Dexon

c. Botron   d. Karathane

Ans. (d) Karathane

328. Nematicides inhibits which enzyme of nervous system in killing of nematodes

a. Kinase   b. Isomerise

c. Phosphatase   d. Acetyl cholinesterase

Ans. (d) Acetyl cholinesterase

329. Who discovered the downey mildew for the first time in India

a. EJ Butler   b. JF Dastur

c. BB Mundakur   d. KR Kirtikar

Ans. (a) EJ Butler

330. Which one of the following is a single cell fungi

a. Yeast   b. Aspergillus

c. Penicillium   d. Alternaria

Ans. (a) Yeast

331. What is the source of agar–agar

a. Bacteria   b. Fungi

c. Mycoplasma   d. Algae

Ans. (d) Algae

332. MLO and spiroplasma are mostly

a. Xylem inhibiting

b. Phloem inhibiting

c. Both a and b

d. Stomata inhibiting

Ans. (b) Phloem inhibiting

333. Mad cow disease is caused by

a. Virion   b. Prion

c. Bacteria   d. MLO

Ans. (b) Prion

334. Most widely used biocontrol agent is

a. Pseudomonas florescence

b. P. putida

c. Bacillus subtilis

d. Clostridium

Ans. (a) Pseudomonas florescence

335. Most widely used fungicide for rust fungi is

a. Vitavax   b. Plantvax
c. Bavistin   d. Dithane M-45

Ans. (b) Plantvax

336. Most widely used fungicide for smut fungi is

a. Vitavax   b. Plantvax
c. Dithane M-45   d. Dithane Z-78

Ans. (a) Vitavax

337. Race specific resistance called

a. Vertical resistance
b. Horizontal resistance
c. Adult plant resistance
d. Apparent resistance

Ans. (a) Vertical resistance

338. When plant showed the partial resistance against all the races of pathogen then it is a type of

a. Horizontal resistance
b. Vertical resistance
c. Induced resistance
d. Non-host resistance

Ans. (a) Horizontal resistance

339. Which is the most recent widely used fungicide for the control of powdery mildew

a. Calaxin
b. Sulphur dust
c. Dithane M-45
d. Apron SD-35

Ans. (a) Calaxin

340. Which fungicide is used against downey mildew

a. Metalaxyl   b. Karathane
c. Oxathind.   Streptomycin

Ans. (a) Metalaxyl

341. Which one of the following can not be detected by ELISA technique

a. Virus   b. Bacteria
c. Viroid   d. Fungus

Ans. (c) Viroid

342. Nuclear polyhedrosis virus is the most effective for the control of

a. Chilo partellus
b. Pectionophora gossypiella
c. Helicoverpa armigera
d. Diacrasia oblique

Ans. (c) Helicoverpa armigera

343. Bacteria can be differentiated from plants and animals on the basis of which of the following characters:

i. Asexual reproduction
ii. Prokaryotic nature of cell organization
iii. Presence of muramic acid in cell wall
iv. Have a cell wall

Choose the correct answer:

a. ii, iii, iv   b. i, ii
c. i, ii, iii   d. iii, iv

Ans. (b) i, ii

344. Which of the following classes represent gram negative (–) becteria?

i. Pseudomonidaceae
ii. Enterobacteriaceae
iii. bacteridaceae
iv. Brucillaceae
v. Achromobacteriaceae

Choose the correct answer

a. i, ii, iii, v   b. iii, iv, v
c. i, ii, iii   d. i, ii, iii, iv,v

Ans. (d) i, ii, iii, iv,v

345. Match the correct pair:

Organisms	Cell wall composition
i. Fungi	c. Cellulose + other Polysaccharides + CaCO$_3$
ii. Algae	b. Mucopeptide
iii. Bacteria	c. Mainly cellulose
iv. Diatoms	d. Cellulose + chitin
v. Plants	e. Cellulose + silica + other polysaccharides

Choose the correct answer:

	I	II	III	IV	V
(a)	b	d	c	e	a
(b)	c	b	d	a	e
(c)	b	c	d	e	a
(d)	a	e	c	d	b

Ans. (a)

346. *Escherichia coli* in the genus *Escherichia* named after Escherich who?

a. Was a great Psycologist
b. Isolated this bacteria in 1885
c. Isolated virus in 1985
d. Was a great Embryologist

Ans. (b) Isolated this bacteria in 1885

347. Which of the following pair is not matched correctly?

Bacterial organelle	Stain used for identification
a. Capsule	Indian ink stain
b. Unusual cell walls	Ziehl Neelasen acid fast stain
c. Spore	Malachite green stain
d. Metachromatic	Sudan black

Ans. (d) Metachromatic   Sudan black

348. Vogues-proskaeur test is a biochemical test used in bacteria for:

a. The presence of cellulose

b. The presence of toxic molecules

c. Test end product of their metabolic processes

d. The presence of specific nitrogen source

Ans. (c) Test end product of their metabolic processes

349. In E. coli fimbriae is 75 to 100 A in thickness and is made up of two parallel protein rods (pilin) with a groove between them. The main function of fimbriae in bacteria is:

a. Conjugation

b. Transduction

c. Translation

d. Transcription

Ans. (a) Conjugation

350. Archaebacteria differ from eubacteria because archaebacteria:

a. Have ester linked lipids

b. Have ether linked lipids

c. Lack muramic acid in cell wall

d. Both a and b

Ans. (d) Both a and b

351. Which of the following is not the characteristic of archaebacteria?

a. These are found in colon (*E. coll*)

b. These are found in high salinity (*Halabacterium*)

c. These are found in hot springs (*Sulpholobus and Phyrococcus*)

d. They produce methane as a result of metabolism (*Methobacterium*)

Ans. (a) These are found in colon (*E. coll*)

352. Mesosomes are the imagination of the plasma membrane in bacteria which helps in:

a. Locomotion	b. Digestion
c. Cell division	d. None of these

Ans. (c) Cell division

353. Eubacteria are frequently divided into two groups – Gram (+) and Gram (–) on the basis of their reaction to a stain devised by Christian Gram in 1884. Gram positive bacteria have:

a. Both gram (+) and gram (-) have similar thickness of peptidoglycan layer

b. Thick layer of peptidoglycan

c. Thin layer of peptidoglycan

d. Thick layer of cellulose

Ans. (d) Thick layer of cellulose

354. Bacterial cell wall is composed of peptidoglycan, a complex of oligosaccharides and proteins. The oligosaccharide component consist of:

a. Linear chain of glucose linked by β (1 – 4) linkage.

b. Linear chains of alternating NAG and NAM linked $\beta(1 – 4)$ linkage

c. Linear chain of alternating NAG and NAM linked $\alpha(1 – 4)$ linkage

d. Linear chain of glucose linked by $\alpha(1 – 4)$ linkage

Ans. (b) Linear chains of alternating NAG and NAM linked $\beta(1 – 4)$ linkage

355. Why peptidoglycan is resistant to the action of proteases?

a. Due to lack of amino acids

b. Due to presence of L-amino acids

c. Due to presence of D-amino acids

d. Due to presence of non-functional proteases

Ans. (c) Due to presence of D-amino acids

356. Large amount of teicoic acid polymer is found in:

a. Green algae	b. Gram negative bacteria
c. Gram positive bacteria	d. Red algae

Ans. (c) Gram positive bacteria

357. Why antibiotic 'penicillin' affects only bacterial cell wall not human, cell wall?

a. Due to presence of L-amino acids

b. Due to presence of D-amino acids

c. Due to presence of NAM which absent in eukaryotes

d. Due to lack of amino acids

Ans. (b) Due to presence of D-amino acids

358. Lysozyme breaks down :

a. Covalent cross-links in the peptidoglycan

b. (1 – 4) linkage between NAM and NAG

c. (1 – 4) linkage between NAM and NAG

d. (1 – 4) linkage between two glucose molecules

Ans. (b) (1 – 4) linkage between NAM and NAG

359. Bacterial cell wall become weak by the use of antibiotic penicillin due to:

a. Inhibition of conjugation

b. Stimulation of lysozyme secretion by penicillin

c. Inhibition of enzyme that forms the covalent cross links in the peptidoglycan

d. Inhibition of transduction

Ans. (c) Inhibition of enzyme that forms the covalent cross links in the peptidoglycan

360. Which of the following enzyme digest peptidoglycan layer in bacterial cell wall?

a. Autolysins   b. Trypsin

c. Rennin   d. Pepsin

Ans. (a) Autolysins

361. Bacteria that are capable of growing in 3M NaCl, called:

a. Aerotolerant   b. Osmotolerant

c. Haplophiles   d. Thermophiles

Ans. (b) Osmotolerant

362. Alkaliphiles bacteria grow at pH 8.5 – 11.5 whereas acidophiles grow at pH:

a. 8.0 – 8.9   b. 0 – 5.5

c. 7.0 – 7.5   d. 12 – 14

Ans. (b) 0 – 5.5

363. Actinomycetes a sub group of filamentous bacteria is:

a. Fuelgen positive   b. Fuelgen negative

c. Gram negative   d. Gram positive

Ans. (d) Gram positive

364. Gram negative bacteria is:

a. *Erysipliilothrix*   b. *Corynebacteria*

c. Spirilla   d. *Lactobacilli*

Ans. (c) Spirilla

365. MDT (mean doubling time) is expressed as (where 'n' is generation number)

a. $MDT = 2 + 2n$ b. $MDT = 2 \times 2^n$

c. $MDT = 2n$ d. $MDT = 2 \% 2n$

Ans. (b) $MDT = 2 \times 2^n$

366. Lodine is used as a sterilant agent because it is a strong:

a. Reducing agent   b. Oxidizing agent

c. Redox agent   d. Heavy toxin

Ans. (b) Oxidizing agent

367. A toxoid is a:

a. Toxin that losses its activity

b. Heavy toxin

c. Potent toxin

d. Harmful toxin

Ans. (a) Toxin that losses its activity

368. The most common type of reproduction in bacteria is:

a. Budding   b. Binary fission

c. Binary   d. Sexual reproduction

Ans. (b) Binary fission

369. Diphtheria toxin is an exotoxin produced by:

a. *Clostridium sp.*   b. *Corynebacterium sp.*

c. *Streptococcus sp.*   d. *Staphylococcus sp.*

Ans. (b) *Corynebacterium sp.*

370. Which of the iron bacteria oxidizes ferrous compounds into ferric compounds

a. *Treponema pallidum*   b. *Leptothrix ochracae*

c. *Bacillus thermophyllus*   d. *Pasturella pestis*

Ans. (b) *Leptothrix ochracae*

371. Lactic acid is produced from pyruvic acid at industrial level by the help of:

a. *Clostridium*   b. *Streptococcus*

c. *Enterobacter*   d. *Staphylococcus*

Ans. (b) *Streptococcus*

372. Microbes use inorganic compounds as electron donar and utilize solar energy are known as:

a. Photo-organotrophs

b. Chemolithotrophs

c. Photolithotrophs

d. Chemo-organotrophs

Ans. (c) Photolithotrophs

373. Endotoxins are toxin chemicals secreted by pathogen inside the host cells, chemically they are:

a. Lipopolysaccharides

b. Proteins

c. Lipids

d. Phospholipids

Ans. (a) Lipopolysaccharides

374. Food poisoning is caused by :

a. *Pseudomonas fragi*

b. *Clostridium nigrificans*

c. *Salmonella typhimurium*

d. All of these

Ans. (d) All of these

375. 'Aggessins' are:

a. Group of diffusible substances or cellular components produced by certain pathogens

b. Substances that activate the host response system

c. Group of chemical compounds resembling hormones

d. None of these

Ans. (a) Group of diffusible substances or cellular components produced by certain pathogens

376. The bacteria oxidizes molecular hydrogen in order to form water in soil is:

a. *Rhizobium noduliformis*   b. *Albugo candida*

c. *Bacillus pentatrophus*   d. *Lactobacillus*

Ans. (c) *Bacillus pentatrophus*

377. Which of the following is true for photolithotrophs?

a. $NO_2 + O_2 \xrightarrow{\text{Nitrobacter}} NO_3$

b. $NH_2 + 3O_2 \xrightarrow{\text{Nitrosomonas}} NO_2 + H^+ + H_2O$

c. $H_2O + CO_2 \xrightarrow{\text{Light}} CH_2O + O_2$

d. $2H_2S + CO_2 \xrightarrow{\text{Nitrosomonas}} CH_2O + H_2O + 2S$

Ans. (c) $H_2O + CO_2 \xrightarrow{\text{Light}} CH_2O + O_2$

378. Which of the following is true?

i. $NO_2 + O_2 \xrightarrow{\text{Nitrobacter}} NO_3$ (Chemolithotroph)

ii. $2CH_3CHOHCH_3 + CO_2 \longrightarrow CH_2O + 2CH_3CCH_3 + H_2O$ (Photo-organotroph)

iii. $H_2O + CO_2 \xrightarrow{\text{Light}} CH_2O + O_2$ (Photolithotroph)

iv. $NH_2 + 3O_2 \xrightarrow{\text{Nitrosomonas}} NO_2 + H^+ + H_2O$

a. ii and iii only   b. i, ii, iii only

c. i and ii only   d. i, ii, iii and iv

Ans. (d) i, ii, iii and iv

379. 'Lecithinase' causes lysis of RBCs and other lipid containing tissues, is produced by:

a. *Clostridium perfringenes*

b. *Streptococcus aureus*

c. *Streptococcus pyogenus*

d. *Aspergillus protein is sold as*

Ans. (b) *Streptococcus aureus*

380. Single cell protein (SCP) containing 50–80% protein is sold as pruteen, brovile and Marmite trade name in various countries. The pruteen is obtained from:

a. Salmonella typhi

b. Mycolbgacterium tuberculosis

c. Mythylophilus methulotropous

d. Pasturella pestis

Ans. (c) Mythylophilus methulotropous

381. Storage granule most often seen in bacterial cell is:

a. Polyglucan granule

b. Poly-hydroxybutyrate

c. Polymetaphosphate

d. All of these

Ans. (d) All of these

382. Bacterial growth in liquid medium follow a typical pattern called bacterial growth curve. The correct sequence of phases in growth curve is:

a. Stationary phase, lag phase, log phase, death phase

b. Log phase, lag phase, stationary phase, death phase

c. Lag phase, log phase, stationary phase, death phase

d. Log phase, stationary phase, lag phase, death phase

Ans. (c) Lag phase, log phase, stationary phase, death phase

383. The technique of three steps treatment of 90 – 100°C for 10 minute with 24 hours gaps in between is called:

a. Radiation   b. Tyndalization

c. Pasteurization   d. Autoclaving

Ans. (b) Tyndalization

384. Streaking plate method and spread plate method is used for:

a. Recombination of bacteria

b. Reproduction of bacteria

c. Isolation of bacterial strain or colonies

d. Sterilization of bacteria

Ans. (c) Isolation of bacterial strain or colonies

385. The number of bacteria in a culture can be estimated by:

a. Using specialist electronic methods

b. Total count

c. Viable count

d. All of the above

Ans. (d) All of the above

386. In pure culture, the cells have arisen from:

a. Gram positive and gram negative bacterium and form hybrid

b. Same original bacterium

c. Different strains of bacterium

d. None of the above

Ans. (b) Same original bacterium

387. Gram positive bacteria retain Gram's stain due to high percent age of

a. Proteins
b. Peptidoglycan
c. Lipoprotein
d. Lipopolysaccharides

Ans. (b) Peptidoglycan

388. Polymetaphosphate, a storage granule acts as a source of:

a. Phosphate
b. Sulphate
c. Sulphur
d. Phosphoric acid

Ans. (a) Phosphate

389. Bacterial capsule surrounding cell wall commonly made up of:

a. Polypetides
b. Polysaccharide
c. Monosaccharide
d. Polyglycogen

Ans. (b) Polysaccharide

390. The cocci bacteria is:

a. *Streptococcus*
b. *Streptomyces*
c. *Staphylococcus*
d. *Sarcina*

Ans. (b) *Streptomyces*

391. Which of the following micro organism is a true homolactic fermentor?

a. Staphylococcus
b. Streptococcus
c. Clostridium
d. Propionobacterium

Ans. (b) Streptococcus

392. The bacteria, bacillus mesenteries is used for the production fo:

a. Pectinase and cellulose
b. Polymerase and invertase
c. Amylase and protease
d. Cellulose and carboxylase

Ans. (c) Amylase and protease

CHECK YOU GRASP

1. 'Lecithinase' causes lysis of RBCs and other lipid containing tissues, is produced by:
   a. *Clostridium perfringenes*
   b. *Streptococcus aureus*
   c. *Streptococcus pyogenus*
   d. *Aspergillus protein is sold as*

2. The bacteria oxidizes molecular hydrogen in order to form water in soil is:
   a. *Rhizobium noduliformis*
   b. *Albugo candida*
   c. *Bacillus pentatrophus*
   d. *Lactobacillus*

3. Example of VAM fungi
   a. *Pisoletecis*
   b. *Sclerotenia*
   c. *Glomus*
   d. *Trichoderma*

4. Lysozyme breaks down:
   a. Covalent cross-links in the peptidoglycan
   b. (1 – 4) linkage between NAM and NAG
   c. (1 – 4) linkage between NAM and NAG
   d. (1 – 4) linkage between two glucose molecules

5. Cubical packets of 8 cells is called in bacteria
   a. Staphylococcus
   b. Diplococcus
   c. Bacillus
   d. Sarcina

6. Bacteria that are capable of growing in 3M NaCl, called:
   a. Aerotolerant
   b. Osmotolerant
   c. Haplophiles
   d. Thermophiles

7. Name the organism which are predatory on bacteria
   a. Virus
   b. Viroid
   c. Bdellovibrios
   d. Prion

8. In 1845, the late blight of potato destroyed the potato crop of Ireland was caused by
   a. Phytophthora infestans
   b. Alternaria solani
   c. Pythium aphanidermatum
   d. Pseudomonas solanacearum

9. In cocoa fermentation the microbial inoclumn used is of
   a. Aspergillus niger
   b. Candida krusei
   c. Rhizopus oryzae
   d. None

10. Bacteriophage M13 contains as its genetic material
    a. ssRNA
    b. dsRNA
    c. ss DNA
    d. ds DNA

11. Brown Leaf spot disease of rice is caused by
    a. Drechslera graminea
    b. Cercospora arachidicola
    c. Xanthomonas oryzae
    d. Pyricularia oryzae

12. The cocci bacteria is:
    a. *Streptococcus*
    b. *Streptomyces*
    c. *Staphylococcus*
    d. *Sarcina*

In case of less than 80% score, go through brief Review and Glance one again from chapter

Key: 1-b 2-c 3-c 4-b 5-d 6-b 7-c 8-a 9-b 10-c 11-a 12-b

11

Bioinformatics

1. Swiss-Model Is available at

   a. ExPASy   b. NCBI

   c. TIGR   d. DDBJ

Ans. (a) ExPASy

2. SEQRES records

   a. Nucleic acid residue in file of Gen Bank

   b. Amino acid or nucleic acid residue each chain of macromolecule at PDB

   c. Amino acid or nucleic acid residues in EMBL

   d. Amino acid or nucleic acid residues in DDBJ sequence file

Ans. (b) Amino acid or nucleic acid residue each chain of macromolecule at PDB

3. The ExPASy is dedicated to the analysis of protein sequences and structure as well as 2-D PAGE This server is maintained by

   a. Swiss Institute of Bioinformatics

   b. European Binformatics Institute

   c. The Institute of Genome Research

   d. Protein information Resource

Ans. (a) Swiss Institute of Bioinformatics

4. A database that classifies protein 3-D structure in a hierarchical scheme of structural classes

   a. CATH   b. PDB

   c. PROSITE   d. SCOP

Ans. (a) CATH

5. Protein data bank is available at

   a. Research collaborator for structural Bioinformatics

   b. Research collaborator for structural Biology

   c. National Biomedical Research Foundation

   d. Expert Protein Analysis System server

Ans. (a) Research collaborator for structural Bioinformatics

6. Deep View can be downloaded from

   a. Expert protein analysis system server

   b. Protein information resource

   c. Molecular modeling database site at NCBI

   d. DNA databank of japan

Ans. (a) Expert protein analysis system server

7. The full form of RCSB is

   a. Research center for structural biology

   b. Research collaboratory for structural bioinformatics

   c. Research center for structural bioinformatics

   d. None of these

Ans. (b) Research collaboratory for structural bio-informatics

8. PIR was established in

   a. 1980   b. 1964

   c. 1984   d. 2000

Ans. (c) 1984

9. Swiss-prot was established in

   a. 1985   b. 1986

   c. 1987   d. 1988

Ans. (b) 1986

10. Prosite is a database for

   a. Searching the pattern or motif

   b. Searching the ligand

   c. Searching for RNA

   d. None of these

Ans. (a) Searching the pattern or motif

11. The database which is a catalogue of human gene and genetic disorder

   a. PRS

   b. SCOP

   c. TIGR

   d. OMIM

Ans. (d) OMIM

12. TIGRFAM is a database of

   a. Protein families based on Hidden Markov Models

   b. Nucleotide families based on HMMs

c. Both nucleotide and protein families based on HMMs

d. None of thesed

Ans. (a) Protein families based on Hidden Markov Models

13. The TIGR Gene Indices are built using

a. Mega BLAST

b. Cap3

c. DNA-prptein search program

d. All of these

Ans. (d) All of these

14. iPro Class is

a. An identical protein classification database in NCBI

b. An identical protein classification database in EBI

c. An identical protein classification database in PIR

d. An identical parasite classification database

Ans. (c) An identical protein classification database in PIR

15. In PDB file the MODRES record

a. Provides descriptions of modification (e.g. chemical or post translational)

b. Provides description of mutation

c. Provides description of translation

d. All of these

Ans. (a) Provides descriptions of modification (e.g. chemical or post translational)

16. In PDB file FORMUL record represent

a. The chemical formula

b. The charge of a non standard group

c. The chemical formula and charge of a non standard group

d. None of these

Ans. (c) The chemical formula and charge of a non standard group

17. The major function of INSDC is

a. Promotion of human genome project

b. Validation of 3D model of proteins with respect to structures solved by either X-ray crystallography or NMR spectroscopy

c. Facilitating exchange of sequence data on a daily basis

d. None of these

Ans. (c) Facilitating exchange of sequence data on a daily basis

18. What does the term 'LOCUS' explain in Gen Bank flat file?

a. Accession number

b. Length of molecule

c. Type of molecule(DNA/RNA)

d. All of these

Ans. (d) All of these

19. Which of the following is similar to 'Organism' of Gen Bank flat file to EMBL data entry formal?

a. OS, OC

b. SO, CO

c. Source

d. Source organism

Ans. (a) OS, OC

20. Comment lime '>' denotes.

a. Origin of sequence in nucleotide flat file

b. End of protein sequence in gene pept

c. Origin of nucleotide sequence in FASTA format

d. Origin of gene sequence in EMBL nucleotide sequence

Ans. (c) Origin of nucleotide sequence in FASTA format

21. What is Readseq?

a. A tool which helps to read and translate nucleotide sequences

b. A tool which converts sequence in one format to another format

c. Database which helps to download nucleotide sequences

d. A tool which reads the nucleotide sequences

Ans. (b) A tool which converts sequence in one format to another format

22. Bank it is

a. Use of informatics for DNA databank manipulation

b. A standalone multiplatform sequence submission program available on NCBI

c. A standalone sequence submission program available on EMBL

d. A web-based sequence submission tool available on NCBI

Ans. (d) A web-based sequence submission tool available on NCBI

23. PMC is

a. A digital archive of peer reviewed journals in life sciences

b. A protein Modelling center available at DDBJ

c. A secondary structure prediction tool

d. Aphylogeny method based on maximum parsimony method

Ans. (a) A digital archive of peer reviewed journals in life sciences

24. Uniport stands for

a. Uniform protein database
b. Universal protein Database
c. Universal Polypeptide Database
d. Unique protein Database

Ans. (b) Universal protein Database

25. Which of the following is the role of MSD?

a. It deals with collection, management, and distribution of data about structures determined by X-ray crystallography, NMR spectroscopy, and 3D electron microscopy
b. It's central, public repository for storing and accessing protein-protein interaction information.
c. It's sequence submission tool at DDBJ site
d. It's sequence retrieval system

Ans. (a) It deals with collection, management, and distribution of data about structures determined by X-ray crystallography, NMR spectroscopy, and 3D electron microscopy

26. In PDB file FORMUL record represents

a. The chemical formula
b. The charge of a non-standard group
c. The chemical formula and charge of a none standard group
d. None of these

Ans. (c) The chemical formula and charge of a none standard group

27. In PDB file the SSBOND record identifies

a. Each disulphide bond in protein and polypeptide structures by identifying the two residues involved in the bond
b. Each hydrogen bond in protein and polypeptide structures by identifying all the residues involved in the bond
c. Each electrostatic bond in protein and polypeptide structure by identifying the tow residues involve in the bond
d. All of these

Ans. (a) Each disulphide bond in protein and polypeptide structures by identifying the two residues involved in the bond

28. In PDB file the SIGUIJ record represent

a. The standard deviations of anisotropic pressure factors scaled by a factor of 10**4 (Abgstrins**2)
b. The standard deviations of anisotropic temperature factors scaled by a factor of 10**4 (Abgstrins**2)

c. The standard deviations of anisotropic temperature and pressure factors scaled by a factor of 10**4 (Abgstrins**2)
d. None of these

Ans. (b) The standard deviations of anisotropic temperature factors scaled by a factor of 104 (Abgstrins**2)**

29. Within NCBI the NSP is

a. A database of structural nucleotide and protein
b. A database of single nucleotide polymorphism
c. A database for major histo-compatiblity complex
d. None of these

Ans. (b) A database of single nucleotide polymorphism

30. The database that deals with cancer disease in NCBI is

a. Cancer gene
b. Oncogene
c. Cancer chromosome
d. None of these

Ans. (c) Cancer chromosome

31. GENSAT database of NCBI is

a. Gene expression atlas of human
b. Gene expression atlas of mouse
c. Gene expression atlas of rice
d. Gene expression atlas of rat

Ans. (b) Gene expression atlas of mouse

32. GlycoMod in ExPASy database predicts

a. Possible oligosaccharide structures that occur on proteins from their experimentally determined masses
b. Possible oligosaccharide structures that occur on DNA from their experimentally determined masses
c. Possible oligosaccharide structures that occur on DNA and proteins from their experimentally determined masses
d. None of these

Ans. (c) Possible oligosaccharide structures that occur on DNA and proteins from their experimentally determined masses

33. In the ExPASy database Target P is used for the prediction of

a. Homologous protein
b. Sub-cellular location
c. Homologous DNA
d. None of these

Ans. (a) Homologous protein

34. The field of bioinformatics

a. Uses biometric algorithms to develop more efficient software

b. Integrates concepts and techniques from information technology and molecular biology

c. Requires complete genome sequences to be useful

d. Has only developed in the last five years

Ans. (b) Integrates concepts and techniques from information technology and molecular biology

35. The principle application of the BLAST family of algorithms is

a. Identifying sequences that are similar to a protein or nucleotide sequence in a biological sequence database

b. Aligning two nucleotide sequences from ene to end

c. Identifying the best possible alignment of two short protein sequence

d. Finding the minimum energy configuration of a polypeptide sequence

Ans. (a) Identifying sequences that are similar to a protein or nucleotide sequence in a biological sequence database

36. At the NCBI website, the default scoring matrix for protein-protein BLAST analysis (BLASTP) is the BLOSUM62 matrix. The most likely reason for this matrix to be selected by default is because

a. It represents a compromise between information content for each residue and the amount of information that contributes to the matrix

b. Only this matrix is appropriate for all protein comparisons

c. It incorporates 62 position-specific scoring patterns

d. Unlike PAM matrices, this matrix is based on explicit phylogenetic information

Ans. (a) It represents a compromise between information content for each residue and the amount of information that contributes to the matrix

37. RID stands for

a. Request identifier
b. Request in demand
c. Review in depth
d. Reservation is done

Ans. (a) Request identifier

38. PHYLIP signifies

a. Phylogeny inference package

b. A person who postulated phylogeny

c. A phylogeny editing tool

d. A bioinformatics language

Ans. (a) Phylogeny inference package

39. The software that follows the global alignment method is

a. CLUSTALW
b. Pile-up
c. T-COFFEE
d. All of these

Ans. (d) All of these

40. What is CINEMA?

a. A molecular viewer

b. Similarity search method

c. Multiple alignment editor

d. Database of 3D structure of protein

Ans. (c) Multiple alignment editor

41. KITSCH, a package in PHYLIP is based on

a. Maximum Likelihood method

b. Distance method

c. Maximum parsimony method

d. None of these

Ans. (b) Distance method

42. Maximum likelihood method is use in molecular phylogeny when

a. There is maximum similarity among the aligned sequences

b. There is minimum similarity among the aligned sequences

c. There is maximum number of hits found in BLAST

d. All the sequences are from same phylum

Ans. (b) There is minimum similarity among the aligned sequences

43. DNA pars is a

a. DNA translation tool

b. Partial DNA sequence

c. Molecular phylogeny tool

d. Multiple alignment tool

Ans. (c) Molecular phylogeny tool

44. The file formate that serves as input for Cn3D, the molecular viewer, is

a. GCG
b. PDB
c. Cn3
d. MOL

Ans. (c) Cn3

45. The green colour in RasMol indicates

a. Sulphur

b. Hydrogen

c. Disulphide bond

d. Hydrogen bond

Ans. (d) Hydrogen bond

46. Saul Needleman and chritan wunsch postulated an algorithm which is useful for

a. Multiple alignment of sequences
b. Global alignment of sequences
c. Local alignment of sequence
d. All of these

Ans. (b) Global alignment of sequences

47. The molecular viewer used for mutation in protein sequence is

a. Deep view   b. Cn3D
c. rasMol   d. pyMol

Ans. (a) Deep view

48. Intra-strands base pairing

a. Stabilizes the structure of DNA
b. Unstabilizes the structure of mRNA
c. Stabilizes the structure of Rrna-Trna
d. Never happens in RNA

Ans. (a) Stabilizes the structure of DNA

49. Clustalw does

a. Local alignment
b. Global alignment
c. Partial alignment
d. Multiple alignment editing

Ans. (d) Multiple alignment editing

50. The variation in DNA sequence that occurs on average once every 300–500 bp are known as

a. Point mutation
b. Polymorphism
c. Insertion
d. Deletion

Ans. (b) Polymorphism

51. A map showing the position of expressed DNA region relative to a particular

Chromosomal region is named as
a. c-DNA map
b. a-DNA map
c. z-DNA map
d. None of these

Ans. (a) c-DNA map

52. RNA polymerase II binds to the transcription initiation site known as

a. Black box   b. White box
c. TAGA box   d. TATA box

Ans. (d) TATA box

53. The program that implements gene structure prediction by using information on homologous protein is

a. ORF gene   b. Profound
c. B Link   d. SIM

Ans. (a) ORF gene

54. Translate is a bio-tool used for

a. Protein mass fingerprinting
b. Translation of nucleotide
c. Identifying the protein function
d. Topology prediction

Ans. (b) Translation of nucleotide

55. The previous name of Swiss PDB viewer was

a. Swiss view   b. Mole view
c. Deep view   d. Modelling view

Ans. (c) Deep view

56. In Swiss PDB viewer the colour of the first element of secondary structure is

a. Red   b. Violet
c. Green   d. White

Ans. (a) Red

57. In Deep View the colour of the last element of secondary structure is

a. Red   b. Green
c. White   d. Violet

Ans. (a) Red

58. The most popular plot, phi-psi plot, for protein conformation is known as

a. Raja raman plot
b. Ram mohan plot
c. Ram chandran plot
d. Ronald ross plot

Ans. (c) Ram chandran plot

59. How many windows are generated for opening RASMOL?

a. One   b. Two
c. Three   d. Four

Ans. (b) Two

60. Vntrs refers to

a. Variable number tandem repeat
b. Variable number of template region
c. Variable number of template recognition site
d. None of these

Ans. (a) Variable number tandem repeat

61. Two genes are said to be paralogous

    a. When they are not orthologous

    b. When there are no evidences of GENE duplication

    c. When two copies of the duplicated gene and their progeny are found in the evolutionary lineage

    d. None of these

Ans. (c) When two copies of the duplicated gene and their progeny are found in the evolutionary lineage

62. The number of edges that meet at every branch nolde of the phylogenetic tree is

    a. Two

    b. Three

    c. Four

    d. Any one of them are possible

Ans. (d) Any one of them are possible

63. If there are nine leaves in a phylogenetic tree then how many nodes are present in this rooted tree?

    a. Eight   b. Ten

    c. Seventeen   d. Twenty

Ans. (d) Twenty

64. Which of the following is not correct?

    a. RNA Data bank was established by Japan

    b. National Biochemical Research Foundation established the Protein Information System in 1984.

    c. National center for bioinformatics Institute was established in USA and serves as primary information databank and provider of information

    d. None of these

Ans. (a) RNA Data bank was established by Japan

65. Which of the following is not correct?

    a. In single letter codes, R denotes guanine or adenine, while Y denotes thymine or cytosine.

    b. Base sequence runs from the 3′ to the 5′ direction

    c. In database, base sequence of ony one strand is listed

    d. The nomenclature system adapted in bioinformatics is based on the recommendations of international Union of pure and applied chemistry.

Ans. (b) Base sequence runs from the 3′ to the 5′ direction

66. Motif is a

    a. Secondary structure

    b. Tertiary structure

    c. Super secondary structure

    d. Quaternary structure

Ans. (b) Tertiary structure

67. Macromolecular crystallographic information file format is the input file format of

    a. Cn3D   b. DALI

    c. SPDV   d. None of these

Ans. (a) Cn3D

68. Database on DNA sequences contain which of the following types of sequence

    a. Genomic DNA and cDNA sequence

    b. EST and GST sequences

    c. Organelle DNA sequence and sequences of other molecules such as t-RNA small RNAs.

    d. All of the above

Ans. (d) All of the above

69. Which of the following is correct about EST sequence?

    a. One of the problems with ESTs is duplication

    b. These sequences are obtained by sequencing only a part of the C-DNA

    c. The sequences are dubbed as tags

    d. All of the above

Ans. (d) All of the above

70. Which of the following is an example of major nucleotide sequence database?

    a. Gene Bank held by NCBI, USA

    b. DNA databank of Japan

    c. Nucleotide sequence database main tained by EMBL

    d. All of the above

Ans. (d) All of the above

71. Which of the following databases is used by ENTREZ for bibliographic or citation search?

    a. PDB   b. TrEMBL

    c. PubMed   d. SWISS-PORT

Ans. (c) PubMed

72. Which of the following software have not been developed for the prediction/detection of genes from genome sequence of eukaryotes?

    a. GENMARK

    b. GENIE

    c. HMM Gene and GRAIL

    d. Gene finder and GENESCAN

Ans. (a) GENMARK

73. Which of the following approaches have been used for the identification of genes?

    a. Northern   b. Exon trapping

    c. Zoo blot   d. All of the above

Ans. (d) All of the above

74. Which of the following programmes can be used for the identification/detection of genes from genome sequence of prokaryotes?

a. Genefinder   b. Geneglamer

c. Genmark   d. None of the above

Ans. (c) Genmark

75. The colour of phosphorus atom is RasMol is

a. White   b. Yellow

c. Red   d. Orange

Ans. (d) Orange

76. The software that takes file input in mmdb format is

a. Cn3D   b. RasMol

c. SPDV   d. PyMoL

Ans. (a) Cn3D

77. The proper order in protein modelling is

a. Loop modelling , side chain modelling, backbone generation

b. Template recognition, alignment correction, backbone generation

c. Model validation, loop modelling, model evaluation

d. Backbone generation, model evaluation, side chain modeling

Ans. (b) Template recognition, alignment correction, backbone generation

78. The key 's' is used in Cn3D for

a. Rotation   b. Zooming in

c. Zooming out   d. Stopping rotation

Ans. (d) Stopping rotation

79. In homology medelling the most suitable BLAST is

a. PSI-BLAST   b. PHI-BLAST

c. GEO-BLAST   d. RP BLAST

Ans. (a) PSI-BLAST

80. The expansion of NMR is

a. Nuclear magnetic resonance

b. Non-magnetic resource

c. Nuclear magnetic resolution

d. Nuclear magnetic resource

Ans. (a) Nuclear magnetic resonance

81. Which of the following bioinformatics tools can be used for the identification of protein motifs and protein domains?

a. BOCKS   b. SMART

c. PRINTS   d. All of the above

Ans. (d) All of the above

82. Which of the following is used for comparing the submitted nucleotide sequence with nucleotide database?

a. BLASTx   b. BLASTt

c. BLAST n   d. t-BLASTn

Ans. (c) BLAST n

83. Commercial software for both protein and nucleotide mutation is

a. DALI   b. PyMoL

c. Biopolymer   d. VAX

Ans. (b) PyMoL

84. The percentage of safe zone in homology modelling is

a. ≥40%   b. ≥25%

c. ≥30%   d. ≥20%

Ans. (c) ≥30%

85. Swiss-model is

a. Protein database

b. Modelling database

c. Commercial modelling software

d. Protein homology modelling server

Ans. (d) Protein homology modelling server

86. CPK is

a. Colin paul Kit

b. Corey pauling Kultum

c. Canning Pam Kokin

d. None of these

Ans. (b) Corey pauling Kultum

87. The commercial software for energy minimization is

a. GROMOS96   b. DISCOVER

c. GROMACS   d. ROSSETA

Ans. (a) GROMOS96

88. Internal evaluation of homology model is done by

a. Porcheck   b. CASP

c. Verfy 3D   d. All of these

Ans. (a) Porcheck

89. Threading is a method of

a. X-ray crystallography

b. Circular dichroism

c. Protein modelling

d. Ab initio protein modeling

Ans. (c) Protein modelling

90. Verify 3D is used for

a. Model optimization
b. Loop modelling
c. External evaluation of model
d. Side-chain modeling

Ans. (c) External evaluation of model

91. Which of the following is used for comparing the submitted nucleotide sequence with amino acid sequence database?

a. BLASTx
b. BLASTt
c. BLAST n
d. t-BLASTx

Ans. (d) t-BLASTx

92. Which of the following is used for comparing the submitted amino acid sequence with nucleotide sequence database?

a. BLASTx
b. BLASTt
c. t-BLAST n
d. t-BLASTx

Ans. (c) t-BLAST n

93. Deep view accepts which of the following input files

a. Only PDB file
b. PDB, Cn3, and text files
c. Cn3, PDB, and Molfiles
d. PDB, Mol, mm CIF, and text files

Ans. (d) PDB, Mol, mm CIF, and text files

94. We can build 3D model of

a. Template
b. Tourism
c. Target
d. Turns of a protein

Ans. (a) Template

95. The alogithem used for energy minimization is Swiss-Model is

a. GROMOS96
b. GROMACS
c. Dnergy M
d. CharmM

Ans. (a) GROMOS96

96. Give the expansion of PHD, the protein secondary structure prediction software

a. Protein helix determination
b. Purely heetic days
c. Profile network from heidelberg
d. Protein of highest dimension

Ans. (c) Profile network from heidelberg

97. Which of the following one is threading software?

a. Libra I
b. PREDATOR

c. MODELLER
d. BUILDER

Ans. (c) MODELLER

98. The whole set of mRNA molecules in one or more population of biological cell in a specific environment is known as

a. Genome
b. Proteome
c. Transcriptome
d. Metabolome

Ans. (c) Transcriptome

99. The universal genetic code was discovered in

a. 1953
b. 1966
c. 1991
d. 1997

Ans. (b) 1966

100. Pdb2cif generates

a. CIF from PDB
b. mmCIF from PDB
c. Pseudo-PDB from PDB
d. All of these

Ans. (b) mmCIF from PDB

101. The first protein to be sequenced is

a. Insulin
b. Haemoglobin
c. Myosin
d. Tannin

Ans. (a) Insulin

102. The first biological sequence database was a

a. Nucleotide sequence database
b. Protein database
c. Transcriptone database
d. None of these

Ans. (b) Protein database

103. Name the database of genetic disorders and traits in animals, other than human and mouse

a. OMIM
b. OMIA
c. Cancer chromosome
d. EMB net

Ans. (b) OMIA

104. Gene expression data retrieval system of NCBI is

a. Entrez
b. GEO
c. SRS
d. Sakura

Ans. (a) Entrez

105. The data of molecular Modelling Database are sourced from

a. Protein information resource
b. Entrez protein
c. Protein data bank
d. UniProt

Ans. (c) Protein data bank

106. GENSAT is

a. A tool to predict genes
b. Atlas of gene expression data of CNS of mouse
c. Atlas of predicted genes within a species
d. None of these

Ans. (b) Atlas of gene expression data of CNS of mouse

107. The proteins showing clear evolutionary relationship are grouped under same

a. Fold
b. Family
c. Super family
d. Domain

Ans. (b) Family

108. Name the database that deals with structure classification

a. SCOP
b. CATH
c. VAST
d. All of these

Ans. (a) SCOP

109. Cn3D is a

a. Molecular file format
b. Molecular viewer
c. Molecular file format conversion
d. All of these

Ans. (b) Molecular viewer

110. Who introduced the concept of distinct species of animals and plants:

a. Johan Ray
b. Carolus Linneeus
c. W. fleming
d. None

Ans. (a) Johan Ray

111. Who said"computers are to bilogy,what mathematics is to physics":

a. T. K. Ottwood
b. Harold Morowitz
c. Charles
d. a and b.

Ans. (b) Harold Morowitz

112. Which is not the application of bioinformatics:

a. Biodiversity
b. DNA Forensic
c. Classes
d. None of these

Ans. (c) Classes

113. In which year DBT launch the BTIS:

a. 1986
b. 1985
c. 1988
d. 1990

Ans. (a) 1986

114. Institute of Microbial Technology related to:

a. Plant tissue culture
b. Animal cell culture
c. Protein modelling
d. Nucleic acid sequencing

Ans. (c) Protein modelling

115. In which year plan recommended to set NBI under DBT:

a. 10th
b. 9th
c. 5th
d. 6th

Ans. (c) 5th

116. Which institute provide distance learning program in bioinformatics in the country:

a. BII
b. IIT
c. None of these
d. Both of these

Ans. (a) BII

117. In which year Switzerland Institute(SBI) of Bioinformatics is established:

a. 30 March, 1998
b. 28 May, 1997
c. 14 April, 1994
d. 11 june, 1999

Ans. (a) 30 March, 1998

118. Which of these is not a protein sequence database:

a. PDB
b. PIR
c. Gene bank
d. Swiss

Ans. (c) Gene bank

119. Global alignment uses algorithm:

a. Needleman-wunsch algorithm
b. Dot Plots
c. DALI
d. PDB

Ans. (a) Needleman-wunsch algorithm

120. FASTA was first described by:

a. Lipmann and pearson
b. Kyte and dolittle
c. None of these
d. Both of these

Ans. (a) Lipmann and pearson

121. TAP tags are useful for:

a. Proteome exploration
b. Protein resolution
c. Genome sequencing
d. Nucleotide sequencing

Ans. (a) Proteome exploration

122. Bioinformatics cannot analyse:

a. Chemical analysis
b. Biomedical analysis
c. Statistical analysis
d. Mathematical analysis

Ans. (c) Statistical analysis

123. URL for NCBI is:

a. www.ncbi.nlm.nih.gov
b. www.ncbi.gov
c. www.ncbi.nlm.gov
d. www.ncbi.nic.in

Ans. (a) www.ncbi.nlm.nih.gov

124. FASTA algorithm was published by:

a. Altschul et al.
b. F.Sangar
c. None
d. Both

Ans. (a) Altschul et al.

125. BLAST's statistical theory was developed by:

a. Samul Karim and Steven Altschul
b. Josheph Sambrook
c. None of these
d. F. sangar

Ans. (a) Samul Karim and Steven Altschul

126. PDB is:

a. Primary database for macromolecules
b. Composite database
c. None
d. Both of these

Ans. (a) Primary database for macromolecules

127. Scop is:

a. Structural database,which identify structural and evolutionary relationships
b. It is primary database
c. None
d. Both

Ans. (a) Structural database, which identify structural and evolutionary relationships

128. CLUSTA family of programs are:

a. Multiple sequence analysis
b. Phylogenetic analysis

c. Both of these
d. None of these

Ans. (c) Both of these

129. In routine work which language is used in bioinformatics:

a. Alphabet-nucleotide
b. Words-gene(pork)
c. Both of these
d. None of these

Ans. (c) Both of these

130. PRINTS are software used for:

a. Identification of functional domains of proteins
b. Detection of t RNA gene
c. None of these
d. Both a and b

Ans. (a) Identification of functional domains of proteins

131. Gene Bank and SWISS PROT are examples of:

a. Primary database
b. Composite database
c. Secondary database
d. None of these

Ans. (a) Primary database

132. Which is the model organism database:

a. GOLD
b. SGD
c. SCOP
d. PAD

Ans. (b) SGD

133. BLAST and FASTA programs is used for:

a. End free space alignment
b. Global similarity
c. Local similarity
d. Both a and b

Ans. (a) End free space alignment

134. BLASTX program is used for:

a. Translate input sequence
b. Translate DNA database
c. None
d. Both of these

Ans. (a) Translate input sequence

135. BLOSUM matrices are used for:

a. Pair wises equence alignment
b. Phylogenetic analysis
c. Protein analysis
d. Both a and b

Ans. (a) Pair wises equence alignment

136. One major difference between BLAST and FASTA is:

a. If requires a preformatted search database
b. BLASTA is word based method
c. FASTA is word based method
d. None of these

Ans. (a) If requires a preformatted search database

137. To match protein quarry against translated nucleotide database you will use:

a. TBLASTX   b. TBLASTY
c. TBLASTR   d. TBLASTZ

Ans. (a) TBLASTX

138. Full form of DDBJ:

a. data Bank of Japan
b. DNA data Bank of Journal
c. DNA data bank of japan
d. None

Ans. (c) DNA data bank of japan

139. Full form of EBI:

a. European Bioinformatics Institute
b. Egypt Bioinformatics Institute
c. None of these
d. Both a and b

Ans. (a) European Bioinformatics Institute

140. SRS is:

a. Sequence retrival system
b. System retrival sequence
c. Sequence retro system
d. None

Ans. (a) Sequence retrival system

141. Database of enzymatic pathway, and biological chemicals is:

a. COG's   b. KEGG
c. SEOP   d. SCOP

Ans. (b) KEGG

142. Which stain can be used for staining gel in proteomics experiment:

a. Silver stain   b. Furoscent stain
c. Both   d. None of these

Ans. (b) Furoscent stain

143. CCMB Institute works in which discipline:

a. Oncogenes   b. Cell transfer
c. Both   d. None of these

Ans. (c) Both

144. India has initiated genome sequencing project of which of the following?

a. Rice   b. Wheat
c. Pigeonpea   d. Tomato

Ans. (c) Pigeonpea

145. Sequence of the 24 human chromosomes was completed in which year?

a. 2002   b. 2003
c. 2006   d. 2009

Ans. (c) 2006

146. Which of the following is correct about genome annotation?

a. DAS is useful in indexing and visualization
b. GAME is a programmed for describing experimental evidence to support annotation
c. Bio Perl 2001 is used for storing-manipuating and visualizing the genome annotation.
d. All of the above

Ans. (d) All of the above

147. Which of the following approach can be used for gene identification?

a. C-DNA selection   b. C-DNA capture
c. Exon trapping   d. All of the above

Ans. (d) All of the above

148. The sequence of a human genome has now many nucleotide pairs?

a. 3.8×10^6 b. 3.0×10^6
c. 3.2×10^6 d. 3.5×10^6

Ans. (c) 3.2×10^6

149. Which of the following is concerned with the development and application of computer hardware and software for acquisition, storage, analysis and visualization of biological information?

a. Bioinformatics
b. Computer science
c. Biotechnology
d. Information technology

Ans. (a) Bioinformatics

150. Which of the following procedure can be used for the identification/discovery of SNPs?

a. Microarray
b. Analyzing the sequence data
c. DNA chip
d. All of the above

Ans. (d) All of the above

151. National biomedical research foundation serves as

a. Primary information data bank
b. Protein information system
c. Both a and b
d. None of these

Ans. (b) Protein information system

152. National biomedical research foundation was established in:

a. 1983   b. 1984
c. 1985   d. 1986

Ans. (b) 1984

153. European molecular biology laboratory endeavours to:

a. Collect, organise and distribute nucleotide sequence data
b. Primary information data bank
c. Protein information system
d. All of these

Ans. (a) Collect, organise and distribute nucleotide sequence data

154. The freeware commonly used for genome assembly is/are

a. Phred   b. Phrap
c. Consed   d. All of these

Ans. (d) All of these

155. National centre of bioinformation was established in:

a. USA   b. Japan
c. England   d. China

Ans. (a) USA

156. Which of the following refers to next gen sequencing?

a. 454 pyro sequencing   b. Illunina sequencing
c. Solid sequencing   d. All of these

Ans. (d) All of these

157. National centre of Bioinformation serves as:

a. Primary information data bank
b. Provides of information
c. Both a and b
d. None of these

Ans. (c) Both a and b

158. The sequencing data is recorded in the form of:

a. PDF   b. RTF
c. SCF   d. DOC

Ans. (c) SCF

159. Whole genome sequencing can be done by:

a. Whole genome shot gun method
b. Hierarchical clone by clone method
c. Both a and b
d. None of these

Ans. (c) Both a and b

160. In Sangers method of sequencing, which of the following is used in chain termination?

a. TAMRA   b. RGG
c. GIIO   d. dd NTP

Ans. (d)

161. Bioinformatics encompasses which of the following:

a. Biology
b. Computer science
c. Information technology
d. All of these

Ans. (d) All of these

162. Sequence retrival system developed by:

a. PAM matrix
b. BLOSUM matrix
c. RNA sequences
d. Thure Etzold

Ans. (d) Thure Etzold

163. The scoring matrix for protein sequences is

a. PAM matrix   b. BLOSUM matrix
c. RNA sequences   d. Thure Etzold

Ans. (a) PAM matrix

164. Which is not correct about printed oligonucleotide chips?

a. These are produced by a light directed printing technology
b. These chips have double stranded oligonucleotides of 20–25 bases
c. Oligonucleotides are synthesized directly onto the chips
d. Each sequence is represented by a set of 20 non overlapping oligonucleotides to reduce false positive

Ans. (b) These chips have double stranded oligonucleotides of 20–25 bases

165. The programme is used to compare a nucleotide sequence with a nucleotide sequence database is;

a. BLASTn   b. BLASTx
c. BLASTp   d. Both a and b

Ans. (a) BLASTn

166. Sequencing of the 24 human chromosomes was completed in which year?

    a. 2000   b. 2002

    c. 2004   d. 2006

Ans. (d) 2006

167. It compare the submitted protein sequence against a protein database is:

    a. BALST n   b. BLASTx

    c. BLAST p   d. tBLSTn

Ans. (c) BLAST p

168. Which is not correct about NIH guidelines?

    a. The first NIH guidelines were prepared in 1975

    b. NIH guidelines were more liberal than the recommendations of the Asilomar conference

    c. The guidelines wrer revised after two year

    d. In 1977, NIH prepared an Environmental Impact Statement

Ans. (b) NIH guidelines were more liberal than the recommendations of the Asilomar conference

169. Which approach can be used for gene identification?

    a. Exon trapping   b. c-DNA capture

    c. c-DNA selection   d. All of these

Ans. (d) All of these

170. shot gum sequencing was conceptualized by:

    a. Giovannoni   b. Young

    c. Michelmore   d. Craig venter

Ans. (d) Craig venter

171. The strategy uses nucleic acid hybridization in colony hybridization or chromosome walking/jumping or is based on PCR is:

    a. Sequence-dependent screening

    b. Sequence-tagged microsatellites sites

    c. Sequence-tagged cite

    d. Single Locus Probe Analysis

Ans. (a) Sequence-dependent screening

172. Which is not correct?

    a. In databases, base sequence of only one strand is listed

    b. Base sequences runs from the 3′ to the 5′ direction

    c. In single letter codes, R denoted guanine or adenine, while Y denotes thymine or cytosine

    d. The nomenclature system adapted in bioinformatics is based on the recommendation of international Union of Pure and Applied chemistry

Ans. (b) Base sequences runs from the 3′ to the 5′ direction

173. First of all c-DNA of the mRNA is produced using the enzymes reverse transcriptase; the cDNA single strand is then used for amplification to obtain cDNA deplexes:

    a. Random amplified polymorphic DNA

    b. Pulsed field gel electrophoresis

    c. Restriction fragment length Polymorphism

    d. Reverse transcription PCR

Ans. (d) Reverse transcription PCR

174. India has initiated genome sequencing project of:

    a. Rice   b. Tomato

    c. Pigeon   d. Human

Ans. (a) Rice

175. Which is not correct?

    a. The public funded Human Genome project employed the clone by clone celera Genomics followed whole genome shot gun approach

    b. Clone by clone approach is based on contigs

    c. In the whole genome shot-gun approach, genome DNA is sheared to obtain 2 to 10 kb fragments, which are then cloned and sequenced from both the ends

    d. Assigning biological functions to the DNA sequencens using a variety of tools and technology is described as structural genome

Ans. (d) Assigning biological functions to the DNA sequencens using a variety of tools and technology is described as structural genome

176. Sequencing of the 24 human chromosome was completed in which year?

    a. 2006   b. 2000

    c. 2004   d. 2010

Ans. (a) 2006

177. The first comprehensive collection of amino acid sequences was compiled in the Atlas of protein sequence and structure by

    a. European Bioinformatics Institute

    b. National Biomedical Research foundation

    c. National Centre for Boinformatics Information

    d. European Molecular Biology Laboratory

Ans. (b) National Biomedical Research foundation

178. Which is not correct?

    a. RecA strains lack recombination

    b. Transposon vectors lacking transposase gene are not able to transpose to other bacteria

c. Auxotrophic mutants can survive in nature

d. Transgenes integrated into plasmids may be transferred to other bacteria

Ans. (c) Auxotrophic mutants can survive in nature

179. The type of regulation necessary during field trials should depend on:

a. Ability of the modified plants to survive in nature

b. Their ability for dispersal and reproduction

c. Their ability to hybridize with crop and weed plants

d. All of these

Ans. (d) All of these

180. Which is not correct about TaqMan Probes?

a. They are oligonucleotides longer than the primers

b. They contain a fluorescent dye usually on the 5' base, and a quenching dye typically on the 3' base

c. When Taq polymerase replicates a tempelate to which a Taq Man probe is paired, its 5' exonuclease activity cleavage the TaqMan probe

d. The fluorescence decreases proportionately to PCR amplification

Ans. (d) The fluorescence decreases proportionately to PCR amplification

181. Which is correct about genome annotation?

a. GAME is a programme for describing experimental evidence to support annotation

b. DAS is useful in indexing and visualization

c. BioPerl 2001 is used for storing, manipulating and visualizing the genome annotation

d. All of these

Ans. (d) All of these

182. Which database is used by ENTREZ for bibliographic or citation search?

a. SWISS PROT
b. PDB
c. TrEMBL
d. PubMed

Ans. (d) PubMed

183. Which is not correct about NIH guidelines?

a. A major revision of the guidelines was effected in 1982

b. In the revision, the containment levels were made more stringent

c. Experiments that were previously prohibited, were changed to category requiring review and approval by NIH

d. In USA, the NIH guidelines are followed by all federal agencies that fund research on recombinant DNA

Ans. (b) In the revision, the containment levels were made more stringent

184. Database on DNA sequence contain which types of sequences?

a. EST and GST sequences

b. Genomic DNA and cDNA sequences

c. Organellar DNA sequences and sequences of other molecular such as tRNA, small RNAs

d. All of the above

Ans. (d) All of the above

185. India has not been involved in sequencing the genomes of which organisms as:

a. Pigeon
b. Rat
c. Pigeonpea
d. Humans

Ans. (d) Humans

186. The rough draft of human genome was announced on:

a. May 26, 2001
b. June 26, 2001
c. July 26, 2001
d. June 26, 2002

Ans. (b) June 26, 2001

187. Which programmes can be used for the identification on/detection of genes from genome sequence of prokaryotes?

a. Glimmer
b. Genmark
c. Genefinder
d. Both a and b

Ans. (d) Both a and b

188. Which is the example of major nucleotide sequence database?

a. DNA databank of JAPAN

b. Nucleotide sequence Database maintained by EMBL

c. Gene Bank Held by NCBI, USA

d. All of these

Ans. (d) All of these

189. Implements the sequential growing strategy of building up the molecular from a single starting block known as the seed by:

a. Grow module
b. Lig Builder
c. POCKET module
d. Link module

Ans. (a) Grow module

190. The binding site of the target proteins and derives the key interaction site within this site is:

a. Grow module
b. Lig Builder
c. POCKET module
d. Link module

Ans. (c) POCKET module

191. Lig Builder programme basically consists of:

a. POCKET   b. GROW

c. LINK   d. None of these

Ans. (a) POCKET

192. Phylogeny usually described:

a. Plant   b. Tree

c. Ferns   d. Algae

Ans. (b) Tree

193. A de novo ligand design program which build ligands from library of organic fragments taking into consideration the structural consist of the target proteins is:

a. Lig Builder   b. POCKET module

c. GROW module   d. Link module

Ans. (a) Lig Builder

194. To introduce a mathematical formulation to determine the potential energy of a molecular called:

a. Microarray

b. Molecular force field

c. Shot gun sequencing strategy

d. Shot gun approach of sequence

Ans. (b) Molecular force field

195. The search tool can be used to match a sequence against the PROSISTE database is:

a. TBLASTN   b. TBLASTX

c. TBLASTE   d. PROMOT

Ans. (d) PROMOT

196. The programme is used to compare a nucleotide sequence with a nucleotide sequence database is:

a. TBLASTN

b. TBLASTX

c. TBLASTE

d. PROMOT

Ans. (b) TBLASTX

197. The step in implementing the algorithm for alignment using dynamic programming is:

a. Matrix initialization   b. Matrixfill

c. Trace back   d. All of these

Ans. (d) All of these

198. The sequence derived database are;

a. Protein   b. TrEMBL

c. Pfam   d. SWISS PORT

Ans. (c) Pfam

199. Secondary data base derived from PDB are the:

a. SCOP   b. PAM

c. PDB   d. Pfam

Ans. (a) SCOP

200. The dot plot was first described by:

a. Gibbs and McIntyre

b. Margaret Dayoff

c. Senger et al.

d. None of these

Ans. (a) Gibbs and McIntyre

CHECK YOU GRASP

1. The universal genetic code was discovered in

a. 1953   b. 1966

c. 1991   d. 1997

Ans. (b) 1966

2. Pdb2cif generates

a. CIF from PDB

b. mmCIF from PDB

c. Pseudo-PDB from PDB

d. All of these

Ans. (b)

3. The first protein to be sequenced is

a. Insulin   b. haemoglobin

c. Myosin   d. Tannin

Ans. (a) Insulin

4. PMC is

a. A digital archive of peer reviewed journals in life sciences

b. A protein Modelling center available at DDBJ

c. A secondary structure prediction tool

d. Aphylogeny method based on Maximum parsimony method

Ans. (a) A digital archive of peer reviewed journals in life sciences

5. Uniport stands for

a. Uniform protein database

b. Universal protein database

c. Universal polypeptide database

d. Unique protein database

Ans. (b) Universal protein database

6. BLASTX program is used for:

a. Translate input sequence

b. Translate DNA database

c. None

d. Both of these

Ans. (a) Translate input sequence

7. BLOSUM matrices are used for:

a. Pair wise sequence alignment

b. Phylogenetic analysis

c. Protein analysis

d. Both a and b

Ans. (a) Pair wise sequence alignment

8. In homology medelling the most suitable BLAST is

a. PSI-BLAST   b. PHI-BLAST

c. GEO-BLAST   d. RP BLAST

Ans. (a) PSI-BLAST

9. Bioinformatics can not analyse:

a. Chemical analysis

b. Biomedical analysis

c. Statistical analysis

d. Mathematical analysis

Ans. (c) Statistical analysis

10. URL for NCBI is:

a. www.ncbi.nlm.nih.gov

b. www.ncbi.gov

c. www.ncbi.nlm.gov

d. www.ncbi.nic.in

Ans. (a) www.ncbi.nlm.nih.gov

In case of less than 80% score, go through brief Review and Glance one again from chapter

Key: 1-b 2-b 3-a 4-a 5-b 6-a 7-a 8-a 9-c 10-a

12

Principle of Genetics and Plant Breeding

1. Mendel's law of segregation, as applied to the behavior of chromosome in meiosis, means that

 a. Paring of homologs will convert one allele into the other, leading to separation of the types

 b. Allels of a gene separate from each other when homologs separate in meiosis I

 c. Genes on the same chromosome will show 50% recombination

 d. Alleles of a gene will be linked and passed on together through meiaosis

Ans. (b) Allels of a gene separate from each other when homologs separate in meiosis I

2. The phenomenon of independent assortment refers to

 a. Expression at the same stage of development

 b. Unlinked transmission of genes in crosses resulting from being located on different chromosomes

 c. Association of an RNA and a protein implying related function

 d. Independent location of genes from each in an interphase cell

Ans. (b) Unlinked transmission of genes in crosses resulting from being located on different chromosomes

3. One of Mendel's pure strains of pea plants had green peas. How many different kinds of egg could such a plant produce with regard to pea colour?

 a. One   b. Two

 c. Three   d. Four

Ans. (a) One

4. List all the different gametes produced by the following individuals AA BB Cc aa Bb Cc

 a. 1. ABC, ABc ; 2. aBC, aBc , abC , abc

 b. 1. AbC, ABc ; 2. ABC, aBc, abC, aBC

 c. 1. ABC, ABC ; 2. aBC, aBc, abc, aBC

 d. 1. ABC, ABc ; 2. aBC, ABc, abc, abC

Ans. (a) 1. ABC, ABc ; 2. aBC, aBc , abC , abc

5. If a diploid cell contains six chromosomes, how many possible random arrangements of homologous could occur during Metaphasse-I?

 a. 4   b. 8

 c. 6   d. 64

Ans. (b) 8

6. 6. Determine the frequency of only one genotype, BBLI ,in the offspring of dihybrid parents (BbLI).

 a. 1/4   b. 1/8

 c. 1/16   d. 1/2

Ans. (b) 1/8

7. 7. If an individual of genotypes AaBbCcDd is test crossed, how many different phenotypes can appear in the progeny?

 a. 16   b. 8

 c. 32   d. 64

Ans. (a) 16

8. If individuals of genotypes AaBbCc are intercrossed, how many different phenotypes can appear their offspring?

 a. 16   b. 8

 c. 32   d. 64

Ans. (b) 8

9. If individual of genotypes AaBbCc are intercrossed, how many different genotypes can Occur in their progeny?

 a. 8   b. 64

 c. 27   d. 9

Ans. (c) 27

10. If individual of genotypes AaBbCc are intercrossed, how many different F_2 phenotypes can appear assuming complete codominance at all loci?

 a. 8   b. 64

 c. 27   d. 9

Ans. (c) 27

11. **A man is heterozygous B/b for one autosomal gene, and he carries a recessive X-linked allele d. What proportion of his sperm will be bd?**

a. 1/4
b. 1/8
c. 1/16
d. 1/2

Ans. (a) 1/4

12. **A trihybrid cross is made between two yeast, both with genotype A/a, B/b, C/c. What proportion of the offspring will be of genotype a/a, b/b, c/c?**

a. 1/8
b. 1/32
c. 1/64
d. 1 /74

Ans. (c) 1/64

13. **When heterozygous black pigs are intercrossed then what is the chance of the first two offspring being black?**

a. 46
b. 1/32
c. 1/64
d. 1/74

Ans. (b) 1/32

14. **Medical geneticists usually abbreviate the normal beta- globin gene as b, and the abnormal gene (in this case) as b^0 .Neither of your patient's parents has beta-thalassemia .Which of these described the most likely genotypes of both parents?**

a. none is b^0 and one in b
b. One is $b^0 b^0$ and one is bb
c. Both are $b^0 b^0$
d. Both are bb^0

Ans. (d) Both are bb^0

15. **If a man of blood group AB marries a woman of blood group A whose father was of blood group O, to what different blood group can this man and woman expect their children to belong?**

a. A, AB, B
b. A, AB
c. AB, O
d. A, O, B

Ans. (a) A, AB, B

16. **In the human ABO blood system, the alleles A and B are dominant to O, what will be the number of different possible genotype?**

a. 4
b. 8
c. 6
d. 12

Ans. (c) 6

17. **A brown mouse is mated with two female blackmice. when each female has produced several litters of young, the first female has had 48 black and the second female has 14 black and 11 brown young. deduce the pattern of inheritance coat colour and the genotype of all the parents (B-Black; b - brown)**

a. Male Bb; female 1, BB; female 2 Bb
b. Male BB; female 1, BB; female 2 Bb
c. Male Bb; female 1, BB; female 2 bb
d. None of the above

Ans. (d) None of the above

18. **Three genes (P, Q and R) are found of three different chromosome. For the following diploid genotypes, describe all of the possible gamete combinations and their predicted ratios.**

P. AABbCC   Q. AaBBCc   R. Aabbcc

a. P. 1ABC: 1AbC   Q. 1ABC: 1ABc: 1aBC: 1aBc
   R. 1Abc: 1abc
b. P. 1ABC: 1Abc   Q. 1abc : 1Abc: 1aBC: 1aBc
   R. 1abc: 1abc
c. P. 1ABC: 1Abc   Q. 1ABC: 1aBc: 1aBC: R. 1Abc:
   1abc
d. P. 1ABC: 1Abc   Q. 1ABC: 1Abc: 1aBC:R. 1Abc:
   1Abc

Ans. (a) P. 1ABC: 1AbC   Q. 1ABC: 1ABc: 1aBC: 1aBc
R. 1Abc: 1abc

19. **A true-breeding pea plant with round and green seeds is correct is crossed to a true -breeding plant with wrinkled and yellow seeds .Round and yellow seeds are the dominant traits .The F_1 plants are allowed to self-fertilize. What are the following probabilities for the F2 generation?**
P. An F2 plant with wrinkled, yellow seeds
Q. An F2 plant with round, yellow seeds

a. P. 2/16   Q. 9/16
b. P. 3/16   Q. 7/16
c. P. 3/16   Q. 9/16
d. Cannot be determined from the information

Ans. (c) P. 3/16 Q. 9/16

20. **In Guinea pig, black coat colour is a dominant trait and white is recessive trait .A black female is test crossed, producing six black offspring. The probability that heterozygous black would do this by chance alone is approximately**

a. 50%
b. 25%
c. 1%
d. Cannot be determined from the information

Ans. (a) 50%

21. What are the minimum progeny population sizes allowing for random union of all kinds of gametes from AaBbCc parent?

    a. 64

    b. 32

    c. 16

    d. 8

Ans. (a) 64

22. A red -flowered tall parent plant (PI) was crossed to a true breeding red-flowered dwarf plant (P2) and half of the progenies obtained was red and tall and the other half red and dwarf. In the next generation, half of all these progenies segregated only for flower colour and the other half segregated only for height . The genotype of the P1 is

    a. Heterozygous for colour and heterozygous for height

    b. Homozygous for colour and heterozygous for height

    c. Heterozygous for colour and homozygous for height

    d. Homozygous for colour and homozygous for height

Ans. (a) Heterozygous for colour and heterozygous for height

23. According to classical genetics, Which of the following statements is true?

    a. Recessive alleles are detected by the phenotype of the F_1 generation

    b. The closer two genes are, the more frequently they recombine

    c. Genes on different autosomes segregate independently

    d. Gene on sex chromosomes segregate with the same pattern as autosomal genes

Ans. (c) Genes on different autosomes segregate independently

24. Assuming the comparable chromosomes in different individuals are genetically dissimilar because of different alleles. How many unique zygotic combinations are possible following fertilization in an organism where n = 3 (Assuming that no crossing over occurs) ?

    a. 8

    b. 16

    c. 64

    d. 216

Ans. (c) 64

25. The colour of flowers of an annual species of plants is controlled by a single locus with two alleles R and r, and the genotypes RR, Rr and rr and red, pink and white respectively. A large number of seeds from individuals with pink flowers were collected and planted on an island, Where because of absence of pollinators, only self-pollination is possible. What will be the most likely outcome after 25 years?

    a. About 50% plants with red flowers 50 % with white flowers

    b. Almost 100% plants with pink flowers

    c. Red, pink, and white flowered plants in a ratio of 1:2:1

    d. Red, pink and white flowered plants in equal proportion

Ans. (c) Red, pink, and white flowered plants in a ratio of 1:2:1

26. Coat colour of dogs depend upon the action of at least two genes. At one locus a dominant epistatic inhibitor of colour pigment (A–) prevents the expression of colour at another independently assorting locus, producing white coat colour. when the recessive condition exists at the inhibitor locus (aa) the alleles of the hypostatic locus may be expressed, aaB-producing black and aabb producing brown. When dihybrid white dogs are together, determine the phenotypic proportions expected in the progeny.

    a. 9 : 7   b. 9 : 3 : 4

    c. 12 : 3 : 1   d. 13 : 3

Ans. (c) 12 : 3 : 1

27. Short hair in rabbits is governed by a dominant gene L and long hair by its recessive allele I. black hair results from the action of the dominant genotype B- and brown from the recessive genotype bb.

    a. In crosses between dihybrid short-haired, black and homozygous short-haired, brown rabbits, genotypic ratio will be 1 : 1 : 1 : 1

    b. In crosses between dihybrid short-haired, black and homozygous short-haired, brown rabbits, phenotypic ratio will be 1 : 1

    c. Expected phenotypic ratio from the cross LIBb x LIbb will be 3 : 3 : 1 : 1

    d. Expected genotypic ratio of LIBb will be ¼

Ans. a, b, c, and d

28. In a cross between two individuals with the genotypes AaBbccDdEeFf and AaBbCCDDeeff, the probability that an offspring will be heterozygous at all these loci is

    a. 0

    b. 1/16

c. 1/32

d. 1/64

Ans. (c) 1/32

29. Two pink-flowered four-o'clocks are crossed to each other. Flower colour is incompletely dominant and giving phenotypic ratio if 1 red : 2 pink : 1 white. What are the following probabilities?
P. The first three plants with while flower
Q. A plant with either white or pink flower

a. P. 1/64 Q. 3/4   b. P.3/16 Q. 1/64

c. P.3/64 Q.9/16   d. P. 1/64 Q.1/64

Ans. (a) P. 1/64 Q. 3/4

30. Which of the following is a mismatch?

a. Phenotypic F_2 ratio of 1 : 4 : 6 : 4 : 1-polygenic inheritance

b. Phenotypic F_2 ratio of 9 : 3 : 4-recessive epistasis

c. Phenotypic F_2 ratio of 1 : 2 : 1-codominance

d. Phenotypic F_2 ratio of 3 : 1-partial dominance

Ans. (d) Phenotypic F_2 ratio of 3 : 1-partial dominance

31. Why would you predict that half of the human babies born will be maies and half will be femaies?

a. Because of the segregation of the X and Y chromosomes during male meiosis

b. Because of the segregation of the X chromosomes during female meiosis

c. Because all eggs contain an X chromosome

d. Because, on average, one- half of all eggs produce females

Ans. (a) Because of the segregation of the X and Y chromosomes during male meiosis

32. Asymmetry between reciprocal crosses is seen in

a. Pleiotropy

b. Sex-linked inheritance

c. Interaction of genes

d. Autosomal inheritance

Ans. (b) Sex-linked inheritance

33. Which of the following is not true autosomal dominant traits?

a. Every affected person should have at least one affected parent

b. Males and females should be equally often affected

c. An affected person has a 50% chance of transmitting the dominant allele to each offspring

d. All the daughters of an affected male will be affected but none of the sons

Ans. (d) All the daughters of an affected male will be affected but none of the sons

34. Albinism is a recessive human trait. If a normal couple produces an albino child, what is the probability that their next child will be albino?

a. 1/4   b. 1/8

c. 1/16   d. 1/64

Ans. (a) 1/4

35. When a man with hypertrichosis marries a normal woman, what % of their sons would be expected to have hairy ears?

a. 50%   b. 100%

c. 0%   d. 25%

Ans. (b) 100%

36. A man with a certain disease marries a normal woman. They have 8 children (4 boys and 4 girls); all of the girls have their father's disease, but none of the boys do. What inheritance is suggested?

a. Autosomal recessive

b. Autosomal dominant

c. Y-linked

d. X-linked

Ans. (d) X-linked

37. Cystic fibrosis is a hereditary disease that affects the respiratory and digestive systems. Cystic fibrosis occurs when two recessive genes (cc) are present. A person with one allele for Cystic fibrosis is called a carrier (Cc) of the disease. If the mother is a carrier of the disease and the father is homozygous dominant, what are chances that their child will be carrier of Cystic fibrosis?

a. 25%   b. 50%

c. 75%   d. 100%

Ans. (b) 50%

38. Which of the following is/are correct about sex – linked recessive inheritance?

a. Most affected individuals are male

b. Affected females come from affected father and affected or carrier mothers

c. The sons of affected females should be affected

d. The trait does not skip generations

Ans. a, b, and c

39. Which of the following is/are not feature (s) of quantitative trait?

a. Characters of degree

b. Continuous variation

c. Polygenic control

d. Discontinuous variation

Ans. (d) Discontinuous variation

40. Which of the following are correct?

    a. Classical Mendelian traits are qualitative in nature
    b. Qualitative traits show discontinuous variations
    c. Qualitative traits are polygenic traits
    d. Qualitative traits are referred to as metric traits

Ans. a and b.

41. Wheat grain colour is controlled by four loci and following qualitative inheritance.

    P. Calculate the number of different F_2 phenotypes in a certain stock of wheat

    Q. Calculate the number of F_2 as extreme as one parent or the other

    a. P-9, Q-1/16   b. P-16, Q-1/256
    c. P-8, Q-1/32   d. P-9, Q-1/256

Ans. (d) P-9, Q-1/256

42. Two pure lines of corn have mean cob lengths of 9 and 3 inches, respectively. The polygenes involved in this trait all exhibit additive gene action. Crossing these two lines is expected to produce a progeny with mean cob length (in inches) of

    a. 12.0   b. 7.5
    c. 6.0   d. 2.75

Ans. (c) 6.0

43. In a plant, height varies from 6 to 36 cm. When 6 cm and 36 cm plants were crossed all F1 plants were 21 cm. In the F2 generation, a continuous range of heights was observed. Most were around 21 cm, and 3 of 200 were 6 cm. Find out how many gene pairs are involved in this mode of inheritance?

    a. 3   b. 4
    c 2   d. 5

Ans. (a) 3

44. If four chromosomes synapse into a cross-shaped configuration during meiotic prophase, the organism is heterozygous for a

    a. Pericentric inversion   b. Delection
    c Translocation   d. Paracentric inversion

Ans. (c) Translocation

45. Philadelphia chromosome is generated by translocation between

    a. Chromosome 18 and chromosome 6
    b. Chromosome 22 and chromosome 9
    c Chromosome 22 and chromosome 3
    d. Chromosome 16 and chromosome 4

Ans. (b) Chromosome 22 and chromosome 9

46. Retinoblastoma is caused by loss of both copies of the RB gene in the chromosome band

    a. 13p11   b. 13q11
    c. 3q14   d. 21q14

Ans. (c) 3q14

47. Position effect is the result of

    a. Mutations
    b. Deletions
    c Inversions
    d. Transversions

Ans. (c) Inversions

48. The bridge-fragment configuration at anaphase-1 is characteristic of

    a. Translocation heterozygote
    b. Paracentric inversion heterozygote
    c Pericentric inversion heterozygote
    d. Duplication heterozygote

Ans. (b) Paracentric inversion heterozygote

49. A mechanism that can cause a gene to move from one linkage group to another is

    a. Translocation   b. Inversion
    c. Crossing over   d. Duplication

Ans. (a) Translocation

50. Pseudodominance may be observed in heterozygotes for

    a. A deletion
    b. A duplication
    c. A reciprocal translocation
    d. More than one of the above

Ans. (a) A deletion

51. Which of the following chromosomal changes is usually the most damaging when in the homozygous condition?

    a. Deletion
    b. Duplication
    c. Translocation
    d. Inversion

Ans. (a) Deletion

52. In a trisomic individual the number of chromosome is

    a. 2n-1
    b. 2n+2
    c. 2n+3
    d. 2n+1

Ans. (d) 2n+1

53. A person with Klinefelter syndrome is considered a

a. Monosomic

b. Triploid

c. Trisomic

d. Delection heterozygote

Ans. (c) Trisomic

54. IF the garden pea has 14 chromosomes in its diploid complement, how many double trisomics could theoretically exist?

a. 6   b. 9

c. 16   d. 21

Ans. (d) 21

55. The condition in which there is too many or one too few chromosomes is called

a. Aneuploidy   b. Polytene

c. Polyploidy   d. Monoploidy

Ans. (a) Aneuploidy

56. Most cases of Down syndrome are caused by the presence of a third copy chromosome 21 associated with the chromosome 21 pair. This genetic condition, known as trisomy 21, is caused by

a. A frame-shift mutation

b. Chromosome nondisjunction

c. Fragile X syndrome

d. Chromosome transloction

Ans. (b) Chromosome transloction

57. Which statement about Downn's syndrome are correct?

a. The frequency increases dramatically in mothers over the age of 40

b. The cause is a non-disjunction when chromosomes do not separate during the first meiotic division

c. The long time lag between onset of meiosis in ovarian tissue and its completion (at ovulation) is most likely the reason for increased incidence in older mothers

d. All the above

Ans. (d) All the above

58. People with klinefelter syndrome have 47 chromosome, including three sex chromosome (XXY).What is the term to describe the aberration that occurs during meiosis that results in abnormal chromosome number

a. Crossing over

b. Non-disjunction

c. Independent assortment

d. Pairing of homologous chromosome

Ans. (b) Non-disjunction

59. The genes abcde are determined to be closely linked on the *E. coli* chromosome. Three random short deletions are created in the region, resulting in the removal of various genes are shown below. Which of the following gene orders is possible based on the deletion analysis?

Deletion 1: genes bde are lost

Deletion 1: genes ac are lost

Deletion 1: genes abd are lost

a. abcde   b. acded

c. bdeac   d. cabde

Ans. (d) cabde

60. Datura plants have been regenerated from anther cultures, endosperm culture and embryo culture. Their respective ploidy levels will be

a. n,2n and 2n   b. n,3n and 2n

c. n,2n and 3nn   d. 2n, 2n and 2n

Ans. (b) n,3n and 2n

61. Diagnosis of chromosome aneuploidy of unborn children is normally done by a combination of amniocentesis, cell culture, and

a. Enzyme assay

b. RRLP analysis

c. Pedigree analysis

d. Karyotyping

Ans. (d) Karyotyping

62. The Hardy- Weinberg law describes

a. Genotype frequencies of a population when evolutionary forces are not acting

b. How sexual reproduction would change the relative gene frequencies in a population

c. How mutations occur and balance each other

d. Genotype frequencies of a population when evolutionary forces are acting

Ans. (a) Genotype frequencies of a population when evolutionary forces are not acting

63. What are the assumptions of Hardy-Weinberg equilibrium?

a. Small population size, random mating, no selection, no migration, no mutation

b. Large population size, random mating, no selection, no migration, no mutation

c. Large population size, random mating, heterozygotes survive the best, no migration, no mutation

d. Large population size, random mating, no migrants enter from other populations,no mutation

Ans. (b) Large population size, random mating, no selection, no migration, no mutation

64. Genetic diversity is required for natural selection to act, but natural selection can reduce or eliminate diversity. What process can restore genetic diversity to a population?

    a. Genetic drift
    b. Mutation
    c. Sexual selection
    d. Stabilizing selection

Ans. (b) Mutation

65. Deviation from the Hardy-Weinberg assumption of infinitely large population size results in

    a. Genetic lethal
    b. Hetrozygote advantage
    c. Consanguinity
    d. Genetic drift

Ans. (d) Genetic drift

66. If to population are merged, each with different frequencies of an allele at a locus, and randomly mating occurs immediately, how long will it take to achieve a hardy-Weinberg equilibrium in the new population ?

    a. One generation
    b. Ten generations
    c. Variable-depends on allele frequencies
    d. The population will never achieve equilibrium

Ans. (a) One generation

67. In a population that is in equilibrium, the proportion of individuals showing the domain trait at a given locus having two alleles is 84%. The frequency of the recessive allele in the population is

    a. 0.4
    b. 0.3
    c. 0.2
    d. 0.16

Ans. (a) 0.4

68. How many A and a alleles are present in a sample of organisms consisting of 10 AA, 15Aa and 4aa individuals? What are the allele frequencies in the sample?

    a. A = 0.6; a = 0.40
    b. A = 0.4; a = 0.60
    c. A = 0.6; a = 0.6
    d. A = 0.4; a = 0.4

Ans. (a) A = 0.6; a = 0.40

69. In a diploid organism, what is the maximum number of alleles that can exist in a population for any given gene?

    a. a.1
    b. b.2
    c. c.4
    d. Unlimited

Ans. (d) Unlimited

70. Cystic fibrosis is an autosomal recessive inherited disease. ITS frequency in newborns is 1 in 1700. One of the following indicates the frequency of the disease carriers

    a. a.0.024
    b. 0.047
    c. 0.976
    d. 0.148

Ans. (b) 0.047

71. Which statement about allele frequencies in not true?

    a. The sum of any set of allele frequency is always 1
    b. If there are two alleles at a locus and we know the frequency of one of them, we can obtain the frequency of the other by subtraction
    c. If an allele is missing from a population, its frequency is 0
    d. If two populations have the same gene pool for a locus, they will have the same proportion of homozygotes at that locus

Ans. (d) If two populations have the same gene pool for a locus, they will have the same proportion of homozygotes at that locus

72. The ratio of phenotypes in F_2 of a monohybrid cross is

    a. 3:1
    b. 1:2:1
    c. 9:3:3:1
    d. 2:1

Ans. (a) 3:1

73. A pure tall Pea was crossed with a pure dwarf Pe a. All the plants of F_1 were found to be tall. This is due to

    a. Dominance
    b. Disappearance of factor for dwarfness in F_1 generation
    c. Segregation of factors
    d. Coordination

Ans. (a) Dominance

74. The monohybrid genotypic ratio 1:2:1 in F_2 generation indicates

    a. Segregation
    b. Independent assortment
    c. Dominance
    d. Incomplete dominance

Ans. (a) Segregation

75. A monohybrid cross is the one in which

    a. Only a single plant is involved for the experiment
    b. A single pair of contrasting characters is considered for the genetic results

c. A hybrid is crossed to a homozygous

d. None of the above

Ans. (b) A single pair of contrasting characters is considered for the genetic results

76. The F₂ generation of a cross produced identical phenotypic and genotypic ratio. It is not an excepted Mendelian result, and can be attributed to

    a. Independent assortment b. Linkage

    c. Incomplete dominance d. None of the above

Ans. (c) Incomplete dominance

77. The law of independent assortment can be related to one of the following

    a. Both homologous chromosomes of each pair are received by a single gamete

    b. The genes present on the same chromosome get randomly redistributed

    c. The non-homologous chromosomes show random distribution during anaphase-1 of meiosis

    d. The exchange of segments between the non-homologous chromosomes

Ans. (c) The non-homologous chromosomes show random distribution during anaphase-1 of meiosis

78. The law of segregation of characters postulated by Mendel can be related to

    a. The presence of two genes for each character in a somatic cell

    b. A gamete receiving only one of the two homologous chromosomes during meiosis

    c. Presence of both genes on the same chromosome

    d. None of the above

Ans. (b) A gamete receiving only one of the two homologous chromosomes during meiosis

79. The factors which represents the contrasting pairs of characters are called

    a. Dominant and recessive

    b. Alleles

    c. Homologous pairs

    d. Determinants

Ans. (b) Alleles

80. The back cross is

    a. A cross between F₁ individual and F₂ individual

    b. A cross between an F₁ individual with another F₁ individual

    c. Cross between F₁ and one of the two parents

    d. Cross between F₂ with one of the parents

Ans. (c) Cross between F₁ and one of the two parents

81. Mendel selected Pea as material for his experiments because

    a. It is an annual with comparatively short life cycle

    b. The flowers are self-pollinated

    c. The number of seeds produced is quite large

    d. All the above

Ans. (d) All the above

82. One of the following did not constitute the seven contrasting pairs of characters noticed by G.J. Mendel in Pea

    a. Height of the plants   b. Shape of the leaves

    c. Shape of pod   d. Colour of pod

Ans. (b) Shape of the leaves

83. In genetics the term test cross means

    a. The crossing of F₁ individual with homozygous recessive

    b. Crossing an F₁ individual with either of the two parents

    c. Crossing an F₁ individual with another F₁ individual

    d. Crossing F₁ individual with that of F₂

Ans. (a) The crossing of F₁ individual with homozygous recessive

84. The first work on genetics was done by

    a. Lamarck   b. Hugo de Vries

    c. Mendel   d. Darwin

Ans. (c) Mendel

85. According to the law of Independent Assortment in a dihybrid was done by

    a. There are four genotypes in F₂

    b. F₂ contains 16 phenotypes

    c. There is a single individual which is homozygous recessive for both the characters

    d. It is not possible to forecast the different phenotypes

Ans. (c) There is a single individual which is homozygous recessive for both the characters

86. The discipline which deals with the study of inheritance of characters is

    a. Darwinism   b. Cytology

    c. Genetics   d. Evolution

Ans. (c) Genetics

87. Who is regarded as the 'Father of Genetics'?

    a. Gregor Johann Mendel b. Morgan

    c. Lamarck   d. Hugo de Vries

Ans. (a) Gregor Johann Mendel

88. The number of different type of gametes produced from a plant with genotype Aa Bb Cc is

    a. 2   b. 8
    c. 4   d. 16

Ans. (b) 8

89. How many types of gametes are excepted from the organism with genotype AABBCC?

    a. One   b. Two
    c. Four   d. Eight

Ans. (a) One

90. How many types of gametes are expected from the plants with genotypes AA, BB, aa, bb?

    a. 7   b. 4
    c. 8   d. 16

Ans. (b) 4

91. A haploid set of all the genes present in a gamete is called

    a. Genotype   b. Phenotype
    c. Genome   d. Linkage group

Ans. (c) Genome

92. A plant with a genotype Aa Bb is crossed with a plant having the genotype aa bb. The genotype of F_1 would be

    a. AaBb, AABB
    b. aabb, aaBb
    c. aaBB, AAbb
    d. AaBb, Aabb, aaBb, abab

Ans. (d) AaBb, Aabb, aaBb, abab

93. Mendel was born in

    a. Australia   b. Heizendorf
    c. Maravia   d. Brunn

Ans. (b) Heizendorf

94. How many types of gametes are expected from a plant with genotype Pp Qq, provided there occurs independent assortment?

    a. 4   b. 8
    c. 2   d. 1

Ans. (a) 4

95. How would you test a Pea plant whether it is a pure or hybrid for tallness?

    a. Cross it with another tall Pea plant of unknown genotype
    b. Cross it with a pure tall Pea plant

    c. Cross with a homozygous dwarf Pea
    d. Cross it with any Pea plant

Ans. (c) Cross with a homozygous dwarf Pea

96. The Mendelian principle which has always stood true is

    a. The law of independent assortment
    b. The law of segregation
    c. The law of dominance
    d. All the above

Ans. (b) The law of segregation

97. Which of the following crosses would produce a genotypic ratio of 1:2:1 in F_2?

    a. AB × AB   b. Ab × ab
    c. Ab × Ab   d. Ab × ab

Ans. (c) Ab × Ab

98. In *Mirabilis jalapa* when two F_1 pink flowered plants were crossed with each other, the F_2 generation produced 40 red, 80 pink and 40 white flowering plants. This is a case of

    a. Duplicate genes
    b. Lethal genes
    c. Incomplete dominance
    d. Epistasis

Ans. (c) Incomplete dominance

99. The term genetics was coined by

    a. Mendel   b. Bateson
    c. Muller   d. Morgan

Ans. (b) Bateson

100. Genotype-phenotype concept was first proposed by

    a. Bateson
    b. Johannsen
    c. Sutton and Boveri
    d. Punnet

Ans. (b) Johannsen

101. At which stage is the fate of genetic constitution of gametes finally decided?

    a. Metaphase – I   b. Anaphase – I
    c. Anaphase – II   d. Interkinesis

Ans. (c) Anaphase – II

102. The phenomenon which defies the independent assortment is

    a. Segregation   b. Crossing over
    c. Dominance   d. Linkage

Ans. (d) Linkage

103. A tobacco plant heterozygous for albinism (a recessive character) is self pollinated and 1200 seeds are subsequently germinated. How many seedlings would have the parental phenotype?

    a. 900   b. 600
    c. 1200   d. 300

Ans. (b) 600

104. Mendel's law were rediscovered by

    a. Lamarck, de Vries and Correns
    b. Hugo de Vries, Correns and Tschermak
    c. Morgan, Beadle and Tatum
    d. Hugo de Vries, Morgan and Correns

Ans. (b) Hugo de Vries, Correns and Tschermak

105. When a yellow mouse was crossed to another yellow mouse, the F_1 generation produces yellow and brown-black mice in the ratio 2:1. The yellow mice are never homozygous. The reason is

    a. Homozygous yellow cannot survive due to lethal effect of genes
    b. Yellow mice are not very suitable to live
    c. There is no formation of zygotes with homozygous yellow constitution
    d. None of the above

Ans. (a) Homozygous yellow cannot survive due to lethal effect of genes

106. A pea with whit flowers was crossed to another pea which is also white flower plant. When selfed the F_2 generation produced purple and white in the ratio 9:7. The reason for the result is that

    a. It is typical monohybrid Mendelian ratio
    b. Purple flower colour is dominant over the white
    c. It is a complementary factor
    d. None of the above

Ans. (c) It is a complementary factor

107. Multiple alleles are present

    a. At different loci in the same chromosome
    b. In different chromosomes
    c. At the same locus in one type of chromosomes
    d. None of the above

Ans. (c) At the same locus in one type of chromosomes

108. An example of the quantitative trait in man is

    a. Hair colour
    b. Colour of eye
    c. Skin colour
    d. Shape of nose

Ans. (c) Skin colour

109. The law of segregation of characters is also called the law of purity of gametes because

    a. Gametes have only one of the two alleles for each character
    b. Gametes cannot be contaminated
    c. Gametes are very different type of cells
    d. It was just another name adopted accidentally

Ans. (a) Gametes have only one of the two alleles for each character

110. A dwarf pea plant was treated with G A. The plant became tall. The treated plant was then crossed with a homozygous tall pe a. The results in F_2 are expected to be

    a. All tall
    b. Tall and dwarf in 3:1 ratio
    c. 50% tall
    d. All dwarf

Ans. (b) Tall and dwarf in 3:1 ratio

111. Number of characters studies by Mendel in Pea was

    a. 5   b. 7
    c. 6   d. 4

Ans. (b) 7

112. The genes for same trait present on nonhomologous chromosomes are

    a. Alleles   b. Linked genes
    c. Multiple alleles d. None of these

Ans. (d) None of these

113. Mendel observed red flowers in F_1 when he crossed red and white because of

    a. Dominance
    b. Recessive gene
    c. Law of independent assortment
    d. Law of segregation

Ans. (a) Dominance

114. The genotypic ratio of a monohybrid cross will be

    a. 3:1   b. 1:1
    c. 1:2:1   d. 2:1

Ans. (c) 1:2:1

115. Mendel formulated the laws of heredity considering seven pairs of contrasting characters in the pea plant. If he had studied an eighth pair, the law which would have been altered is

    a. Law of segregation
    b. Law of dominance

c. Law of independent assortment

d. Law of unit characters

Ans. (c) Law of independent assortment

116. Mendel was successful in formulating the laws of inheritance whereas his predecessors were not because

a. He studied one clear-cut character at a time

b. The characters studied by him were present on separate chromosomes

c. Of the right choice of material

d. He kept accurate records of his experiments

Ans. (a) He studied one clear-cut character at a time

117. Appearance of hidden character in some progeny of F_2 population indicates

a. Law of purity of gametes

b. Law of independent assortment

c. Law of dominance

d. None of the above

Ans. (a) Law of purity of gametes

118. Mendel's law of segregation is based upon the F_2 ratio of

a. 1:2   b. 9:3:3:1

c. 1:2:1   d. 3:1

Ans. (d) 3:1

119. Mendel is popular for postulating

a. Origin of species   b. Cell theory

c. Linkage theory   d. Laws of inheritance

Ans. (d) Laws of inheritance

120. 'Like begets like' an important and universal phenomenon of life, is due to

a. Eugenics   b. Inheritance

c. Dominance   d. Crossing over

Ans. (b) Inheritance

121. Why were pea plants more suitable than dogs for Mendelian experiments?

a. Pea plants can be self-pollinated

b. All pea plants are diploid

c. There were no pedigree records of dogs

d. Dogs have many genetics traits

Ans. (a) Pea plants can be self-pollinated

122. A cross between unlike, organisms is called

a. Test-cross   b. Back-cross

c. Heterosis   d. Hybrid

Ans. (d) Hybrid

123. Genes do not occur in pairs in

a. Zygote   b. Somatic cell

c. Endosperm cells   d. Gametes

Ans. (d) Gametes

124. If dwarf pea plant was treated with GA_3 it grew as tall as the pure tall pea plant. If this treated plant is crossed with a pure tall plant the phenotypic ratio F_1 is likely to be

a. All tall

b. All dwarf

c. 50% tall and 50% dwarf

d. 75% tall and 25% dwarf

Ans. (a) All tall

125. A modified dihybrid mendelian ratio of 9:3:4 indicates

a. Supplementary genes

b. Complementary genes

c. Lethal genes

d. Epstatic genes

Ans. (a) Supplementary genes

126. Segregation of genes take place during

a. Metaphase

b. Anaphase

c. Prophase

d. Embryo formation

Ans. (b) Anaphase

127. A cross between hybrid and a parent is known as

a. Test cross   b. Back cross

c. Monohybrid cross   d. Reciprocal cross

Ans. (b) Back cross

128. A cross between offspring and recessive parent is

a. Monohybrid cross   b. Back cross

c. Test cross   d. Reciprocal cross

Ans. (c) Test cross

129. In an experiment on pea plant, pure plants with yellow round seeds (YYRR) were crossed with plants producing green wrinkled seeds (yyrr). What will be phenotypic ratio of F_1 progeny?

a. 9 yellow round : 3 round green : 3 wrinkled yellow: 1 green wrinkled

b. All yellow round

c. 1 round yellow : 1 round green : 1 wrinkled yellow: 1 wrinkled green

d. All wrinkled green

Ans. (b) All yellow round

130. Genetics deals with

a. Heredity and variations
b. Heredity
c. Mutations
d. Nuclear and cytoplasmic inheritance

Ans. (a) Heredity and variations

131. When a wheat variety of red kernels (homozygous for two nonallelic and independent dominant genes) is crossed with white kernelled wheat (homozygous for two recessive nonallelic independent genes), the phenotypic ratio in F_2 generation would be

a. $9:7$
b. $1:10:4:1$
c. $1:4:6:4:1$
d. $1:2:4:2:4:2:1$

Ans. (c) $1:4:6:4:1$

132. ABO blood grouping in humans is an example of

a. Polygenic inheritance
b. Multifactor inheritance
c. Pleiotropic gene
d. Multiple alleles

Ans. (d) Multiple alleles

133. In multiple allele system a gamete possesses

a. Two alleles
b. Three alleles
c. One allele
d. Several allele

Ans. (c) One allele

134. ABO blood grouping shows

a. Codominant genes
b. Polygenes
c. Dominant-recessive genes
d. Both codominant and dominant recessive genes

Ans. (d) Both codominant and dominant recessive genes

135. A pleiotropic gene is one which

a. Affects one character
b. Affects more than one character
c. Supplements the effect of another gene
d. Requires another gene for expression

Ans. (b) Affects more than one character

136. Sum total of all the genetic information in the breeding members of a population at a given time is known as

a. Gene pool
b. Genetic clone
c. Genome
d. Genetic drift

Ans. (a) Gene pool

137. The spread of genes from one breeding population to another by migration which may result in changes in gene frequency is called

a. Genetic drift
b. Gene flow
c. Gene frequency
d. None of the above

Ans. (b) Gene flow

138. Hb^A and Hb^S alleles of normal and sickle celled RBC are

a. Dominant-recessive alleles
b. Polygenic alleles
c. Codominant alleles
d. Multiple alleles

Ans. (c) Codominant alleles

139. A genetic clone is

a. Plants produced by asexual means
b. Hybrid produced by sexual means
c. Homozygous plant produced by sexual means
d. Heterozygous plant produced by sexual means

Ans. (a) Plants produced by asexual means

140. A pure tall plant is reared in a soil poor in nutrition and reached the size of dwarf plant. If this plant is selfed, the phenotype in the F_1 generation is most likely to be

a. All tall plants
b. 50% tall and 50% dwarf
c. All dwarf
d. Data insufficient

Ans. (a) All tall plants

141. A pleiotropic gene is

a. I^A
b. Hb^S
c. Hb^A
d. I^B

Ans. (b) Hb^S

142. Dominant gene for tallness is T and for yellow colour is Y. A plant heterozygous for both the traits is selfed, then the ratio of pure homozygous dwarf and green offspring would be

a. 1/4
b. 4/16
c. 3/16
d. 1/16

Ans. (d) 1/16

143. A gene that shows its effect on more than one character is

a. Polygene
b. Pleiotropic gene
c. Multifactor gene
d. Multiple gene

Ans. (b) Pleiotropic gene

144. **A dihybrid ratio of 1:4:6:4:1 is obtained instead of 9:3:3:1. This is an example of**
    a. Complementary genes
    b. Supplementary genes
    c. Polygenic inheritance
    d. Pleiotropic genes

Ans. (c) Polygenic inheritance

145. **In a dihybrid cross, F_2 phenotypic ratio is 13:3. It is case of**
    a. Complementary genes
    b. Epistatic genes
    c. Multigenic inheritance
    d. Incomplete dominance

Ans. (b) Epistatic genes

146. **Epistatic gene differs from dominant gene in**
    a. Epistatic gene is nonallelic
    b. Epistatic gene never expresses itself independently
    c. Epistatic and hypostatic genes are present at different loci
    d. All the above

Ans. (d) All the above

147. **Medel was**
    a. Plant breeder
    b. Cytologist
    c. Physiologist
    d. Taxonomist

Ans. (a) Plant breeder

148. **Mendel published his research under the title of**
    a. Laws of heredity
    b. Experiments in plant hybridization
    c. Hybridization experiments on Pea
    d. My experiments on particulate inheritance

Ans. (b) Experiments in plant hybridization

149. **The scientist who proposed particulate concept of inheritance was**
    a. Darwin   b. Galton
    c. Mendel   d. Garrod

Ans. (c) Mendel

150. **Hugo de Vries, a rediscoverer of Mendel's work belonged to**
    a. Holland   b. Austria
    c. Germany   d. England

Ans. (a) Holland

151. **Tschermak-Seysenegg, a rediscoverer of Mendel's work belonged to**
    a. USA   b. Spain
    c. Austria   d. Australia

Ans. (c) Austria

152. **Carl Correns, a rediscoverer of Mendel's work, was**
    a. American   b. German
    c. Austrian   d. Spanish

Ans. (b) German

153. **Siblings are**
    a. Sons and daughters of same parents
    b. Individuals formed through asexual means
    c. Individuals from interspecific cross
    d. Mutants

Ans. (a) Sons and daughters of same parents

154. **Offspring are individuals developed as a result of**
    a. Vegetative multiplication
    b. Asexual reproduction
    c. Sexual reproduction
    d. All the above

Ans. (c) Sexual reproduction

155. **Checkerboard method of calculations was developed by**
    a. Mendel   b. Bateson
    c. Punnet   d. Morgan

Ans. (c) Punnet

156. **An individual having similar unit factors of a character is**
    a. Heterozygote   b. Homozygote
    c. Dominant   d. Recessive

Ans. (b) Homozygote

157. **Punnet square is used to know**
    a. Outcome of a cross
    b. Probable result of a cross
    c. Types of gametes
    d. Result of meiosis

Ans. (b) Probable result of a cross

158. **Allele is**
    a. Segment of gene
    b. Form of a gene
    c. Special kind of gene
    d. A muton

Ans. (b) Form of a gene

159. Repeated selfing produces

a. Heterozygosity
b. Homozygosity
c. Homozygosity in some and heterozygosity in other traits
d. Pure hybrids

Ans. (b) Homozygosity

160. YyRR is crossed with yyRR. The progeny will be

a. 1 YyRR : 1 yyRR
b. 3 YyRR : 1 yyRR
c. 1 YyRR : 3 yyRR
d. YyRR only

Ans. (a) 1 YyRR : 1 yyRR

161. AaBb individual produces 2 million gametes. How many of them would carry both the recessive alleles (ab)

a. 1.5 million
b. 1.0 million
c. 0.5 million
d. 0.25 million

Ans. (c) 0.5 million

162. A double homozygous yellow round plant of Pea is crossed with green wrinkled plant. The offspring shall be of

a. One type
b. Two types
c. Four types
d. Several types

Ans. (a) One type

163. A dihybrid cross is made between YYrr and yyRR. In F_2 generation the ratio of parental to recombinant phenotype is

a. 9 : 7
b. 6 : 10
c. 10 : 6
d. 7 : 9

Ans. (b) 6 : 10

164. Percentage of pure breeding F_2 individuals of a monohybrid cross would be

a. 75%
b. 50%
c. 25%
d. 12.5%

Ans. (b) 50%

165. Double homozygous individuals in F_2 generation of a dihybrid cross would be

a. 1/16
b. 2/16
c. 6/16
d. 9/16

Ans. (b) 2/16

166. Ratio between completely homozygous dominant and homozygous recessive individuals of a dihybrid cross is

a. 1 : 1
b. 2 : 2
c. 6 : 10
d. 10 : 6

Ans. (a) 1 : 1

167. Ratio of parental and recombinant phenotypes in a dihybrid cross would be

a. 8 : 8
b. 6 : 10
c. 10 : 6
d. 9 : 7

Ans. (c) 10 : 6

168. Which mendelian principle will not operate if two genes under study are close together

a. Paired unit factors
b. Dominance
c. Segregation
d. Independent assortment

Ans. (d) Independent assortment

169. In a monohybrid cross the ratio of F_2 true breeding dominant and true breeding recessive would be

a. 50 : 50
b. 25 : 25
c. 75 : 25
d. 25 : 75

Ans. (b) 25 : 25

170. A single heterozygous yellow wrinkled seeded Pea plant shall produce gametes

a. YR only
b. yr only
c. Yr and yr
d. YR and yR

Ans. (c) Yr and yr

171. A couple with curly haired husband and straight haired wife have all their children curly haired because

a. Both are heterozygous
b. Husband is homozygous and wife is heterozygous
c. Husband is heterozygous while wife is homozygous
d. Both are homozygous

Ans. (d) Both are homozygous

172. Genes P and Q are both required in dominant state for normal hearing. A deaf couple has all children with normal hearing. The probable genotype for the couple is

a. PPqq × ppQQ
b. PPqq × PPqq
c. PpQq × ppqq
d. PPqq × ppQq

Ans. (a) PPqq × ppQQ

173. Name the scientist who converted Mendel's conclusions into principles of heredity

a. De Vries
b. Tschermak-seysenegg
c. Carl Correns
d. T.H. Morgan

Ans. (c) Carl Correns

174. Pure tall pea plant can be differentiated from hybrid tall pea plant by

a. Selfing and finding the progeny tall
b. Test cross with dwarf plant and finding the progeny tall
c. Selfing and test crossing to find the progeny of both tall and dwarf plants
d. Both a and b

Ans. (d) Both a and b

175. F_1 plants crossed with dominant individuals will yield a progeny of

a. All recessive
b. All dominants
c. Dominant and recessive in the ratio of 1 : 1
d. Dominant and recessive in the ratio of 3 : 1

Ans. (b) All dominants

176. Round seed trait (R) is dominant over wrinkled (r) seed trait in Pe a. Heterozygous round seeded plant (Rr) is crossed with wrinkled seeded plant (rr). What is the possibly progeny?

a. 302 round : 102 wrinkled
b. 210 round : 95 wrinkled
c. 105 round : 99 wrinkled
d. 103 round : 315 wrinkled

Ans. (c) 105 round : 99 wrinkled

177. A dihybrid yellow round seeded plant (YyRr) is crossed to another yellow round seeded plant. The progeny is also yellow round seeded plant. What is the genotype of the second plant?

a. YyRr
b. YYRR
c. YyRR
d. yyRr

Ans. (b) YYRR

178. A yellow round seeded pea plant is crossed with green wrinkled seeded pea plant. Four phenotypes appeared in the progeny in the ratio of 1 : 1 : 1 : 1. The genotype of the two are

a. YyRr and yyrr
b. YYRR and yyrr
c. YYRr and yyrr
d. YyRR and yyrr

Ans. (a) YyRr and yyrr

179. The ratio of 1 : 1 : 1 : 1 is obtained in case of

a. Monohybrid cross
b. Monohybrid test cross
c. Dihybrid cross
d. Dihybrid test cross

Ans. (d) Dihybrid test cross

180. Position of a gene on chromosome is called

a. Locus
b. Factor
c. Cistron
d. Nucleosome

Ans. (a) Locus

181. A recessive character in Pea is

a. Red flower
b. Round seed
c. Green cotyledons
d. Tall plant

Ans. (c) Green cotyledons

182. Mendel was lucky and could discover a law of heredity because he selected traits which

a. Possessed linkage
b. Crossed independently
c. Had complete dominance
d. Had incomplete dominance

Ans. (b) Crossed independently

183. Phenotype is influenced by

a. Environment
b. Development
c. Ageing
d. All the above

Ans. (d) All the above

184. Some gene loci on two homologous chromosomes produce different phenotypes. They bear

a. Homozygous alleles
b. Heterozygous alleles
c. Two different genes
d. Pleiotropic genes

Ans. (b) Heterozygous alleles

185. In a dihybrid test cross, the proportion of individuals showing recessive phenotypes would be

a. 1/16
b. 7/16
c. 1/4
d. 3/4

Ans. (d) 3/4

186. The number of genotypes produced by gametes Y and y would be

a. 1
b. 12
c. 3
d. 4

Ans. (c) 3

187. A phenotypic ratio not obtained by Mendel was

a. 3:1
b. 1:2:1
c. 1:1:1:1
d. 9:3:3:1

Ans. (b) 1:2:1

188. Pea plant with double hybrid yellow round seeds (YyRr) is crossed with plant having single hybrid green round seeds (yyRr). The progeny shall be

a. 3:3:1:1
b. 1:1:1:1
c. 9:3:3:1
d. 3:1:3:1

Ans. (d) 3:1:3:1

189. Trihybrid ratio is

a. 27:9:9:9:3:3:3:1
b. 27:9:9:6:6:3:3:1
c. 1:6:15:20:15:6:1
d. 36:6:6:6:3:3:3:1

Ans. (a) 27:9:9:9:3:3:3:1

190. Number of gamete types produced by genotype Aa Bb Cc Dd will be

a. 4
b. 8
c. 16
d. 32

Ans. (c) 16

191. First generation after a cross is

a. First filial generation
b. F_1 generation
c. Second filial generation
d. Both a and b

Ans. (d) Both a and b

192. F_2 generation is produced as a result of

a. Crossing F_1 individuals with dominant individuals
b. Crossing F_1 individuals with recessive individuals
c. Crossing F_1 individuals amongst themselves
d. All the above

Ans. (c) Crossing F_1 individuals amongst themselves

193. Which is incorrect in Mendelian characters?

Character	Dominant	Recessive
a. Pod colour	Green	Yellow
b. Seed shape	Round	Wrinkled
c. Flower position	Terminal	Axillary
d. Shape of pod	Full	Constricted

Ans. (c) Flower position   Terminal   Axillary

194. F_2 generation of a dihybrid cross possesses one or both the dominant traits in proportion of

a. 1/16
b. 6/16
c. 9/16
d. 15/16

Ans. (d) 15/16

195. What is incorrect in the following Mendelian traits

a. Height	Tall	Dwarf
b. Seed colour	Green	Yellow
c. Flower position	Axillary	Terminal
d. Flower colour	Violet	White

Ans. (b) Seed colour   Green   Yellow

196. In Shepherd's Purse, the fruit shape is controlled by

a. Supplementary genes
b. Complementary genes
c. Duplicate genes
d. Polymeric genes

Ans. (c) Duplicate genes

197. A pure breeding triangular fruit bearing plant of shepherd's Purse is crossed with ovoid fruit bearing plant. The ratio of two types of plants in F_2 generation would be

a. 3:1
b. 1:2:1
c. 13:3
d. 15:1

Ans. (d) 15:1

198. 9:6:1 F_2 generation ratio is obtained in case of

a. Polymeric genes
b. Pleiotropic genes
c. Supplementrary genes
d. Recessive epistasis

Ans. (a) Polymeric genes

199. Two plants of Summer Squash both having circular fruits are crossed. F_1 plants had discoid fruits. F_2 generation has 3 types of fruits, discoid, circular and long in the ratio of

a. 9:3:4
b. 9:6:1
c. 12:3:1
d. 7:6:3

Ans. (b) 9:6:1

200. Recessive epistasis is shown by

a. Flower colour in Sweat Pea
b. Fruit colour of Summer Singh
c. Coat colour Mice
d. Shape of comb in poultry

Ans. (c) Coat colour Mice

201. The ratio of 2 : 1 is observed in case of
    a. Suppressor gene
    b. Dominant-recessive epistasis
    c. Complementary gene
    d. Lethal gene

Ans. (d) Lethal gene

202. Mendel's law of segregation, as applied to the behavior of chromosome in meiosis, means that
    a. Paring of homologs will convert one allele into the other, leading to separation of the types
    b. Allels of a gene separate from each other when homologs separate in meiosis I
    c. Genes on the same chromosome will show 50% recombination
    d. Alleles of a gene will be linked and passed on together through meiaosis

Ans. (b) Allels of a gene separate from each other when homologs separate in meiosis I

203. The phenomenon of independent assortment refers to
    a. Expression at the same stage of development
    b. Unlinked transmission of genes in crosses resulting from being located on different chromosomes
    c. Association of an RNA and a protein implying related function
    d. Independent location of genes from each in an interphase cell

Ans. (b) Unlinked transmission of genes in crosses resulting from being located on different chromosomes

204. One of Mendel's pure strains of pea plants had green peas. How many different kinds of egg could such a plant produce with regard to pea colour?
    a. One
    b. Two
    c. Three
    d. Four

Ans. (a) One

205. List all the different gametes produced by the following individuals
    1. AA BB Cc
    2. aa Bb Cc
    a. 1. ABC, ABc ; 2. aBC, aBc , abC , abc
    b. 1. AbC, ABc ; 2. ABC, aBc, abC, aBC
    c. 1. ABC, ABC ; 2. aBC, aBc, abc, aBC
    d. 1. ABC, ABc ; 2. aBC, ABc, abc, abC

Ans. (a) 1. ABC, ABc ; 2. aBC, aBc , abC , abc

206. If a diploid cell contains six chromosomes, how many possible random arrangements of homologous could occur during Metaphasse-I?
    a. 4   b. 8
    c. 6   d. 64

Ans. (b) 8

207. Determine the frequency of only one genotype, BBLI ,in the offspring of dihybrid parents (BbLI).
    a. 1/4   b. 1/8
    c. 1/16   d. 1/2

Ans. (b) 1/8

208. If an individual of genotypes AaBbCcDd is test crossed, how many different phenotypes can appear in the progeny?
    a. 16   b. 8
    c. 32   d. 64

Ans. (a) 16

209. If individuals of genotypes AaBbCc are intercrossed, how many different phenotypes can appear their offspring?
    a. 16   b. 8
    c. 32   d. 64

Ans. (b) 8

210. If individual of genotypes AaBbCc are intercrossed, how many different genotypes can occur in their progeny?
    a. 8   b. 64
    c. 27   d. 9

Ans. (c) 27

211. If individual of genotypes AaBbCc are intercrossed, how many different F_2 phenotypes can appear assuming complete codominance at all loci?
    a. 8
    b. 64
    c. 27
    d. 9

Ans. (c) 27

212. A man is heterozygous B/b for one autosomal gene, and he carries a recessive X-linked allele d. What proportion of his sperm will be bd?
    a. 1/4
    b. 1/8
    c. 1/16
    d. 1/2

Ans. (a) 1/4

213. A trihybrid cross is made between two yeast, both with genotype A/a, B/b, C/c. What proportion of the offspring will be of genotype a/a, b/b, c/c?

    a. 1/8

    b. 1/32

    c. 1/64

    d. 1 /74

Ans. (c) 1/64

214. When heterozygous black pigs are intercrossed then what is the chance of the first two offspring being black?

    a. 46   b. 1/32

    c. 1/64   d. 1/74

Ans. (b) 1/32

215. Medical geneticists usually abbreviate the normal beta- globin gene as b, and the abnormal gene (in this case) as b^0 .Neither of your patient's parents has beta–thalassemi a Which of these described the most likely genotypes of both parents?

    a. One is b^0 and one in b

    b. One is $b^0 b^0$ and one is bb

    c. Both are $b^0 b^0$

    d. Both are bb^0

Ans. (d) Both are bb^0

216. If a man of blood group AB marries a woman of blood group A whose father was of blood group O, to what different blood group can this man and woman expect their children to belong?

    a. A, AB, B   b. A, AB

    c. AB, O   d. A, O, B

Ans. (a) A, AB, B

217. In the human ABO blood system, the alleles A and B are dominant to O, what will be the number of different possible genotype?

    a. 4   b. 8

    c. 6   d. 12

Ans. (c) 6

218. A brown mouse is mated with two female blackmice. When each female has produced several litters of young, the first female has had 48 black and the second female has 14 black and 11 brown young. Deduce the pattern of inheritance coat colour and the genotype of all the parents (B-Black ; b - brown)

    a. Male Bb; female 1, BB; female 2 Bb

    b. Male BB; female 1, BB; female 2 Bb

    c. Male Bb; female 1, BB; female 2 bb

    d. None of the above

Ans. (d) None of the above

219. Three genes (P, Q and R) are found of three different chromosome .For the following diploid genotypes, describe all of the possible gamete combinations and their predicted ratios.

    P. AABbCC   Q. AaBBCc   R. Aabbcc

    a. P. 1ABC: 1AbC   Q. 1ABC: 1ABc: 1aBC: 1aBc
        R. 1Abc: 1abc

    b. P. 1ABC: 1Abc   Q. 1abc : 1Abc: 1aBC: 1aBc
        R. 1abc: 1abc

    c. P. 1ABC: 1Abc   Q. 1ABC: 1aBc: 1aBC:
        R. 1Abc: 1abc

    d. P. 1ABC: 1Abc   Q. 1ABC: 1Abc: 1aBC:
        R. 1Abc: 1Abc

Ans. (a) P. 1ABC: 1AbC Q. 1ABC: 1ABc: 1aBC: 1aBc
**   R. 1Abc: 1abc**

220. A true -breeding pea plant with round and green seeds is correct is crossed to a true -breeding plant with wrinkled and yellow seeds. Round and yellow seeds are the dominant traits. The F_1 plants are allowed to self-fertilize. What are the following probabilities for the F2 generation?

    P. An F2 plant with wrinkled, yellow seeds
    Q. An F2 plant with round, yellow seeds

    a. P. 2/16   Q. 9/16

    b. P. 3/16   Q. 7/16

    c. P. 3/16   Q. 9/16

    d. Cannot be determined from the information

Ans. (c) P. 3/16   Q. 9/16

221. In Guinea pig, black coat colour is a dominant trait and white is recessive trait. A black female is test crossed, producing six black offspring. The probability that heterozygous black would do this by chance alone is approximately

    a. 50%

    b. 25%

    c. 1%

    d. Cannot be determined from the information

Ans. (a) 50%

222. What are the minimum progeny population sizes allowing for random union of all kinds of gametes from AaBbCc parent?

    a. 64   b. 32

    c. 16   d. 8

Ans. (a) 64

223. **A red -flowered tall parent plant (PI) was crossed to a true breeding red-flowered dwarf plant (P2) and half of the progenies obtained was red and tall and the other half red and dwarf. In the next generation, half of all these progenies segregated only for flower colour and the other half segregated only for height . The genotype of the P1 is**

    a. Heterozygous for colour and heterozygous for height
    b. Homozygous for colour and heterozygous for height
    c. Heterozygous for colour and homozygous for height
    d. Homozygous for colour and homozygous for height

    Ans. (a) Heterozygous for colour and heterozygous for height

224. **According to classical genetics, Which of the following statements is true?**

    a. Recessive alleles are detected by the phenotype of the F_1 generation
    b. The closer two genes are, the more frequently they recombine
    c. Genes on different autosomes segregate independently
    d. Gene on sex chromosomes segregate with the same pattern as autosomal genes

    Ans. (c) Genes on different autosomes segregate independently

225. **Assuming the comparable chromosomes in different individuals are genetically dissimilar because of different alleles. How many unique zygotic combinations are possible following fertilization in an organism where n = 3 (Assuming that no crossing over occurs) ?**

    a. 8   b. 16
    c. 64   d. 216

    Ans. (c) 64

226. **The colour of flowers of an annual species of plants is controlled by a single locus with two alleles R and r, and the genotypes RR, Rr and rr and red, pink and white respectively. A large number of seeds from individuals with pink flowers were collected and planted on an island. Where because of absence of pollinators, only self -pollination is possible. What will be the most likely outcome after 25 years?**

    a. About 50% plants with red flowers 50% with white flowers
    b. Almost 100% plants with pink flowers

    c. Red, pink, and white flowered plants in a ratio of 1:2:1
    d. Red, pink and white flowered plants in equal proportion

    Ans. (c) Red, pink, and white flowered plants in a ratio of 1:2:1

227. **Coat colour of dogs depend upon the action of at least two genes. At one locus a dominant epistatic inhibitor of colour pigment (A-) prevents the expression of colour at another independently assorting locus, producing white coat colour. When the recessive condition exists at the inhibitor locus (aa) the alleles of the hypostatic locus may be expressed, aaB-producing black and aabb producing brown. When dihybrid white dogs are together, determine the phenotypic proportions expected in the progeny.**

    a. 9 : 7   b. 9 : 3 : 4
    c. 12 : 3 : 1   d. 13 : 3

    Ans. (c) 12 : 3 : 1

228. **Short hair in rabbits is governed by a dominant gene L and long hair by its recessive allele I. black hair results from the action of the dominant genotype B- and brown from the recessive genotype bb.**

    a. In crosses between dihybrid short-haired, black and homozygous short-haired, brown rabbits, genotypic ratio will be 1 : 1 : 1 : 1
    b. In crosses between dihybrid short-haired, black and homozygous short-haired, brown rabbits, phenotypic ratio will be 1 : 1
    c. Expected phenotypic ratio from the cross LIBb x LIbb will be 3 : 3 : 1 : 1
    d. Expected genotypic ratio of LIBb will be ¼

    Ans. a, b, c, and d

229. **In a cross between two individuals with the genotypes AaBbccDdEeFf and AaBbCCDDeeff, the probability that an offspring will be heterozygous at all these loci is**

    a. 0   b. 1/16
    c. 1/32   d. 1/64

    Ans. (c) 1/32

230. **Two pink-flowered four-o'clocks are crossed to each other. Flower colour is incompletely dominant and giving phenotypic ratio if 1 red : 2 pink: 1 white. What are the following probabilities?**

    P. The first three plants with while flower
    Q. A plant with either white or pink flower

    a. P. 1/64 Q. 3/4
    b. P.3/16 Q. 1/64

c. P.3/64 Q.9/16

d. P. 1/64 Q.1/64

Ans. (a) P. 1/64 Q. 3/4

231. Which of the following is a mismatch?

a. Phenotypic F_2 ratio of 1 : 4 : 6 : 4 : 1-polygenic inheritance

b. Phenotypic F_2 ratio of 9 : 3 : 4-recessive epistasis

c. Phenotypic F_2 ratio of 1 : 2 : 1-codominance

d. Phenotypic F_2 ratio of 3 : 1-partial dominance

Ans. (d) Phenotypic F_2 ratio of 3 : 1-partial dominance

232. Why would you predict that half of the human babies born will be maies and half will be femaies?

a. Because of the segregation of the X and Y chromosomes during male meiosis

b. Because of the segregation of the X chromosomes during female meiosis

c. Because all eggs contain an X chromosome

d. Because, on average, one- half of all eggs produce females

Ans. (a) Because of the segregation of the X and Y chromosomes during male meiosis

233. Asymmetry between reciprocal crosses is seen in

a. Pleiotropy

b. Sex-linked inheritance

c. Interaction of genes

d. Autosomal inheritance

Ans. (b) Sex-linked inheritance

234. Which of the following is not true autosomal dominant traits?

a. Every affected person should have at least one affected parent

b. Males and females should be equally often affected

c. An affected person has a 50% chance of transmitting the dominant allele to each offspring

d. All the daughters of an affected male will be affected but none of the sons

Ans. (d) All the daughters of an affected male will be affected but none of the sons

235. Albinism is a recessive human trait. If a normal couple produces an albino child, what is the probability that their next child will be albino?

a. 1/4

b. 1/8

c. 1/16

d.1/64

Ans. (a) 1/4

236. When a man with hypertrichosis marries a normal woman, what %of their sons would be expected to have hairy ears?

a. 50%

b. 100%

c. 0%

d. 25%

Ans. (b) 100%

237. A man with a certain disease marries a normal woman. They have 8 children (4 boys and 4 girls); all of the girls have their father's disease, but none of the boys do. What inheritance is suggested?

a. Autosomal recessive

b. Autosomal dominant

c. Y-linked

d. X-linked

Ans. (d) X-linked

238. Cystic fibrosis is a hereditary disease that affects the respiratory and digestive systems. Cystic fibrosis occurs when two recessive genes (cc) are present. A person with one allele for Cystic fibrosis is called a carrier (Cc) of the disease. If the mother is a carrier of the disease and the father is homozygous dominant, what are chances that their child will be carrier of Cystic fibrosis?

a. 25%

b. 50%

c. 75%

d. 100%

Ans. (b) 50%

239. Which of the following is/are correct about sex – linked recessive inheritance?

a. Most affected individuals are male

b. Affected females come from affected father and affected or carrier mothers

c. The sons of affected females should be affected

d. The trait does not skip generations

Ans. a, b, and c

240. Which of the following is/are not feature (s) of quantitative trait?

a. Characters of degree

b. Continuous variation

c. Polygenic control

d. Discontinuous variation

Ans. (d) Discontinuous variation

241. Which of the following are correct?

a. Classical Mendelian traits are qualitative in nature

b. Qualitative traits show discontinuous variations

c. Qualitative traits are polygenic traits

d. Qualitative traits are referred to as metric traits

Ans. (a and b)

242. Wheat grain colour is controlled by four loci and following qualitative inheritance.

P. Calculate the number of different F_2 phenotypes in a certain stock of wheat

Q. Calculate the number of F_2 as extreme as one parent or the other

a. P-9, Q-1/16   b. P-16, Q-1/256
c. P-8, Q-1/32   d. P-9, Q-1/256

Ans. (d) P-9, Q-1/256

243. Two pure lines of corn have mean cob lengths of 9 and 3 inches, respectively. The polygenes involved in this trait all exhibit additive gene action. Crossing these two lines is expected to produce a progeny with mean cob length (in inches) of

a. 12.0   b. 7.5
c. 6.0   d. 2.75

Ans. (c) 6.0

244. In a plant, height varies from 6 to 36 cm. When 6 cm and 36 cm plants were crossed all F1plants were 21 cm. In the F2 generation, a continuous range of heights was observed. Most were around 21 cm, and 3 of 200 were 6 cm. Find out how many gene pairs are involved in this mode of inheritance?

a. 3   b. 4
c. 2   d. 5

Ans. (a) 3

245. If four chromosomes synapse into a cross-shaped configuration during meiotic prophase, the organism is heterozygous for a

a. Pericentric inversion   b. Delection
c. Translocation   d. Paracentric inversion

Ans. (c) Translocation

246. Philadelphia chromosome is generated by translocation between

a. Chromosome 18 and chromosome 6
b. Chromosome 22 and chromosome 9
c. Chromosome 22 and chromosome 3
d. Chromosome 16 and chromosome 4

Ans. (b) Chromosome 22 and chromosome 9

247. Retinoblastoma is caused by loss of both copies of the RB gene in the chromosome band

a. 13p11
b. 13q11
c. 13q14
d. 21q14

Ans. (c) 13q14

248. Position effect is the result of

a. Mutations   b. Deletions
c. Inversions   d. Transversions

Ans. (c) Inversions

249. The bridge-fragment configuration at anaphase-1 is characteristic of

a. Translocation heterozygote
b. Paracentric inversion heterozygote
c. Pericentric inversion heterozygote
d. Duplication heterozygote

Ans. (b) Paracentric inversion heterozygote

250. A mechanism that can cause a gene to move from one linkage group to another is

a. Translocation
b. Inversion
c. Crossing over
d. Duplication

Ans. (a) Translocation

251. Pseudo-dominance may be observed in heterozygotes for

a. A deletion
b. A duplication
c. A reciprocal translocation
d. More than one of the above

Ans. (a) A deletion

252. Which of the following chromosomal changes is usually the most damaging when in the homozygous condition?

a. Deletion
b. Duplication
c. Translocation
d. Inversion

Ans. (a) Deletion

253. In a trisomic individual the number of chromosome is

a. 2n-1   b. 2n+2
c. 2n+3   d. 2n+1

Ans. (d) 2n+1

254. A person with Klinefelter syndrome is considered a

a. Monosomic
b. Triploid
c. Trisomic
d. Delection heterozygote

Ans. (c) Trisomic

255. IF the garden pea has 14 chromosomes in its diploid complement, how many double trisomics could theoretically exist?

a. 6
b. 9
c. 16
d. 21

Ans. (d) 21

256. The condition in which there is too many or one too few chromosomes is called

a. Aneuploidy
b. Polytene
c. Polyploidy
d. Monoploidy

Ans. (a) Aneuploidy

257. Most cases of Down syndrome are caused by the presence of a third copy chromosome 21 associated with the chromosome 21 pair. This genetic condition, known as trisomy 21, is caused by

a. A frame-shift mutation
b. Chromosome nondisjunction
c. Fragile X syndrome
d. Chromosome transloction

Ans. (b) Chromosome nondisjunction

258. Which statement about Downn's syndrome are correct?

a. The frequency increases dramatically in mothers over the age of 40
b. The cause is a non-disjunction when chromosomes do not separate during the first meiotic division
c. Affected individuals have an extra autosome
d. The long time lag between onset of meiosis in ovarian tissue and its completion (at ovulation) is most likely the reason for increased incidence in older mothers

Ans. (All)

259. People with klinefelter syndrome have 47 chromosome, including three sex chromosome (XXY).What is the term to describe the aberration that occurs during meiosis that results in abnormal chromosome number

a. Crossing over
b. Non-disjunction
c. Independent assortment
d. Pairing of homologous chromosome

Ans. (b) Non-disjunction

260. The genes abcde are determined to be closely linked on the *E. coli* chromosome. Three random short deletions are created in the region, resulting in the removal of various genes are shown below. Which of the following gene orders is possible based on the deletion analysis?

Deletion 1: genes bde are lost
Deletion 1: genes ac are lost
Deletion 1: genes abd are lost

a. abcde
b. acded
c. bdeac
d. cabde

Ans. (d) cabde

261. Datura plants have been regenerated from anther cultures, endosperm culture and embryo culture. Their respective ploidy levels will be

a. n,2n and 2n
b. n,3n and 2n
c. n,2n and 3nn
d. 2n, 2n and 2n

Ans. (b) n,3n and 2n

262. Diagnosis of chromosome aneuploidy of unborn children is normally done by a combination of amniocentesis, cell culture, and

a. Enzyme assay
b. RRLP analysis
c. Pedigree analysis
d. Karyotyping

Ans. (d) Karyotyping

263. The Hardy-Weinberg law describes

a. Genotype frequencies of a population when evolutionary forces are not acting
b. How sexual reproduction would change the relative gene frequencies in a population
c. How mutations occur and balance each other
d. Genotype frequencies of a population when evolutionary forces are acting

Ans. (a) Genotype frequencies of a population when evolutionary forces are not acting

264. What are the assumptions of Hardy-Weinberg equilibrium?

a. Small population size, random mating, no selection, no migration, no mutation
b. Large population size, random mating, no selection, no migration, no mutation
c. Large population size, random mating, heterozygotes survive the best, no migration, no mutation
d. Large population size, random mating, no migrants enter from other populations,no mutation

Ans. (b) Large population size, random mating, no selection, no migration, no mutation

265. Genetic diversity is required for natural selection to act, but natural selection can reduce or eliminate diversity. What process can restore genetic diversity to a population?

a. Genetic drift
b. Mutation
c. Sexual selection
d. Stabilizing selection

Ans. (b) Mutation

266. Deviation from the Hardy-Weinberg assumption of infinitely large population size results in

a. Genetic lethal
b. Hetrozygote advantage
c. Consanguinity
d. Genetic drift

Ans. (d) Genetic drift

267. If to population are merged, each with different frequencies of an allele at a locus, and randomly mating occurs immediately, how long will it take to achieve a hardy–Weinberg equilibrium in the new population ?

a. One generation
b. Ten generations
c. Variable-depends on allele frequencies
d. The population will never achieve equilibrium

Ans. (a) One generation

268. In a population that is in equilibrium, the proportion of individuals showing the domain trait at a given locus having two alleles is 84%. The frequency of the recessive allele in the population is

a. 0.4
b. 0.3
c. 0.2
d. 0.16

Ans. (a) 0.4

269. How many A and a alleles are present in a sample of organisms consisting of 10 AA, 15Aa and 4aa individuals? What are the allele frequencies in the sample?

a. A = 0.6; a = 0.40
b. A = 0.4; a = 0.60
c. A = 0.6; a = 0.6
d. A = 0.4; a = 0.4

Ans. (a) A = 0.6; a = 0.40

270. In a diploid organism, what is the maximum number of alleles that can exist in a population for any given gene?

a. 1
b. 2
c. 4
d. Unlimited

Ans. (d) Unlimited

271. Cystic fibrosis is an autosomal recessive inherited disease. ITS frequency in newborns is 1 in 1700. One of the following indicates the frequency of the disease carriers

a. 0.024
b. 0.047
c. 0.976
d. 0.148

Ans. (b) 0.047

272. Which statement about allele frequencies in not true?

a. The sum of any set of allele frequency is always 1
b. If there are two alleles at a locus and we know the frequency of one of them, we can obtain the frequency of the other by subtraction
c. If an allele is missing from a population, its frequency is 0
d. If two populations have the same gene pool for a locus, they will have the same proportion of homozygotes at that locus

Ans. (d) If two populations have the same gene pool for a locus, they will have the same proportion of homozygotes at that locus

CHECK YOU GRASP

1. Mendel's law of segregation is based upon the F$_2$ ratio of

   a. 1:2   b. 9:3:3:1

   c. 1:2:1   d. 3:1

2. Mendel is popular for postulating

   a. Origin of species   b. Cell theory

   c. Linkage theory   d. Laws of inheritance

3. The monohybrid genotypic ratio 1:2:1 in F$_2$ generation indicates

   a. Segregation

   b. Independent assortment

   c. Dominance

   d. Incomplete dominance

4. A monohybrid cross is the one in which

   a. Only a single plant is involved for the experiment

   b. A single pair of contrasting characters is considered for the genetic results

   c. A hybrid is crossed to a homozygous

   d. None of the above

5. In a trisomic individual the number of chromosome is

   a. 2n-1   b. 2n+2

   c. 2n+3   d. 2n+1

6. A person with Klinefelter syndrome is considered a

   a. Monosomic

   b. Triploid

   c. Trisomic

   d. Delection heterozygote

7. Mendel's law were rediscovered by

   a. Lamarck, de Vries and Correns

   b. Hugo de Vries, Correns and Tschermak

   c. Morgan, Beadle and Tatum

   d. Hugo de Vries, Morgan and Correns

8. Ratio of parental and recombinant phenotypes in a dihybrid cross would be

   a. 8 : 8   b. 6 : 10

   c. 10 : 6   d. 9 : 7

9. Which mendelian principle will not operate if two genes under study are close together

   a. Paired unit factors

   b. Dominance

   c. Segregation

   d. Independent assortment

10. How many types of gametes are excepted from the organism with genotype AABBCC?

   a. One   b. Two

   c. Four   d. Eight

11. Repeated selfing produces

   a. Heterozygosity

   b. Homozygosity

   c. Homozygosity in some and heterozygosity in other traits

   d. Pure hybrids

12. YyRR is crossed with yyRR. The progeny will be

   a. 1 YyRR : 1 yyRR   b. 3 YyRR : 1 yyRR

   c. 1 YyRR : 3 yyRR   d. YyRR only

In case of less than 80% score, go through brief Review and Glance one again from chapter

Key: 1-d 2-d 3-a 4-b 5-d 6-c 7-b 8-c 9-d 10-a 11-b 12-a

13

Environmental Biotechnology

1. Bioaccumulation/ biomagnifications may occurs due to which of the following reason?

a. Consumption of these organisms by other organisms leads to further accumulation in the lipid deposits of the body.

b. The xenobiotics compounds are recalcitrant and lipids soluble

c. Both a and b is correct

d. None of these

Ans. (c) Both a and b is correct

2. Environment consists of which of the following?

a. Sum total of abiotic factor

b. Sum total of biotic factor

c. Both a and b minus humans

d. Both a and b are correct

Ans. (c) Both a and b minus humans

3. Which of the following abiotic components of environment contributes in various way to fulfilment of human needs?

a. Soil

b. Water

c. Air

d. All of the above

Ans. (d) All of the above

4. Which of the following constitutes environmental biotechnology?

a. Technology generate less waste

b. Technology for nonbiodegradable

c. Waste disposal

d. None of the above

Ans. (c) Waste disposal

5. Which of the following constitutes called 'front of pipe' technology?

a. Waste disposal

b. Technology generating less waste

c. Both a and b

d. Only a is correct

Ans. (d) Only a is correct

6. Which of the following constitutes called 'end of pipe' technology?

a. Waste treatment

b. Water disposal

c. Water deposition

d. All of the above

Ans. (a) Waste treatment

7. Water analysis is done to achieve which of the following objective?

a. No need to protect aquatic flora and fauna.

b. To maintain and improve the quality of water for various uses like recreation, irrigation, etc.

c. No need to control the pollution level of water bodies

d. All of the above

Ans. (b) To maintain and improve the quality of water for various uses like recreation, irrigation, etc.

8. Which of the following properties are studied to determine water quality?

a. Chemical properties

b. Aroma properties

c. Colour properties

d. None of these

Ans. (a) Chemical properties

9. Which of the following is the contribution of biotechnology to waste treatment and environmental management?

a. Technology for degradation and conversion of readily biodegradable wastes

b. Cleaner technologies of production, which generate less waste and pollutants.

c. Development of more sensitive and rapid detection techniques for a variety of pollutants.

d. All of the above

Ans. (d) All of the above

10. Which of the following statements are correct about wastes and pollutants?

a. House building and domestic activities generate only non-biodegradable waste.

b. Manufacturing industries using biological materials generate wastes o biological substance. Which are biodegradable.

c. Transport is a minor contributor to atmospheric pollution

d. Manufacturing industries using biological materials generate non biodegradable waste

Ans. (b) Manufacturing industries using biological materials generate wastes o biological substance. Which are biodegradable.

11. **Xenobiotics compounds may be recalcitrant due to which of the following reasons?**

a. Their smaller molecular size prevents their entry into microbial cells.

b. Lack of permease needed for their transport in to microbial

c. They are recognised as substrate by the existing degradative enzyme.

d. All of the above

Ans. (b) Lack of permease needed for their transport in to microbial

12. **Recalcitrant xenobiotics compounds are highly stable due to the presence of which of the following substitution groups?**

a. Halogens and carbamyl groups

b. Immuno and ethoxy group

c. Floro and nitrate group

d. All of the above

Ans. (a) Halogens and carbamyl groups

13. **Which of the following hazards is associated with xenobiotics?**

a. Certain halogenated hydrocarbons have been shown to be carcinogenic

b. Many xenobiotics are recalcitrant and persist in the environment

c. At low concentration, they may cause various skin problems and reduce reproductive

d. All of the above

Ans. (d) All of the above

14. **Chemical wastes may be classified into which of the following?**

a. Non-biodegradable b. Calcitrant

c. Both a and b d. None of these

Ans. (a) Non-biodegradable

15. **Which of the following disease spread through contaminated water/food?**

a. Tuberculosis b. Typhoid

c. Black fever d. All of the above

Ans. (b) Typhoid

16. **Which of the following is not an example of physical pollutants?**

a. Heavy metal

b. Radiation

c. Mechanical stress

d. Sound pollution

Ans. (a) Heavy metal

17. **Presence of coliform bacteria in water is indicative of contamination by mammalian excreata ad suggestive of the presence of which of the following pathogenic bacteria?**

a. Shigella

b. Vibrio cholera

c. Salmonella

d. All of the above

Ans. (d) All of the above

18. **Water analysis permits which of the following?**

a. Determination of polluting effects of various effluents and wastes discharged in water course

b. Determination of its suitability for various uses.

c. Development of water quality objectives and strands

d. All of the above

Ans. (d) All of the above

19. **Which of the following pollutants pose immediate threat to humans and is included in the black list?**

a. Organophosphates, cyanides and asbestos.

b. Heavy metals, metalloids and compounds containing them

c. Oil and hydrocarbons from crude oils

d. All of the above

Ans. (d) All of the above

20. **Various approaches to waste treatment may be grouped into which of the following categories?**

a. Aerobic digestion

b. Bioreactor

c. Technology generating less waste

d. None of these

Ans. (a) Aerobic digestion

21. **Among the given microorganisms, which one is the most commonly found in aerobic digestion systems?**

a. Bacteria b. Protozoa

c. Algae d. Fungi

Ans. (a) Bacteria

22. Which of the following is correct about biofertilizers?

a. In the two phase bio-filters, the biological agents are immunobilized on the membrane on the side of liquid phase.

b. Due to lack of control on the biomass unpredictable results of bioconversion of gases is obtained in the solid support system

c. These devices consist of either a solid support or a two-has system

d. All of the above

Ans. (d) All of the above

23. Which of the following statements are correct about liquid wastes?

a. They are treated by only anaerobic digestion

b. The main objectives of treatment are to enhance the amount of organic material and to inactivate pathogenic organisms.

c. Agriculture use of sludge is limited by the presence of heavy metals, exotic xenobiotics, and pathogenic microorganisms.

d. All of the above

Ans. (c) Agriculture use of sludge is limited by the presence of heavy metals, exotic xenobiotics, and pathogenic microorganisms.

24. Landfill sites can be useful in which of following ways?

a. As a source of organic fertilizers.

b. As a source of methane gas

c. Reclamation of derelict sites to develop

d. All of the above

Ans. (c) Reclamation of derelict sites to develop

25. In case of water quality, the quality parameter of biological properties includes which of the following?

a. Total coccus form bacteria

b. Faccal streptococci counts

c. Clorela count

d. All of the above

Ans. (b) Faccal streptococci counts

26. Bioremediation of inorganic contaminants is

a. Microorganisms   b. Plant species

c. Xerophytic species   d. None of the above

Ans. (b) Plant species

27. Solid waste is collected and may be pre-treated in some way before being placed in the pit. The pre-treatment may be which of the following?

a. Incineration

b. Sorting of the wastes

c. Mechanical pulverization

d. All of the above

Ans. (d) All of the above

28. The water from landfills may contains which of the following?

a. BOD value of 1000–2000.

b. Sodium up to 1000 mg/l

c. Total solid content upto 6000–7000 mg/l

d. COD value of 200–300.

Ans. (c) Total solid content upto 6000–7000 mg/l

29. The various parameters used to determine the level of pollution in water bodies, usually, determine which of the following?

a. Amount of important inorganic nutrient

b. Amount of waste matter present in the water

c. Numbers of bacteria per millilitre of waste water

d. All of the above

Ans. (a) Amount of important inorganic nutrient

30. Which of the following statements is correct about landfill management?

a. The risk of damage from landfill leachate may be avoided by lining the pit with an impermeable material.

b. The risk due to methane can be removed by burning or tapping

c. The risk of fires, offensive odours and increased vector population may be circumvented by covering the waste water.

d. All of the above

Ans. (d) All of the above

31. Which of the following parameter is used to determined the level of pollution in water bodies like rivers?

a. Ammonical nitrogen and phosphate content

b. Biochemical and chemical oxygen demand

c. Suspended solid

d. All of the above

Ans. (d) All of the above

32. Which of the following statement are correct?

a. Measurements of chlorine in water are based on colorimetric assay

b. BOD estimates the amount of biologically oxidisable organic matter present in water

c. COD is an estimate of the chemically oxidisable inorganic matter present in water

d. All of the above

Ans. (b) BOD estimates the amount of biologically oxidisable organic matter present in water

33. Recalcitrant xenobiotics compounds can be grouped into which of the following types?

a. Synthetic polymers   b. Polysaccharides

c. Alkylbenzyl nitrate   d. All of the above

Ans. (a) Synthetic polymers

34. Which of the following waste water treatment is an anaerobic process?

a. Sludge treatment   b. Tertiary treatment

c. Primary treatment   d. All of the above

Ans. (a) Sludge treatment

35. Preliminary treatment for waste water is necessary to prevent which of the following?

a. Interference with subsequent process

b. Damage to pump

c. Cogging of pipeline

d. All of the above

Ans. (d) All of the above

36. Which of the following is correct about aerobic digestion of waste water?

a. Bacteria are responsible for the removal of about 10–20% of the BOD

b. Bacterial population may be more common organism

c. Bacterial population may be less than 100 cell/ml.

d. All of the above

Ans. (b) Bacterial population may be more common organism

37. Practical application of microbes for xenobiotics degradation is facilitated by which of the following?

a. Maintenance of the xenobiotics compounds at toxic levels.

b. Provision of microbial population

c. Supply of sufficient nutrient

d. Both b and c

Ans. (d) Both b and c

38. Rotating biological contactor offer which of the following advantage?

a. Large scale application

b. Very high maintenance

c. Low land requirements

d. All of the above

Ans. (c) Low land requirements

39. During determination of water quality, which of the following chemical properties are measured?

a. Total chlorine and phosphate

b. Total insecticide

c. BOD and COD

d. All of the above

Ans. (c) BOD and COD

40. Aeration in the digester vessel is achieved by which of the following?

a. Introducing pure CO_2 as a fine stream of bubbles.

b. Chemical stirring

c. Generating coarse air bubble stream from a system of pipes

d. None of these

Ans. (c) Generating coarse air bubble stream from a system of pipes

41. The quality of treated effluent from the digester depends mainly on which the following?

a. Residence time

b. Organic loading rate

c. Sludge loading rate

d. All of the above

Ans. (d) All of the above

42. NO_3^- is removed from water by the action of which of the following bacteria?

a. Streptococcus   b. Micrococcus

c. Nitrobactor   d. Nitrosomonas

Ans. (b) Micrococcus

43. Which of the following statement are correct about Denitrification?

a. Denitrification is often achieved by alternating aerobic and anaerobic condition

b. Denitrifying bacteria are aerobic

c. Denitrification bacteria convert NO^{-2} to NO^{-3}

d. Denitrification may also produce various oxides of nitrogen in addition of Cl_2

Ans. (a) Denitrification is often achieved by alternating aerobic and anaerobic condition

44. Sewage contains which of the following pathogenic organisms?

a. Bacteria causing typhoid, cholera, diarrhoea

b. Viruses causes cholera, diarrhoea

c. Protozoa causes tetanus

d. All of the above

Ans. (a) Bacteria causing typhoid, cholera, diarrhoea

45. Protozoa are represented in waste water by which of the following?

a. Ascaris form   b. Pseudopodia

c. Lopopodia   d. Amoebal forms

Ans. (d) Amoebal forms

46. Efficiency of anaerobic digestion can be enhanced by which of the following?

a. By recycling the active biomass
b. By limiting the biomass loss to a rate compatible with high population density in the digester.
c. By using solid support to retain biomass
d. All of the above

Ans. (d) All of the above

47. Bioremediation of organic contaminants in primarily based on which of the following?

a. Microorganisms artificially present at the site
b. Microbial inoculants developed in the laboratory and introduced at the site
c. Suitable plants not planted at the site
d. None of these

Ans. (b) Microbial inoculants developed in the laboratory and introduced at the site

48. Oil spills cause severe damage to the ecosystem and pose which of the following threats?

a. Water pollution due to evaporation
b. Fire
c. Air water pollution due to percolation
d. All of the above

Ans. (b) Fire

49. Which of the following statement is not correct?

a. Oilzapper has not been effective in field trials
b. In india, a consortium of bacterial species has developed to combat oilspills and oily sludge; the inoculants is aptly called oilzapper
c. Inoculation with oilzapper reduced oil sludge contamination in soil to merely 0.5 ub 360 dyas from the initial 13.14%
d. The U.S. Environment protection Agency and the exxon company used microorganisms to clean up Alaskan beaches contaminated by the Valdez oil spill

Ans. (a) Oilzapper has not been effective in field trials

50. The anaerobic digestion process involves a wide variety of organisms which digest the organic molecules, such as lipids, protein, carbohydrates, etc. into mainly which of the following?

a. CH_4 and CO_2
b. NO_2 and CO_3
c. SO_4 and CO
d. SO_3 and CO_2

Ans. (a) CH_4 and CO_2

51. Biofilms contain a complex community of organisms, which degrade coarbohydrates, proteins, lipids etc. Into which of the following?

a. PO^{-3} b. SO_2
c. CO_2 d. NO_2

Ans. (c) CO_2

52. Which of the following heterotropic bacteria are responsible for oxidation of organic matter?

a. Pesticides leach into water bodies, where many of them are subjected to biomagnifications
b. They contain different numbers of halogen atoms in the place of He atoms
c. They used as a solvent, in condenser units of cooling system
d. The C1-C2 haloalkane escape in to the atmosphere where they destroys the protective ozone layer

Ans. (b) They contain different numbers of halogen atoms in the place of He atoms

53. Which of the following heterotrophic bacteria are responsible for oxidation of organic molecules?

a. Shigella and Aerobactor
b. Pseudomonas and Escherichia
c. Streptococcus and salmonelia
d. All of the above

Ans. (d) All of the above

54. Which of the following is correct about alkylbenzyl sulphonates?

a. Sulphonate group present at both end resists microbial degradation
b. At present, alkylbenzyl sulphonates are bio-degraded by β-oxidation from their alkyl group
c. These are not surface active detergents
d. All of these

Ans. (b) At present, alkylbenzyl sulphonates are biodegraded by β-oxidation from their alkyl group

55. Phytoremediation has which of the following inherent technical technical limitation?

a. The site must be sufficiently large for easy plant cultivation
b. The contamination must be present within the root zones of actively growing plants.
c. It takes much longer than do dig and dump techniques.
d. All of the above

Ans. (d) All of the above

56. For phytoremediation of flyash, seedlings of which of the following trees are established at abandoned flyash pond/dams?

a. Seqoia
b. Dabargia siso
c. Popular
d. Cinchona

Ans. (c) Popular

57. Continued exposure of microorganisms to xenobiotics compounds can often lead to the evolution of metabolic processes needed to wholly or partly degrade the xenobiotics. These capabilities may arise due to which of the following?

a. Translation
b. Termination
c. Transfer of plasmid-borne genes
d. Transcription

Ans. (c) Transfer of plasmid-borne genes

58. Alicyclic hydrocarbons are present naturally in which of the following?

a. Wax from bee
b. Microbial lipid
c. Safflower oil
d. All of the above

Ans. (b) Microbial lipid

59. Which of the following is correct about oxidation of aromatic hydrocarbons?

a. These are oxidized by oxidoreductase to catechol
b. These are not oxidized by oxidoreducase to catechol
c. Catechol if further metabolised by metering cleavage pathway to yield 2-hydroxymyconic semialdehyde
d. None of these

Ans. (a) These are oxidized by oxidoreductase to catechol

60. Which of the following is not related to green house gas?

a. CFC
b. CO_2
c. O_2
d. CH_4

Ans. (c) O_2

61. Which of the following statements are correct about aliphatic hydrocarbons?

a. Biodegradation of n-alkane is catalyzed by oxygenase to produce carboxylic acid.
b. Saturated aliphatics are easier to degrade than unsaturated ones.
c. They may be saturated or unsaturated
d. All of the above

Ans. (d) All of the above

62. Flurode pollution mainly affected which of the following?

a. Liver
b. Brain
c. Teeth
d. Stomach

Ans. (c) Teeth

63. Which of the following statement are correct about aromatic hydrocarbons?

a. Catechol is further metabolised by two separate pathways called ortho-clevage pathway and meta-clevage pathway
b. Benzene is degraded by the ortho cleavage pathway
c. They are oxidised by di-oxygenases to catechol.
d. All of the above

Ans. (d) All of the above

64. Biochemical oxygen demand measures which of the following?

a. Water pollution
b. Dissolved O2 needed by microbes to decompose organic waste.
c. Oxygen need to support microorganism growth
d. Industrial pollution

Ans. (b) Dissolved O2 needed by microbes to decompose organic waste.

65. The aerobic degradation of halogenated aromatic compounds usually involves which of the following?

a. Cleavage of the ring by ortho- or meta cleavage
b. Elimination of the halogen from the straight chain product
c. Degradation
d. All of the above

Ans. (d) All of the above

66. Smog is the product of the which of the following?

a. Smoke +fog
b. Fog + carbon
c. Smoke +water
d. Water + carbon

Ans. (a) Smoke +fog

67. Green house effect is related to which of the following?

a. Global warming
b. Noise pollution
c. Water pollution
d. Global afforestation

Ans. (a) Global warming

68. The national Institute of Oceanography is presently situated at

a. Kerala   b. Calicut
c. Goa   d. Cochin

Ans. (c) Goa

69. Mycorrhizae help in the uptake of

a. Potassium   b. Phosphorus
c. Nitrate   d. Boron

Ans. (b) Phosphorus

70. Chaparral vegetation is found in which area?

a. Deccan plateau
b. Coastal India
c. Mediterranean areas
d. Between equator and temperature

Ans. (c) Mediterranean areas

71. The residence time of N2O is atmosphere is approximately

a. 15 years   b. 150 years
c. 15 weeks   d. 15 days

Ans. (b) 150 years

72. Which elemental cycle has no atmospheric reservoir?

a. Sulphur   b. Carbon
c. Nitrogen   d. Phosphorus

Ans. (d) Phosphorus

73. Muscovite is example of which group of minerals?

a. Feldspar   b. Ferromagnesium
c. Quartz   d. Mica

Ans. (d) Mica

74. Highest porosity is found in

a. Sand   b. Clay
c. Gravel   d. Silt

Ans. (b) Clay

75. Solubility of gases in water can be calculated by using

a. Darcy's law   b. Henry's law
c. Avagadro's law d. Stoke's law

Ans. (b) Henry's law

76. The main constituent of biogas is

a. H_2 b. H_2S
c. N_2 d. CH_4

Ans. (d) CH_4

77. The actual global average surface air temperature is about

a. 331 K
b. 288 K
c. 18°C
d. 21°C

Ans. (b) 288 K

78. The ministry of environment was set up in

a. 1970   b. 1980
c. 1975   d. 1985

Ans. (b) 1980

79. Age of earth is approximately

a. 3.5 billion
b. 4.5 billion
c. 4.5 million
d. 3.5 million

Ans. (b) 4.5 billion

80. Among the following which gas is found in maximum concentration in atmosphere?

a. Rn   b. Xe
c. Kr   d. Ar

Ans. (d) Ar

81. Ventilation coefficient is:

a. Maximum mixing depth divided by average wind speed.
b. Product of maximum mixing depth and maximum wind speed.
c. Maximum mixing height divided by maximum wind speed
d. Product of maximum mixing depth and average wind speed

Ans. (d) Product of maximum mixing depth and average wind speed

82. Mosquito repellent coil/ mats contain

a. Paraquat
b. BHC
c. Toxaphene
d. Derivatives of allethrin

Ans. (d) Derivatives of allethrin

83. The concentration of CO_2 in atmosphere is increasing at the rate of about

a. 4%   b. 2%
c. 0.4%   d. 0.2%

Ans. (c) 0.4%

84. 1 Dobson unit at standard temperature and pressure is equal to ozone column thickness of

a. 1mm
b. 10 mm
c. 100 mm
d. 0.01 mm

85. Who is the director of centre for science and Environment

a. Anil Agarwal
b. Sunita Narayan
c. Menka Gandhi
d. Medha Patekar

Ans. (b) Sunita Narayan

86. Which CFC was discovered first?

a. CFC –11
b. CFC – 12
c. CFC – 114
d. CFC – 11n5

Ans. (b) CFC – 12

87. The concentration of ozone is found maximum in

a. Trophosphere
b. Upper stratosphere
c. Lower stratosphere
d. Mesosphere

Ans. (c) Lower stratosphere

88. The national Institute of Oceanography is presently situated at

a. Kerala
b. Calicut
c. Goa
d. Cochin

Ans. (c) Goa

89. The normal lapse rate of temperature per kilometre is

a. 6.4°C
b. 4.6°C
c. 10°C
d. 9°C

Ans. (a) 6.4°C

90. The albedo of the earth as a whole is

a. 25%
b. 50%
c. 30%
d. 10%

Ans. (c) 30%

91. Atmospheric humidity is measured by

a. Radiometer
b. Hygrometer
c. Hydrometer
d. Micrometer

Ans. (b) Hygrometer

92. The origin of simplest life is attributed to

a. Proteozoic Era
b. Cambrian Era
c. Archaezoic Era
d. None of the above

Ans. (c) Archaezoic Era

93. The maximum permissible limit of free residual chlorine in water is

a. 2 ppm
b. 0.02 ppm
c. 0.2 ppm
d. 20 ppm

Ans. (c) 0.2 ppm

94. Radiosonde is used to study

a. Earth's albedo at surface
b. Estimate pollutants in air
c. Atmospheric moisture content
d. Upper atmosphere's conditions

Ans. (d) Upper atmosphere's conditions

95. Which of the following enzymes is involved in the primary carboxylation in C_4 plants?

a. RUBP carboxylase
b. PEP
c. Oxygenase
d. None of the above

Ans. (b) PEP

96. The compound used for artificial rain making/cloud seeding is

a. Dry ice
b. Ag I
c. HgCl2
d. Both a and b

Ans. (b) Ag I

97. How many agro-climatic zones are found in India?

a. 15
b. 16
c. 17
d. 18

Ans. (a) 15

98. About 50% of the atmosphere lies below

a. 5.6 km
b. 10 km
c. 15 km
d. 30 km

Ans. (a) 5.6 km

99. After methane and carbon dioxide which gas is found in highest concentration in biogas?

a. CO
b. H_2
c. N_2
d. H_2S

Ans. (b) H_2

100. The target organ of cadmium toxicity :

a. Lung
b. Liver
c. Kidney
d. Bones

Ans. (c) Kidney

101. Nalgonda technique is used for

a. Chloride
b. Fluoride
c. Bromide
d. Cadmium

Ans. (b) Fluoride

102. The process used for removal of water hardness is

a. Zeolite process
b. Haber's process
c. Ostwald process
d. None of these

Ans. (a) Zeolite process

103. Who gave the term ecosystem and when?

a. A.G. Tansley (1935)
b. A.G. Tansley (1925)
c. E.P. Odum (1935)
d. E.P.Odum (1925)

Ans. (a) A.G. Tansley (1935)

104. IPCC came into exist in

a. 1978
b. 1968
c. 1988
d. 1998

Ans. (c) 1988

105. The first international conference on environmental education held in

a. Tbilisi
b. New Delhi
c. Bombay
d. Turkey

Ans. (b) New Delhi

106. Kyoto protocol came into force on

a. 16 Feb. 2004
b. 16 Feb. 2005
c. 16 Feb. 2002
d. 16 Feb. 2000

Ans. (c) 16 Feb. 2002

107. Indian institute of petroleum in situated at

a. New Delhi
b. Goa
c. Dehradun
d. Mumbai

Ans. (c) Dehradun

108. Which of the following is mainly responsible for eutrophication?

a. Phosphate
b. Nitrate
c. Carbonate
d. Sulphate

Ans. (a) Phosphate

109. The atmospheric layer reflecting radio waves is called

a. Homosphere
b. Ionosphere
c. Ozonosphere
d. None of these

Ans. (c) Ozonosphere

110. The specific heat of water is:

a. 1 cal/gm/°C
b. 4.18cal/gm/°C
c. 10 cal/gm/°C
d. 1 joule/gm/°C

Ans. (a) 1 cal/gm/°C

111. The first biosphere reserve in India was

a. Sundarban
b. Nanda devi
c. Nilgiri
d. Nokrek

Ans. (c) Nilgiri

112. In which year biodiversity act was proposed?

a. 2000
b. 2002
c. 2004
d. 1998

Ans. (a) 2000

113. Headquater of UNEP is situated at

a. Kenya
b. Switzerland
c. U.S.A
d. Britain

Ans. (a) Kenya

114. At which temp. Density of water is found maximum?

a. 0°C
b. 100°C
c. 15°C
d. 4°C

Ans. (d) 4°C

115. The important GHG mainly released from paddy field is:

a. CO_2
b. N_2O
c. CH_4
d. None of the above

Ans. (c) CH_4

116. What is the studies of tree as individuals in relation to their environment known as ?

a. Forest ecology
b. Forest synecology
c. Forest Autecology
d. All of the above

Ans. (c) Forest Autecology

117. Demography is the statistical study of

a. Human society
b. Human population
c. Human settlement
d. Human life

Ans. (b) Human population

118. The pH of normal rain is

a. 6.5
b. 5.6
c. 4.6
d. 3.6

Ans. (b) 5.6

119. Which harmful gas is emitted by masonry building materials, even ground water?

a. H_2S
b. Radon
c. Ammonia
d. CO_2

Ans. (b) Radon

120. Which is the most abundant of all the hydrocarbon pollutants in the atmosphere?

a. Propane
b. Methane
c. Butane
d. Benzene

Ans. (b) Methane

121. Which oil-tanker accident first alerted the public of the grave problem of oil spills in oceans

a. Agro merchant
b. Ocean eagle
c. Exon valdez
d. Torrey canyon

Ans. (d) Torrey canyon

122. The process of preparing compost with the help of earth worm is known as

a. Composting
b. Bioslury
c. Vermin composting
d. Maturing

Ans. (c) Vermin composting

123. Mycorrhizae is the association of

a. Higher plants and fungi
b. Algae and fungi
c. Lower plants and fungi
d. Both a and b

Ans. (a) Higher plants and fungi

124. When was Ganga action plan launched?

a. June 1985
b. December 1985
c. May 1984
d. July 1984

Ans. (a) June 1985

125. Largest salt water lake in India is :

a. Lonar
b. Chilka
c. Sambhar
d. Wullar

Ans. (b) Chilka

126. The main pollutant of London smog was

a. SO_2
b. NO_2
c. PAN
d. Ozone

Ans. (a) SO_2

127. Which detector for DDT should be used in gas chromatography?

a. Electron capture detector
b. Flame ionised detector
c. Thermal conductivity detector
d. None of the above

Ans. (a) Electron capture detector

128. In which of the following, inverted pyramid of biomass is found?

a. Grassland ecosystem
b. Pond ecosystem
c. Desert ecosystem
d. Forest ecosystem

Ans. (b) Pond ecosystem

129. Which term represents the sum total of life on earth?

a. Biomass
b. Gaia
c. Biosphere
d. Biome

Ans. (c) Biosphere

130. Any living thing that successfully competes with people for food space, of other essential needs is called:

a. Virus
b. Bug
c. Parasite
d. Pest

Ans. (d) Pest

131. Of the following environmental assessment terms, tell which one deals exclusively with the carbon content of the environment?

a. BOD
b. COD
c. TOC
d. POC

Ans. (c) TOC

132. The dominance of a new genetic from as a result of environment change is called:

a. Adaptation
b. Natural selection
c. Succession
d. Synergism

Ans. (b) Natural selection

133. What does the term overkill deal with?

a. Pesticidal poisoning
b. Soil erosion
c. Nuclear holocaust
d. Global warming

Ans. (c) Nuclear holocaust

134. What is a chemical substance or physical agent capable of inducing inheritable genetic change called?

a. Carcinogen
b. Mutagen
c. Teratogen
d. Tumorogen

Ans. (b) Mutagen

135. When lakes become acidic due to acid rain, this is added to counteract the acidity in

a. Soil
b. Sand
c. Lime
d. None of the above

Ans. (c) Lime

136. Which technique can map the concentration of SO_2 over a whole town by operation Gadget from one location?

a. LIDAR
b. Spectrophotometer
c. Gas chromatography
d. Mass spectroscopy

Ans. (a) LIDAR

137. Air pollution can be controlled and reduced considerably, but which one of the following factors comes in its way?

a. Politics
b. Economics
c. Manpower
d. Geography

Ans. (b) Economics

138. Photocopying and other electrical equipment produce one of the following pollutants?

a. Methane
b. Ozone
c. Hydrogen
d. Nitrogen oxides

Ans. (b) Ozone

139. Who formulated the ecological concept of the pyramid of numbers?

a. Charles Elton
b. Paul R. Ehrlich
c. Paul colivaus
d. All of the above

Ans. (a) Charles Elton

140. Where was the Mitti bachao movement launched in India?

a. Thane, Maharashtra
b. Mysore, Karnataka
c. Darbhanga, Bihar
d. Hooshangabad, M.P

Ans. (d) Hooshangabad, M.P

141. When was the use of DDT banned for agricultural purposes in India?

a. 1962
b. 1985
c. 1974
d. 1971

Ans. (b) 1985

142. For the production of biogas, the Indian biogas plant need:

a. Fire wood
b. Cattle dung
c. Agricultural waste
d. Kerosene

Ans. (c) Agricultural waste

143. Which forest area in India was first brought under control and protection?

a. Malabar
b. Konkan
c. Garhwal
d. Sunderbans

Ans. (a) Malabar

144. When was the first national forest policy formulated?

a. 1948
b. 1980
c. 1964
d. 1952

Ans. (d) 1952

145. Which plant is known as the gasoline plant?

a. Salvadora persica
b. Sterculia feetida
c. Thevetia peraviana
d. Euphoribia lathyris

Ans. (d) Euphoribia lathyris

146. When did the three mmile island disaster occur?

a. 1972
b. 1979
c. 1980
d. 1976

Ans. (b) 1979

147. Flyash is the environmental pollutant generated by

a. Thermal power plant
b. Oil refinery
c. Fertilizer plant
d. Strip mining

Ans. (a) Thermal power plant

148. Which of the following is known as liquid gold?

a. Water
b. Petroleum
c. Mercury
d. Mustard oil

Ans. (b) Petroleum

149. In denitrification process the nitrogen is released in the form of

a. NH_3
b. N_2
c. N_2O
d. Both a and b

Ans. (d) Both a and b

150. Who coined the term symbiosis?

a. A.G. Tansley
b. De Bary
c. Clements
d. Mc Dougall

Ans. (b) De Bary

151. Which type of symbiosis is obligatory?

a. Mutualism
b. Protocooperation
c. Commensalism
d. Amensalism

Ans. (a) Mutualism

152. Concept of hyper volume niche was given by

a. Grinnel
b. Clement
c. Hutchinson
d. Odum

Ans. (c) Hutchinson

153. Vehicular pollution emits mainly

a. SO2
b. CO
c. NO
d. Ozone

Ans. (b) CO

154. Of the following classes of beings, tell which one is least sensitive to nuclear radiation's

a. Single celled organism
b. Amphibian
c. Repliles
d. Birds

Ans. (a) Single celled organism

155. Which region of the seas and occans are the most polluted?

a. Estuarine
b. Coastal
c. Sea depths
d. Coral

Ans. (b) Coastal

156. Of the following types of nuclear bombs, tell which one was tested on a pacific atoll?

a. Atom bomb
b. Hydrogen bomb
c. Neutron bomb
d. None of these

Ans. (b) Hydrogen bomb

157. Which were the first living beings to establish themselves on rocky slopes?

a. Toads
b. Grasses
c. Lichens
d. Frogs

Ans. (c) Lichens

158. What is lost when one organism consume other?

a. Food
b. Water
c. Energy
d. Chemicals

Ans. (c) Energy

159. Which category of wastewater dosen't require seeding during a BOD test?

a. Distillery spentwash
b. Dyeing unit effluent
c. Domestic sewage
d. Pulp and paper mill effluent

Ans. (c) Domestic sewage

160. Permanent hardness of water is caused by:

a. Carbonates and chlorides
b. Bicarbonates and sulphates
c. Carbonates and bicarbonates
d. Chlorides and sulphates

Ans. (d) Chlorides and sulphates

161. The most commonly used method for desalination of water is

a. Distillation
b. Reverse osmosis
c. Electrodialysis
d. Flash evaporation

Ans. (b) Reverse osmosis

162. Elemental chlorine is widely used in

a. Metallurgy
b. Water purification
c. Process industry
d. Deodorants

Ans. (c) Process industry

163. The single largest class of insecticides of total registered pesticides in the world is

a. Organochlorine
b. Organophosphate
c. Carbamate
d. Pyrethroids

Ans. (b) Organophosphate

164. Cup anemmommeter is used for measuring:

a. Water evaporation
b. Wind speed
c. Wind direction
d. Water flow

Ans. (b) Wind speed

165. Which type o humus is acidic in nature?

a. Mor
b. Mull
c. Moder
d. All of the above

Ans. (a) Mor

166. Lambert's and Beer's law is used in

a. Spectrophotometer
b. Chromatography
c. Potentiometer
d. pH meter

Ans. (a) Spectrophotometer

167. Law of minimum was given by

a. Shelford
b. Liebig
c. Blackman
d. Clement

Ans. (b) Liebig

168. When was project higer launched by India?

a. 1972
b. 1973
c. 1978
d. 1974

Ans. (b) 1973

169. Increasing skin cancer and rate of mutation are the result of which of the following?

a. CO pollution
b. CO_2 pollution
c. Ozone depletion
d. Acid rain

Ans. (c)

170. Which of the following diseases is caused by eating fish inhabiting mercury contaminated water?

a. Osteosclerosis
b. Brain fever

c. Osteosclerosis

d. Minamata disease

Ans. (d) Minamata disease

171. The atmosphere of metro cities is polluted by which of the following?

a. House hold wastes

b. Automobile exhausts

c. Radioactive fallout

d. Pesticide

Ans. (b) Automobile exhausts

172. Depletion of ozone layer is caused by which of the following?

a. CFC

b. SO_2

c. CO_2

d. Both a and b

Ans. (d) Both a and b

173. Which of the following decibels of sound becomes hazardous noise pollution?

a. >80

b. >100

c. >120

d. >150

Ans. (a) >80

174. Which of the following associates with the blood haemoglobin more rapidly than oxygen?

a. CO

b. NO_2

c. SO_2

d. CO_2

Ans. (a) CO

175. Attack of asthama in certain persons may be due to which of the following?

a. Exposure to all type of pollen grains

b. Exposure to hot temperature

c. Exposure to cold temperature

d. All of the above

Ans. (c) Exposure to cold temperature

176. Which of the following plants can be used as indicator of SO_2 pollution of air?

a. Hornworts

b. Fern

c. Liverworts

d. Lichen

Ans. (d) Exposure to cold temperature

177. Which of the following green house gases is being generated by agriculture field?

a. Ammonia

b. Nitrous oxide

c. Sulphur oxide

d. SO_3

Ans. (b) Nitrous oxide

178. Which of the following gases contributes the maximum to the green house effect?

a. CO

b. N_2O

c. CFC

d. CH_4

Ans. (d) CH_4

179. Ozone day is observed on which of the following ?

a. 5 June

b. 1 December

c. 16 December

d. 23 December

Ans. (c) 16 December

180. Which of the following poses the greatest risk?

a. Biogas plants

b. Nuclear plants

c. Thermal power plant

d. Hydroelectric plants

Ans. (b) Nuclear plants

181. Which of the following is an example of a renewable resource?

a. Microorganism

b. Animals

c. Plants

d. All of the above

Ans. (d) All of the above

182. Which of the following is an example of non renewable resources?

a. Natural gas

b. Petroleum

c. Both a and b

d. Biological agents

Ans. (c) Both a and b

183. Ozone depletion in the stratosphere will cause which of the following

a. Increased incidence of skin cancer

b. Global warming

c. Increased sea level

d. All of the above

Ans. (d) All of the above

184. Maximum deposition of DDT will occur in which of the following?

a. Fish

b. Sea gull

c. Crab

d. Phytoplankton

Ans. (b) Sea gull

185. Ozone layer of upper atmosphere is being destroyed by which of the following?

a. Soot

b. Smoke

c. CFC

d. Smog

Ans. (c) CFC

186. Bioremediation of organic waste is generally based on which of the following?

a. Plant species   b. Bacteria
c. Animal species   d. All of the above

Ans. (b) Bacteria

187. Which of the following is the most ecofriendly?

a. Biogas plant   b. Thermal plant
c. Nuclear plant   d. All of the above

Ans. (a) Biogas plant

188. The term nuclear war associated with

a. Water pollution   b. Soil pollution
c. Radioactive pollution   d. Noise pollution

Ans. (c) Radioactive pollution

189. Most dangerous radioactive pollutant is

a. St^{90} b. Ca^{40}
c. S^{32} d. P^{32}

Ans. (a) St^{90}

190. Algal bloom in a lake

a. Kills fshes and other organisms
b. Increase CO3 level
c. Lead to O2 depletion
d. All of these

Ans. (d) All of these

191. Secondary pollutant is

a. CO   b. O_2
c. SO_2 d. PAN

Ans. (a) CO

192. Chemical causes bone cancer and degeneration of tissue

a. Ca-40   b. Str-90
c. C-14   d. I-131

Ans. (b) Ca-40

193. A pollutant is any substance, chemical or other factor that changes

a. The natural balance of our environment
b. The natural wildlife of our region
c. The natural flora of our environment
d. None of these

Ans. (a) The natural balance of our environment

194. The chief source of pollutant H_2S is

a. Oil refineries
b. Automobiles

c. Thermal power plants
d. Decaying vegetation and animal matter

Ans. (d) Decaying vegetation and animal matter

195. Black foot disease in human is caused by

a. Fluorine   b. Cd
c. SPM   d. Arsenic

Ans. (d) Arsenic

196. The antiknock agent added to unleaded petrol s

a. Tetramethyl lead
b. Tetraethyl lead
c. Dibromo ethane
d. Methyl tertiary butyl ether

Ans. (b) Tetraethyl lead

197. Lichens like Usnea is an indicator of

a. CO_2 b. CO
c. NO   d. SO_2

Ans. (d) SO_2

198. Ozone hole over antarctica was first detected by

a. Framan et al.   b. Augus
c. Molina and Molina   d. Molina and Rowland

Ans. (a) Framan et al.

199. Leukemia is caused by

a. Iodine   b. Ca-40
c. Sr-90   d. Caesium

Ans. (c) Sr-90

200. 3–4 benzopyrene causes

a. Leukemia   b. Cytosilicosis
c. Lung cancer   d. Tuberculosis

Ans. (c) Lung cancer

201. Osteoporosis will be caused by pollutant

a. Chlorine
b. Bromine
c. Fluorine
d. None of the above

Ans. (c) Fluorine

202. Kyoto conference s connected with

a. Reduction in use energy
b. Limiting production of CO_2 and other green house gases
c. Developing alternative to ODS
d. None of these

Ans. (b) Limiting production of CO_2 and other green house gases

203. Component of living cell affected by pollutant SO_2 is

a. Cell wall
b. All cell membrane system
c. Nucleus
d. None of these

Ans. (b) All cell membrane system

204. The threshold of normal human hearing lies between

a. 50–60 db
b. 120–140 db
c. 30–40 db
d. 160–180 db

Ans. (b) 120–140 db

205. SPM causes

a. Skin disease
b. Respiratory disease
c. Bone deformities
d. All of the above

Ans. (b) Respiratory disease

206. Montreal protocol was signed in (reduction in CFC)

a. 1990
b. 1987
c. 1978
d. 1993

Ans. (b) 1987

207. Ozone hole is widest in

a. Equator
b. Antarctica
c. North pole
d. North temperate area

Ans. (b) Antarctica

208. BOD is related to

a. Organic pollutant
b. Inorganic pollutant
c. Detergents
d. Putrescibility

Ans. (a) Organic pollutant

209. In metro cities, the automobile causes air pollution

a. 70%
b. 80%
c. 60%
d. 50%

Ans. (b) 80%

210. Climate of the world is threatened by

a. Increasing concentration of atmospheric oxygen
b. Increase amount of atmospheric CO_2
c. Decrease amount of atmospheric CO_2
d. None of the above

Ans. (b) Increase amount of atmospheric CO_2

211. Green house gases are

a. Transparent to both large and short waves
b. Absorb of solar radiation for warming the atmosphere of earth
c. Absorbs of large-wave radiations from earth
d. Transparent to emission from earth for passage into outerspace

Ans. (c) Absorbs of large-wave radiations from earth

212. Classical smog was first observed in

a. London
b. New York
c. Tokyo
d. Sydney

Ans. (a) London

213. Montreal protocol which calls for appropriate action to protect the ozone layer from human activities, was passed in the year

a. 1982
b. 1984
c. 1987
d. 1990

Ans. (c) 1987

214. Pulmonary oedema is caused by

a. Hydrocarbon
b. Carbon oxide
c. Nitrogen oxide
d. SO2

Ans. (a) Hydrocarbon

215. The blue baby syndrome result from

a. Excess of dissolved oxygen
b. Methaemoglobin
c. Excess of TDS
d. Excess of chloride

Ans. (b) Methaemoglobin

216. Common indicator organism of water pollution is

a. Cholera vibro
b. Salmonella typhi
c. E. coli
d. None of the above

Ans. (c) E. coli

217. Which of the following pair is mismatch

a. Fossil fule burning-release of CO_2
b. Nuclear power-radioactive wastes
c. Solar energy-green house effect
d. Biomass burning-release of CO_2

Ans. (c) Solar energy-green house effect

218. Limit of BOD prescribed by Central pollution control board for the discharge of Industrial and municipal waste waters in to natural surface water, is

a. <50 ppm
b. <100 ppm
c. <10 ppm
d. <5ppm

Ans. (c) <10 ppm

219. Bhopal gas tragedy of 1984 took place because methyl isocyanate reacted with

    a. DDT   b. CO_2

    c. SO_2 d. Water

Ans. (d) Water

220. Fluoride pollution mainly affected

    a. Brain   b. Heart

    c. Teeth   d. Kidney

Ans. (c) Teeth

221. Polluted water do not contains

    a. Water hyacinth   b. Sewage fungus

    c. Cyanobacteria   d. Stone fly larvae

Ans. (d) Stone fly larvae

222. Melanin protects us from

    a. IR rays   b. X-rays

    c. UV rays   d. Visible rays

Ans. (c) UV rays

223. Intensity of sound n normal conversation is

    a. 10–20 db

    b. 20–30 db

    c. 30–60 db

    d. 60–70 db

Ans. (c) 30–60 db

224. Green house effect is related to

    a. Global warming

    b. Cultivation of vegetables in houses

    c. Development of terrace gardens

    d. Increased growth of green algae

Ans. (a) Global warming

225. Pollution related occupational hazard is

    a. Silicosis   b. Asthma

    c. Leprosy   d. Pneumoconiosis

Ans. (d) Pneumoconiosis

226. Amospheric content of CO2 s

    a. 0.36%   b. 0.036%

    c. 0.0036%   d. 3.6%

Ans. (b) 0.036%

227. Highest DDT deposition shall occur in

    a. Crab   b. Sea gull/birds

    c. Phytoplankton   d. Eel

Ans. (b) Sea gull/birds

228. Carbon monoxide, emitted by automobile prevents transport of oxygen in body due to

    a. Preventing reaction between oxygen and haemoglobin

    b. Destruction of haemoglobin

    c. Forming stable compound with haemoglobin

    d. None of the above

Ans. (c) Forming stable compound with haemoglobin

229. Which green house gas other than methane is being produced by agriculture fields?

    a. Sulphur oxide   b. Nitrous oxide

    c. Sulphur dioxide   d. Ammonia

Ans. (b) Nitrous oxide

230. In coming years, skin related disorder will become more common due to

    a. Depletion of ozone layer

    b. Air pollution

    c. Water pollution

    d. Excessive use of detergent

Ans. (a) Depletion of ozone layer

231. Phosphate pollution is caused by

    a. Agriculture fertilizer

    b. Sewage and agriculture fertilizer

    c. Phosphate rock and sewages

    d. Weathering of phosphate rocks only

Ans. (b) Sewage and agriculture fertilizer

232. MIC and Chernobyl tragedies occurred at

    a. Bhopal 1983, Ukraine 1984

    b. Bhopal 1984, Ukraine 1988

    c. Bhopal 1986, Ukraine 1988

    d. Bhopal 1984, Ukraine 1988

Ans. (c) Bhopal 1986, Ukraine 1988

233. Country contributed maximum to hole formation in ozone layer is

    a. Australia   b. USA

    c. Germany   d. Japan

Ans. (b) USA

234. Which of the following is normally not an important atmospheric pollutant and remains constant?

    a. SO_2

    b. CO

    c. NO

    d. CO_2

Ans. (d) CO_2

235. **Which of the following is an environment related disorder with the correct main cause?**

    a. Blue baby syndrome due to heavy use of nitrogenous fertilizers in the area
    b. Black lung disease found mainly in worker in stone quarries and crushers
    c. Skin cancer mainly in people exposed to benzene and methane
    d. All of the above

Ans. (b) Black lung disease found mainly in worker in stone quarries and crushers

236. **Pollutant released by jet planes is**

    a. Smog
    b. Aerosol
    c. Colloid
    d. Fog

Ans. (b) Aerosol

237. **Mottling of teeth s due to presence of an element in drinking water**

    a. Fluorine
    b. Chlorine
    c. Boron
    d. Mercury

Ans. (a) Fluorine

238. **Pollution is rising due to**

    a. Pollution explosion
    b. Rain
    c. Research institute
    d. Automobile and industries

Ans. (d) Automobile and industries

239. **Catalytic converter in vehicle is used for controlling**

    a. Water pollution
    b. Air pollution
    c. Soil pollution
    d. Radioactive pollution

Ans. (b) Air pollution

240. **Sudden mass death of fish is more likely to occurs in**

    a. Oligotrophic lake
    b. Oxalotrophic lake
    c. Eutrophic lake
    d. Mesotrophic lake

Ans. (c) Eutrophic lake

241. **The chemical that contribute to the destruction of ozone layer of the earth's surface is**

    a. Chlorofluorocarbon
    b. Carbon mono oxide
    c. Sulphur dioxide
    d. Mercury

Ans. (a) Chlorofluorocarbon

242. **Minimata and itai-itai disease are due to toxicity of**

    a. Mercury and lead
    b. Mercury and strontium
    c. Mercury and tin
    d. Mercury and cadmium

Ans. (d) Mercury and cadmium

243. **Carbon monoxide kills because of the destruction of structure**

    a. Cytochrome
    b. Phytochrome
    c. Haemoglobin
    d. None of the above

Ans. (c) Haemoglobin

244. **In Bhopal gas tragedy gas methyl isocyanate is a**

    a. Organo phosphate
    b. Carbamate
    c. Organochlorides
    d. None of the above

Ans. (b) Carbamate

245. **The loss of species in the tropical countries is mainly due to**

    a. Soil erosion
    b. Urbanization
    c. Deforestation
    d. Pollution

Ans. (c) Deforestation

246. **Ozone hole cause**

    a. More UV rays come to earth
    b. Reduction in the rate of photosynthesis
    c. Global warming
    d. All of the above

Ans. (a) More UV rays come to earth

247. **It is said, the Taj Mahal may be destroyed due to**

    a. Flood in Yamuna river
    b. Air pollutants (SO_2) released from oil refinery of Mathura
    c. Decomposition of marble as a result of high temperature
    d. All of the above

Ans. (b) Air pollutants (SO_2) released from oil refinery of Mathura

248. **Treatment of polluted water is carried out with the help of**

    a. Ferns
    b. Phytoplankton
    c. Fungi
    d. Lichens

Ans. (b) Phytoplankton

249. The number of ecological hot spot in the world is

    a. 15   b. 35

    c. 25   d. 45

Ans. (c) 25

250. Number of ecological hotspot in India are

    a. 1   b. 3

    c. 5   d. 2

Ans. (d) 2

251. A pollutant is any substance, chemical or other factor that changes

    a. The natural balance of our environment

    b. Natural flora of a place

    c. Natural geochemical cycles

    d. Natural wild life of a region

Ans. (a) The natural balance of our environment

252. Lichens are imp. In the studies on atmospheric pollution because they

    a. Efficiently purify the atmosphere

    b. Can readily multiply polluted atmosphere

    c. Can also grow in greatly polluted atmosphere

    d. Are very sensitive to pollutants like SO_2

Ans. (d) Are very sensitive to pollutants like SO_2

253. Which of the following is normally not an atmospheric pollutant

    a. Hydrocarbons

    b. SO_2

    c. CO_2

    d. CO

Ans. (c) CO_2

254. Which of the following is rich source of energy but never causes atmospheric pollution

    a. Solar energy

    b. Wood

    c. Coal

    d. Nuclear energy

Ans. (a) Solar energy

255. Some effects of SO_2 and its transformation products on plkants include

    a. Plasmolysis

    b. Golgi body destruction

    c. Chlorophyll destruction

    d. None

Ans. (c) Chlorophyll destruction

256. BOD stands for

    a. Biotic community

    b. Chemical oxygen demand

    c. Biochemical oxygen demand

    d. Growing algae in large tanks

Ans. (c) Biochemical oxygen demand

257. D.D.T. is a

    a. Antibiotic

    b. Biogradable pollutant

    c. Non biogradable pollutant

    d. None

Ans. (c) Non biogradable pollutant

258. If water pollution continues at its present rate, it will eventually

    a. Make nitrate molecules unavailable to water plants

    b. Make oxygen molecules unavailable to water plants

    c. Prevent precipitation

    d. None

Ans. (b) Make oxygen molecules unavailable to water plants

259. In a polluted lake the index of pollution is

    a. Frog   b. Daphnia

    c. Artemia   d. None

Ans. (b) Daphnia

260. All the following contribute to pollution except

    a. Nuclear power plants

    b. Thermal power plants

    c. Hydroelectric power project

    d. Automobiles

Ans. (c) Hydroelectric power project

261. Some reliable indicators of air pollutants (SO_2 gases) are

    a. Neem tree and Eichornia

    b. Lichens and mosses

    c. Green algae and aquatic liverworts

    d. Ferns and cycas

Ans. (b) Lichens and mosses

262. U.V. rays prove lethal due to inactivation of

    a. Minerals, air and water

    b. Carbohydrates, fats and vitamins

    c. Proteins, pigments and nucleic acid

    d. Water, oxygen and carbon dioxide

Ans. (c) Proteins, pigments and nucleic acid

263. Radioactive strontium as aresult of radioactive fall out is

   a. Sr^{90} b. Sr^{80}

   c. Sr^{95} d. Sr^{85}

Ans. (a) Sr^{90}

264. Exposure of plants to high fluoride conc. result in necrosis or chlorosis characteristic in

   a. Leaf tip and leaf marging

   b. Only mid rib of lamina

   c. Petiole but not in lamina

   d. Stem tips only

Ans. (a) Leaf tip and leaf marging

265. Major pollution causing agent is

   a. Animals   b. Man

   c. Hydrocarbon gases   d. None

Ans. (b) Man

266. Biological treatment of water pollution is done with the help of

   a. Fungi   b. Lichens

   c. Phytoplanktons   d. None

Ans. (c) Phytoplanktons

267. Effect of pollution is first and most marked on

   a. Natural balance of our environment

   b. Natural gaseous cycle

   c. Natural geo-chemical cycle

   d. Natural flora of a place

Ans. (a) Natural balance of our environment

268. Which one of the following radiations is nonionising and has more specific biological effects than others

   a. Beta rays

   b. Gamma rays

   c. U.V. rays

   d. X-rays

Ans. (c) U.V. rays

269. Pollutant from motor car exhaust that causes mental diseases is

   a. SO_2 b. NO_2

   c. Hg   d. Pb

Ans. (d) Pb

270. Air pollution is maximum caused by

   a. Sewage and pesticides

   b. Automobile exhausts and chemicals from industries

   c. House hold detergents and pesticides

   d. Industrial effluents

Ans. (b) Automobile exhausts and chemicals from industries

271. Which of the following statement is incorrect?

   a. Lichens are affected by SO_2

   b. N_2 and Mg can pollute water

   c. All pollutants are not waste

   d. CO is the major environmental pollutant

Ans. (b) N_2 and Mg can pollute water

272. Which of the following does not cause pollution?

   a. Thermal power project

   b. Nuclear energy project

   c. Automobiles

   d. Hydro-electric schemes

Ans. (d) Hydro-electric schemes

273. Species that occur in different geographical regions reported by special barrier are

   a. Allogenic   b. Sympatic

   c. Autogenic   d. Allopartic

Ans. (d) Allopartic

274. UVradiations from sunlight causes the reaction that produces

   a. Fluorides   b. Ozone

   c. SO_2 d. CO

Ans. (b) Ozone

275. Which of the following atmospheric pollutant is not produced by exhaust of motor vehicle in Delhi

   a. CO

   b. SO_2

   c. Flyash

   d. Hydrocarbon gases

Ans. (c) Flyash

276. The component of a living cell affected by the pollutant SO_2 is

   a. Plasmodesmata

   b. Cell wall

   c. All cell membrane system

   d. Nucleus

Ans. (c) All cell membrane system

277. The molecular action of UV light is mainly reflected through

   a. Formation of sticky metaphase

   b. Formationpyrimidine

c. Phytodynamic action

d. Destruction of hydrogen bonds between DNA strands

Ans. (d) Destruction of hydrogen bonds between DNA strands

278. **National Environmental Planning Engineering Organization at Nagpur is engaged in the problem of environmental pollution**

    a. ICAR
    b. CPHERI
    c. NEERI
    d. CSIR

Ans. (c) NEERI

279. **National institute of oceanography is situated at**

    a. Panaji
    b. Mumbai
    c. Chennai
    d. Lucknow

Ans. (a) Panaji

280. **The ultimate environmental hazard to mankind is**

    a. Nuclear winter
    b. Noise pollution
    c. Water pollution
    d. Air pollution

Ans. (a) Nuclear winter

281. **Thermal pollution of water bodies is due to**

    a. Discharge of waste from mining
    b. Discharge of agricultural run of
    c. Discharge of heat from power plants
    d. Discharge of chemical from industries

Ans. (c) Discharge of heat from power plants

282. **Spraying D.D.T. on crops produce pollution of**

    a. Air and water only
    b. Air, soil and water
    c. Air and soil only
    d. Air only

Ans. (b) Air, soil and water

283. **The atmospheric pollutant is caused by**

    a. N_2
    b. CO_2
    c. CO
    d. O_2

Ans. (c) CO

284. **Water pollution is caused by**

    a. Industrial effluents
    b. Growth of phytoplanktons
    c. Rain
    d. Decay of bodies of acquatic animals

Ans. (a) Industrial effluents

285. **Rhizosphere is denoted to soil which is**

    a. Subjected to the influence of plant rhizoids
    b. Attached to root surface only

c. Attached to surface of root hair only

d. Subjected to the influence of plant root

Ans. (d) Subjected to the influence of plant root

286. **CO is a pollutant because**

    a. Combines with oxygen
    b. Inactivates nerves
    c. Inhibits glycolysis
    d. Combines with haemoglobin

Ans. (d) Combines with haemoglobin

287. **Decomposition of domestic waste under natural processes is known as**

    a. Thermal pollution
    b. Industrial pollution
    c. Biogradable pollution
    d. Non biogradable pollution

Ans. (c) Biogradable pollution

288. **Increase in the percentage of fauna and decrease in the flora may be dangerous because it enhances**

    a. Percentage of radioactive pollution
    b. Percentage of oxygen
    c. Percentage of disease
    d. Percentage of CO_2

Ans. (d) Percentage of CO_2

289. **In cities like Delhi pollution can be controlled to some extent**

    a. By cleanliness of city proper and less use of insecticides
    b. By proper disposal of organic wastes of industries and sewage
    c. By broader roads and factories away from city proper
    d. By all the above means

Ans. (d) By all the above means

290. **Burning of fossil fuels is the main cause of**

    a. Nitric oxide pollution
    b. Nitrogen oxide pollution
    c. Nitrous oxide pollution
    d. Sulphur dioxide pollution

Ans. (d) Sulphur dioxide pollution

291. **Water pollution is caused by or which one of the following is most important water pollutant**

    a. Ammonia
    b. Pesticides
    c. Detergents
    d. Industrial wastes or effluents

Ans. (d) Industrial wastes or effluents

292. Air pollution causing production of photochemical oxidants include

   a. Oxygen, chlorine, nitric acid fumes

   b. Nitric oxide, Nitrous oxide and nitric acid fumes

   c. O_3, SO_2, Cl_2

   d. SO_2, CO_2, CO

Ans. (b) Nitric oxide, Nitrous oxide and nitric acid fumes

293. When UV rays fall on the plant cell wall, which one of the following pigment helps in prevention against the damage of the cells

   a. Phycobillins   b. Xanthophylls

   c. Carotenoids   d. Chlorophyll

Ans. (c) Carotenoids

294. Gases commonly referred as green house gases are

   a. CH_4, N_2, CO_2 and NH_3

   b. N_2, CO_2, NH_3, NO_2 and O_2

   c. CFC, N_2, CO_2 and NH_3

   d. CFC, CO_2, CH_4 and NO_2

Ans. (d) CFC, CO_2, CH_4 and NO_2

295. Lead is considered as

   a. Soil pollutant

   b. Water pollutant

   c. Air pollutant

   d. Radioactive pollutant

Ans. (c) Air pollutant

296. Which of the following gas when combines with Hb of the blood forms a toxic substance

   a. CO_2 b. CH_4

   c. O_2 d. CO

Ans. (d) CO

297. Attacks of asthma in certain seasons may be due to

   a. Eating of some seasonal vegetables

   b. Exposure to cold temp.

   c. Inhalation of certain air borne pollens

   d. Absence of oxygen in the air, due to increased rate of photosynthesis

Ans. (c) Inhalation of certain air borne pollens

298. The maximum biological magnification of DDT through food web is seen in

   a. Algae

   b. Bacteria

   c. Higher plants

   d. Man

Ans. (d) Man

299. Which one of the following groups of plants can caused as indicators of SO_2 pollution of air

   a. Ferns   b. Horn works

   c. Epiphytic lichens   d. Liverworts

Ans. (c) Epiphytic lichens

300. Which of the following groups of parts of electromagnetic radiations are listed in increasing order of wavelengths

   a. Cosmic rays-> infra red ->radio waves -> ultraviolet -> X rays -> gamma rays

   b. infra red ->radio waves -> ultraviolet -> X rays -> gamma rays -> Cosmic rays

   c. Cosmic rays -> gamma rays -> X rays -> ultraviolet -> infra red radiations -> radio waves

   d. Light -> infra red radiations -> Cosmic rays -> radio waves -> gamma rays -> ultraviolet

Ans. (c) Cosmic rays -> gamma rays -> X rays -> ultraviolet -> infra red radiations -> radio waves

301. Which of the following enhances BOD of water

   a. Sand   b. Moss

   c. Algae   d. Sugar mill effluent

Ans. (d) Sugar mill effluent

302. Which of the following when inhaled dissolve in blood Hb more rapidly than

   a. CO

   b. SO_2

   c. O_3

   d. Nitrous oxide

Ans. (a) CO

303. Thermocline refers to

   a. Vegetation of alpine region

   b. Region in a lake where there is maximum fall in temp.

   c. Transitional zone between two vegetational types

   d. Region in a lake where there is freezing temp.

Ans. (b) Region in a lake where there is maximum fall in temp.

304. It is said that Taj may be destroyed due to

   a. Air pollutants released from oil refinery of Mathura

   b. Decomposition of marble as aresult of high temp.

   c. Flood in Yamuna river

   d. All

Ans. (a) Air pollutants released from oil refinery of Mathura

305. Pollutant from motor car exhaust that causes mental disease is

   a. Pb
   b. Hg
   c. SO_2
   d. NO_2

Ans. (a) Pb

306. Smog is a common pollutant in places having

   a. Low temp.
   b. High temp.
   c. Excessive ammonia in the air
   d. Excessive SO_2 in the air

Ans. (c) Excessive ammonia in the air

307. Which causes water pollution

   a. 2,4 D and pesticides
   b. Smoke
   c. Automobile exhaust
   d. Aeroplanes

Ans. (a) 2,4 D and pesticides

308. Pollution can be controlled by

   a. Sewage treatment
   b. Manufacturing electrically operated vehicles
   c. By checking atomic blasts
   d. All

Ans. (d) All

309. Air pollution is not caused by

   a. Thermal power plant
   b. Diesel engine
   c. Hydro electric power station
   d. Pollen grain

Ans. (c) Hydro electric power station

310. CO is harmful to human being because

   a. It decreases CO_2 conc.
   b. It completes O_2 to combine with Hb
   c. It is carcinogenic
   d. It depletes O_3

Ans. (d) It depletes O_3

311. Which pf the following is the cheap source of water and soil pollution

   a. Mining
   b. Agroindustry
   c. Thermal power station
   d. All

Ans. (d) All

312. Spraying of pesticides is an example of

   a. Point sources water pollution
   b. Defuse water pollution
   c. Both
   d. None

Ans. (b) Defuse water pollution

313. The effect of gaseous pollutant on human health depends mainly on

   a. Their ionisation potential
   b. Their atomic size
   c. Their solubility in water
   d. All

Ans. (c) Their solubility in water

314. Acid rain occurs in areas where

   a. Citrus plant are grown
   b. There are large plantation of eucalyptus
   c. There are large plantation of pine plants
   d. There are big industry and the atmosphere is polluted with SO_2

Ans. (d) There are big industry and the atmosphere is polluted with SO_2

315. As compared to tape water, BOD of water pollution with sewage

   a. High   b. Plane area
   c. Deserts   d. None

Ans. (a) High

316. Terracing is technique of farming in

   a. Hilly area   b. Plane area
   c. Deserts   d. None

Ans. (a) Hilly area

317. Presence of SO_2 in atmosphere is indicated by

   a. Moss   b. Liverworts
   c. Lichen   d. Fern

Ans. (c) Lichen

318. Checking of reradiation heat by atmospheric dust, water vapour, ozone, CO_2 etc. Is known as

   a. Green house effect   b. Radioactive effect
   c. Ozone layer effect   d. Solar effect

Ans. (a) Green house effect

319. Photochemical smog is related to pollution of

   a. Soil   b. Water
   c. Noise   d. Air

Ans. (d) Air

320. Existence of coal and petroleum may be detected with the study of

a. Palaeobotany
b. Ecology
c. Bacteriology
d. Economic botany

Ans. (a) Palaeobotany

321. Most imp causative pollutant of soil may be

a. Plastics
b. Iron junks
c. Detergents
d. Glass junks

Ans. (c) Detergents

322. Sounds above what level considered hazardous noise pollution

a. Above 120 dB
b. Above 30 dB
c. Above 100 dB
d. Above 80 dB

Ans. (d) Above 80 dB

323. Often in water bodies subjected to sewage pollution, fishes die because of the

a. Pathogens released by the sewage
b. Clogging of their gills by solids substances
c. Reduction in dissolved oxygen caused by microbial activity
d. Foul smell

Ans. (c) Reduction in dissolved oxygen caused by microbial activity

324. Which one is the major sources of pollution in metropolitan cities

a. Radioactive substances
b. Automobiles
c. Industries
d. Pesticides

Ans. (b) Automobiles

325. Which one among the following is lightly to have the highest levels of DDT deposition on its body

a. Eel
b. Crabs
c. Seagull
d. Phytoplanktons

Ans. (c) Seagull

326. Which one of the following isotopes is most dangerous to Homo sapiens

a. Cs-137
b. I-131
c. P-32
d. Sr-90

Ans. (d) Sr-90

327. In mineral bay, Japan which of the following animals remained free from minamata disease

a. Cats
b. Rabbits
c. Dogs
d. Pigs

Ans. (b) Rabbits

328. Taj mahal is threatened due to the effect of

a. Chlorine
b. SO_2
c. O_2
d. H_2

Ans. (b) SO_2

329. Which of the following radioactive isotopes is used in the detection thyroid cancer

a. I-131
b. C-14
c. Ur-238
d. P-32

Ans. (a) I-131

330. When huge amount of sewage is dumped into the river the BOD will

a. Increase
b. Remain unchanged
c. Slightly decrease
d. Decrease

Ans. (a) Increase

331. CO is a pollutant because it

a. Inactivates nerves
b. Combine with oxygen
c. Inhibit glycolysis
d. Combines with haemoglobin

Ans. (d) Combines with haemoglobin

332. Which of the following is responsible for atmospheric pollution

a. C^{14}
b. Sr^{90}
c. P^{32}
d. S^{35}

Ans. (b) Sr^{90}

333. Which is the cause of air pollution

a. Pesticides
b. Smoke
c. Noise
d. Chemical discharge

Ans. (b) Smoke

334. It is advised to consume iodised salt to escape a disease called

a. Tuberculosis
b. Goitre
c. Measles
d. Hydrophobia

Ans. (b) Goitre

335. Increase asthamatic attacks in certain seasons are related to

a. Expose to cold temperature
b. Inhalation of certain air borne pollens
c. Eating of some seasonal vegetables
d. Absence of O_2 in air due to increased rate of photosynthesis

Ans. (b) Inhalation of certain air borne pollens

336. Which of these is mismatched
a. Fossil fuel burning - CO₂ gives off
b. Biomass burning - CO₂ gives off
c. Solar energy - green house effect
d. Nuclear power - radio active wastes

Ans. (c) Solar energy - green house effect

337. Photocopying machines and other electrical equipment produce one of the following
a. Methane
b. Nitrogen dioxide
c. Ozone
d. Hydrogen sulphide

Ans. (c) Ozone

338. Tropical rain forest destruction is extremely serious because
a. Tropical soil cannot support agriculture for long
b. Large tracts of forest absorb CO₂, reducing the threat of global warming
c. It will lead to global warming biological diversity
d. All of these

Ans. (d) All of these

339. Acid deposition causes
a. Acid indigestion in humans
b. Lakes and forests to die
c. The green house effect to lesson
d. All

Ans. (b) Lakes and forests to die

340. Nuclear radiation can caused one of the following disease to eyes when expose to them
a. Trachoma
b. Retinitis
c. Cataract
d. All

Ans. (c) Cataract

341. Which disease in children is caused by the intensive use of nitrate fertilizer
a. Jaundice
b. Septicaemia
c. Mumps
d. Nathemoglobinemia

Ans. (d) Nathemoglobinemia

342. Sound pollution can be controlled by
a. Sound proof buildings
b. Traffic control
c. Adequate urban planning and road design
d. All

Ans. (d) All

343. Which of the following metals causes systemic poisioning in man
a. Pb
b. Zn
c. Mn
d. Se

Ans. (a) Pb

344. Which of the following damages WBC, bone marrows and lymph nodes
a. Cs
b. Sr⁹⁰
c. Ca⁴⁰
d. I¹³¹

Ans. (d) I¹³¹

345. Excessive inhalation of maganese cause
a. Anaemia
b. Gout
c. Diphtheria
d. Pneumonia

Ans. (d) Pneumonia

346. Harmful UV radiations coming from the sun cause
a. Skin cancer
b. Lung cancer
c. Mouth cancer
d. Liver cancer

Ans. (a) Skin cancer

347. Which of the following is non renewable source
a. Forest
b. Coal
c. Sunlight
d. Water

Ans. (b) Coal

348. In big cities, air pollution is due to
a. Burning of fossil fuels
b. Thermal power plants
c. Sewage
d. Suspended particles

Ans. (a) Burning of fossil fuels

349. Which one of the following is most poisonous
a. C
b. CO₂
c. SO₂
d. CO

Ans. (d) CO

350. Biodegradable pollutants is
a. Sewage
b. Asbestos
c. Plastic
d. All

Ans. (a) Sewage

351. Minamata disease s caused by
a. Air pollution
b. Water pollution
c. Soil pollution
d. All

Ans. (b) Water pollution

352. In social forestry programme which slogan was adopted

    a. Society for clean environment
    b. A tree for each child
    c. Save globe
    d. Save environment

Ans. (b) A tree for each child

353. The congress grass/carrot grass that causes allergy arrived in an India is 1956. It is

    a. Opuntia dilleri
    b. Parthenium hysterophorus
    c. Eichornia crassipes
    d. Sorghum halepens

Ans. (b) Parthenium hysterophorus

354. Excess atmospheric CO_2 increases green house effected as

    a. Reduce cloud formation
    b. Ppt. Dust
    c. Reduces atmospheric pressure
    d. Is opaque to infrared rays

Ans. (d) Is opaque to infrared rays

355. The news paper contains one of the following toxic material

    a. Pb   b. Cd
    c. Mg   d. Hg

Ans. (a) Pb

356. One of the best method to reduce air pollution is growing of plants capable of fixing oxides of N, C and S and radioactivity. Which plants has maximum power of absorbing CO_2 and oxide of N in a polluted areas

    a. Daucos carrota
    b. Bobinta pseudoacacia
    c. Phaseolus vulgaris
    d. Coleus indica

Ans. (b) Bobinta pseudoacacia

357. Which aquatic animals has been released on a large scale in the Ganga to rid it of waste flesh

    a. Dolphin   b. Gharial
    c. Turtle   d. Fishes

Ans. (c) Turtle

358. Pheumoconiosis caused by

    a. CO   b. SO_2
    c. Industrial dust   d. Air dust

Ans. (c) Industrial dust

359. CO can be absorbed by plants like

    a. Carrot   b. Bean
    c. Coleus   d. All

Ans. (d) All

360. Which of the following is not produce by motor vehicle

    a. CO_2 b. SO_2
    c. Fly ash   d. Hydrocarbon gases

Ans. (c) Fly ash

361. Radioactivity is absorbed by plants like

    a. Ginkgo   b. Lichens
    c. Both a and b   d. Pines

Ans. (c) Both a and b

362. Nitrogen oxide can be absorbed by plants like

    a. Quercus   b. Pinus
    c. Junipes   d. All

Ans. (d) All

363. It is advised not to have brick kiln near fruit orchard to

    a. Protect the orchard from operation of trunks and used for transporting fruits
    b. Save trees from soil erosion
    c. Save trees from poisonous fumes (H2F2) of smoke from brick kiln chimneys
    d. Save guard trees from large labour pollution

Ans. (c) Save trees from poisonous fumes (H2F2) of smoke from brick kiln chimneys

364. Harmful UV radiations cause

    a. Lung cancer   b. Mouth cancer
    c. Liver cancer   d. Skin cancer

Ans. (d) Skin cancer

365. Xeroderma pigmentation is

    a. Tanning of skin to light
    b. Spots formed by rays
    c. Sensitivity of skin to UV rays
    d. Both a and b

Ans. (c) Sensitivity of skin to UV rays

366. An isotope that causes damage to RBC, bone marrow. Spleen, lymph nodes and causes skin cancer is

    a. Cs^{137} b. I^{127}
    c. I^{131} d. Sr^{90}

Ans. (a) Cs^{137}

367. Fish eating birds like sea gulls are endangered because

a. DDT in them is carcinogenic

b. Chlorinated hydrocarbons interfere with their reproduce ability

c. Chlorinated hydrocarbons like DDT cause mutations

d. All

Ans. (d) All

368. The conc. of DDT is maximum in the breast muscles of birds that eat

a. Sea fish   b. Flesh

c. Sea plants   d. All

Ans. (a) Sea fish

369. Lichens have disappeared from cities because they are highly susceptible to

a. NO_2 b. SO_2

c. N_3 d. CO_2

Ans. (b) SO_2

370. Which disease in children are due to intensive use of nitrate fertilizers

a. Mumps

b. Cyanosis (blue baby)

c. Methaemoglobianaemia

d. Both b and c

Ans. (d) Both b and c

371. Which harmful item was discussed in Rachel Carson's 'Silent spring' book on damage of wildlife

a. DDT   b. CO_2

c. CFC   d. PCB

Ans. (a) DDT

372. Forests are destroyed mainly by

a. Acid rains

b. Soil pollutions

c. Water borne pollutants

d. Air pollution

Ans. (a) Acid rains

373. Deficiency of fluoride in drinking water caused

a. Goiter

b. Skeletal fluorosis

c. Dental caries

d. Dental fluoris

Ans. (c) Dental caries

374. The chrnobyl disaster in USSR was caused on 26.4.1986 by a

a. Nuclear weapon accident

b. Nuclear test

c. Nuclear reactor

d. Nuclear waste disposal leak

Ans. (c) Nuclear reactor

375. Taj mahal is being destroyed by

a. Nuclear pollution   b. Water pollution

c. Air pollution   d. Both b and c

Ans. (c) Air pollution

376. Electrostatic scrubbers meant to absorb pollutants also produce

a. CO_2 b. SO_2

c. Ozone   d. Dust

Ans. (c) Ozone

377. What is the major source of harmful radiations in the house

a. Colour TV   b. Oven

c. Heater   d. Tube light

Ans. (a) Colour TV

378. Which of the following is not a water pollutant but present in ordinary tap water

a. Cr   b. F

c. Cl   d. Ba

Ans. (c) Cl

379. Noise is unwanted sound above 80 dB. It is slow poison causes

a. Dialates cerebrall blood vessels and eyes

b. High blood pressure and deafness

c. Headache and high cholesterol level

d. All

Ans. (d) All

380. Water pollutant gas has adversely affected the flower growing industry in Los Angeles

a. N_2O b. CO_2

c. SO_2 d. Ozone

Ans. (d) Ozone

381. Coal burning heaters or stoves produce a hazardous gas which suffocates living being even to death

a. CO   b. CO_2

c. SO_2 d. H_2S

Ans. (a) CO

382. Which gas is pollutant and beneficial to life

    a. CO_2 b. O_2
    c. CH_4 d. Ozone

Ans. (d) Ozone

383. Photocopying and other electrical equipment produce

    a. H_2S b. Ozone
    c. CH_4 d. N_2O

Ans. (b) Ozone

384. Sometimes secondary pollutants like ozone, PAN, HNO_2, H_2SO_4 formed from primary pollutants are more toxic than primary pollutants. This phenomenon of increased toxicity in pollutants is called

    a. Green house effect   b. Synergism
    c. Biomagnifications   d. Eutrophication

Ans. (b) Synergism

385. Ceramic crokery of substandard quality could become a source of pollutant if food taken in it. This pollutant is

    a. Cr   b. Hg
    c. Pb   d. Cd

Ans. (d) Cd

386. Which satellite recorded the presence of an ozone hole

    a. LANDSAT-3   b. GOES
    c. NIMBUS-7   d. TIROS-N

Ans. (c) NIMBUS-7

387. Fly ash is the pollutant generated by

    a. Oil refinery
    b. Fertilizer plant
    c. Thermal power plant
    d. Mining

Ans. (c) Thermal power plant

388. The incomplete combustion of fossil fuel and motor vehicles produce large amount of CO. Which city has maximum conc. of CO in India?

    a. Calcutta   b. Delhi
    c. Chennai   d. Mumbai

Ans. (a) Calcutta

389. Protists are least sensitive to nuclear radiations but more sensitive are

    a. Toads   b. Birds
    c. Reptiles   d. Mammals

Ans. (d) Mammals

390. Most polluted city of India and world are

    a. Mumbai in India and Paris in world
    b. Kolkata in India and Tokyo in world
    c. Delhi in India and New York in world
    d. None

Ans. (b) Kolkata in India and Tokyo in world

391. Which part of the body is first be affected by nuclear radiation

    a. Brain   b. Liver
    c. Bone marrow   d. Lunges

Ans. (c) Bone marrow

392. The most serious pollutant to rubber tyres is

    a. CO   b. O_3
    c. CO_2 d. NO_2

Ans. (b) O_3

393. Of the following different occupations of women workers, tell which were first to die of cancer from nuclear radiations

    a. Air hostesses
    b. Nurses handling X-rays machines
    c. Painters of luminous watch dials
    d. Assemblers of colour TV parts

Ans. (c) Painters of luminous watch dials

394. Mumbai shows highest level of ...... in air

    a. Oxides of nitrogen   b. Smog
    c. Oxides of carbon   d. Oxides of sulphur

Ans. (d) Oxides of sulphur

395. Osteoporosis will be caused by pollutant

    a. F   b. Cl
    c. Br   d. None

Ans. (a) F

396. Highest level of oxides of nitrogen (NO and NO_2) in air is recorded in

    a. Mumbai   b. Chennai
    c. Bangalore   d. Calcutta

Ans. (d) Calcutta

397. When was NEPA (National Environmental Policy Act) enforce in India

    a. 1959
    b. 1970
    c. 1969
    d. 1968

Ans. (c) 1969

398. When did the water (prevention and control of pollution) Act came into operation in India

   a. 1976   b. 1974

   c. 1972   d. 1969

Ans. (b) 1974

399. Ganga Action Plan to restore the quality of the river Ganga was launched in

   a. 1981   b. 1982

   c. 1985   d. 1998

Ans. (c) 1985

400. The example of natural pollution is

   a. DDT   b. SO_2

   c. Smoke   d. Volcanoes

Ans. (d) Volcanoes

401. Ecological backlash (ecological bomerang) is

   a. Heat emission due to bomb explosion

   b. Production of adverse ecological effect by a previously useful chemical

   c. Production of useful ecological effect by a previously useful chemical

   d. None

Ans. (b) Production of adverse ecological effect by a previously useful chemical

402. Cadmium damages

   a. Liver and kidneys   b. Stomach

   c. Heart   d. Lungs

Ans. (a) Liver and kidneys

403. Of the four following metropolitan Indian cities, where polluted air hanges above like a cloud

   a. Delhi   b. Chennai

   c. Mumbai   d. Calcutta

Ans. (a) Delhi

404. Which causes fibrosis in lungs

   a. Asbestos   b. DDT

   c. CFC   d. Lead

Ans. (a) Asbestos

405. Where did the first recoreded incident of release of hazardous waste occur in India

   a. Kanpur (UP)

   b. Bhopal (MP)

   c. Thane (Maharashtra)

   d. Monghyr (Bihar)

Ans. (c) Thane (Maharashtra)

406. Of the following types of microbes, which one has been genetically altered to protect crops from frost, marine pollution, organic wastes etc

   a. Thiobacillus   b. Klebsilla

   c. Escherichia   d. Pseudomonas

Ans. (d) Pseudomonas

407. Leaking of methyl isocyanate (MIC) caused the biggest industrial disaster of the recent times in 1984 (Bhopal tragedy), what did the industrial plant manufacture when the leakage occurred

   a. Pesticides   b. Cement

   c. Explosives   d. Fertilizers

Ans. (a) Pesticides

408. In polluted water, index of pollution is

   a. Daphnia   b. BOD

   c. MPN   d. All

Ans. (a) Daphnia

409. Which organism in cases of colour changes after the industrial revolution is quoted as the most striking example of Industrial melanism and natural selections as result of environment change

   a. Dot moth

   b. Speckled wood

   c. Spotted lady bird

   d. Peppered moth

Ans. (d) Peppered moth

410. Match the following-

   a. Acid rain   i. Biological amplification

   b. DDT   ii. Mineral pollution

   c. BOD   iii. Smog

   d. Eutrophication   iv. Sewage pollution

   e. PAN   v. SO_2

Codes:

	A	B	C	D	E
1.	v	i	iv	ii	iii
2.	iii	i	v	iv	ii
3.	ii	iv	v	i	iii
4.	iv	v	i	ii	iii

Ans. (a) Acid rain   i. Biological amplification

411. Sewage and garbage in water kill fish due to

   a. High BOD

   b. Increase in bacteria and decrease in oxygen

   c. Increase in bacterial activity

   d. Decrease in bacteria and Increase in BOD

Ans. (b) Increase in bacteria and decrease in oxygen

412. Sewage water can be made fit drinkable/recycling with the help of

a. Micro-organisms
b. Hydrophytes
c. Fishes
d. Alum and sodium hypochlorite

Ans. (a) Micro-organisms

413. Eutrophication is maximum in

a. Bottom layers of deep lakes
b. Upper layers of deep lakes
c. Bottom layers of shallow lakes
d. Upper layers of shallow lakes

Ans. (a) Bottom layers of deep lakes

414. Sewage stimulates activity of osmotrophs (decomposers). A high content of which refers to water pollution

a. Fungi
b. E. coli and Beggiatoa
c. Diatoms and Oscillatoria
d. All

Ans. (d) All

415. The increased productivity of lakes and streams brought about by nutrient enrichment particularly by NO_3^- and PO_4^- of detergents is known as

a. Biochemical oxygen demand
b. Biomagnification
c. Green house effect
d. Eutrophication

Ans. (d) Eutrophication

416. The amplification of DDT in the various trophic level is known as

a. Pollution
b. Biomagnification
c. Green house effect
d. Eutrophication

Ans. (b) Biomagnification

417. A disease caused by eating fish contaminated by industrial waste containing mercury compounds is known as

a. Minamata disease
b. Hiroshima disease
c. Osteoschlerosis
d. Bright's disease

Ans. (a) Minamata disease

418. Which oil tanker accident (occurred in march 1967) first alerted the public of the grave problem of oil spills in oceans

a. Torrey Canyon
b. Ocean Eagle
c. Beagle
d. Agromerchant

Ans. (a) Torrey Canyon

419. In a photochemical smog which gas causes eye and mucous membrane irritant

a. O_3
b. SO_2
c. CO
d. N_2O

Ans. (a) O_3

420. The major source of pollution upto 80% of total air pollution in metropolitan cities is due to

a. Pesticides
b. Radioactivity and noise
c. Industries
d. Automobiles

Ans. (d) Automobiles

421. Which pollutant gas is released by Cud chewing ruminants

a. CO_2
b. CO
c. NO_2
d. CH_4

Ans. (d) CH_4

422. Which regions of seas or oceans are the most polluted

a. Coastal
b. Sea depths
c. Estuarine
d. Coral reefs

Ans. (a) Coastal

423. Most abundant pollutant in the atmosphere among hydrocarbons is

a. Butane
b. Benzpyrene
c. Propane
d. Methane

Ans. (d) Methane

424. Fluorides stop or reduce photosynthesis and cause chlorosis of tip and margin of leaves by

a. Combining with phytol tail of chlorophyll
b. Combining with Mg^{++} of chlorophyll
c. Combining with CHO group of chlorophyll
d. Combining with CH_3 of chlorophyll

Ans. (b) Combining with Mg^{++} of chlorophyll

425. Peeling of ozone umbrella (which protects us from UV rays) is made by

a. CO_2
b. PAN
c. CFMs
d. Coal burning

Ans. (c) CFMs

426. The most published oil disaster is

a. Release of petrochemicals in Goa by Zuari chemicals

b. Wreck of Tanker in 1967

c. Blow out of an oil well at Santa Barbara

d. Explosion in Brauni oil refinery

Ans. (b) Wreck of Tanker in 1967

427. PAN is a secondary pollutant and is found in

a. Herbicide   b. Pesticide

c. Fertilizer   d. Smog

Ans. (d) Smog

428. Ozone increases

a. Respiration   b. Transpiration

c. Photosynthesis   d. Both a and b

Ans. (d) Both a and b

429. Eutrophication of water bodies leading to the killing of fishes is mainly due to

a. Nonavailability of essential minerals

b. Nonavailability of oxygen

c. Nonavailability of light

d. Nonavailability of food

Ans. (b) Nonavailability of oxygen

430. In stratosphere, bulk of the UV rays are absorbed by

a. CO_2 b. N_2

c. O_3 d. Water vapours

Ans. (c) O_3

431. The compound mainly responsible for pollution which caused the ill famed Bhopal gas tragedy was

a. NH_4OH b. CH_3NH_2O

c. CH_3NCO d. $CHCl_3$

Ans. (c) CH_3NCO

432. Among the following environment pollutants, which has the problem of biomagnification

a. SO_2 b. O_3 and CO_2

c. NO_3 d. Hg fungicides

Ans. (d) Hg fungicides

433. An increase in atmospheric level of automobile exhaust gases does not lead to

a. Pb pollution

b. Particulate air pollution

c. O_3 pollution

d. O_3 depletion

Ans. (d) O_3 depletion

434. Which of the following gases was primarily responsible for the 1984 Bhopal gas tragedy

a. Methane   b. Methyl cyanide

c. Hydrogen cyanide   d. Methyl isocyanate

Ans. (d) Methyl isocyanate

435. Depletion of the ozone layer in the stratosphere is caused by

a. Hydrocarbons   b. Nitrogen dioxide

c. Carbon monoxide   d. Polychlorobiphenyls

Ans. (d) Polychlorobiphenyls

436. When exposed to sulphur dioxide gas, teh green colour of the plant leaves will be changed into

a. Red   b. Violet

c. Indigo   d. Yellow

Ans. (a) Red

437. How does acid ppt affect plants

a. It releases H^+ ions , thereby increasing the rate of photophosphorylation in green cells

b. It ppt organic acids in palisade cells of leaves, thereby inhibiting respiration

c. It injures foliage leading to reduction in photosynthesis, biomass and occasionally death

d. It ppt toxic nutrients in soil leading to growth inhibition in trees

Ans. (c) It injures foliage leading to reduction in photosynthesis, biomass and occasionally death

438. Which one of the following statement is correct

a. Up to 15 km above the earth's surface ozone is beneficial to life but CFCs are harmful

b. Beyond about 20 km above the earth's surface presence of ozone is vital to life on earth and CFCs are beneficial

c. Beyond about 20 km above the earth's surface presence of ozone is vital to life on earth, but CFC are harmful

d. Up to 15 km above the earth's surface both ozone and CFCs are harmful to life

Ans. (c) Beyond about 20 km above the earth's surface presence of ozone is vital to life on earth, but CFC are harmful

439. The protective ozone shield is to found in the

a. Hydrosphere

b. Ionosphere

c. Stratosphere

d. Iroposphere

Ans. (c) Stratosphere

440. Which of the following statement regarding the maintenance of carbon cycle in the biosphere are correct

i. Plants utilise solar energy to convert CO_2 and water into cellular materials and produce oxygen that animals consume

ii. Oxygen produced by the plants during carbon assimilation is not a by product

iii. Energy used by an animal comes from the oxidation plant material releasing CO_2 and water

iv. All decaying organic matter on the earth is ultimately degraded by molds and bacteria to yield CO_2 that escape into the atmosphere

Select the correct answer:

a. i, iii and iv   b. i, iii and iv

c. i and ii   d. i, ii, iii and iv

Ans. (b) i, iii and iv

441. Water pollution is best assessed by determining

a. DO and acidity

b. DO and BOD

c. BOD and turbidity

d. Hardness and alkalinity

Ans. (c) BOD and turbidity

442. Green house gases are called such because they

a. Are produced in green house

b. Prevent the escape of heat waves reradiated from the earth's surface

c. Are used in warming plants growth chambers

d. Help in maintaining atmospheric O_2 and CO_2 balance

Ans. (b) Prevent the escape of heat waves reradiated from the earth's surface

443. Measurement of the rate of O_2 consumption in unit volume of water over a period of time is done to find out

a. Biogas generation

b. BOD

c. Biosynthetic pathways

d. Fermentation

Ans. (b) BOD

444. CO is a major pollutant of

a. Water

b. Air

c. Noise

d. Soil

Ans. (b) Air

445. The worst environment hazards were created by accidents in nuclear power plant and MIC gas tragedy respectively in

a. Russia in 1990 and Bhopal in 1986

b. Ukraine in 1998 and USA in 1994

c. Bhopal in 1984 and Russia in 1990

d. Ukraine in 1986 and Bhopal in 1984

Ans. (d) Ukraine in 1986 and Bhopal in 1984

446. Increasing skin cancer and higher mutation rates are generally the consequences of

a. CO_2 b. Ozone depletion

c. Ozone biome   d. Acid rains

Ans. (b) Ozone depletion

447. Sudden mass death of fishes from oxygen depletion is more likely in case of

a. Eutrophic lake   b. Mesotrophic lake

c. Oligotrophic lake   d. Oxalotrophic lake

Ans. (a) Eutrophic lake

448. Acid rains occur when atmosphere is heavily polluted with

a. CO, CO_2 b. SO_2, NO_2

c. Ozone   d. Smoke particles

Ans. (b) SO_2, NO_2

449. Sewage drained into water bodies kill fishers because

a. Excessive CO_2 is added in water

b. It gives off a bad smell

c. It removes the competition with fishes to dissolved oxygen

d. It increase competition with fishes to dissolved oxygen

Ans. (d) It increase competition with fishes to dissolved oxygen

450. The basic component of the smog may be

a. O_3 b. PAN

c. O_3 and PAN   d. PPN and PBN

Ans. (c) O_3 and PAN

451. Which of the following type of pollution causes the out break of jaundice

a. Air

b. Thermal

c. Water

d. Land

Ans. (c) Water

452. Man made radioactive element Sr^{90} accumulates in the body through

   a. Breathing   b. Drinking water

   c. Food chain   d. Contaminated soil

Ans. (c) Food chain

453. Ozone day is observed on

   a. January 30   b. April 21

   c. September 16   d. December 25

Ans. (c) September 16

454. Air pollution effects are usually found on

   a. Leaves   b. Stems

   c. Roots   d. Flowers

Ans. (a) Leaves

455. Water pollution

   a. Increases oxygenation

   b. Decreases turbidity

   c. Increases turbidity and deoxygenation

   d. Increases photosynthesis

Ans. (c) Increases turbidity and deoxygenation

456. Most harmful types of environment pollutants are

   a. Non biodegradable chemicals

   b. Human organic wastes

   c. Wastes from feed lots

   d. Natural nutrients present in excess

Ans. (a) Non biodegradable chemicals

457. Phosphate pollution is caused by

   a. Phosphate rocks only

   b. Agricultural fertilizer only

   c. Sewage and phosphate rocks

   d. Sewage and Agricultural fertilizers

Ans. (d) Sewage and Agricultural fertilizers

458. Formation of ozone hole is maximum over

   a. India   b. Europe

   c. Antartica   d. Africa

Ans. (c) Antartica

459. The carbon dioxide contents in atmospheric air is about

   a. 0.034%

   b. 0.34%

   c. 3.34%

   d. 6.5%

Ans. (a) 0.034%

460. In coming years skin related disorders will be more common due to

   a. Pollution in air

   b. Depletion of ozone layer

   c. Use of detergents

   d. Water pollution

Ans. (b) Depletion of ozone layer

461. The most common indicator organisms that represents polluted water is

   a. E. coli   b. P. Typhi

   c. C. vivrio   d. Entamoeba

Ans. (a) E. coli

462. An environmentalist associated with Chipko movement is

   a. Sunder lal Bahuguna

   b. Medha Patekar

   c. Acharya Vinoba Bhave

   d. Baba Amte

Ans. (a) Sunder lal Bahuguna

463. Which of the following are the nature's cleaner

   a. Producers

   b. consumers

   c. Symbionts

   d. Decomposers

Ans. (d) Decomposers

464. Noise pollution is meqasured in

   a. Decibels   b. Tonns

   c. Pikograms   d. Kilograms

Ans. (a) Decibels

465. The term biomagnifications refers to

   a. Increase in the conc. of nondegradable pollutants as they pass through food chain

   b. Increase in population size

   c. Growth of organisms due to food consumption

   d. Blowing up of environmental issues by man

Ans. (a) Increase in the conc. of nondegradable pollutants as they pass through food chain

466. One of the imp. effects of SO$_2$ and its transformation products on plants is

   a. Plasmolysis

   b. Destruction of chlorophyll

   c. Destruction of Golgi bodies

   d. Destruction of cell wall

Ans. (b) Destruction of chlorophyll

467. Major pollutant present in the jet plaqne emission is

a. CCl_4 b. SO_2
c. CO d. FC

Ans. (d) FC

468. Sewage water is purified for recycling by the action of

a. Light b. Micro-organisms
c. Aquatic plants d. Fishes

Ans. (b) Micro-organisms

469. Spraying of DDT on crops produces pollution of

a. Soil and water b. Air and soil
c. Crops and air d. Air and water

Ans. (b) Air and soil

470. Which one is not dangerous not for life

a. Biopollutants
b. Ozone layers
c. Nuclear blast
d. Deforestation

Ans. (b) Ozone layers

471. If there was no CO_2 in the earth's atmosphere, the temp of earth's surface would be

a. Dependent on the amount of oxygen in the atmosphere
b. Higher than the present
c. Less than the present
d. The same

Ans. (c) Less than the present

472. Which one of the following organism is used as indicator of water quality

a. Beggiota b. Chlorella
c. Azospirillum d. Escherichia

Ans. (d) Escherichia

473. A sewage treatment process in which a portion in the waste is recycled into the beginning of the process is called

a. Cyclic treatment
b. Primary treatment
c. Activated sludge treatment
d. Tertiary treatment

Ans. (c) Activated sludge treatment

474. Life can not originate from inorganic materials at present because of

a. High degree of environment pollution
b. A very high amount of oxygen in the atmosphere

c. Very low atmospheric temp.
d. Absence of raw material

Ans. (b) A very high amount of oxygen in the atmosphere

475. Photochemical smog always contain

a. O_3 b. CH_4
c. CO d. None

Ans. (a) O_3

476. The depletion of ozone layer is due to the

a. Oxides of N_2 b. Oxides of C
c. Oxides of S d. None

Ans. (a) Oxides of N_2

477. Central Arid Zone Research Institute (CAZRI) is situated in

a. Jaiselmer b. Hisar
c. Jodhpur d. Karnal

Ans. (c) Jodhpur

478. The following may be used as an index of pollution in water body

a. Daphnia b. Typha
c. Trapa d. All

Ans. (a) Daphnia

479. Ozone hole refers to

a. Reduction in thickness of ozone layer in stratosphere
b. Reduction in ozone thickness in troposphere
c. Hole in the ozone layer
d. Increased conc. of ozone

Ans. (a) Reduction in thickness of ozone layer in stratosphere

480. Grambusia fish is an example by

a. Biocontrol b. Parasitism
c. Hyperparasitism d. None

Ans. (a) Biocontrol

481. Ozone umbrella is affected by

a. CFM b. CO_2
c. CH_4 d. CH_3NC

Ans. (a) CFM

482. In 1984, the Bhopal gas tragedy was caused by the leaking of

a. CO b. CO_2
c. NO_2 d. CH_3NC

Ans. (d) CH_3NC

483. Which one of the following is secondary air pollutant

a. SO_2 b. CO_2
c. PAN   d. Aerosol

Ans. (c) PAN

484. A labour working in a cement factory may have chances of suffering from

a. Bone marrow cancer
b. Cardiac disease
c. Asbestosis
d. Cystosilicosis

Ans. (d) Cystosilicosis

485. Acid rain

a. Is due to excess SO_2
b. Is due to excess CO_2
c. Is due to excess O_2
d. Is a natural phenomenon

Ans. (a) Is due to excess SO_2

486. Smog is a combination of

a. Air and water   b. Fire and water
c. Smoke and fog   d. Water and smoke

Ans. (c) Smoke and fog

487. Pollution caused by persistent pesticides is relatively more dangerous to which type of organisms

a. Top carnivores   b. Producres
c. Herbivores   d. First level carnivores

Ans. (a) Top carnivores

488. At present the most significant cause dwindling biodiversity is probably

a. Biological magnification of DDT
b. Global warming
c. The deterioration of ozone layer
d. The destruction of habitat

Ans. (d) The destruction of habitat

489. Which of this is a pollution related occupational health hazard

a. Fluorosis   b. Silicosis
c. Pneumoconiosis   d. Asthma

Ans. (c) Pneumoconiosis

490. Ozone layer is disturbed by

a. Super bonic jets
b. Large no. of automobiles

c. Large no. of factories
d. None

Ans. (a) Super bonic jets

491. Pollution is an unavoidable consequence of

a. Industrialization   b. Population
c. Urbanisation   d. Deforestation

Ans. (c) Urbanisation

492. Which of the following does not cause pollution

a. CO_2 b. SO_2
c. H_2 d. CO

Ans. (a) CO_2

493. Water pollution is caused by

a. Ammonia   b. Phytoplankton
c. Industrial effluents   d. Smoke

Ans. (c) Industrial effluents

494. Relative biological effectiveness (RBE) is usually referred to damages caused by

a. High temp.   b. Low temp.
c. Radiation   d. Pollution

Ans. (c) Radiation

495. The indiscriminate use of chemical fertilisers and pesticides may cause pollution of

a. Air   b. Soil
c. Water   d. All

Ans. (d) All

496. Air pollution is caused by excess of

a. Dinitrogen   b. Hydrogen
c. Water vapour   d. None

Ans. (d) None

497. Large quantities CO produced by gas heaters, charcoal stoves, coal mines etc. Usually prove fatal as the pollutant

a. Is carcinogenic   b. Impairs respiration
c. In combustible   d. None

Aas. (b) Impairs respiration

498. The removal of lead and its products from petrol used in automobiles is necessary because lead

a. Causes cancer of skin
b. Impairs respiration
c. Hampers Hb formation
d. All

Ans. (c) Hampers Hb formation

499. Photochemical combination of hydrocarbons and nitrogen oxides emitted by automobiles produces health threatening

  a. Acid rains   b. CFC

  c. Fly ash   d. Smog

Ans. (d) Smog

500. Water becomes polluted due to presence or addition of

  a. Inorganic substances   b. Organic substances

  c. Biological agents   d. All

Ans. (d) All

501. Which the pollutant flow is conveyed in well defined channels as municipal or industrial waste it is called

  a. Diffuse source   b. Non point source

  c. Point source   d. All

Ans. (c) Point source

502. the polluting strength of community waste water is usually characterised by its

  a. BOD   b. CFC

  c. MIC   d. ABS

Ans. (a) BOD

503. BOD stands for

  a. Biological growth database

  b. Biological oxygen demand

  c. Biological and organic diversity

  d. None

Ans. (b) Biological oxygen demand

504. Municipal waste, containing human and animal excreta, food residues, detergents etc. And rich in bacteria and organic substances, is called

  a. Sewage   b. Sewar

  c. Sewerage   d. None

Ans. (a) Sewage

505. Eutrophication of water bodies is associated with water

  a. Hole   b. Hyacinth

  c. Lily   d. None

Ans. (b) Hyacinth

506. Nuclear reactor malfunction in any country is a case of concern for

  a. The reactor's employees and neighbours

  b. The entire human population

  c. Some enlightened persons world wide

  d. Some developed and developing countries

Ans. (a) The reactor's employees and neighbours

507. An American plant which has become a troublesome aquatic weed in India is

  a. Typha latifolia   b. Trapa bispinosa

  c. Cyperus rotundus   d. Eicchornia crassipes

Ans. (b) Trapa bispinosa

508. Most inhabitants of calcutta suffer from bronchitis. It is due to excess

  a. Polluted soil   b. Polluted air

  c. Impurity of water   d. Adulteration of food

Ans. (d) Adulteration of food

509. Which one of the following is not pollutant

  a. CO   b. CO_2

  c. SO_2 d. NO_2

Ans. (b) CO_2

510. Peeling of ozone umbrella is due to

  a. Coal burning   b. PAN

  c. CFCs   d. CO_2

Ans. (b) PAN

511. Pollutant released by jet planes is

  a. Fog   b. Aerosol

  c. Smog   d. Colloid

Ans. (b) Aerosol

512. Anxiety and stress are caused by

  a. Noise pollution   b. Water pollution

  c. Air pollution   d. Nuclear pollution

Ans. (a) Noise pollution

513. Environmental pollution affects

  a. Man only

  b. Plants only

  c. Biotic components

  d. Biotic and abiotic components of environment

Ans. (d) Biotic and abiotic components of environment

514. Green muffler is related to pollution of

  a. Soil

  b. Water

  c. Noise

  d. Air

Ans. (c) Noise

515. Water pollution is due to

a. Industrial effluents
b. Sewage and other wastes
c. Agricultural discharges
d. All

Ans. (d) All

516. CFCs are polluting agents. They are produced by

a. Thermal power plant   b. Diesel trucks
c. Acid batteries   d. Jet planes

Ans. (d) Jet planes

517. Water is treated with chlorine to

a. Kill germs
b. Remove hardness
c. Remove suspended particles
d. Increase oxygen content

Ans. (a) Kill germs

518. Water blooms are formed by

a. Water Hyacinth   b. Planktonic algae
c. Hydrilla   d. Lemna

Ans. (b) Planktonic algae

519. Mottling of teeth is due to presence of an element in drinking water

a. B   b. Cl
c. F   d. Hg

Ans. (c) F

520. Aerosols decrease primary productivity by

a. Competing with CO_2
b. Preventing N_2 fixation
c. Reducing photosynthesis
d. Decreasing O_2 conc.

Ans. (c) Reducing photosynthesis

521. Methane gas producing field is

a. Cotton field
b. Ground nut field
c. Paddy field
d. Wheat field

Ans. (c) Paddy field

522. A person has impaired nervous system and signs of madness due to continued intake of metal contaminated water. The metal is

a. Mn   b. Pb
c. Ca   d. Hg

Ans. (b) Pb

523. As it passes into food chain, the conc. of DDT

a. Remains same
b. Increases
c. Decreases
d. Unpredictable

Ans. (b) Increases

524. Acid rain is caused due to

a. Sulphur dioxide and nitrous oxide emission from the combustion of fossil fuel
b. High conc. of carbon dioxide in the atmosphere which forms carbonic acid
c. High conc. of Cl which forms hydrochloric acid
d. None

Ans. (a) Sulphur dioxide and nitrous oxide emission from the combustion of fossil fuel

525. Electrostatic precipitators are extensively employed to control

a. Water pollution
b. Air pollution
c. Radioactive pollution
d. None

Ans. (b) Air pollution

526. Cyclone collectors are nowadays commonly used to control

a. Air pollution with special reference to dust particles
b. Radioactive pollution
c. Water pollution in general
d. Water pollution with special reference to Ganga Action plan

Ans. (a) Air pollution with special reference to dust particles

527. Air pollution causing photochemical oxidants production include

a. Oxygen, chlorine, fuming nitric acid
b. Ozone, peroxyacetyl nitrate, aldehydes
c. Nitrous oxide, nitric acid fumes, nitric oxide
d. Carbon monoxide, sulphur dioxide

Ans. (b) Ozone, peroxyacetyl nitrate, aldehydes

528. The protective ozone layer of stratosphere itself requires protection from indiscriminate use of

a. Fungicides, insecticides, bactericides and medicines
b. Aerosols and high flying jets
c. Ballons and turboprop aeroplanes
d. Atomic explosions and industrial wastes

Ans. (b) Aerosols and high flying jets

529. The effect of today's radioactive fall out probably be more harmful to children of future generation than to children now living because

a. Mutated genes are frequently recessive
b. Susceptibility to radiation increases with age
c. Infant are more susceptible to radiation
d. Contamination of milk supply is not cumulative

Ans. (a) Mutated genes are frequently recessive

530. In cities like Mumbai and Calcutta the major air pollutants are

a. Algal spores and marsh gas
b. Hydrocarbons and hot air
c. CO and oxides of sulphur
d. Ozone

Ans. (c) CO and oxides of sulphur

531. SO_2 and NO_2 cause pollution by increasing

a. Buffer action
b. Alkalinity
c. Acidity
d. None

Ans. (c) Acidity

532. Threat for the existence of human beings is

a. Deforestation
b. High population and pollution
c. Low forest
d. High population

Ans. (b) High population and pollution

533. Acid rains are caused by- Or. recent reports of acid rain in some industrial cities are due to the effect of atmospheric pollution by

a. Excessive release of CO in atmosphere by incomplete combustion of coke, charcoal and other carbonaceous fuels in paucity of oxygen
b. Excessive release of NH_3 by industrial plants and coal gas
c. Excessive release of CO_2 by burning of fuels like wood and charcoal cutting of forests and increased animal population
d. Excessive release of NO_2 and SO_2 in atmosphere by burning of fossil fuels

Ans. (d) Excessive release of NO_2 and SO_2 in atmosphere by burning of fossil fuels

534. Indicator plant which can be used to indicate atmospheric pollution by SO_2 are

a. Climbers like Cucurbia
b. Moss plants like Sphagnum
c. Grasses like Deschampsia
d. Lichens like Usnea

Ans. (d) Lichens like Usnea

535. One of the most dangerous radioactive pollutant is – Or. Which radioactive pollutant accumulates in bones

a. Ca -40
b. S -35
c. P -3
d. Sr -90

Ans. (d) Sr -90

536. Generally speaking, the atmosphere in big cities is polluted most by

a. Pesticides residues
b. Automobile exhaust
c. Household waste
d. Radioactive fall out

Ans. (b) Automobile exhaust

537. Which of the following disease caused or agrevated by pollution

a. Haemophilia
b. Rheumatism
c. Scurvy
d. Bronchitis

Ans. (d) Bronchitis

538. Ozone layer in stratosphere is destroyed by or which one of the chemical is responsible for the reduction of ozone content of the atmosphere

a. SO_2
b. CFC
c. Photochemical smog
d. HCl

Ans. (b) CFC

539. Which of the following changes would be likely to make terrestrial life on this planet impossible

a. Disappearance of moon
b. Change in the orbit of the earth from an ellipse to a circle
c. Change in atmosphere permitting all the solar radiation reaching the upper atmosphere to penetrate to the surface of the earth
d. Decrease in mean annal temp. By 10°C

Ans. (c) Change in atmosphere permitting all the solar radiation reaching the upper atmosphere to penetrate to the surface of the earth

540. Sewage water can be purified for recycling with the action of

a. Fishes
b. Micro-organisms
c. Penicillium
d. Aquatic plants

Ans. (b) Micro-organisms

541. Biologist celebrate 5th June as

a. World population day
b. World environment day
c. World hygiene day
d. Darwin birthday

Ans. (b) World environment day

542. Gas released during Bhopal gas tragedy was

a. Methyl isocyanate
b. Potassium isothiocyanate
c. Ethyl isothiocyanate
d. Sodium isothiocyanate

Ans. (a) Methyl isocyanate

543. Which one of the following element is the critical limiting factor in the function of ecosphere because of its irretrievable loss into the ocean

a. Fe   b. Mg
c. Ca   d. P

Ans. (d) P

544. Major aerosol pollutant present in the jet plane emission is

a. CO   b. CCl_4
c. FC   d. SO_2

Ans. (c) FC

545. Minamata disease is a pollution related disease which results from

a. Release human organic waste into drinking water
b. Release of industrial waste mercury into fishing water
c. Accumulation of arsenic into atmosphere
d. Oil spills into sea

Ans. (b) Release of industrial waste mercury into fishing water

546. The presence of O_3 n the atmosphere of earth

a. Hinders higher rate of phothosynthesis
b. Helps in checking and penetration of ultra violet rays to earth
c. Has been responsible for increasing the average global temperature in recent
d. Is advantageous since it supplies O_2 for people travelling in jets

Ans. (b) Helps in checking and penetration of ultra violet rays to earth

547. Which of the following is non renewable resource

a. Wild life   b. Water
c. Coal deposits   d. Forests

Ans. (c) Coal deposits

548. From the following which is the best source of renewable energy

a. Cattles   b. Trees
c. Petroleum   d. Coal

Ans. (b) Trees

549. Of the following sources of energy which one is the non-conventional source

a. Coal
b. Petroleum
c. Solar radiation
d. Electricity from nuclear power plants

Ans. (c) Solar radiation

550. There is no life on moon because there is no

a. Water
b. Oxygen
c. Nitrogen
d. Carbon

Ans. (a) Water

551. A depleting source of energy is

a. Water
b. Wind
c. Sun light
d. Fossil fuels

Ans. (d) Fossil fuels

552. Geothermal energy is

a. Renewable, conventional source of energy
b. Non renewable, non-conventional source of energy
c. Renewable, non conventional source of energy
d. Non-renewable, conventional source of energy

Ans. (b) Non renewable, non-conventional source of energy

553. Today concentration of green house gases is high because is

a. Use of refrigeration
b. Increased combustion of oil and coal
c. Deforestation
d. All of the above

Ans. (d) All of the above

554. Green house effect is

a. To grow vegetable is green
b. To grow more and more green plants in green garden
c. To maintain heat of radiation by CO_2
d. To reduce the green light from sun light which is received by the earth

Ans. (c) To maintain heat of radiation by CO_2

555. Green house effect is

a. Moisture layer in the atmosphere
b. Ozone layer in the atmosphere

c. Infra red waves reaches to earth

d. Increased in temperature due to increased in CO_2 concentration of atmosphere or CO_2 layer in the atmosphere

Ans. (d) Increased in temperature due to increased in CO_2 concentration of atmosphere or CO_2 layer in the atmosphere

556. **Phytotron is a device by which**

a. Electrons are bombarded

b. Plants are grown in controlled environment

c. Proton are librated

d. Mutations are produced in plants

Ans. (b) Plants are grown in controlled environment

557. **The race gas which is produced in rice paddies and is associated with global warming is**

a. Chlorine

b. Methane

c. CO_2

d. Hydrogen sulphide

Ans. (b) Methane

558. **Which is not a green house gas**

a. CO_2

b. CH_4

c. Freon

d. Hydrogen

Ans. (d) Hydrogen

559. **Green house effect is related to**

a. Global warming

b. Global green algae

c. Cultivation of green plants

d. Cultivation of vegetable in house

Ans. (a) Global warming

560. **Carbon dioxide in atmosphere air amount to about**

a. 0.3%

b. 3%

c. 0.03%

d. 0.003%

Ans. (c) 0.03%

561. **Earth summit at Rio dejanerio was related**

a. Soil fertility

b. Conservation of genetic resource of plants and animals

c. Survey of the land

d. None of the above

Ans. (b) Conservation of genetic resource of plants and animals

562. **The stratospheric ozone depletion leads to**

a. Increased in the incidence of skin cancer

b. Forest fire

c. Global warming

d. None of the above

Ans. (a) Increased in the incidence of skin cancer

563. **Which of the following country hosted the first world earth summit on conservation of environment**

a. India

b. Spain

c. Peru

d. Brazil

Ans. (d) Brazil

564. **Which one of the following is a renewable source of energy**

a. Petroleum

b. Coal

c. Nuclear fuel

d. Trees

Ans. (d) Trees

565. **Which of the following is non conventional source of energy**

a. Tidal energy

b. Wind energy

c. Solar energy

d. All of the above

Ans (d) All of the above

566. **Inexhaustible but limited source of energy is**

a. Nuclear fuels

b. Products of lakes

c. Products of oceans

d. Fossil fuels

Ans. (a) Nuclear fuels

567. **Petroleum is a**

a. Non renewable source

b. A rebewable source

c. A synthetic product

d. A unconvenient source

Ans. (a) Non renewable source

568. **Which of the following is non renewable source**

a. Mineral

b. water

c. forest

d. solar energy

Ans. (a) Mineral

569. **Ozone layer is disturbed by**

a. Supersonic jets

b. Large number of automobiles

c. Large number of factories

d. None of the above

Ans. (a) Supersonic jets

570. **Phytotron is a facility to**

a. Induce mutation

b. Grow plants under disease free conditions

c. Conserve endangered species

d. Grow plants under controlled condition

Ans. (d) Grow plants under controlled condition

571. L.P.G cooking gas is

a. Law pressure gas   b. Biogas
c. Fossil fuel   d. Low price gas

Ans. (c) Fossil fuel

572. Green house effect is enhanced in the environment by the gas

a. CO_2 b. CO
c. Fluorocarbon   d. Methane

Ans. (a) CO_2

573. Which of the following gases can depleted the ozone layer in the upper atmosphere

a. Sulphur dioxide   b. Methane
c. Carbon monoxide   d. Ammonia

Ans. (b) Methane

574. Which of the following gases contributes maximum to the green house effect on the earth

a. Freon   b. Methane
c. Carbon dioxide   d. Chlorofluorocarbon

Ans. (c) Carbon dioxide

575. Which of these is a true statement

a. Global warming is of no immediate concern
b. Since gases not derived from fossile fuel combustion are involved, reduction in fossil fuel burning will not help the green house effect
c. Global warming is so imminent that nothing can be done
d. Reduction in fossil fuel burning will lessen the green house effect

Ans. (d) Reduction in fossil fuel burning will lessen the green house effect

576. Heating of earth surface is due to

a. Air pollution   b. Water
c. Soil   d. All of the above

Ans. (a) Air pollution

577. Layer of ozone is present in

a. Stratosphere
b. Trophosphere
c. Thermosphere
d. Mesosphere

Ans. (a) Stratosphere

578. Earth is protected from dangerous U.V radiation by

a. Oxygen layer
b. CO_2 layer
c. Ozone layer
d. Photochemical smog layer

Ans. (c) Ozone layer

579. A natural resource that has inherent capacity to replenish is called

a. Non renewable resource
b. Renewable resource
c. Exhaustible resource
d. Inexchaustible resource

Ans. (b) Renewable resource

580. Which of the following resources is going to be exhausted by the end of this century

a. Tin   b. Gold
c. Lead   d. All of the above

Ans. (d) All of the above

581. For the production of biogas, the biogas plant requires

a. Agriculture waste   b. Cattle dung
c. Kerosene   d. Fire wood

Ans. (b) Cattle dung

582. The inexhaustive non conventional source of energy is/are

a. Sun tides
b. Solar radiation
c. Wind power
d. All of the above

Ans. (d) All of the above

583. Minerals, metals and fossil fuels are

a. Renewable resources
b. Biodegradable resources
c. Non renewable resources
d. Renewable as well as non-renewable resources

Ans. (c) Non renewable resources

584. Which of the following is most non renewable source

a. Water   b. Wild life
c. Coal and minerals   d. Forest

Ans. (c) Coal and minerals

585. Which of the following is a renewable resource

a. Soil
b. Water
c. Forest and wild life
d. All of the above

Ans. (d) All of the above

586. The renewable source is

a. Wild life species
b. Agriculture products
c. Trees
d. Both b and c

Ans. (d) Both b and c

587. Nitrogen fixation occurs in

a. Some herbaceous plant and legumes
b. Legumes and some bacteria
c. Some bacteria, cyanobacteria and legumes
d. All green plants

Ans. (c) Some bacteria, cyanobacteria and legumes

588. Both power and manure is provided by

a. Biogas plants
b. Thermal plants
c. Nuclear plants
d. Hydroelectric plants

Ans. (a) Biogas plants

589. Excess atmospheric CO_2 increases green house effect as CO_2

a. Reduce cloud formation
b. Precipitate dust
c. Reduces atmospheric pressure
d. Is opaque to infrared rays

Ans. (d) Is opaque to infrared rays

590. Green house gases are CO_2, CH_4, CFC, NO_2 and halons. These are

a. Transparent to emission from earth fro passage into spaces
b. Absorber of long wave radiation like infrared emitted from earth surface
c. Transparent to solar infrared radiation earth
d. Absorber of solar radiation for warming of atmosphere

Ans. (b) Absorber of long wave radiation like infrared emitted from earth surface

591. Where is NEERI located at

a. Cochin
b. Shimla
c. Nagpur
d. Banglore

Ans. (c) Nagpur

592. Green house effect is due to

a. CO_2
b. CO
c. NO_2
d. None of these

Ans. (a) CO_2

593. Which is most effective in warming atmosphere

a. CFCs
b. Methane
c. CO_2
d. Nitrogen oxide

Ans. (b) Methane

594. A biogeochemical cycle without an atmospheric component is

a. Carbon
b. Phosphorus
c. Nitrogen
d. Sulphur

Ans. (c) Nitrogen

595. Beijerinck discovered

a. Nodule formation in legume
b. Nitrogen fixation
c. Bacillus radicicola
d. Both a and c

Ans. (d) Both a and c

596. The source of methane pollution is

a. Marshes
b. Paddy field
c. Cattle and other herbiovores
d. All of the above

Ans. (d) All of the above

597. One hectare of good forest picks up CO_2 and release O_2 respectively

a. 30000 kg and 60000 kg
b. 30000 kg and 10000 kg
c. 10000 kg and 25000 kg
d. 8000 kg and 10000 kg

Ans. (b) 30000 kg and 10000 kg

598. Carbondioxide content of atmosphere has increased in the past 150 years from

a. 0.2 to 0.3 PPM
b. 0.027 to 0.034 PPM
c. 20 to 35 PPM
d. 270 to 340 PPM

Ans. (d) 270 to 340 PPM

599. Fertiliser obtained from sea birds along the coast of chile and peru is

a. Guano
b. Dung
c. Bone meal
d. Urea

Ans. (a) Guano

600. Which has a sedimentary cycle

a. Sulphur
b. Carbon
c. Water
d. Nitrogen

Ans. (a) Sulphur

601. Pseudomonas is an important component of nitrogen cycle. It

a. Changes ammonium nitrogen to nitrate state
b. Fixes elemental nitrogen
c. Produces elemental nitrogen
d. Transfers nitrogen

Ans. (c) Produces elemental nitrogen

602. Which one of the following statement is correct

a. Upto about 15 km above the earth's surface ozone is beneficial to life but CFC are harmful
b. Beyond about 20 km above the earth's surface, presence of ozone is vital to life on the earth and CFC are beneficial
c. Beyond about 20 km above the surface1 of earth, ozone vital to life on the earth but CFC are harmful
d. Upto about 15 km above the earth surface both ozone and CFC are harmful to life

Ans. (c) Beyond about 20 km above the surface of earth, ozone vital to life on the earth but CFC are harmful

603. Rise of atmosphere temperature because of high concentration of CO2 is known as

a. Pollution
b. Green house effect
c. Ecotone
d. Biomagnifications

Ans. (b) Green house effect

604. Nonbiological nitrogen fixation is

a. Rhizobial
b. Electrochemical and photochemical
c. Cyanobacterial
d. None of these

Ans. (b) Electrochemical and photochemical

605. Lithosphere is reservoir of

a. CO_2
b. N_2
c. Phosphorus
d. Carbon

Ans. (c) Phosphorus

606. Water cycle is made up of two overlapping cycles

a. Oceanic and fresh water cycles
b. Global and biological cycles
c. Ground water and atmospheric cycle
d. Surface water and atmospheric cycle

Ans. (b) Global and biological cycles

607. Sedimentary cycle having a small gaseous component is found is

a. Carbon
b. Sulphur
c. Nitrogen
d. Phosphorus

Ans. (b) Sulphur

608. Of the total fresh water, ground water constitutes

a. 44.2%
b. 10%
c. 22.4%
d. 90%

Ans. (c) 22.4%

609. Percentage of fresh water in the hydrosphere is

a. 33%
b. 30%
c. 13%
d. 3%

Ans. (d) 3%

610. Percentage of fresh water found in lakes, pounds swamps, streams and rivers is

a. 0.36%
b. 7.7%
c. 22.4%
d. 77.2%

Ans. (a) 0.36%

611. Maximum energy in world is used by the country

a. U.K.
b. Japan
c. America
d. China

Ans. (c) America

612. Peak concentration of ozone in the tratosphere lies at a height of sphere

a. 50 km
b. 40 km
c. 25 km
d. 10 km

Ans. (c) 25 km

613. Guano is the major source

a. Sulphur
b. Nitrogen
c. Phosphorus
d. Zinc

Ans. (c) Phosphorus

614. Stratosphere is characterised by

a. Rise in temperature with height
b. Fall in temperature
c. Lack of water vapours and dust particle
d. Both a and c

Ans. (d) Both a and c

615. Under ground water is

a. Renewable resource
b. International resource
c. Non-renewable resource
d. Mixed resource

Ans. (a) Renewable resource

616. Green house effect refers to

a. Global warming caused by increasing CO_2
b. Ozone hole

c. Increased chlorofluorocarbon

d. Plant grown in green houses

Ans. (a) Global warming caused by increasing CO_2

617. Green house effect with respect to global climate change refers to:

a. Cooling of the earth

b. Warming of earth

c. Increased rainfall and greenery

d. Desertification

Ans. (b) Warming of earth

618. NEERI is

a. National Environmental Engineering Research Institute

b. National Ecological Engineering Research Institute

c. National Eugenics Engineering Research Institute

d. National Ethological Engineering Research Institute

Ans. (a) National Environmental Engineering Research Institute

619. The region of earth comprising water forms

a. Hydrosphere

b. Lithosphere

c. Biosphere

d. None of the above

Ans. (a) Hydrosphere

620. The organisms which live in the bottom of lake are called

a. Phytoplankton

b. Zooplankton

c. Nekton

d. Benthos

Ans. (d) Benthos

CHECK YOU GRASP

1. **Component of living cell affected by pollutant SO₂ is**
   a. Cell wall
   b. All cell membrane system
   c. Nucleus
   d. None of these
   Ans. (b) All cell membrane system

2. **The threshold of normal human hearing lies between**
   a. 50–60 db   b. 120–140 db
   c. 30–40 db   d. 160–180 db
   Ans. (b) 120–140 db

3. **Landfill sites can be useful in which of following ways?**
   a. As a source of organic fertilizers.
   b. As a source of methane gas
   c. Reclamation of derelict sites to develop
   d. All of the above
   Ans. (c) Reclamation of derelict sites to develop

4. **In case of water quality, the quality parameter of biological properties includes which of the following?**
   a. Total coccus form bacteria
   b. Faccal streptococci counts
   c. Clorela count
   d. All of the above
   Ans. (b) Faccal streptococci counts

5. **Bioremediation of inorganic contaminants is**
   a. Microorganisms   b. Plant species
   c. Xerophytic species d. None of the above
   Ans. (b) Plant species

6. **Pulmonary oedema is caused by**
   a. Hydrocarbon   b. Carbon oxide
   c. Nitrogen oxide   d. SO₂
   Ans. (a) Hydrocarbon

7. **The blue baby syndrome result from**
   a. Excess of dissolved oxygen
   b. Methaemoglobin
   c. Excess of TDS
   d. Excess of chloride
   Ans. (b) Methaemoglobin

8. **Common indicator organism of water pollution is**
   a. Cholera vibro
   b. Salmonella typhi
   c. *E. coli*
   d. None of the above
   Ans. (c) *E. coli*

9. **Smog is the product of the which of the following?**
   a. Smoke + fog
   b. Fog + carbon
   c. Smoke + water
   d. Water + carbon
   Ans. (a) Smoke + fog

10. **Green house effect is related to which of the following?**
    a. Global warming
    b. Noise pollution
    c. Water pollution
    d. Global afforestation
    Ans. (a) Global warming

11. **The national Institute of Oceanography is presently situated at**
    a. Kerala   b. Calicut
    c. Goa   d. Cochin
    Ans. (c) Goa

12. **Mycorrhizae help in the uptake of**
    a. Potassium   b. Phosphorus
    c. Nitrate   d. Boron
    Ans. (b) Phosphorus

In case of less than 80% score, go through brief Review and Glance one again from chapter

Key: 1-b 2-b 3-c 4-b 5-b 6-a 7-b 8-c 9-a 10-a 11-c 12-b

14

Biostatistics

1. **We can transform the original data before applying the ANOVA technique using change of:**
   - a. Origin
   - b. Scale
   - c. Origin and scale both
   - d. All the three

   Ans. (d) All the three

2. **Who is considered as father of statics?**
   - a. Pearson
   - b. Boddington
   - c. RA fisher
   - d. AL bowley

   Ans. (c) RA fisher

3. **When statistics is used in plural sense it means**
   - a. Statistical method
   - b. Collect statistics
   - c. Both a and b
   - d. None of these

   Ans. (b) Collect statistics

4. **Select the two dimension diagrams of data representation**
   - a. Cubes
   - b. Pictures
   - c. Squares
   - d. Rectangular bodies

   Ans. (c) Squares

5. **Which measure of central tendency is applied for calculation of regression and correlation coefficient?**
   - a. Mode
   - b. Median
   - c. Geometric mean
   - d. Arithmetic mean

   Ans. (d) Geometric mean

6. **Which measure of central tendency requires data arrangement in ascending or descending order for its estimation?**
   - a. Median
   - b. Mode
   - c. Arithmetic mean
   - d. None of these

   Ans. (a) Median

7. **The intelligency, ability or efficiency can be measured by use of**
   - a. Mode
   - b. Median
   - c. Weighted HM
   - d. Geometrc mean

   Ans. (b) Median

8. **Which measure of central tendency is especially suited inb the field of business?**
   - a. Mode
   - b. Median
   - c. Arithmetic
   - d. Harmonic mean

   Ans. (a) Mode

9. **The result drawn from ANOVA based on transformed data is:**
   - a. Same as based on original data
   - b. Different from original data
   - c. More efficient than based on original data
   - d. Less efficient than based on original data

   Ans. (a) Same as based on original data

10. **For two factors A and B being dependent, the statistical model with one observation per cell can be written as:**
    - a. $Y_{ij} = \mu + \alpha_{ij} + r_{ij} + e_{ij}$
    - b. $Y_{ij} = \mu + \beta_i + r_{ij} + e_{ij}$
    - c. $Y_{ij} = \mu + \alpha_l + \beta_j + r_{ij} + e_{ij}$
    - d. $Y_{ij} = \mu + \alpha_l + \beta_j + e_{ij}$

    Ans. (c) $Y_{ij} = \mu + \alpha_l + \beta_j + r_{ij} + e_{ij}$

11. **For the interaction $r_{ij} = A_i B_j$ to be present in the two way classified data, we have:**
    - a. $\alpha_i + \beta_j \neq r_{ij}$
    - b. $\alpha_i + \beta_j = r_{ij}$
    - c. $\alpha_i + \beta_j > 2^\sim r_{ij}$
    - d. $\alpha_i + \beta_j < 2^\sim r_{ij}$

    Ans. (a) $\alpha_i + \beta_j \neq r_{ij}$

12. **The functional form for M.S. A can be written as:**
    - a. $M.S. A = \sigma_e^2 + {}^\sim (a_i^2) + \mu(\beta_j^2)$
    - b. $M.S. A = \sigma_e^2 + {}^\sim (a_i^2)$
    - c. $M.S. A = \sigma_e^2 + \mu (\beta_j^2)$
    - d. $M.S. A \, \epsilon\$\% - \sigma_e^2 + {}^\sim (a_j^2)$

    Ans. (b) $M.S. A = \sigma_e^2 + {}^\sim (a_i^2)$

13. The functions form for M.S.B can be written as:

a. $M.S. A = \sigma_e^2 + \tilde{} (a_i^2)$
b. $M.S. A = \sigma_e^2 + \tilde{} (a_i^2) + \mu (\beta_j^2)$
c. $M.S. A = \sigma_e^2 + \mu (\beta_j^2)$
d. $M.S. A < 2^{\tilde{}} \varepsilon_e^2 + \tilde{} (a_j^2) + \mu (\beta_j^2)$

Ans. (c) $M.S. A = \sigma_e^2 + \mu (\beta_j^2)$

14. If the null hypothesis Ho: $\alpha_i = 0$, is true then $\tilde{} (\alpha_i^2)$ will be:

a. $\tilde{} (\alpha_i^2) + = 1$
b. $\tilde{} (\alpha_i^2) = 1$
c. $\tilde{} (\alpha_i^2) = 0$
d. $\tilde{} (\alpha_i^2) = 0$

Ans. (c) $\tilde{} (\alpha_i^2) = 0$

15. If Ho ($\alpha_i^2 = 0$), is found to be non significant then E. (M.S.A.) will:

a. Give an unbiased estimate of σ_e^2
b. Not give an unbiased estimate of σ_e^2
c. Not give a biased estimate of σ_e^2
d. Give a biased estimate of σ_e^2

Ans. (a) Give an unbiased estimate of σ_e^2

16. If in two way classified data, Ho: $\beta_j = 0$ is found non significant then E. (M.S.B.) will:

a. Give an unbiased estimate of σ_e^2
b. Not give an unbiased estimate of σ_e^2
c. Not give a biased estimate of σ_e^2
d. Give a biased estimate of σ_e^2

Ans. (a) Give an unbiased estimate of σ_e^2

17. Out of three designs, C.R.D., R.C.B.D. and L.S.D., the simplest design is:

a. L.S.D.　　　b. R.C.B.D.
c. C.R.D.　　　d. None

Ans. (c) C.R.D.

18. To apply C.R.D. the experimental material should:

a. Not be homogenous
b. Be homogenous
c. Not be non homogenous
d. Both (b) and (c)

Ans. (d) Both (b) and (c)

19. Two basic principles followed C.R.D. are:

a. Randomization and local control
b. Randomization and replication
c. Randomization and local control
d. Randomization and regularity

Ans. (b) Randomization and replication

20. C.R.D. permits the complete flexibility in:

a. No and randomization replications
b. No of treatment and replication
c. No of treatment and randomization
d. All the above three

Ans. (d) All the above three

21. The most frequent occurred value of data or whose frequency is maximum is known as

a. Median　　　b. GM
c. AM　　　d. Mode

Ans. (d) Mode

22. In a symmetrical distribution of data which pair s correct

a. Mean = median > mode
b. Mean > median > mode
c. Mean = median = mode
d. None of these

Ans. (c) Mean = median = mode

23. Geometric mean of a given series is always less than its

a. Arithmetic mean
b. Weighed harmonic mean
c. Weighted mean
d. Harmonic mean

Ans. (a) Arithmetic mean

24. If any items of the series is zero, which mean of central tendency become zero

a. Arithmetic mean　　　b. Geometric mean
c. Harmonic mean　　　d. None of these

Ans. (b) Geometric mean

25. When we want average of rates f change or ratios or index number, which measure of central tendency is suitable

a. Mode
b. Median
c. Geometric mean
d. Arithmetic mean

Ans. (c) Geometric mean

26. To calculate the average woud be suitable to calculate the size of agriculture holding

a. Mode
b. Median
c. Weighted HM
d. Weighed AM

Ans. (a) Mode

27. Which type of average would be suitable to calculate the size of agricultural holding

a. Median   b. Arithmetic mean

c. Geometric mean   d. Mode

Ans. (d) Mode

28. Which is the simplest measure of dispersion?

a. Range   b. Mean deviation

c. Variance   d. Standard deviation

Ans. (a) Range

29. The principle which assures that extraneous factors do not influence continuously one factor is:

a. Replication   b. Randomization

c. Local control   d. Regularity

Ans. (b) Randomization

30. The design which provides maximum number of possible d.f to estimate is the:

a. R.C.B.D.   b. C.R.D.

c. L.S.D.   d. B.I.B.D.

Ans. (b) C.R.D.

31. The sensibility or precision of an experiment in case of a small experiment is permitted in:

a. L.S.D.   b. C.R.D.

c. R.C.B.D.   d. Both (a) and (c)

Ans. (b) C.R.D.

32. In methodological studies like physics chemistry cookery, in same green house experiment the design applicable is:

a. L.S.D.   b. R.C.B.D.

c. C.R.D.   d. B.I.B.D.

Ans. (c) C.R.D

33. In C.R.D. the two treatment (i,j) being replicated (r_i, r_j) times, the S.E. (x•I – x•,) will be estimated by:

a. $2eS\sqrt{\left[\dfrac{1}{r_i}+\dfrac{1}{r_j}\right]}$ b. $\sqrt{S_e^2\left[\dfrac{1}{r_i}+\dfrac{1}{r_j}\right]}$

c. $S_e^2\sqrt{\left[\dfrac{1}{r_i}+\dfrac{1}{r_j}\right]}$ d. $S_e^2\sqrt{\left[\dfrac{1}{r_i}+\dfrac{1}{r_j}\right]}$

Ans. (b) $\sqrt{S_e^2\left[\dfrac{1}{r_i}+\dfrac{1}{r_j}\right]}$

34. The number of basic principles followed in R.C.B.D. is equal to:

a. 1   b. 2

c. 3   d. 5

Ans. (c) 3

35. Analysis of R.C.B.D. is analogous to the analysis of:

a. One way classified data

b. Two way classified data with one observation per cell.

c. Incomplete three way classified data

d. None of the above

Ans. (b) Two way classified data with one observation per cell.

36. In R.C.B.D., the randomization is done:

a. Separately within each block

b. Independently within each block

c. Not independently within each block

d. As (a) and (b) both

Ans. (d) As (a) and (b) both

37. In R.C.B.D. the object is to keep the experimental error:

a. Within each block as high as possible

b. Within each block as small as possible

c. Between two adjacent block as small as possible

d. Both (b) and (c)

Ans. (d) Both (b) and (c)

38. Mean deviation is the least when calculated about

a. Median

b. Mode

c. Arithmetic mean

d. Geometric mean

Ans. (a) Median

39. If all the variate values are the same (e.g. 8,8,8), the standard deviation will be

a. 0   b. 1

c. 2   d. 3

Ans. (a) 0

40. The coefficient of variation can be calculated by using the formula

a. Square root of standard deviation/Arithmetic mean × 100

b. Standard deviation/arithmetic mean × 100

c. Standard deviation/geometric mean × 100

d. None of these

Ans. (b) Standard deviation/ arithmetic mean × 100

41. Unit less measure of dispersion is

    a. CV   b. Range

    c. Mean deviation   d. Mode deviation

Ans. (a) CV

42. The first central moment is always

    a. 4   b. 2

    c. 0   d. 1

Ans. (c) 0

43. The second central moment (about the arithmetic mean) is always equal to

    a. Mean deviation   b. Variance

    c. Standard deviation   d. Both b and c

Ans. (b) Variance

44. When a frequency distribution is not symmetrical about the mean it is said to be

    a. Kurtosis   b. Skewed

    c. Moment   d. None of these

Ans. (b) Skewed

45. When the distribution of data continuous, whch distribution is applicable

    a. Binomial   b. Norma distribution

    c. Poisson   d. Both b and c

Ans. (b) Norma distribution

46. The curves which are very highly peaked and have the value of b2 > 3 are called

    a. Patykurtic   b. Mesokurtic

    c. Eptokurtic   d. All of the above

Ans. (c) Eptokurtic

47. In case of m observation missing in R.C.B.D., with the number of treatments and replications as (t, r) respectively the error d.f. will be equal to:

    a. $(r-1)(t-1) + m$ b. $(r-1)(t-1) - m$

    c. $(rt-1-m)$ d. $(rt-1) - (m-1)$

Ans. (b) $(r-1)(t-1) - m$

48. If R.C.B.D. is conducted as R.C.D. with the same experimental material then M.S. (C.R.D.) will be worked out from the expression:

    a. $\dfrac{n_r s_t^2 + (n_r n_e) se^2}{(n_r + n_t + n_e)}$

    b. $\dfrac{n_r s_r^2 + (n_t n_e) se^2}{(n_r + n_t + n_e)}$

    c. $\dfrac{n_r s_r^2 + (n_r n_e) se^2}{(n_r + n_t + n_e)}$

    d. $\dfrac{n_t s_r^2 + (n_r n_e) se^2}{(n_r + n_t + n_e)}$

Where (n_r, n_t, s_e^2) have usual meaning.

Ans. (c) $\dfrac{n_r s_r^2 + (n_r n_e) se^2}{(n_r + n_t + n_e)}$

49. For more than two observations missing in R.C.B.D., to estimate them, the technique used is known as:

    a. Bartllet's missing plot technique

    b. Fisher's missing plot technique

    c. Kemthorn's missing plot technique

    d. Cochran and cox's missing plot technique

Ans. (a) Bartllet's missing plot technique

50. In R.C.B.D., the treatment M.S. will give an unbiased estimate of σ_e^2 when:

    a. Block effect is declared significant

    b. Treatment effect is declared non-significant

    c. Treatment effect is declared significant

    d. Block effect is declared non significant

Ans. (b) Treatment effect is declared non-significant

51. In R.C.B.D. the block M.S. will provide an unbiased estimate of σ_e^2 when:

    a. Block effect is declared significant

    b. Treatment effect is declared non-significant

    c. Treatment effect is declared significant

    d. Block effect is declared non significant

Ans. (d) Block effect is declared non significant

52. If in case of some extra replication in R.C.B.D., the two treatments (t_1 and t_2) are replicated (r_1 and r_2) time with error M.S. as s_e^2 then S.E. ($\tilde{t}_1 - \tilde{t}_2$) will be estimated by:

    a. $s_e^2 \sqrt{\left[\dfrac{1}{r_1} + \dfrac{1}{r_2}\right]}$ b. $2s_e \sqrt{\left[\dfrac{1}{r_1} + \dfrac{1}{r_2}\right]}$

    c. $s_e^2 \sqrt{\left[\dfrac{1}{r_1} + \dfrac{1}{r_2}\right]}$ d. $\sqrt{2s_e^2 \left[\dfrac{1}{r_1} + \dfrac{1}{r_2}\right]}$

Ans. (a) $s_e^2 \sqrt{\left[\dfrac{1}{r_1} + \dfrac{1}{r_2}\right]}$

53. In agricultural field experiment where fertility contour map is not known then a suitable design applicable is the:

a. R.C.B.D.   b. C.R.D.

c. L.S.D.   d. B.I.B.D.

Ans. (c) L.S.D.

54. In L.S.D., the experimental material of heterogeneous nature is controlled simultaneously in:

a. Two parallel directions

b. Two perpendicular directions

c. Incomplete three way classifications

d. Both (b) and (c)

Ans. (d) Both (b) and (c)

55. Normal distribution is due to the work of

a. SD poisson

b. Demoivre

c. LAPACE and Gauss

d. None of these

Ans. (b) Demoivre

56. Binomial distribution is a very useful distribution for dealing with which variates

a. Continuous   b. Discrete

c. CV   d. None of these

Ans. (b) Discrete

57. The mean of the binomial distribution is

a. np   b. pn

c. npq   d. none of these

Ans. (a) np

58. The arithmetic mean of he poisson distribution is

a. m   b. 1/m

c. 4/m   d. 8/m

Ans. (a) m

59. Arithmetic mean and variance are always equal in

a. Binomial

b. Normal distribution

c. Poisson distribution

d. All of these

Ans. (c) Poisson distribution

60. The hypothesis of no difference s known is

a. Composite hypothesis

b. Null hypothesis

c. Alternative hypothesis

d. Simple hypothesis

Ans. (b) Null hypothesis

61. The probability of committing type I error is known as

a. Test of significance

b. Composite hypothesis

c. Level of significance

d. Sampling

Ans. (c) Level of significance

62. The statical procedure for estimating whether the difference under stude s significant or non significant s known

a. Standard error

b. Test of significance

c. Level of significance

d. Sampling

Ans. (a) Standard error

63. Which test is used to test of significance of the difference between two mean?

a. t-test   b. z-test

c. f- test   d. None of these

Ans. (b) z-test

64. In a m x m, L.S.D. the number of experimental units is equal to:

a. m   b. m^2

c. m^3 d. (m-1) (m-2)

Ans. (b) m^2

65. In case of four treatments being A, B, C, D for L.S.D. the following layout plan is correct:

a. A B C D
   D A B C
   B C D A
   C D A B

b. A B C D
   D A B C
   C D A B
   D A B C

c. D A B C
   A B C D
   B C D A
   C B C D

d. Both (a) and (b)

Ans. (d) Both (a) and (b)

66. The number of basic principle followed in L.S.D. is equal to:

a. 1   b. 2

c. 3   d. 4

Ans. (c) 3

67. L.S.D. is arranged in:

a. One way classified in

b. Two way classified data

c. Incomplete three way classified in

d. The way classified data

Ans. (c) Incomplete three way classified in

68. In an incomplete 3 way layout plan of order m x m, the number of experimental unit is:

a. m

b. m^2

c. m^3

d. (m-1) (m-2)

Ans. (b) m^2

69. In L.S.D., a suitable approximate number of treatment is from:

a. (4 to 10)

b. (5 to 10)

c. (7 to 10)

d. (5 to 8)

Ans. (b) (5 to 10)

70. In m x m, L.S.D., the error d.f. is equal to:

a. (m-1) (m+1)

b. m (m-1)

c. (m-1) (m-2)

d. m (m-2)

Ans. (c) (m-1) (m-2)

71. The suitable linear model for m × m, L.S.D. is:

a. $y_{ijk} = \mu + \alpha_i + \beta_j + e_{ijk}$

b. $y_{ijk} = \mu + \alpha_i + t_k + e_{ijk}$ (i = j = k = 1,2.....m)

c. $y_{ijk} = \mu + \alpha_i + \beta_j + t_k + e_{ij}$

d. $y_{ijk} = \mu + \alpha_i + \beta_j + t_k + e_{ijk}$

Ans. (d) $y_{ijk} = \mu + \alpha_i + \beta_j + t_k + e_{ijk}$

72. In an incomplete 3 way layout experiment, the three factors responsible for variation in observation are:

a. Row, Column and Blocks

b. Row, Column and replication

c. Row, Column and treatment

d. Row, treatment and blocks

Ans. (c) Row, Column and treatment

73. In 7 × 7, L.S.D., the error d.f. is equal to:

a. 42

b. 36

c. 35

d. 30

Ans. (d) 30

74. Error S.S. in L.S.D. using the some experimental material will be:

a. Less than that in C.R.D.

b. Same as in C.R.D. and R.C.B.D.

c. Less than that in R.C.B.D.

d. Both (a) and (c)

Ans. (d) Both (a) and (c)

75. The error M.S. in L.S.D. using the same experimental material will be:

a. Less than that in R.C.B.D.

b. Same as in R.C.B.D. and R.C.R.D.

c. Less than that in C.R.D. and R.C.B.D.

d. Greater than that in R.C.B.D.

Ans. (c) Less than that in C.R.D. and R.C.B.D.

76. For the validity of probability statements about the treatment differences in an experimental design, the suitable principles used is:

a. Local control

b. Randomization

c. Replication

d. None

Ans. (b) Randomization

77. S.S. due to contrast Y = $T_1 - T_2 + T_4 - T_3$ where each treatment total (Ti) is the sum of 5 observations is equal to:

a. $\dfrac{Y^2}{16}$

b. $\dfrac{Y^2}{25}$

c. $\dfrac{Y^2}{20}$

d. $\dfrac{Y^2}{15}$

Ans. (b) $\dfrac{Y^2}{25}$

78. In an I.B.D., the number of treatments under study is:

a. Less than block size

b. Equal to block size

c. Greater than block size

d. Equal to number of blocks

Ans. (c) Greater than block size

79. Student's t-test is used when sample size is .... and population standard deviation is not known

a. Large

b. Small

c. Both

d. None of these

Ans. (b) Small

80. For paired observation, which test s used for testing the significance of a mean difference

a. t-test

b. f-test

c. z-test

d. Paired t-test

Ans. (d) Paired t-test

81. the comparison of two means from independent samples which test is applicable
  - a. f-test
  - b. z-test
  - c. t-test
  - d. None of the above

Ans. (c) t-test

82. The value of χ^2 ranges from which range and s always positive
  - a. −1 to +1
  - b. 0 to 2
  - c. 0 to ∞
  - d. None of these

Ans. (c) 0 to ∞

83. For calculation of χ^2, N should be at least
  - a. 10
  - b. 20
  - c. 50
  - d. 100

Ans. (c) 50

84. For χ^2 test no theoretical cell frequency should be small, it should be at least
  - a. 8
  - b. 5
  - c. 7
  - d. 10

Ans. (b) 5

85. χ^2 test is applied for
  - a. Testing the expectation of ratio
  - b. Genetic problem and detection of linkage
  - c. Testing of independence of attribute
  - d. All of the above

Ans. (d) All of the above

86. The validity of correlation coefficient is tested by
  - a. Z-test
  - b. χ^2 test
  - c. t-test
  - d. f-test

Ans. (c) t-test

87. The range of correlation coefficient lies between
  - a. +1 to −1
  - b. −1 to +1
  - c. 0 to 1
  - d. None of the above

Ans. (b) −1 to +1

88. The validity of regression coefficient is tested by
  - a. χ^2-test
  - b. t-test
  - c. z-test
  - d. Both b and c

Ans. (d) both b and c

89. A set of parameters of B.I.B.D. is:
  - a. v, b , r, λ
  - b. v, b, k, λ
  - c. v, b , r, k, λ
  - d. v, b, λ, k

Ans. (c) v, b , r, k, λ

90. In B.I.B.D., each pair of treatment (say t_i, t_j, i ≠ j) occurs together in:
  - a. λ number of block
  - b. (λ −1) number of block
  - c. (λ +1) number of block
  - d. None of the three

Ans. (a) λ number of block

91. The inequality b >2~ k is known as:
  - a. Kemthorn's in equality
  - b. Fisher's in equality
  - c. Cochran 8 cox inequality
  - d. Neyman's inequality

Ans. (b) Fisher's in equality

92. For the existence of B.I.B.D., the parametric relations are:
  - a. Only sufficient conditions
  - b. Only necessary conditions
  - c. Necessary and sufficient conditions
  - d. Not necessary conditions

Ans. (b) Only necessary conditions

93. In case of λ = r in B.I.B.D., then B.I.B.D. reduces to:
  - a. Complete block design
  - b. Randomized block design
  - c. Complete randomized design
  - d. Both (a) and (b)

Ans. (d) Both (a) and (b)

94. For any B.I.B.D., if λ = r, k will be:
  - a. Equal to number of blocks
  - b. Equal to number of replications
  - c. Equal to number of treatments
  - d. Both (a) and (b)

Ans. (c) Equal to number of treatments

95. If in a B.I.B.D., any two blocks intersect at a constant number of treatment (say λ), then design is said to be:
  - a. Asymmetrical
  - b. Symmetrical
  - c. Complete design
  - d. Unconfounded design

Ans. (b) Symmetrical

96. A given I.B.D., is also a:
  - a. Balanced design
  - b. Connected design
  - c. Confounded design
  - d. Both (a) and (b)

Ans. (d) Both (a) and (b)

97. For a given B.I.B.D., there exists:

a. Complementary design
b. Residual design
c. Both (a) and (b)
d. None

Ans. (c) Both (a) and (b)

98. The designs R.C.B.D. and L.S.B., both are:

a. Balanced designs   b. Connected designs
c. Orthogonal designs   d. All the three

Ans. (d) All the three

99. Coefficient of determination is a square of

a. Regression coefficient
b. Correlation coefficient
c. Both a and b
d. None of the above

Ans. (b) Correlation coefficient

100. The range of multiple correlation coefficient lies between

a. 0 to ∞   b. −1 to +1
c. 0 to +1   d. −∞ to +∞

Ans. (c) 0 to +1

101. The significance of multiple correlation is tested by

a. F-test   b. Z-test
c. T-test   d. None of these

Ans. (a) F-test

102. The repetition of the treatment under investigation is know is

a. Local control
b. Randomization
c. Replication
d. None of the above

Ans. (c) Replication

103. The allocation of the treatment to the different experimental units in a random manner is knows as

a. Replication   b. Randomization
c. Local control   d. None of these

Ans. (b) Randomization

104. The principle of making use of greater homogeneity in groups of experimental units to reduce the experimental error is referred as

a. Local control   b. Replication
c. Randomization   d. Sampling

Ans. (a) Local control

105. What are the basic principles of field experimentation

a. Replication   b. Randomization
c. Local control   d. All of these

Ans. (d) All of these

106. The completely randomized design is appropriate when the experimental material is

a. Unlimited and homogenous
b. limited and heterogeneous
c. Unlimited and heterogeneous
d. None of the above

Ans. (c) Unlimited and heterogeneous

107. Local control is not applied for the design

a. SPD   b. LSD
c. RBD   d. CRD

Ans. (d) CRD

108. When the fertility gradient of the field is in one direction, which design s appropriate

a. RBD   b. SPD
c. LSD   d. CRD

Ans. (a) RBD

109. When the fertility gradient of the field goes in two directions, which design is most appropriate

a. RBD   b. LSD
c. SPD   d. CRD

Ans. (b) LSD

110. The efficiency factor of a B.I.B.D. is:

a. Less than 1.0   b. Greater than 1.0
c. Greater than 2.0   d. None of three

Ans. (a) Less than 1.0

111. The basic purpose of ANOVA technique is to test the homogeneity of several:

a. Population means
b. Population correlation
c. Population variances
d. None of the three

Ans. (a) Population means

112. The ANOVA technique was introduced first time in agricultural data by:

a. Prof. P.C. Mahalanobis
b. Prof. R.A. Fisher
c. Prof. P.V. Suchatme
d. Prof. C.R. Rao

Ans. (b) Prof. R.A. Fisher

113. The ANOVA technique is now frequently used in testing the linearity of:

a. Fitted correlation coefficient
b. Fitted regression line
c. Fitted regression coefficient
d. Correlation ratio n

Ans. (b) Fitted regression line

114. ANOVA technique is also used in testing in significance of:

a. Correlation ratio
b. Correlation coefficient
c. Regression coefficient by
d. Homogeneity of variance

Ans. (a) Correlation ratio

115. In ANOVA model, the different components of variance should follow:

a. Multiplicative law
b. Additive law
c. Probabilistic law
d. Large sample theory

Ans. (b) Additive law

116. In ANOVA model the error term e_{ij} should be distributed as:

a. Randomly
b. Independently
c. Normally
d. All the three

Ans. (d) All the three

117. The error term e_{ij} in ANOVA model have:

a. Mean zero
b. Constant variance σ_e^2
c. Same variance
d. All the three

Ans. (d) All the three

118. In ANOVA model, the constant error variance σ_e^2 is estimated unbiasedly by:

a. Error M.S.
b. Treatment M.S.
c. Replication M.S.
d. Both (a) and (c)

Ans. (a) Error M.S.

119. In ANOVA model, the variates y_{ij} should be:

a. Homosedastic
b. Heterogeneous
c. Of equal variance
d. Both (a) and (c)

Ans. (d) Both (a) and (c)

120. The normality of variates y_{ij} in ANOVA model is necessary to apply the:

a. The t statistic
b. F statistic
c. π^2 statistic
d. Z statistic

Ans. (b) F statistic

121. The d.f. due to various sources of variation in ANOVA model, should follow the:

a. Probabilistic law
b. Multiplicative law
c. Additive law
d. None

Ans. (c) Additive law

122. If the Ho is true then theoretically the value of F statistic becomes:

a. Equal to 1.0
b. Greater than 1.0
c. Less than 1.0
d. Equal to as

Ans. (a) Equal to 1.0

123. If the null hypothesis Ho in ANOVA is declared significant then theoretically the value of F statistic becomes:

a. Equal to 1.0
b. Greater than 1.0
c. Less than 1.96
d. Greater than 1.96

Ans. (b) Greater than 1.0

124. If s_t^2 and σ_e^2 are the treatment and error M.S. in ANOVA model then the ratio s_t^2 / σ_e^2 follow:

a. X^2 distribution with $(t-1)$d.f
b. F distribution with $(t-1)$ and $(n-1)$ d.f
c. Student's t distribution with $(t-1)$ d.f
d. Z distribution

Ans. (a) X^2 distribution with $(t-1)$d.f

125. If $(s_e^2 \, \sigma_e^2)$ are the error M S with $(n-t)$ d.f and error variance respectively then the ratio will follow:

a. Student's t distribution with $(t-1)$ d.f
b. F distribution with $(t-1)$ and $(n-1)$ d.f
c. X^2 distribution with $(t-1)$ d.f
d. Normal distribution with mean zero and variance unity

Ans. (c) X^2 distribution with $(t-1)$ d.f

126. If $(s_e^2 \, \sigma_e^2)$ are treatment and error M.S. with $(t-1)$, $(n-1)$ d.f respectively than the ratio (s_t^2/s_e^2) will follow:

a. F distribution with $(t-1)$ and $(n-1)$ d.f
b. X^2 distribution with $(t-1)$ d.f
c. Student's t distribution with $(t-1)$ d.f
d. Normal distribution as N (0,1)

Ans. (b) X^2 distribution with $(t-1)$ d.f

127. In ANOVA model, to define the F statistic, the effect due to treatment and error term must follow the:

a. Normal distribution
b. X^2 distribution
c. Mean X^2 distribution
d. Z distribution

Ans. (a) Normal distribution

128. F statistic is defined as the ratio of two:
- a. Dependent mean X^2 statistics
- b. Independent mean X^2 statistics
- c. Two independent sample mean squares
- d. Both (a) and (c)

Ans. (b) Independent mean X^2 statistics

129. In randomized block design, how many treatments can be adopted without any loss of efficiency
- a. 10
- b. 15
- c. 20
- d. 25

Ans. (c) 20

130. How many number of treatments can be adopted in LSD
- a. 5 to 8
- b. 5 to 12
- c. Both a and b
- d. None of the above

Ans. (c) Both a and b

131. When there are several factors with different levels to be experimented simultaneously with the same level of precision, which design is most appropriate
- a. LSD
- b. CRD
- c. RBD
- d. Factorial factor

Ans. (d) Factorial factor

132. When the experimental material is very less and number of genotypes are very large, which design is most suited
- a. RBD
- b. LSD
- c. Split plot design
- d. Augmented design

Ans. (d) Augmented design

133. In the experiment, a treatment requires large area and b treatment requires smaller area, which design s most appropriate
- a. RBD
- b. LSD
- c. Split plot design
- d. Augmented design

Ans. (c) Split plot design

134. The minimum error degree of freedom should be at least
- a. 5
- b. 10
- c. 12
- d. 18

Ans. (c) 12

135. The values of regression coefficient lies between
- a. −1 to +1
- b. −∞ to +∞
- c. −∞ to +1
- d. 0 to +1

Ans. (b) −∞ to +∞

136. The well known ANOVA technique is the technique in fact an analysis of:
- a. Variance
- b. Sum of square
- c. Mean sum of square
- d. Both (b) and (c)

Ans. (d) Both (b) and (c)

137. A model in which each of the factor has fixed effect and only effect of error term is of random nature, is known as:
- a. Mixed effect model
- b. Random effect model
- c. Fixed effect model
- d. Both (a) and (c)

Ans. (c) Fixed effect model

138. A model in which some factors have fixed effect and others have random effect, is known as:
- a. Mixed effect model
- b. Random effect model
- c. Fixed effect model
- d. Both (b) and (c)

Ans. (a) Mixed effect model

139. A random effect model has:
- a. All factors along with error term are of random nature
- b. Some factor are of random and others are of fixed effect
- c. All factor are of random nature except error term
- d. None of the term

Ans. (a) All factors along with error term are of random nature

140. The main objective of fixed effect model is to estimate the:
- a. Effect of different factors
- b. Variability of different factors
- c. Variance of different factors
- d. Both (b) and (c)

Ans. (a) Effect of different factors

141. In random effect model, the main objective is to estimate the:
- a. Mean effect of different factors
- b. The variability among the effects of different factors
- c. The variance among effects due to different factors
- d. Both (b) and (c)

Ans. (d) Both (b) and (c)

142. When a set of observations are classified over different levels of only one factor then such type of classification, is known as:
- a. Two way classification
- b. One way classification
- c. Multi way classification
- d. Both (a) and (c)

Ans. (a) Two way classification

143. Complete randomized design is an example of:

a. Two way classification
b. One way classification
c. Multi way classification
d. Both (a) and (c)

Ans. (b) One way classification

144. When a set of observations are classified with respect to two factors simultaneously at different levels then such classification is known as:

a. Two way classification
b. Multi way classification
c. Both (a) and (b)
d. None of the three

Ans. (a) Two way classification

145. Randomized complete block design is an example of:

a. One way classification
b. Two way classification
c. Multi way classification
d. Both (a) and (b)

Ans. (b) Two way classification

146. The model for one way classification is written as:

a. $Y_{ij} = \beta_i + e_{ij}$, $(i = 1,2,.....t, j=1,2, ..., ni)$
b. $Y_{ij} = \mu + \beta_i + e_{ij}$ $(i = 1,2,.....t.\ j=1,2, ..., ni)$
c. $Y_{ij} = \mu + \beta_i + \alpha_i + e_{ij}$ $(i= 1,2......t, j = 1,2, ... ni)$
d. None of the above

Ans. (b) $Y_{ij} = \mu + \beta_i + e_{ij}$ $(i = 1,2,.....t.\ j= 1,2, ..., ni)$

147. In question 29, the $\hat{a}_i$ can be estimated through:

a. $\beta_i = \dfrac{1}{n_i} \sum\limits_{j=1}^{n} y_{ij}$

b. $\beta_i = \dfrac{1}{t} \sum\limits_{i=1}^{t} y_{ij}$

c. $\beta_i = \left\langle \dfrac{1}{n_i} \sum\limits_{j=1}^{ni} y_{ij} - \dfrac{1}{n} \sum\limits_{i}^{t} \sum\limits_{j=1}^{ni} y_{ij} \right\rangle n_i$

d. $\beta_i = \dfrac{1}{n_i} \sum\limits_{j=1}^{ni} y_{ij} - \mu$

Ans. (d) $\beta_i = \dfrac{1}{n_i} \sum\limits_{j=1}^{ni} y_{ij} - \mu$

148. Let S_A^2 denotes the mean square due to factor A then we have:

a. $E(S_A^2) = \sigma_e^{\ 2} + \varphi\ (Ai, i = 1,2, ...t\ )$
b. $E(S_A^2) = \sigma_e^{\ 2} - \varphi\ (Ai, i = 1,2, ...t\ )$

c. $E(S_A^2) = \sigma_e^2 + \mu\ (Ai, i = 1,2, ...t\ )$
d. Both (a) and (c) where φ and μ are variance like functions of (A is,)

Ans. (d) Both (a) and (c) where φ and μ are variance like functions of (A is,)

149. When the null hypothesis Ho is true in case of one way classified data, treatment mean square gives:

a. An unbiased estimate of σ_e^2
b. A biased estimate of σ_e^2
c. A consistant estimate of σ_e^2
d. None of the above

Ans. (a) An unbiased estimate of σ_e^2

150. If in question 32, $E(S^2_A) = \sigma_e^2 + \varphi\ (Ai, i = 1,2, ...t)$ is true in case of under Ho, then the value of $\varphi\ (A_{is})$ is:

a. Equal to
b. Equal to zero
c. Greater than zero
d. Less than zero

Ans. (b) Equal to zero

151. In this question if Ho is declared significant then the value of ö (A_{is}) will be:

a. Greater than zero
b. Less than zero
c. Equal to
d. Nothing can said with surety

Ans. (a) Greater than zero

152. In C.R.D. with r replication the C.D between two treatment means $(t\tilde{}_i,\ t\tilde{}_i)$ will be given by:

a. $C\,D\,(t_i, t_i) = t \propto \sqrt{\dfrac{s_e^2}{2r}}$

b. $C\,D\,(t_i, t_i) = t \propto \sqrt{\dfrac{2s_e^2}{r}}$

c. $C\,D\,(t_i, t_i) = t \propto \sqrt{\dfrac{rs_e^2}{2}}$

d. $C\,D\,(t_i, t_i) = t \propto \sqrt{\dfrac{s_e^2}{2r}}$

Ans. (b) $C\,D\,(t_i, t_i) = t \propto \sqrt{\dfrac{2s_e^2}{r}}$

153. In the split plot experiment, the main factor A and subfactor B are studied in the:

a. Factorial experiment
b. Same experiment
c. Two simple experiment
d. Latin square design

Ans. (b) Same experiment

154. The main factor A requires:

    a. Smaller plot design   b. Squared plot design

    c. Larger plot size   d. Sub plot

Ans. (c) Larger plot size

155. The sub plot treatment B requires:

    a. Larger plot size   b. Smaller plot size

    c. Sub plots   d. Both (b) and (c)

Ans. (d) Both (b) and (c)

156. In split plot experiment, the subfactor B is allotted to the split plots:

    a. Within blocks   b. Between blocks

    c. Between rows   d. Between columns

Ans. (a) Within blocks

157. In split plot experiment, the factors allotted to plots within blocks are known as:

    a. Subfactors   b. Split plot treatment

    c. Interactions   d. Both (a) and (b)

Ans. (d) Both (a) and (b)

158. In split plot experiment, the factors allotted to blocks within replication, are known as:

    a. Main plot treatment   b. Whole plot treatment

    c. Both (a) and (b)   d. Subplot treatment

Ans. (c) Both (a) and (b)

159. In factorial experiment, all the treatment combinations of two or more than two factors are allotted at random to the:

    a. Plots within blocks

    b. Block within replications

    c. Split plot within main

    d. Split plots within replications

Ans. (a) Plots within blocks

160. In split plot experiment, the maximum importance is given to the:

    a. Main factor A   b. Sub factor B

    c. Interaction A B   d. Interaction RA

Ans. (c) Interaction A B

161. In split plot experiment, the precision of interaction AB is:

    a. Equal to that of A

    b. Equal to that of B

    c. More than that of A and B both

    d. Less than that of A and B

Ans. (c) More than that of A and B both

162. In ordinary 2^2 factorial experiment in R.C.B.D., the interaction effect AB will be estimated with precision:

    a. Equal to that of A

    b. Less than that of A

    c. Equal to that of A and B both

    d. More than that of A and B both

Ans. (c) Equal to that of A and B both

163. In split plot experiment, the subplot treatment is:

    a. Different from main plot treatment

    b. Different from whole plot treatment

    c. Same as split plot treatment

    d. All the (a), (b) and (c) are correct

Ans. (d) All the (a), (b) and (c) are correct

164. In split plot experiment if main plot error variance and sub plot error variance are as σ_a^2 and σ_b^2 respectively then the error term n_{ij} for the main factor A is distributed as:

    a. $n_{ij} \sim N(o, \sigma_b^2)$ b. $n_{ij} \sim N(\mu, \sigma_a^2)$

    c. $n_{ij} \sim N(o, \sigma_a^2)$ d. $n_{ij} \sim N(\mu, \sigma_b^2)$

Ans. (c) $n_{ij} \sim N(o, \sigma_a^2)$

165. in question 12, the error term e_{ijk} occurring in subplot treatment B, is distributed as:

    a. $e_{ijk} \sim N(\mu, \sigma_b^2)$ b. $e_{ijk} \sim N(o, \sigma_a^2)$

    c. $e_{ijk} \sim N(\mu, \sigma_a^2)$ d. $e_{ijk} \sim N(o, \sigma_b^2)$

Ans. (d) $e_{ijk} \sim N(o, \sigma_b^2)$

166. In a split plot experiment, between the main plot error Ea and subplot error Eb, the following relation exists:

    a. Ea < Eb   b. Ea = Eb

    c. Ea > Eb   d. None

Ans. (c) Ea > Eb

167. The correlation coefficient remains unaffected by change of

    a. Scale   b. Origin

    c. Both a and b   d. None of these

Ans. (c) Both a and b

168. The regression coefficient are independent of change of

    a. Origin

    b. Scale

    c. Both a and b

    d. None of these

Ans. (a) Origin

169. When the value of correlation coefficient is 1 then two variable are

    a. Highly correlated   b. Perfectly correlated

    c. Partially correlated   d. Uncorrelated

Ans. (b) Perfectly correlated

170. The correlation coefficient is the geometric mean between two

    a. Regression coefficient

    b. Standard deviation

    c. Median

    d. Mode

Ans. (a) Regression coefficient

171. The R rank correlation was suggested by

    a. C Spearman   b. SD poisson

    c. Laplace and Gauss   d. James Bernoulli

Ans. (a) C Spearman

172. Poisson distribution deals with

    a. Continuous   b. Discrete variable

    c. Both a and b   d. None of these

Ans. (b) Discrete variable

173. The variation due to uncontrolled factor is spoken as

    a. Experimental error   b. Standard error

    c. Treatment effects   d. All of these

Ans. (a) Experimental error

174. In the field experimentation, local control is used for

    a. Diminution of error

    b. Validity of estimate of error

    c. Validity of treatment effects

    d. All of these

Ans. (a) Diminution of error

175. The accuracy of a measurement signifies the closeness with which a estimate approaches the

    a. Average value

    b. True value

    c. Both a and b

    d. None of the above

Ans. (b) True value

176. Which test is applied for the test of significance between the two variances

    a. T-test   b. Z-test

    c. χ^2-test   d. f-test

Ans. (d) f- test

177. Which transformation is most appropriate for percentages?

    a. Arc sine   b. Logarithmic

    c. Square root   d. None of these

Ans. (c) Square root

178. If there are 5 treatments with 4 replication to each, the error degree of freedom for CRD will be

    a. 5   b. 10

    c. 15   d. 20

Ans. (c) 15

179. Which design provides maximum number of degrees of freedom for the estimation of error as compared with other design for the given number of experimental

    a. LSD   b. CRD

    c. RBD   d. Augmented design

Ans. (b) CRD

180. Which design is most appropriate for the laboratory experiments?

    a. RBD   b. LSD

    c. CRD   d. None of these

Ans. (c) CRD

181. If there are 5 varieties and 4 replication to each, the error degree of freedom for RBD will be

    a. 10   b. 14

    c. 12   d. 16

Ans. (c) 12

182. If there are 6 levels of moisture regime and 6 replications each, the error degree of freedom for LSD will be

    a. 10   b. 20

    c. 30   d. 40

Ans. (b) 20

183. When we want to conduct a experiment on a long strip of land, which design will be preferred

    a. SPD   b. CRD

    c. RBD   d. LSD

Ans. (d) LSD

184. Which design gives precision high enough to reduce the standard error to less than 1%?

    a. Strip plot design   b. CRD

    c. RBD   d. LSD

Ans. (d) LSD

185. In confounding, the precision on the main effect and certain interaction of lower order

a. Increases
b. Decreases
c. Remain same
d. None of the above

Ans. (a) Increases

186. In confounding, generally which order of interaction is confounded

a. Higher order
b. First order
c. Lower order
d. Second order

Ans. (a) Higher order

187. If 4 levels of sowing dates are laid out in main plot, 5 levels of nitrogen applied in subplot and they are replicated three times, then what will be the degree of freedom from error

a. 16
b. 32
c. 64
d. 54

Ans. (b) 32

188. Selected the most appropriate design when all factor are not of equal importance in experimentation

a. Split plot design
b. Strip plot design
c. LSD
d. Augmented

Ans. (a) Split plot design

189. In split plot experiment, the d,f. for the error Ea is equal to:

a. $(r-1)(q-1)$
b. $(r-1)(p-1)$
c. $(p-1)(q-1)$
d. $(p-1)$

Ans. (b) $(r-1)(p-1)$

190. In split plot experiment the d.f. for interaction AB is equal to:

a. $(r-1)(q-1)$
b. $(r-1)(p-1)$
c. $(p-1)(q-1)$
d. $p(q-1)$

Ans. (c) $(p-1)(q-1)$

191. In split plot experiment the d.f for the error E_b is equal to:

a. $p(r-1)(q-1)$
b. $r(p-1)(q-1)$
c. $q(r-1)(p-1)$
d. None

Ans. (a) $p(r-1)(q-1)$

192. The F_A statistic defined for main plot treatment A is distributed as:

a. $F_A \sim {}^F (q-1), (r-1)(p-1)$
b. $F_A \sim {}^F (p-1), (r-1)(p-1)$
c. $F_A \sim {}^F (p-1), p(r-1)(p-1)$
d. $F_A \sim {}^F (q-1), p(r-1)(q-1)$

Ans. (b) $F_A \sim {}^F (p-1), (r-1)(p-1)$

193. The F_B statistic defined for sub factor B is distributed as:

a. $F_B \sim {}^F (q-1), (r-1)(p-1)$
b. $F_B \sim {}^F (q-1), (p-1)(q-1)$
c. $F_B \sim {}^F (q-1), p(r-1)(q-1)$
d. $F_B \sim {}^F (p-1), (r-1)(q-1)$

Ans. (c) $F_B \sim {}^F (q-1), p(r-1)(q-1)$

194. F_{AB} statistic defined for interaction AB in split plot experiment is distributed as:

a. $F_{AB} \sim {}^F (p-1)(q-1), p(r-1)(q-1)$
b. $F_{AB} \sim {}^F (p-1)(r-1), r(p-1)(q-1)$
c. $F_{AB} \sim {}^F (p-1)(q-1), q(r-1)(p-1)$
d. $F_{AB} \sim {}^F (r-1)(q-1), p(r-1)(q-1)$

Ans. (a) $F_{AB} \sim {}^F (p-1)(q-1), p(r-1)(q-1)$

195. The estimate of S.E. (Between two A means) is equal to:

a. $\sqrt{\dfrac{2E_a}{rp}}$
b. $\sqrt{\dfrac{2E_a}{rq}}$

c. $\sqrt{\dfrac{2E_a}{pq}}$
d. $\sqrt{\dfrac{2E_b}{pq}}$

Ans. (b) $\sqrt{\dfrac{2E_a}{rq}}$

196. The estimate of S.E. (Between two B means) is equal to:

a. $\sqrt{\dfrac{2E_b}{rq}}$
b. $\sqrt{\dfrac{2E_b}{pq}}$

c. $\sqrt{\dfrac{2E_b}{rq}}$
d. $\sqrt{\dfrac{2E_a}{rp}}$

Ans. (c) $\sqrt{\dfrac{2E_b}{rq}}$

197. The estimate of S.E. (Between two B means are the same level of A) is:

a. $\sqrt{\dfrac{2E_b}{r}}$
b. $\sqrt{\dfrac{2E_a}{r}}$

c. $\sqrt{\dfrac{2E_b}{p}}$
d. $\sqrt{\dfrac{2E_b}{q}}$

Ans. (a) $\sqrt{\dfrac{2E_b}{r}}$

198. S.E. (Different between two A means at the same level of B or different levels of B) is equal to:

a. $\sqrt{2\left[\dfrac{(q-1)E_b + E_a}{rq}\right]}$

b. $\sqrt{2\left[\dfrac{(q-1)E_b + E_a}{rp}\right]}$

c. $\sqrt{\left[\dfrac{(p-1)E_b + E_a}{rp}\right]}$

d. $\sqrt{\left[\dfrac{(p-1)E_b + E_a}{rq}\right]}$

Ans. (a) $\sqrt{2\left[\dfrac{(q-1)E_b + E_a}{rq}\right]}$

199. The replicated experiment designed to compare a number of parent plants w.r.t. some attribute under study is known as:

a. Progeny row trial
b. Compact family block design
c. Split plot design
d. Randomized complete block design

Ans. (a) Progeny row trial

200. The mass selection technique was adopted to select the plants showing superior genetic values in:

a. Plant breeding experiment
b. Agronomy's experiment
c. Crop cutting experiment
d. Experiment on plant protection

Ans. (a) Plant breeding experiment

201. 'A progeny row trial' adopted as an improved technique over mass selection technique was investigated by:

a. Agronomists
b. Plant breeders
c. Entomologists
d. Crop physiologists

Ans. (b) Plant breeders

202. In a progeny row trial each plot consists of a single row and all the seeds of the row belong to the:

a. Same parent plant
b. Progeny plant
c. Different parent plant
d. Different plant of F2 generation

Ans. (a) Same parent plant

203. Let there be p progenies and r replications with ki plants in each plot. Then d.f. for progeny is equal to:

a. (r-1)
b. (p-1)
c. r(p-1)
d. p(r-1)

Ans. (b) (p-1)

204. A progeny row trial is carried out in a simple:

a. C.R.D.
b. R.B.D.
c. L.S.D.
d. Compact family block design

Ans. (b) R.B.D.

205. In question 122, the error (plot error) d.f. is equal to:

a. (ki-1)
b. r (p-1)
c. (r-1) (p-1)
d. p (r-1)

Ans. (c) (r-1) (p-1)

206. In a layout described in question 5 the d.f. for pooled plant error is equal to:

a. (ki-1)
b. (ki-1)
c. p (ki-1)
d. (r-1) (p-1)

Ans. (b) (ki-1)

207. A progeny row trial has been found suitable for the crop:

a. Wheat
b. Cotton
c. Sorghum
d. All the three crop

Ans. (d) All the three crop

208. If the progenies tried in an experiment belong to a number of families then the type of comparison made in:

a. The comparison between different families
b. Comparison between progenies within family
c. Comparison between families within progenies
d. Both (a) and (b)

Ans. (d) Both (a) and (b)

209. A layout suitable for studies as considered in question 10, is known as:

a. R.B.D.
b. Split plot design
c. Progeny row trial
d. Compact family block design

Ans. (d) Compact family block design

210. In a compact family block design the progenies belonging to the same family are sown side by side in a family:

a. Main plot
b. Sub plot
c. Row
d. Block

Ans. (a) Main plot

211. In a compact family block design, the family plots are randomized in:

 a. Each main plot
 b. Each block
 c. Each sub plot
 d. Each row

Ans. (b) Each block

212. The progeny plots are randomized within the:

 a. Main plots
 b. Family plots
 c. Sub plots
 d. Both (a) and (b)

Ans. (b) Family plots

213. Compact family block design is analogous to the:

 a. R.C.B.D.
 b. L.S.D.
 c. Split plot design
 d. Strip plot design

Ans. (c) Split plot design

214. For f families, p progenies in each family and r replications, in compact family block design the error d.f. for main plot is equal to:

 a. (r-1) (p-1)   b. (r-1) (f-1)
 c. (p-1) (f-1)   d. p(r-1) (f-1)

Ans. (b) (r-1) (f-1)

215. In a compact family block design as discussed in question 16, the d.f. for progenies within family is equal to:

 a. p (f-1)   b. f (p-1)
 c. r (p-1)   d. r (f-1)

Ans. (b) f (p-1)

216. As described in question 16, the d.f. for sub plot error is equal to:

 a. (fpr-1)
 b. r (p-1) (f-1)
 c. p (r-1) (f-1)
 d. f (r-1) (p-1)

Ans. (a) (fpr-1)

217. In compact family block design, the subplot treatments are:

 a. Different for all the main plots
 b. Same for all the main plots
 c. Same for all the blocks
 d. Different for all the blocks

Ans. (a) Different for all the main plots

218. S.E. (Difference between two progeny means taken from two different families) is equal to:

 a. $\sqrt{\dfrac{2}{r}\left[\dfrac{E_a+(p+1)E_b}{r}\right]}$ b. $\sqrt{2\left[\dfrac{E_a+(p+1)E_b}{r}\right]}$

 c. $\sqrt{\dfrac{r}{2}\left[\dfrac{E_a+(p+1)E_b}{p}\right]}$ d. $\sqrt{\dfrac{2}{r}\left[\dfrac{E_a+(p+1)E_b}{p}\right]}$

Ans. (a) $\sqrt{\dfrac{2}{r}\left[\dfrac{E_a+(p+1)E_b}{r}\right]}$

219. To test the homogeneity of error variances obtained from family to fanmily, the appropriate test has been suggested by:

 a. Prof. R.A. Fisher
 b. Prof. Kemthorn
 c. Prof. Bartlett
 d. Prof. R.C. Mahalanobis

Ans. (c) Prof. Bartlett

220. The ANOVA s a tool by which total variation may be split up into several physically assignable components was defined by

 a. Horace secrist   b. RA fisher
 c. Karl pearson   d. AL Bowley

Ans. (b) RA fisher

221. During experimentation, we lost some information and we want to get idea about these values, which technique will be useful

 a. Seed plot technique
 b. Uniformity
 c. Missing plot technique
 d. Field plot technique

Ans. (c) Missing plot technique

222. Indian Agricultural Statistical Research Institute is established at

 a. Luck now   b. Kanpur
 c. New Delhi   d. Kolkata

Ans. (c) New Delhi

223. A measure of the peakness or convexity of a curve is known as

 a. Ogive
 b. Kurtosis
 c. Skewness
 d. Histogram

Ans. (b) Kurtosis

224. The square of the standard deviation is known as the

a. Mean deviation
b. Variance
c. Standard deviation
d. Coefficient of variance

Ans. (b) Variance

225. Which measure of central tendency is appropriate for index number?

a. Mode
b. Arithmetic mean
c. Geometric mean
d. Median

Ans. (c) Geometric mean

CHECK YOU GRASP

1. A progeny row trial is carried out in a simple:

   a. C.R.D.

   b. R.B.D.

   c. L.S.D.

   d. Compact family block design

2. If in case of some extra replication in R.C.B.D., the two treatments (t_1 and t_2) are replicated (r_1 and r_2) time with error M.S. as s_e^2 then S.E. ($t_1 - t_2$) will be estimated by:

   a. $s_e^2 \sqrt{\dfrac{1}{r_1} + \dfrac{1}{r_2}}$ b. $2s_e \sqrt{\dfrac{1}{r_1} + \dfrac{1}{r_2}}$

   c. $2s_e^2 \sqrt{\dfrac{1}{r_1} + \dfrac{1}{r_2}}$ d. $2s_e^2 \sqrt{\dfrac{1}{r_1} + \dfrac{1}{r_2}}$

3. The result drawn from ANOVA based on transformed data is:

   a. Same as based on original data

   b. Different from original data

   c. More efficient than based on original data

   d. Less efficient than based on original data

4. In L.S.D., a suitable approximate number of treatment is from:

   a. (4 to 10)

   b. (5 to 10)

   c. (7 to 10)

   d. (5 to 8)

5. The number of basic principle followed in L.S.D. is equal to:

   a. 1   b. 2

   c. 3   d. 4

6. In m x m, L.S.D., the error d.f. is equal to:

   a. (m-1) (m+1)   b. m (m-1)

   c. (m-1) (m-2)   d. m (m-2)

7. In agricultural field experiment where fertility contour map is not known then a suitable design applicable is the:

   a. R.C.B.D.   b. C.R.D.

   c. L.S.D.   d. B.I.B.D.

8. A model in which some factors have fixed effect and others have random effect, is known as:

   a. Mixed effect model

   b. Random effect model

   c. Fixed effect model

   d. Both (b) and (c)

9. Out of three designs, C.R.D., R.C.B.D. and L.S.D., the simplest design is:

   a. L.S.D.   b. R.C.B.D.

   c. C.R.D.   d. None

10. In a m x m, L.S.D. the number of experimental units is equal to:

   a. m   b. m^2

   c. m^3 d. (m-1) (m-2)

In case of less than 80% score, go through brief Review and Glance one again from chapter

Key: 1-b   2-a   3-a   4-b   5-c   6-c   7-c   8-a   9-c   10-b

UNIT 2
Practice Model Paper for Biotechnology

Model Test Paper 1

1. **Among the following enzymes which is not involved in DNA replication process**
   a. RNA polymerase
   b. DNA polymerase
   c. Ligase
   d. Helicase

2. **Among the following which mutagen induces formation of thymidine dimmers in DNA**
   a. Nitrous oxide
   b. Ethylmethyl sulphate
   c. UV light
   d. Ethydium bromide

3. **An operon is inducible means**
   a. The operon is for catabolic process
   b. The operon is for anabolic process
   c. There is another operator in the system
   d. None of these

4. **Bacterial DNA polymerase I can cause nick translation. This property of the enzyme is due to**
   a. $3' \rightarrow 5'$ exonuclease activity
   b. $3' \rightarrow 5'$ polymerase activity
   c. $5' \rightarrow 3'$ exonuclease activity
   d. $5' \rightarrow 3'$ polymerase activity

5. **Biologically not common but sometimes playing regulatory role in gene expression, the DNA is**
   a. B-form
   b. Z-form
   c. E-form
   d. All of the above

6. **CAAT box and GC box are component of the promoter of**
   a. Halo bacteria
   b. Arabidopsis
   c. Mycoplasma
   d. Bacteria

7. **During DNA synthesis frame reading is form**
   a. $3' - 5'$
   b. $5' - 3'$
   c. Both simultaneously
   d. None of these

8. **During glycosylation of protein the oligosaccharide groups are modified by**
   a. Glycosidase
   b. Glycosyl transferases
   c. Proteases
   d. None of these

9. **During meiosis centromere divides at**
   a. Metaphase
   b. Anaphase
   c. Teleophase
   d. Anaphase II

10. **During meiosis cohesion protein is broken down at**
    a. Anaphase I
    b. Anaphase II
    c. metaphase
    d. interkinesis

11. **During photoreactivation reaction DNA photolyase utilizes**
    a. Red light
    b. Blue light
    c. Far red light
    d. Green light

12. **Bacteria protect themselves from viruses by fragmenting viral DNA upon entry with**
    a. Methtylase
    b. Endonucleases
    c. Ligases
    d. Exonucleases

13. **Which of the following tools of recombinant DNA technology is incorrectly paired with its use?**
    a. Restriction enzyme–Production of RFLPs
    b. DNA ligase-enzyme that cuts DNA, creating the sticky ends of restriction fragments
    c. DNA polymerase–used in a polymerase chain reaction to amplify section of DNA
    d. Reverse transcriptase–production of cDNA from mRNA

14. **T4 polynucleotide kinase is used for**
    a. Labelling 3'ends of DNA
    b. Labeling 5'ends of DNA
    c. Creating blunt ends of DNA
    d. Dephosphorylation of DNA

411

15. **You have cut the genome of a double–stranded viral genome with a restriction endonuclease and electrophoresed the products on an agarose gel. You observe only one band on the gel, equivalent to the size of the genome. This is because**

    a. There are no introns in the genome

    b. The introns contain the recognition sites and have already been spliced out

    c. All of restriction fragments are too small to detect

    d. Restriction endonucleases do not cut RNA, and this virus has a dsRNA genome

16. **A southern transfer of E.coil DNA after complete digestion with EcoRI was probed with labeled cDNA probe of a gene which occurs only once in the *E.coil* genome. If the gene contains one EcoR1 cleavage site near its center, the number of radioactive bands you are most likely to find on autoradiography would be**

    a. 0   b. 1

    c. 2   d. 3

17. **The substrate for restriction enzyme is**

    a. Single stranded RNA

    b. Partially double stranded RNA

    c. Cell wall proteins

    d. Double stranded DNA

18. **Two restriction enzymes A and B have eight and four base pairs as their recognition sites respectively .The ratio of the number of fragments that they will generate on restriction digestion of a genomic DNA of *E. coli* is approximately**

    a. 4 : 8   b. 8 : 4

    c. 1 : 64   d. 1 : 256

19. **Restriction endonucleases are enzymes that**

    a. Cleave the 5' terminal nucleotides from duplex DNA molecules

    b. Make sequence-specific cuts in both strands of duplex DNA molecules

    c. Promote circularization of the duplex DNA molecule by removal of the 5' terminal nucleotides

    d. None of these

20. **Which of the following sequences is most likely to be a restriction enzyme recognition site?**

    a. CGGCTT

    b. CGCCGC

    c. GTAATG

    d. GTCGAC

21. **Yeast artificial chromosomes (YAC) is used for**

    a. Cloning large segments genomic of DNA

    b. Cloning only yeast genomic sequences

    c. Cloning of only cDNA sequences

    d. All DNA except plant DNA sequences

22. **For cloning a DNA fragment larger than 100 Kb, which of the following vector system would be suitable?**

    a. Plasmid

    b. Cosmid

    c. Yeast artificial chromosome

    d. Lambda bacteriophage

23. **Expression vector contain a sequence, not normally found in other vector that is known as**

    a. A ribosome–binding site

    b. An ori site

    c. A multiple–cloning site

    d. An antibody–resistant marker

24. **What is the approximate length of DNA between two COS sites that can be packed by a lambda packing extract?**

    a. 10 Kb   b. 15 Kb

    c. 25 Kb   d. 45 Kb

25. **Which statement correctly describes sequential steps in cDNA in DNA cloning?**

    a. Reverse transcription of mRNA, second strand synthesis, cDNA end modification, ligation to vector

    b. mRNA preparation, cDNA synthesis using reverse transcription, second strand synthesis using terminal transferase, ligation to vector

    c. mRNA synthesis using RNA polymerase ,reverse transcription of mRNA, second strand synthesis ligation to vector

    d. Double stranded cDNA synthesis, restriction enzyme digestion, addition of linkers, ligation to vector

26. **ncers of eukaryotic gene may have a special form of DNA called**

    a. A-DNA   b. C-DNA

    c. B-DNA   d. Z-DNA

27. **Epinephrine plays its role in glycogenolysis by**

    a. Activating glycogen synthase

    b. Activating phophorylase kinase

    c. Inactivating adenylyl cyclase

    d. None of these

28. **Epinephrine promotes glycogenolysis there by**

   a. Hydrolysizing cAMP
   b. Synthesizing c-AMP
   c. Inactivating G-protein
   d. Inactivating Adenylyl cyclase

29. **Eukaryotic chromosomes are transcriptionally most active during**

   a. Prophase
   b. Metaphase
   c. Anaphase
   d. Interphase

30. **Eukaryotic organisms lack**

   a. DNA photolyase
   b. DNA glycosylase
   c. AP endonuclease
   d. Excinucleases

31. **Which statement is not true for DNA transcription?**

   a. Template strand is used as coding strand
   b. Transcription is in 5'–3' direction
   c. Template strand and m-RNA have complementary
   d. None of these

32. **Genetic code is not degenerate for**

   a. Leucine
   b. Isoleucine
   c. Glycine
   d. Cysteine

33. **Guide RNA are involved in**

   a. Cutting event of m-RNA
   b. RNA editing
   c. End modification of hn-RNA
   d. Splicing

34. **Histones are replaced by protamines in**

   a. Nerve cell
   b. Muscle cell
   c. Heart cell
   d. Sperm cell

35. **Holiday junction are formed during**

   a. DNA replication
   b. DNA repair
   c. Chromosomal aberration
   d. Recombination

36. **Holiday structure is used to explain**

   a. Site specific recombination
   b. Homologous recombination
   c. Gene transfer
   d. Nonhomologous recombination

37. **In B-DNA the distance between two base pair is**

   a. 0.24
   b. 0.35
   c. 0.34
   d. 0.45

38. **In cell-cycle centrioles replicate in**

   a. G1- phase
   b. G2-phase
   c. S-phase
   d. M-phase

39. **In cell cycle which of the following is usually not a check point?**

   a. G2- check point
   b. G1- check point
   c. S- check point
   d. None of these

40. **In prokaryotes, the lagging primers are removed by...**

   a. 3' to 5' exonuclease
   b. DNA ligase
   c. DNA polymerase I
   d. DNA polymerase III

41. **The essential initiator protein at the E.Coli origin of replication is**

   a. DnaA
   b. DnaB
   c. DnaC
   d. DnaE

42. **Which phase would a cell enter if it was starved of mitogens before the R point?**

   a. G1
   b. S
   c. G2
   d. G0

43. **Prokaryotic plasmids can replicate in yeast cells if they contain a cloned yeast**

   a. ORC
   b. CDK
   c. ARS
   d. RNA

44. **The net product/s of non-cyclic electron flow in photosynthesis is /are:**

   a. ATP
   b. O_2
   c. $NADH_2$
   d. All of these

45. **In cyclic flow of electrons during photosynthesis, the electrons from ferredoxin are accepted by:**

   a. Ferrodoxin
   b. Plastoquinone
   c. Cytochromes
   d. Plastocyanin

46. **In photosynthesis, the energy released by the protons when they diffuse across the thylakoid membrane in to the stroma is used to produce:**

   a. NAD
   b. $NADH_2$
   c. ATP
   d. AMP

47. **The highest amount of protein in the biome is:**

   a. Rubisco
   b. Zein
   c. Phytochrome
   d. Gliadin

48. **Photolysis of water occurs in association of :**

   a. PSII
   b. PSI
   c. Both PSI andPSII
   d. Stroma

49. PSI in photosynthesis plays an important role in:
   a. Reduction of $NADPH_2$
   b. Reduction of NADP
   c. Release of O_2 from water
   d. None of these

50. Which elements play important role in photolysis of water?
   a. Mg and Cl
   b. Mg and Mo
   c. Mn and Cl
   d. Fe and Mg

51. In photosynthetic bacteria, the electron donor is:
   a. H_2O
   b. H_2S
   c. O_2
   d. Ferredoxin

52. The assimilatory power in photosynthesis are:
   a. ATP
   b. ADP
   c. $NADPH_2$ and ATP
   d. $NADPH_2$ and ADP

53. Which colour of light is absorbed during bacterial photosynthesis?
   a. Orange
   b. Far red
   c. Red
   d. Blue

54. Amplification of genes involves
   a. Removal of histones from DNA to allow transcription of gene
   b. Multiple duplications of gene via replication
   c. Multiplication of extra chromosomal elements only
   d. Invertebrate genomes only

55. Full expression of lac operon requires
   a. Lactose and cAMP
   b. Allolactose and cAMP
   c. Lactose
   d. Allolactose

56. Which one of the following partial diploids will express β-galactosidase constitutively?
   a. F′ lacO^c lacZ$^+$/lacO$^+$ lacZ$^+$
   b. F′ lacO$^-$ lacZ$^+$/lacI$^+$ lacZ$^+$
   c. F′ lacO$^+$ lacZ$^+$/lacI$^-$ lacZ$^+$
   d. F′ lacO^c lacZ$^-$/lacO$^+$ lacZ$^+$

57. Synthesis of β-galactosidase will be constitutive in a strain with the genotype
   a. I$^+$ Z$^+$ Y$^+$
   b. I$^-$ Z$^+$ Y$^+$
   c. I$^+$ Z$^-$ Y$^+$
   d. I$^+$ Z$^+$ Y$^-$

58. The scientists involved in discovery of DNA as chemical basis of heredity were
   a. Hershey and Chase
   b. Griffith and Avery
   c. Avery, Mac Leod and Mc Carty
   d. Watson and Crick

59. One turn of DNA possesses
   a. One base pair
   b. Two base pairs
   c. Five base pairs
   d. Ten base pairs

60. Number of codons in the genetic triplet code is
   a. 4
   b. 16
   c. 32
   d. 64

61. Initiation codons for protein synthesis are
   a. UUU and GGG
   b. AAU and UAA
   c. AUG and GUA
   d. GUG and AUG

62. Termination codons for protein synthesis are
   a. AUU, AUG and GUU
   b. UGA, UAA and UAG
   c. UAU, UAG and UUA
   d. AAA, UUU and UGA

63. The two antiparallel strands of DNA are
   a. Equidistant and run in $5 \rightarrow 3$ direction
   b. Equidistant and run in $5 \rightarrow 3$ and $3 \rightarrow 5$ directions
   c. Unequal and run in opposite directions
   d. Unequal and diverge from each other

64. The process of multiplication of DNA from DNA is known as
   a. Replication
   b. Duplication
   c. Transcription
   d. Translation

65. The first stable compound formed during photosynthesis in C_3 plant is:
   a. PEP
   b. PCAL
   c. RuBP
   d. PGA

66. A process which involves more than one organelle is:
   a. Translation
   b. Transcription
   c. Photorespiration
   d. Photosynthesis

67. How many turns of Calvin cycle are taken to produce one hexose molecule?
   a. 3
   b. 4
   c. 5
   d. 6

68. In C₄ plants, calvin cycle occurs in:

a. Stroma of bundle sheath chloroplast

b. Mesophyll of chloroplast

c. Grana of bundle sheath chloroplast

d. None of these

69. In 2DE, separation is done on the basis of

a. Charge

b. Mass

c. Both charge and mass

d. None of these

70. For first dimensional separation in 2DE, the gels used include

a. Polyacrylamide with IPG

b. Polyacrylamide with SDS

c. Normal poilyacrylamide

d. None of these

71. Genome of the smallest cterium, Mycoplasma genitelium codes for

a. 498 protein

b. 456 protein

c. 1022 protein

d. 479 protein

72. Which of the following genomics technology is being used extensively in diagnostics?

a. Gradient PCR

b. qRT-PCR

c. Automated sequencing

d. None of these

73. The private company that produced human genome sequence is

a. Genetic computer group

b. Affymetrix

c. Celera Genomics

d. Applied Biosystem

74. EcoRI was discovered by

a. J.Hedgepeth, H.M. Goodman and H.W.Boyer

b. S.cohen and H.W.Boyer

c. W. Arber and D. Nathans

d. None of these

75. The restriction enzyme used by Cohen and Boyer to create recombinant DNA molecule was

a. Hind III

b. Hind II

c. Sma I

d. Eco RI

76. Sma 1 is a

a. Sticky end hexacutter

b. Blunt end hexacutter

c. Sticky end tetracutter

d. Blunt end tetracutter

77. Taq 1 is a

a. Sticky end tetracutter

b. Blunt end hexacutter

c. Blunt end tetracutter

d. Sticky end hexacutter

78. Which of the following restriction enzyme is methylation insensitive?

a. Sma 1

b. Eco RI

c. Sau 3A

d. Hind III

79. Baculovirus vectors are

a. ds DNA

b. ss DNA

c. ds RNA

d. ss RNA

80. SV 40 vector are

a. ds DNA

b. ds RNA

c. ss DNA

d. ss RNA

81. Retroviral vectors are

a. ds RNA

b. ss DNA

c. ds DNA

d. ss RNA

82. Vectors based on BPV have plasmid components of

a. Cosmid vectors

b. pBR322

c. pUC vector

d. pBluescript vector

83. Which of the following is a retroviral vector used in animal cloning?

a. MLV

b. EBV

c. BPV

d. SV 40

84. Higher specific hybridization I sobserved in

a. Spotted microarray

b. Oligo microarray

c. Both of these

d. None of these

85. In silico chip designing is possible in

a. Spotted microarray

b. Oligo microarray

c. Both of these

d. None of these

86. MPSS technique was developed by

a. R.S.Yalow and S.A. Berson

b. E. Engvall and P.Periman

c. Brenner et al.

d. None of these

87. Fluorescence based sequencing is used in

a. MPSS

b. SAGE

c. ELISA

d. RNA dot blot

88. Tags and anti-tags are used in

a. SAGE
b. MPSS
c. Two hybrid system
d. None of these

89. Which enzyme is not proteinaceous

a. Isozyme
b. Ribozyme
c. Holozyme
d. Trypsin

90. Ribozyme is

a. RNA without sugar
b. RNA without phosphate
c. RNA having enzyme activity
d. RNA with extra phosphate

91. NADP is

a. An enzyme
b. A part of soluble RNA
c. A part of transfer RNA
d. A coenzyme

92. FAD or FMN is a coenzyme; which vitamin is incorporated in its structure

a. Vitamin B_1
b. Vitamin B_2
c. Vitamin B_6
d. Vitamin C

93. The nature of coenzyme is

a. Non proteinaceous
b. Proteinaceous
c. Both a and b
d. None of the above

94. During enzyme activity, the coenzyme

a. Acts as a donor or acceptor of atoms which are added to or removed from the substrates
b. Are important in oxidation-reduction reactions

c. Both a and b
d. None of the above

95. Which of the following are coenzymes

a. NAD, NADP, FAD, FMN
b. Vitamin, Fe, Cu
c. $NADPH_2$, Ca, Co
d. NAD, K, CoA

96. R.Q. of germinating caster seed is:

a. 1
b. >1
c. <1
d. 2

97. The glycolate metabolism occurs in:

a. Mitochondria
b. Lysosomes
c. Peroxisomes
d. Ribosome

98. Oxidative phosphorylation involves simulataneous oxidation and phosphorylation to finally produce:

a. ATP
b. NAD
c. FAD
d. FADH

99. The activity of enzyme hexokinase, which catalyse glucose to glucose 6-posphate. Is inhibited by glucose 6-phosphate, it is an example of:

a. Competitive inhibition
b. Non competitive inhibition
c. Feedback allosteric inhibition
d. None of these

100. An example of polycistronic enzyme is:

a. Pepsin
b. Rennin
c. Papin
d. RNA polymerase

ANSWERS OF MODEL PAPER 1

1. a	2. c	3. a	4. c	5. b	6. b	7. a
8. b	9. d	10. b	11. b	12. b	13. b	14. b
15. d	16. c	17. d	18. d	19. b	20. d	21. a
22. c	23. a	24. d	25. a	26. d	27. b	28. b
29. d	30. a	31. a	32. c	33. b	34. d	35. d
36. b	37. c	38. c	39. c	40. c	41. a	42. d
43. c	44. d	45. b	46. c	47. a	48. a	49. b
50. c	51. b	52. c	53. b	54. b	55. b	56. b
57. b	58. c	59. d	60. d	61. d	62. b	63. b
64. a	65. d	66. c	67. d	68. a	69. c	70. a
71. d	72. b	73. c	74. a	75. d	76. b	77. a
78. c	79. a	80. a	81. a	82. b	83. a	84. a
85. b	86. c	87. a	88. b	89. b	90. c	91. d
92. b	93. a	94. c	95. a	96. c	97. c	98. b
99. c	100. d					

Model Test Paper 2

1. Genetic code was discovered by
- a. Nirenberg and Mathei
- b. Novick and Szilard
- c. Kornberg
- d. Willkins

2. Site of protein synthesis
- a. Lysosome
- b. Peroxisome
- c. Ribosome
- d. Splisosome

3. Dr. Hargobind Khorana has been awarded Noble Prize for research on
- a. Oral contraceptives
- b. Hormones
- c. Genetic code
- d. Immunology

4. There are 64 codons in genetic code dictionary because
- a. There are 64 type of tRNAs found in the cell
- b. There are 44 meaningless and 20 codons for amino acids
- c. There are 64 amino acids to be coded
- d. Genetic code is triplet

5. Genetic code was deciphered through chemical synthesis of trinucleotides by
- a. Watson and Crick
- b. Beadle and Tatum
- c. Briggs and King
- d. M.W. Nirenberg

6. Nirenberg synthesized a mRNA containing 34 poly-adenine (A-A-A-A-A-A......) and found a polypeptide formed of 11 polylysine. It proved that the genetic code for lysine is
- a. Lone adenine
- b. A-A doublet
- c. A-A-A triplet
- d. Many adenines

7. Khorana and his colleagues synthesized an RNA molecule with ripening sequence of UG N-bases (UGUGUGUGUGUG). It produced a tetrapeptide with altering sequence of cystien and valine. It proves that codon for cysteine and valine is
- a. UGG and GUU
- b. UUG and GGU
- c. UGU and GUG
- d. GUG and UGU

8. Dr. H.G. Khorana deciphered first the triplet codon of
- a. Serine and isoleucine
- b. Phenylalanine and methionine
- c. Threonine and histidine
- d. Tyrosine and tryptophan

9. 5ˆ end of the tRNA always ends in the base
- a. Adenine
- b. Guanine
- c. Cytosine
- d. Thymine

10. UGA in the yeast mitochondria codes for
- a. Stop signal
- b. Tryptophan
- c. Glutamine
- d. Aspartic acid

11. The amount of which of these is least in a cell
- a. mRNA
- b. rRNA
- c. tRNA
- d. Nothing can be said definitely

12. The genetic code is
- a. Universal
- b. Nearly universal
- c. Similar in the members of a genus
- d. Different for every species

13. For cloning a DNA fragment larger than 100 Kb, which of the following vector system would be suitable?
- a. Plasmid
- b. Cosmid
- c. Yeast artificial chromosome
- d. Lambda bacteriophage

14. Expression vector contain a sequence, not normally found in other vector that is known as
- a. A ribosome-binding site
- b. An ori site
- c. A multiple-cloning site
- d. An antibody-resistant marker

15. What is the difference between a PAC and a BAC?

a. One has ampicillin and another has kanamycin resistance marker

b. One is plasmid-based vector and the other is derived a yeast chromosome

c. One is derived from the E.coli F- plasmid and other is derived from bacteriophage P1

d. One is derived from bacteriophage P1 and other is derived from bacteriophage

16. For a plasmid to be a cloning vector, the minimum numbers of elements required are

a. Origin of replication, multiple cloning site, selection marker

b. Origin of replication, multiple cloning site, selection marker, promoter

c. Origin of replication, multiple cloning site, selection marker, translation start site

d. Origin of replication, multiple cloning site, promoter

17. Technique of pyrosequencing was described first by

a. F. Sanger5   b. A.R. Coulson

c. D.J. Harrison   d. E. D. Hyman

18. Idea of capillary array electrophoresis for sequencing was developed by

a. F. Sanger   b. A.R.Coulson

c. D.J. Harrison   d. E. D. Hyman

19. In pyrosequencing, light energy is released by the action of

a. ATP sulfurylase   b. Luciferase

c. Both of these   d. None of these

20. Which of the following is true

a. It involves chain termination method

b. It can sequencing large DNA fragments

c. It involves chain extension by DNA polymerase

d. Pyrosequencing uses a fluorescent detection process

21. RNAi was first reported in

a. A. thaliana   b. D. melanogaster

c. C. elegans   d. Human

22. The technique of radioimmunoassay was developed by

a. R.S.Yalow and S.A. Berson

b. E. Engvall and P. Periman

c. Both of them

d. None of these

23. The okazaki fragments consist of :

a. DNA + RNA   b. DNA + PRIMER

c. DNA ONLY   d. RNA ONLY

24. The amino acid is attached to t-RNA in its.

a. 5′ end

b. 3′end

c. Varies from place to place

d. Anticodon end

25. Which one is the most stable kind of RNA found in a cell?

a. r RNA   b. t RNA

c. m RNA   d. hn RNA

26. The enzyme primase is infact:

a. DNA polymerase I   b. RNA polymerase

c. Helicase   d. Topoisomerase

27. The role of sigma factor in transcription is:

a. Initiation   b. Elongation

c. Termination   d. Translocation

28. The initiator codon is:

a. UUU   b. AUG

c. UGA   d. GGG

29. In eukaryotes, m RNA is formed by:

a. DNA   b. RNA

c. hn RNA   d. All of these

30. DNA is transcribed by some viral RAN using the enzyme:

a. Endonuclease   b. RNA polymerase

c. Reverse transcriptase d. Helicase

31. Constitutive genes are those genes which are active:

a. During differentiation stages

b. During developmental stage

c. Throughout life time

d. At any stage of life

32. Enzymes synthesised in lac operon are:

a. Lactase, permease and glactosidase

b. Permease, glactase and lactase

c. Permease, galactosidse and transacetylase

d. None of these

33. **In lac operon model, an operon consists of :**
    a. One operator gene and one structural gene
    b. One promoter gene and one structural gene
    c. Regulator gene, promoter gene and operator gene
    d. None of these

34. **In tryptophan operon, a repressor consists of co-repressor and apo-repressor. These two are made up of:**
    a. Tryptophan and protein
    b. RNA and tryptophan
    c. DNA and tryptophan
    d. RNA and protein

35. **The colinearity hypothesis indicates that:**
    a. The sequence of nucleotides in gene correlates with the sequence of amino acids in protein
    b. Genes are arranged linearly in both strands of DNA
    c. Genes afe arranged linearly in both strands of RNA
    d. None of these

36. **Which is the most short lived RNA?**
    a. r RNA
    b. m RNA
    c. t RNA
    d. None of these

37. **The annealing temperature, at which the primers attach to the template, can be calculated by determining the melting temperature (Tm)of the primer template hybrid. What will be Tm of the primer 5'-AGACTCAGAGAGAACCC-3'**
    a. 50°C
    b. 52°C
    c. 102°C
    d. 43°C

38. **Efficient expression of a heterologous protein product is influenced by**
    a. Transcriptional efficiency
    b. Copy number of the plasmid
    c. Codon bias
    d. All of the above

39. **Which of the following is not a potential problem associated with expressing a eukaryotic, protein coding nuclear gene in prokaryotic cells?**
    a. Lack of an intron-splicing mechanism in prokaryotes
    b. Differences in the translation intiation codons used by eukaryotic cells and prokaryotic cells
    c. Stability of mRNA in prokaryotic cells
    d. Differences in transcriptional signals between eukaryotic cells and prokaryotic cells

40. **Which of the following conditions prevent efficient expression of foreign gene cloned in E.coli?**
    a. The foreign gene might contain introns
    b. Foreign gene might contain sequence that act as termination signals in E.coli
    c. Codon bias
    d. All of the above

41. **A reporter gene**
    a. A acts as repressor
    b. Allows gene expression to be readily measured
    c. Enhances mRNA stability
    d. Interacts with RNA polymerase

42. **Most common reporter whose product can be directly visualized in transformed cells is**
    a. NPTII (Neomycim phosphotransferase)
    b. CAT (choramphniol acetyl transferase)
    c. β-galactosidase
    d. GFP (green fluorescent protein)

43. **A linear DNA fragment is (100%) labeled at one end and has 3 restriction sites for EcoRI. If it is partially digested by EcoRI so that all possible fragments are produced, how many of these fragments will be labeled and how many will not be labeled?**
    a. 4 labeled ; 6 unlabeled
    b. 4 labeled ; 4 unlabeled
    c. 3 labeled ; 5 unlabeled
    d. 3 labeled ; 3 unlabeled

44. **Restriction endonucleases hydrolyzes polynucleotide from**
    a. Only the 5'end
    b. From either terminal
    c. At an internal phosphodiester bond
    d. A phosphodiester bond within a specific sequence

45. **Bacteria protect themselves from viruses by fragmenting viral DNA upon entry with**
    a. Methtylase
    b. Endonucleases
    c. Ligases
    d. Exonucleases

46. **Which of the following tools of recombinant DNA technology is incorrectly paired with its use?**
    a. Restriction enzyme-Production of RFLPs
    b. DNA ligase-enzyme that cuts DNA, creating the sticky ends of restriction fragments

c. DNA polymerase-used in a polymerase chain reaction to amplify section of DNA

d. Reverse transcriptase-production of cDNA from mRNA

47. The ratio of enzyme to substrate molecules can be as low as

a. 1 : 100,000   b. 1 : 500,000
c. 1 : 10,000   d. 1 : 1,000

48. Vitamin B$_2$ is component of coenzyme:

a. Pyridoxal phosphate   b. TPP
c. NAD   d. FMN/FAD

49. K$_m$ value of enzyme is substrate concentration at

a. ½ V$_{max}$ b. 2 V$_{max}$
c. ½ V$_{max}$ d. 4 V$_{max}$

50. Part of enzyme which combines with nonprotein part to form functional enzyme is

a. Apoenzyme   b. Coenzyme
c. Prosthetic group   d. None of these

51. Who got Nobel Prize in 1978 for working on enzymes?

a. Koshland   b. Arber and Nathans
c. Nass and Nass   d. H.G. Khorana

52. Site of enzyme synthesis in a cell is

a. Ribosomes   b. RER
c. Golgi bodies   d. All of these

53. The fruit when kept is open, tastes bitter after 2 hours because of

a. Loss of water from juice
b. Decreased concentration of fructose in juice
c. Fermentation by yeast
d. Contamination by bacterial enzymes

54. Hexokinase (Glucose + ATP → Glucose-6–P + ADP) belongs to the category:

a. Transferases   b. Lysases
c. Oxidoreductases   d. Isomerases

55. During the functioning of biosensor, which of the following sequences of event occurs?

a. Enzymatic/cellular reaction → detector → transducer
b. Enzymatic/cellular reaction → transducer → detector
c. Enzymatic/cellular reaction → pressure gauge → time
d. Enzymatic/cellular reaction → vibrator → mechanical signal

56. An immobilized enzyme being used in continuous plug flow reactor exhibits an effectiveness factor (η) of 1.2. The value of η being greater than one could be apparently due to one of the following reasons. Identify the correct reasons.

a. The enzyme follows substrate inhibited kinetics with intern pore diffusion initiation
b. The enzyme experiences external film diffusion limitation
c. The enzyme follows sigmoid kinetic
d. The immobilized enzyme is operationally unstable

57. The degree of inhibition for non-competitive inhibition of an enzyme catalyzed reaction

a. Increase with increase substrate concentration
b. Reaches a maxima with increase in substrate concentration and then decreases
c. Is independent of substrate concentration
d. Decreases with increase in substrate concentration

58. An enzyme following Michaelis-Menten kinetics with V$_m$ = 2.5 mmol m^{-3}s^{-1} and km = 5.0 mM was used to carry out the reaction in a batch stirred reactor. Starting with an initial substrate concentration of 0.1 M, the time required for 50% conversion of the substrate will be about

a. 01 hr   b. 06 hr
c. 02 hr   d. 12 hr

59. The maximum reaction velocity (V$_m$) for an enzyme catalyzed reaction was experimentally measured at two different temperatures of following results were obtained

Temperature, °C	27	37
V$_m$ mmolm^{-3}s^{-1}	2.25	4.50

The energy of activation for the reaction is
a. 12834 cal mol^{-1}
b. 25668 cal mol^{-1}
c. 6417 cal mol^{-1}
d. 19251 cal mol^{-1}

60. Transcription is

a. Synthesis of DNA on RNA
b. Synthesis of RNA on DNA
c. Production of proteins on RNA
d. Replication of DNA

61. Enzyme necessary for transcription is (or transcription of DNA is aided by)

a. DNA polymerase
b. RNA polymerase
c. Endonuclease
d. RNAase

62. A DNA strand is directly involved in the synthesis of all the following *except*:

a. tRNA molecule   b. mRNA molecule
c. Another DNA strand   d. Protein synthesis

63. The mRNA is formed

a. In the nucleus
b. By free ribosomes
c. From the ribosomes on endoplasmic reticulum
d. From DNA in nucleus

64. In which of the following places, messenger RNA is found in a living cell?

a. Inside the endoplasmic reticulum
b. Inside the mitochondria
c. Inside the nucleus but outside the nucleolus
d. Inside the nucleolus

65. Which is the correct sequence of code transfer involved in the formation of a polypeptide?

a. DNA, tRNA, rRNA, mRNA
b. rRNA, DNA, mRNA, tRNA
c. mRNA, tRNA, DNA, amino acids
d. DNA, mRNA, tRNA, amino acids

66. The formation of polyribosomes from ribosomes is done in the presence of

a. Na^+ ions   b. K^+ ions
c. Ca^{++} ions   d. Mg^{++} ions

67. In protein synthesis, the codon used as a start signal is

a. AUG   b. UGA
c. GUA   d. UAG, UAA

68. If the DNA strand has the nitrogenous base sequence ATT GCC, the mRNA will have

a. ATT GCA   b. ATC GCC
c. UGG ACC   d. UAA CGG

69. If the sequence of bases in DNA is ATTCGATG, then the sequence of bases in its transcript will be

a. GUAGCUUA   b. UAAGCUAC
c. CAUCGAAU   d. AUUCGAUG

70. From a DNA template with the sequence CTGATAGC, the mRNA sequence formed would be

a. GUCTUTCG
b. GACUAUCG
c. UACTATCU
d. GAUTATUG

71. The function of a non-sense codon is

a. To release polypeptide chain from tRNA
b. To form an unspecified amino acid
c. To terminate the message of gene controlled protein synthesis
d. To convert a sense DNA into non-sense DNA

72. Termination of chain growth in protein synthesis is brought about by

a. UUG, UGC, UCA   b. UCG, GCG, ACC
c. UAA, UAG, UGA   d. UUG, UAG, UCG

73. Each codon present on mRNA and anticodon present on tRNA is composed of

a. One N base only
b. A set of two N base
c. A set of three N base
d. A set of three out of U, C, A, G

74. Lac operon in *E. coli* consists of three structural genes. Out of these, one codes for transacetylase. The function of transacetylase is

a. To carry lactose into the cell
b. To convert lactose into glucose
c. To convert lactose into galactose
d. Not known

75. In split genes, the coding sequence are called

a. Cistrons   b. Operons
c. Exons   d. Introns

76. Restriction enzyme are used in genetic engineering because

a. They can cut DNA at specific base sequence
b. They are proteolytic enzymes which can degrade harmful proteins
c. They are nucleases that cut DNA at variable sites
d. They can join different DNA fragments

77. A piece of DNA, cut by a restriction enzyme, forms bonds with other DNA molecules which have

a. Been fragmented by the same restriction enzyme
b. Unpaired bases
c. Plasmid components
d. Methyl groups attached to them

78. It is preferable to use yeasts rather than bacteria as recipient cells for recombination of eukaryotic DNA because

a. Yeast can produce restriction enzymes
b. Yeast can excise introns from the RNA transcript

c. Yeast can remove methyl groups

d. Yeast can reproduce at a faster rate

79. A bacterium modifies its DNA by adding methyl groups to the DNA. It does so to

a. Clone its DNA

b. Be able to transcribe many genes simultaneously

c. Turn its gene on

d. Protect its DNA from its own restriction enzymes

80. The operon model of gene regulation and organization in prokaryotes was proposed by

a. Jacob and Monod

b. Beadle and Tatum

c. Meselson and Stahl

d. Wilkins and Franklin

81. Which site of a tRNA molecule hydrogen binds to an mRNA molecule?

a. Codon

b. Anticodon

c. 5′ end of the tRNA molecule

d. 3′ end of the tRNA molecule

82. Which one of the following is not a second messenger?

a. PIP_3

b. Mn^{+2}

c. C-AMP

d. Ca^{+2}

83. Which one of the following is not associated with eukaryotic transcription?

a. RNA polymerase-III

b. RNA polymerase-II

c. Poly (a) polymerase

d. None of these

84. Which one of the following is not the component of extra cellular matrix?

a. Major histocompatibilty complex

b. Glycoproteins

c. Proteoglycoans

d. Collagens

85. The basic structural unit of the metaphase chromosome is

a. 10 nm filament

b. 50 nm filament

c. 300 nm filament

d. 30 nm filament

86. The basis for the blocking action of the alkaloid colchicines on the division is

a. G_1 phase

b. S phase

c. M phase

d. G_0 phase

87. the biologically active proteasome is

a. 20S

b. 30S

c. 26S

d. 50S

88. The biologically predominant form of DNA is

a. Left handed B-DNA

b. Right handed A-DNA

c. Left handed A-DNA

d. Right handed B-DNA

89. The protein complex 'dicer' is involved in

a. Gene silencing

b. Transcription

c. Translation

d. Protein sorting

90. The protein of Golgi complex which contain irregular cisternae and tubules is known as

a. Intercisternal Golgi

b. Cis Golgi

c. Trans Golgi

d. Medial Golgi

91. The region where RNA polymerase binds to promoter in prokaryotes is called

a. Hogness box

b. Homeo box

c. Pribnow box

d. Shine-Dalgrano box

92. The shortening of eukaryotic chromosome during replication is prevented by

a. Telomerase

b. Ligase

c. Reverse transcriptase

d. RNA polymerase

93. Which one of the following hormones binds to intracellular receptor?

a. Insulin

b. Estrogen

c. Glucagon

d. Growth hormone

94. The Tm of DNA can be calculated using the formula: Tm = 69.1 + 0.41 (GC) where GC is the percent of guanine + cytosine. A double stranded DNA has 27% adenine. Its Tm is:

a. 79°C

b. 80.73°C

c. 95.50°C

d. 88°C

95. The type of intercellular signalling in which one cell can communicate with anoter over long distances is called

a. Autocrine

b. Paracrine

c. Juxtacrine

d. Endocrine

96. Turn over number of an enzyme depends on its

a. Concentration of enzyme

b. Size of enzyme

c. Number of active sites

d. Molecular weight

97. Which has coenzyme activity

a. Purine

b. Pyrimidine

c. Urease

d. Both a and b

98. Which one is not a simple enzyme

a. Amylase

b. Pepsin

c. Urease

d. Dehydrogenase

99. UbQ (ubiquinone) is

a. Activator

b. Protein cofactor

c. Non protein coenzyme

d. Protein coenzyme

100. The enzyme used to dissolve blood clot in coronary artery is

a. Thrombokinase

b. Rennin

c. Streptokinase

d. Tyrosinase

ANSWERS OF MODEL PAPER 2

1. a	2. c	3. c	4. d	5. d	6. c	7. c
8. a	9. b	10. d	11. a	12. b	13. c	14. a
15. c	16. a	17. c	18. c	19. c	20. c	21. c
22. a	23. c	24. b	25. d	26. a	27. a	28. b
29. c	30. c	31. c	32. c	33. b	34. a	35. a
36. b	37. b	38. d	39. b	40. d	41. b	42. c
43. a	44. d	45. b	46. b	47. a	48. d	49. d
50. c	51. a	52. b	53. d	54. c	55. b	56. c
57. b	58. b	59. a	60. b	61. b	62. d	63. d
64. c	65. d	66. d	67. a	68. d	69. b	70. b
71. c	72. c	73. d	74. d	75. c	76. a	77. a
78. b	79. d	80. a	81. b	82. a	83. c	84. a
85. d	86. c	87. c	88. d	89. a	90. d	91. c
92. a	93. b	94. d	95. d	96. c	97. c	98. d
99. c	100. c					

Model Test Paper 3

1. PCR was invented by:

a. A. Kornberg (1952)
b. Nirenberg (1879)
c. Kary Mullis (1984)
d. Watson and crick (1953)

2. The temperature needed to denature DNA would also denature norma DNA polymerase. The polymerase used in PCR is:

a. Both 'a' and 'b'
b. Pwo DNA polymerase
c. Taq DNA polymerase
d. RNA polymerase

3. Taq DNA Polymerse is isolated from:

a. Mycobacterium tuberculosis
b. Bacillus thermophillus
c. Thermos aquaticus
d. Bacillus thermophillus

4. DNA sequencing method is:

a. Kary Mullis method
b. Sanger Dideoxy method
c. Maxam Gilbert method
d. Both 'a' and 'b'

5. Which of the following technique is used to separate the proteins?

II. Ion exchange chromatograph
II. Isoelectric focusing
III. Gel electorphoresis
IV. Gel filtration chromatography

Choose the correct answer:
a. I, II, III only
b. II and III only
c. I and II only
d. I, II, III, IV

6. Protoplasm fusion can be achieved by which of the following method?

I. PEG
II. Electric current
III. Sandi virus
IV. Ph and temperature shock

a. III and IV only
b. II and III only
c. I and II only
d. I, II, III and IV

7. Restriction endonuclease is ?

a. Hind-III
b. EcoR-1
c. Bamb-H$_1$
d. all of these

8. Pbr-322 is a:

a. Plasmid
b. cosmid
c. Phage
d. bacteriophage

9. Edman's degradation technique is used for sequencing:

a. Fats
b. proteins
c. Carbohydrates
d. nucleic acids

10. The most commonly used to detected the presence of HIV is :

a. FIA
b. RIA
c. ELISA
d. HPLC

11. Template dependent enzyme is :

a. RNA polymerase
b. DNA- polymerase
c. DNA ligase
d. Oligonucleotide

12. Polymerase chain reaction is used for :

a. DNA-amplification
b. DNA recombination
c. DNA-repair
d. DNA identification

13. Individual cells can be indentified by using:

a. Rate zonal centrifugation
b. Flow cytometry
c. Marker enzyme
d. Equilibrium density gradient centrifugation

14. Biolistic PDS-1000 is:

a. An antibiotic
b. A gene therapy operation
c. An important cell fusion technique
d. An instrument used to transfer DNA to wide range of cells and tissues

15. The recognition site for EcoR-I a restricted endonuclease enzyme is:

a. 5′ GTT AAC 3′
   3′ CAA TTG 5′

b. 5′ AAG CTT 3′
   3′ TTC GAA 5′

c. 5′ GAA TCC 3′
   3′ CTT AAG 5′

d. 5′ CC GG 3′
   3′GG CCS 5′

16. Polyacrylamide gel electrophoresis is used for :

a. Joining the two DNA fragments
b. Separation of fragments differing by a few base pairs
c. Separation of large DNA molecules (whole chromosomes)
d. Joining the two amino acids

17. PFGE stands for:

a. Pigment Fragmented Gel Electrophoresis
b. Pulsed Field Gel Electrophoresis
c. Poly Fragment Gel Electrophoresis
d. Pulsed Fragmented gel Electrophoresis

18. RIA stands for:

a. Repeated Immuno Assay
b. Regulated Immuno Assay
c. Radio Immuno Assay
d. Regular Immuno Assay

19. NMR stand for:

a. Nuclear magnetic resonance
b. Nuclear mobidity rate
c. Nuclear management region
d. Nuclear material resource

20. CHEFE stands for:

a. Charged change homogeneous Electric Field Electrophoresis
b. Charged hanger electron field electrophoresis
c. Contour clamped homogeneous electric field electrophoresis
d. All of the above

21. The terminator technology was coined by

a. Syngenta
b. Monsanto
c. RAFI
d. None of these

22. The promoter used in terminator technology was

a. LEA
b. SV 40
c. TA 29
d. CaMV 35S

23. Access factor for E.coli K12 is

a. 10^{-3} b. 10^{-2}
c. 10^{-1} d. 10^{-4}

24. Which of the following is not true for GLSP?

a. Host should be non pathogenic
b. The vector should not have resistance marker
c. The carrier organism should be non pathogenic
d. Shuttle vector can not be used

25. Which of the following experiments are exempted from detailed biosafety analysis?

a. Self cloning experiments
b. Experiments involving plant pathogens
c. Experiments involving animal pathogens
d. Agrobacterium mediated transformation

26. Cloning of GRAS organisms fall in the

a. Category I experiment
b. Category II experiment
c. Category III experiment
d. None of these

27. Field testing of transgenic crop for release as a variety is done by

a. ICAR   b. DBT
c. GEAC   d. MoEF

28. The Indian company not involved in Bt-cotton variety production

a. Ankur seeds
b. Indoi-American Hybrid Seed Company
c. Mayhco
d. Rasi Seeds

29. Rooty locus of T-DNA codes for

a. Tryptophan monooxygenase
b. Indoleacetamide hydrolase
c. Indole pentenyl transferase
d. Nopaline synthase

30. Shooty locus of T-DNA indicate genes

a. iaaH
b. iaaM
c. Both of these
d. None of these

31. Number of genes prescent in vir region of T-DNA is

a. 25   b. 20
c. 15   d. 10

32. Size of Ti-plasmid is about

a. 100 bp   b. 100 kb

c. 200 kb   d. 200 bp

33. Hairy root phenotype is caused by

a. A. Rhizogenes   b. A. Tumefaciens

c. Both of these   d. None of these

34. Better expression of vir genes takes place at

a. Alkaline pH   b. Acidic pH

c. Neutral pH   d. None of these

35. Octopine is converted by Agrobacterium to produce

a. Pyruvate and arginine   b. Glucose and Alanine

c. Sucrose and nopaline   d. Glucose and arginine

36. In binary plasmid for T-DNA transfer, the direct repeats of T-DNA

a. Are trans to vir region

b. Are absent

c. Are about 50 bp

d. Are present in duplicate copies

37. During infection, the Agrobacterium cell show

a. Phototropic movement

b. Nastic movement

c. Chemotactic movement

d. No movement

38. During transfer T-DNA remains as

a. Naked, single stranded

b. Naked double stranded

c. SsDNA-Protein complex

d. dsDNA-protein complex

39. Acetpsuromgpme at lower concentration acts as

a. Regulator of operon

b. Chemoattractant

c. Inhibitor of host-Agrobacterium ecognition

d. Inducer of T-DNA excision

40. Technique of floral dip for transformation was developed by

a. S.J. clough and A.F.Bent

b. J.R.Kikkert

c. Both of these

d. None of these

41. The DNA fingerprinting process involves

a. Chain terminators

b. Degenerate oligonucleotides

c. VNTR loci

d. RFLPs

42. Restriction fragment length polymorphism (RFLP) is

a. The technique used to fingerprint patterns of inheritance

b. The different in the restriction maps between the two alleles in a diploid cell

c. The different in the restriction maps between two individuals of one species

d. The different in the restriction maps between two individuals of one species

43. Which of the following could not possibly give rise to restriction fragment length polymorphism (RFLP)?

a. A missense mutation within the protein coding region of a gene

b. A silent mutation within the protein coding region of a gene

c. A single base change within the intron sequence of a gene

d. An error in RNA splicing that mistakenly removes an exon during RNA processing

44. RFLP analysis can be used to distinguish between alleles based on differences in

a. Restriction enzyme recognition sites between the alleles

b. The amount of DNA amplified from the alleles during PC R

c. The ability of the alleles to be replicated in bacterial cells

d. The proteins expressed from the alleles

45. Positional cloning refers to

a. Using a selection procedure to clone a cDNA

b. Isolating a gene by PCR using primers from another species

c. Isolating a gene from a specific tissue in which it is being expressed

d. Mapping a gene to a chromosomal region and then identifying and cloning a genomic copy of he gene from the region

46. Which of the following genes is defective in patients suffering from severe combined immunodeficiency syndrome (SCID)

a. CFTR

b. Adenosine deaminase

c. Ribonucleotide reductase

d. α2-microoglobin

47. A mouse in which one particular gene has been replaced by its inactivated from generated in vitro is called

a. Transgenic mouse   b. Knockout mouse

c. Nude mouse   d. Mutant mouse

48. The principle of the yeast two-hybrid system is

a. The detection of protein-protein interactions by assembling a functional factor from twob detection proteins

b. The detection of protein-protein interactions in a pair of hybrid yeast strains

c. The detection of protein-protein interactions by studying the hybridization of two cDNA sequence

d. The detection of protein-protein interactions between phage coat protein and target proteins

49. Vacuum infiltration method of transformation was developed by

a. J. R. Kikkert

b. G.Hansen and M.D. Chilton

c. J. C. Sanford

d. N. Bechtold et al.

50. Concept of biolistic transformation was given by

a. J. R. Kikkert

b. G.Hansen and M.D. Chilton

c. J. C. Sanford

d. None of these

51. The method of pollen tube transformation was developed by

a. J. R. Kikkert

b. G.Hansen and M.D. Chilton

c. Z. X. Luo and R. Wu

d. None of these

52. Pollen tube transformation was first reported in

a. Wheat   b. Rice

c. Brassica   d. Arubulopsis

53. A. Rhizogenes infects

a. Monocots only

b. Gymnosperms

c. Dicots only

d. Both a and c

54. The gene expressing hairy root phenotype in A. Rhizogenes is

a. ipt   b. ocs

c. rol   d. nos

55. a gene of A. Rhizogenes that con induce male sterility is

a. rolC   b. rolA

c. rolB   d. ocs

56. The techniqye of liposome mediated transformation in plant was developed by

a. A. Deshayes et al   b. A. Crossway et al.

c. I. Potrykus   d. J. D. Liu

57. During Electroporation the potential of electric current passed is

a. 2–5 kv   b. 10–20 kv

c. 20–30 kv   d. None of these

58. More number of stable transformants can be obtained by

a. Lipofection   b. Electroporation

c. Laser beam   d. Agrobacterium

59. Diameter of gene guns are about

a. 2000–4000 nm   b. 200–400 nm

c. 20–40 nm   d. 2–4 nm

60. Silicon carbide fiber was used for gene delivery in plants by

a. H. F. Kaeppler et al.   b. A. Deshayes et al.

c. J. C. sanfrd   d. None of these

61. Di-isopropyl fluorophosphates (DEF) reacts with serine proteases stoichiometrically and irreversibly and therefore is a

a. Competitive inhibitor

b. Non-competitive inhibitor

c. Uncompetitive inhibitor

d. Repressor

62. In non-competitive inhibition

a. The concentration of active enzyme molecules is reduced

b. V_{max} is increased

c. The concentration of active enzyme molecules is unchanged

d. The apparent K_m is increased

63. In an enzyme assay in which substrate concentration is much lower then K_m, the rate

a. Approaches V_{max}

b. Shows zero-order kinetics

c. It proportional to substrate concentration

d. Is independent of enzyme concentration

64. Isoenzymes

a. Are enzymes that exist in more than one amino acid sequence in the same species

b. Cannot ne distinguished in a geiven species except immunologically

c. By definition must have the same amino aicd composition

d. Are single polypeptide chains that differ by an amino acid replacement

65. Which of the following is not a component of coenzyme A?

a. Adenylic acid   b. Pantothenic acid

c. Cysteamine   d. Acetic acid

66. As a coenzyme, pyruvate decarboxylase requires

a. Coenzyme A

b. NAD$^+$

c. FMN

d. Thiamine pyrophosphate

67. Dehydrogenases use as coenzymes all of the following *except*:

a. NAD$^+$ b. NADP

c. FAD   d. Ferriprotoporphyrin

68. Which of the following is an essential cofactor in carboxylation reactions?

a. Coenzyme A   b. Biotin

c. CTP   d. Lipoic acid

69. The enzyme that catalyses the reaction $2H_2O \rightarrow 2H_2O + O_2$ is a

a. Dehydrogenase   b. Peroxidase

c. Catalase   d. Hydrolase

70. Which enzyme will cleave leucyl-glycyl-proline to leucine and glycyl-proline?

a. Carboxypeptidase

b. Glycylglycyl peptidase

c. Aminopeptidase

d. Chymotrypsin

71. An enzyme of saliva that hydrolyzes starch is

a. Pepsin   b. β-Amylase

c. Lysozyme   d. α-Amylase

72. The isoenzymes of lactate dehydrogenase

a. Demonstrate the evolutionary development of this enzyme

b. Range from monomers to tetramers

c. Differ only in a single amino acid

d. Exist in 5 forms depending upon the content of M and H monomers

73. The nerve gas, DFP, has been a useful reagent in enzyme chemistry. At the active site of many hydrolytic enzymes of DFP combines with

a. Histidine   b. Serine

c. Lysine   d. Aspartate

74. The isocitrate dehydrogenase reaction is analogous to (performs the same type of chemical reaction)

a. Pyruvate dehydogenase

b. α-ketoglutarate dehydrogenase

c. α-hydroxyacyl-CoA dehydrogenase

d. 6-phosphogluconate dehydrogenase

75. Antimetabolites act by

a. Competitive inhibition when they combine irreversibly with an enzyme

b. Competitive inhibition when they combine reversibly with an enzyme

c. Non-competitive inhibition if there is no relation between degree of inhibition and substrate concentration

d. Lactate dehydrogenase

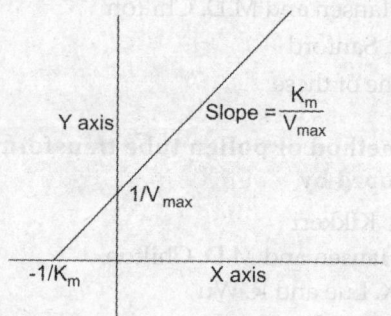

76. K_m and V_{max} can be determined from the Lineweaver – Burk plot of the Michaelis – Menton equation shoen below. Where V is the reaction velocity at substrate concentrations S, the X-axis experimental data are expressed as

a. 1/V   b. V

c. 1/S   d. S

77. All the following gastrointestinal enzymes are secreted as inactive zymogens (proenzymes) *except*:

a. Ribonuclease

b. Pepsin

c. Trypsin

d. Chymotrypsin

78. Which enzyme has the greatest specificity for peptide bonds on the carboxyl side of a cationic amino acid side chain?

   a. Carboxypeptidase
   b. Trypsin
   c. Rennin
   d. Pepsin

79. Which of the following statements about myosin is true?

   a. It is a spherically symmetric molecule
   b. It is low in α-helix content
   c. It is a zinc-requiring enzyme
   d. It is an actin-binding protein

80. If an enzyme behaves according to classic Michaelis-Menton kinetics, from a double reciprocal plot of velocity versus substrate concentration, the value for the Michaelis constant (K_m) of the substrate can be determined graphically as the

   a. Slope of curve
   b. Point of infection of the curve
   c. Absolute value of the intercept of the curve with the X-axis
   d. Reciprocal of the absolute value of the intercept of the curve with the Y-axis

81. Which of the following oxidation-reduction systems has the highest redox potential?

   a. Fumarate/succinate
   b. $NAD^+/NADH$
   c. Fe^{+++} Cytochrome a/Fe^{++}
   d. Fe^{+++} Cytochrome b/Fe^{++}

82. Dinitrophenol would be most likely to inhibit cell function by disrupting

   a. TCA cycle
   b. Glycolysis
   c. Hepatic gluconeogenesis
   d. Oxidative phosphorylation

83. DNA is denatured by:

   a. Acid
   b. Alkali
   c. Heat
   d. All of these

84. Synthesis of RNA molecule is terminated by a signal by a signal which is recognized by :

   a. δ-factor
   b. p-(Rho) factor
   c. α-factor
   d. σ-factor

85. The carbon atoms at positions 4 and 5 and the N atom at position 7 of purine base are supplied from:

   a. Valine
   b. Glycine
   c. Alanine
   d. Serine

86. All α-amino acids are optically active *except:*

   a. Glycine
   b. Alanine
   c. Serine
   d. Phenylalanine

87. In many proteins, the hydrogen bonding produces a regular coiled arrangement called:

   a. γ-helix
   b. β-helix
   c. α-helix
   d. δ-helix

88. a-helix is stabilized by:

   a. Disulphide bond
   b. Covalent bond
   c. Ionic bond
   d. Hydrogen bond

89. The distance travelled per turn of α-helix is:

   a. 0.54 nm
   b. 0.44 nm
   c. 0.34 nm
   d. 0.64 nm

90. The space covered by each amino acid residue of α-helix is:

   a. 0.25 nm
   b. 0.18 nm
   c. 0.15 nm
   d. 0.35 nm

91. Glutamate dehydrogenase is a:

   a. Dimer
   b. Monomer
   c. Tetramer
   d. All of these

92. When egg albumin is coagulated (by heating)

   a. Only tertiary structure is changed
   b. Only primary structure is changed
   c. Secondary and tertiary structures are changed
   d. Only secondary structure is changed

93. Oxidative conversion of many amino acids to their corresponding α-keto acids occurs in mammalian:

   a. Adipose tissue
   b. Pancreae
   c. Intestine
   d. Liver and kidney

94. Synthesis of glutamine is accompanied by the hydrolysis of:

   a. ATP
   b. ADP
   c. TPP
   d. Creatine phosphate

95. In brain, the major mechanism for removal of ammonia is the formation of:

   a. Asparagines
   b. Aspartate
   c. Glutamine
   d. Glutamic acid

96. The metabolism of protein is integrated with that of carbohydrate and fat through:

   a. Malate
   b. Oxaloacetate
   c. Isocitrate
   d. Citrate

97. Sulphur of sulphur containing amino acid is removed as:

a. SO_2

b. $BaSO_4$

c. H_2SO_4

d. SO_3

98. Transamination is a:

a. Physical process

b. Irreversible process

c. Reversible process

d. None of these

99. Which of the following can not undergo transamination?

a. Threonine

b. Alanine

c. Serine

d. Valine

100. The process of transamination requires:

a. FAD

b. ATP

c. NAD^+

d. PLP

ANSWERS OF MODEL PAPER 3

1. c	2. a	3. c	4. d	5. d	6. b	7. d
8. a	9. b	10. c	11. b	12. a	13. b	14. d
15. c	16. b	17. b	18. c	19. a	20. c	21. c
22. a	23. a	24. d	25. a	26. a	27. a	28. b
29. c	30. c	31. a	32. c	33. a	34. b	35. a
36. a	37. c	38. c	39. b	40. a	41. c	42. c
43. d	44. a	45. d	46. b	47. b	48. a	49. d
50. c	51. b	52. b	53. c	54. c	55. b	56. a
57. a	58. d	59. a	60. a	61. b	62. a	63. c
64. a	65. d	66. d	67. d	68. b	69. c	70. c
71. d	72. c	73. b	74. d	75. b	76. c	77. a
78. b	79. d	80. d	81. c	82. d	83. d	84. b
85. b	86. c	87. c	88. d	89. a	90. c	91. c
92. c	93. d	94. a	95. c	96. b	97. c	98. c
99. a	100. d					

Model Test Paper 4

1. **Intrachain hydrogen bonding in α-helix occurs between**
   a. 1 and 6 amino acid
   b. 1 and 4 amino acid
   c. 1 and 3 amino acid
   d. 2 and 4 amino acid

2. **Introns is a region of the chromosomal DNA**
   a. That is a part of a gene that is transcribed but is removed during maturation of the transcript
   b. That is located between two adjacent genes
   c. That is located at the centromere
   d. None of these

3. **Ionophores are used as antibiotics because they**
   a. Equilibriate concentration gradient across the membrane for a particular solute
   b. Are competitive inhibitor of pyruvate dehydrogenase
   c. Cause ionization of enzymes involved in metabolic reactions
   d. Inhibit transcription

4. **JAK-STAT pathway is governed by**
   a. Ion channel linked receptor
   b. Tyrosine kinase receptor
   c. Monomeric G-protein linked reception
   d. Heterotrimeric G-protein linked receptor

5. **Karyotype shows 45 chromosome appear normal male, due to**
   a. Translocation
   b. Inversion
   c. Deletion
   d. Non disjunction

6. **Which sequence is the best target for damage by UV radiation**
   a. AGGCAAA   b. AGGCAAA
   c. GUAAAAU   d. CTTTTGA

7. **Kinetochore is a proteinaceous structure of centromere. It is important for cell division because**
   a. It causes spindle formation
   b. Microtubules attach to kinetochore during separation of chromosome
   c. It causes spindle formation
   d. None of these

8. **Lactose operon is both negatively and positively regulated, this means that lactose is used**
   a. Along with glucose
   b. After glucose has been used
   c. Preferentially
   d. All of these

9. **Which one of the following ion channels is an example of second messenger gated ion channel**
   a. K+ channel   b. Na+ channel
   c. Ca++ channel   d. Cl- channel

10. **Lipid bilayer can be formed by phospholipids which have variable head groups and fatty acyl chains. The fluidity of the membrane will depend on**
    a. Only the nature of head groups
    b. Only the length of the fatty acid chains irrespective of the extent of unsaturation
    c. Only unsaturation irrespective of the length of the fatty acid chain
    d. Length and degree of unsaturation of fatty acid chain

11. **Lipid bilayer fluid mosaic model is not applicable to the plasma membrane of**
    a. Bacteria   b. Oleosomes
    c. Mitochondria   d. Ribosome

12. **Low pH of the lysosomal compartment is maintained by**
    a. Luminal acid production
    b. Glycolysis
    c. H+ ATPase the membrane
    d. Electron transport

13. **Which one of the following transporters enables eukaryotic cells to pump out a large number of dufferent drugs and other foreign compounds?**
    a. ABC transporter
    b. H+ pumps
    c. Na+/K+ pumps
    d. Aquaporins

14. **Lysozyme has no effect on archaeal cell because**
    a. It works on cell wall and archael cell lacks it
    b. It works on β-1,3 glycosidic bond and this bond is not found in archael cell wall
    c. It works on β-1,4 linkage and archaeal cell lack point
    d. None of these

15. **Mad 2 protein acts at mitotic spindle assembly check point of cell cycle. It attached at**
    a. Randomly any region of chromosome
    b. Centromeric region of chromosome
    c. Telomeric region of chromosome
    d. Secondary construction

16. **Maltose is disaccharide of**
    a. Glucose + galactose
    b. Glucose + maltose
    c. Glucose + fructose
    d. Glucose + Glucose

17. **Mannose-6-phosphate receptor is found in**
    a. Lysosome
    b. Ribosome
    c. ER
    d. Trans golgi network

18. **Membrane channels**
    a. Commonly contain amphipathic α-helix
    b. Allow substrates to flow only from outside to inside the cell
    c. Are opened or closed only as a result of a change in the transmembrane potential
    d. None of these

19. **Membrane potential is controlled by**
    a. Ligand-gated ion channel
    b. Second messenger-gated ion channels
    c. Voltage gated ion channel
    d. Pressure sensitive ion channels

20. **Membrane of which of the following organelles are contiguous**
    a. Golgi and plasma membrane
    b. Golgi and lysosome
    c. ER and Golgi
    d. Nucleus and ER

21. **Mercaptoethanol can break**
    a. Ionic bond
    b. Hydrogen bond
    c. Disulphide bond
    d. Hydrophobic interactions

22. **Mesokaryotic cells have**
    a. Nucleus with nuclear membrane but lacks histones
    b. Nuclear membrane and histone
    c. Nucleus without nuclear membrane
    d. None of these

23. **Methotrexate is used as anticancer drug because**
    a. It blocks cytokinesis
    b. It inhibits synthesis of dNTPs
    c. It stabilizes in G0 phase
    d. It blocks mitosis

24. **MGMT is a "sucide enzyme" it is involved in**
    a. Direct DNA repair
    b. Mismatch DNA repair
    c. Genetic recombination
    d. Excision DNA repair

25. **Mitochondria is involved in all of the following except?**
    a. TCA cycle
    b. ATP production
    c. Fatty acid biosynthesis
    d. Apoptosis

26. **Mitosis promoting factor is**
    a. Cyclin independent protein kinase
    b. Cyclin dependent protein kinase
    c. Complex of cyclin protein
    d. Complex of securing and proteasome

27. **Movement of solute through the cell membrane against the concentration gradient is termed active transport and occurs when**
    a. Energy is utilized for this purpose
    b. A metal ion, Ca++ is bound to it
    c. Facilitated by hydrolysis of ATP
    d. It is transported with a carrier protein

28. **MPF acts at**
    a. S-phase
    b. M-phase
    c. G2/M phase
    d. G1/S phase

29. Multidrug resistance transporter protein is an example of

a. P-type ATPase
b. ABC-transporter
c. G-type ATPase
d. V-type ATPase

30. Mutation which changes a triplet is called

a. Nonsense mutation
b. Neutral mutation
c. Missense mutation
d. Silent mutation

31. Na+/K+ pump is an example of

a. Uniporter
b. Symporter
c. Antiporter
d. None of these

32. Native form of DNA is called

a. A-DNA
b. B-DNA
c. C-DNA
d. Z-DNA

33. Neomycin in bacterial protein synthesis

a. Inhibits binding of amino acyl t-RNA to ribosome
b. Inhibits initiation of translation and causes misreading
c. Inhibits interaction between t-RNA and m-RNA
d. Inhibits interaction between r-RNA and t-RNA

34. Nieman-Pick disease and Gaucher syndrome occurs due to loss of enzyme from

a. Proteasomes
b. Lysosomes
c. Endosomes
d. Microbodies

35. Nitric oxide receptor is

a. Membrane bound and ion channel linked
b. Membrane bound and enzyme linked
c. Membrane bound and G-Protein linked
d. Cytosolic

36. Nucleosome consist of

a. H2A, H2B, H3, H4 and 200bp
b. Two H2A, H2B, H3, H4, non-histone protein and 200 bp
c. Two H2A, H2B, H3, H4, H1 and 200bp
d. Two H2A, H2B, H3, H4 and 200bp

37. Okazaki fragments are

a. Found on the lagging strand
b. Found on the leading strand
c. Synthesized in the 3′ to 5′ direction
d. None of these

38. O-linked glycosylation of protein occurs in

a. Golgi body
b. Lysosome
c. Endoplasmic reticulum
d. Cytosol

39. Which one of the following transport mechanisms across the membrane is not an active process?

a. Uptake of glucose by erythrocytes
b. Uptake of fructose by intestinal epithelial cells
c. Uptake of glucose by intestinal epithelial cells
d. None of these

40. One of the major transmembrane proteins in a tight junction is

a. Adherin
b. Claudin
c. Lectin
d. Integrin

41. Operons are found in prokaryotes but they are also reported in an eukaryote that is

a. Drosophila
b. Maize
c. Caenorhabditis elegans
d. Arabidopsis thaliana

42. Oubain is a potent inhibitor of

a. H^+ pump
b. Na^+ ion channel
c. Na^+/K^+ channel
d. Na^+/Ca^{++} channel

43. Parietal cells are found in

a. Liver
b. Kidney
c. Stomach
d. Heart

44. Pattern of shell coiling in fresh water snails is an example of

a. Maternal effect
b. Cytoplasmic effect
c. Infectious inheritance
d. Mendelian inheritance

45. Pemphigoid is an autoimmune disease in which the patient develops antibodies against proteins in

a. Na+ ion channel
b. Cl- ion channel
c. Hemidesmosomes
d. Desmosomes

46. Peptidyl transferase activity is contained

a. Within the small ribosomal subunit
b. Within t-RNA
c. Within the large ribosomal subunit
d. Within both large and small subunits of ribosome

47. Which one of the following statements is true for prokaryotic cell?

a. Hey always divide mitotically
b. Their signalling system involves two component system
c. Their cytoskeleton consists only of microtubules
d. Their end membrane system consists only of ER and mesosome

48. Pertussis toxin causes

a. ADP-ribosylation of $G_{s\alpha}$

b. Ceasation of GTPase activity of $G_{s\alpha}$

c. Hydrolysis of cAMP

d. ADP-ribosylation of $G_{s\alpha}$

49. Phagocytes kill harmful bacteria by

a. Complement   b. Endocytosis

c. Inflammation   d. T-cell stimulation

50. Phosphatidyl serine is usually found in

a. Inner leaflet of lipid bilayer

b. Outer leaflet of lipid bilayer

c. It is randomly distributed in both leaflets of lipid bilayer

d. None of these

51. Phospholipase C is found in

a. ER membrane

b. Tonoplast

c. Plasma membrane of an eukaryotic cell

d. Outer membrane of mitochondria

52. Plant cells communicate through

a. Plasmodesmata   b. Desmosomes

c. Cell wall   d. Gap junction

53. Plasmids differ from transposons because plasmids

a. Move from chromosome to chromosome

b. Can self-replicate outside the cell

c. Carry genes for antibiotic resistance

d. Become inserted in to chromosome

54. Plasmodesmata of plant cells are similar to the animal's

a. Adherens junctions   b. Desmosomes

c. Gap junctions   d. Tight junctions

55. Podophyllotoxin is used to treat cancer. It prevents cell division by inhibiting

a. Cohesion breakdown

b. Cyclin synthesis

c. Cdks

d. Polymerization of microtubules

56. Point mutation in which there is deletion or addition of one base pair is termed as

a. Transversion

b. Transition

c. Frame shift mutation

d. Deletion

57. Polyadenylation is a post-transcriptional phenomenon. It was proved after the discovery of

a. AAUAAAA signal sequences in m-RNA

b. Terminal sequences in template DNA

c. Template independent poly (A) polymerase

d. None of these

58. Polyadenylation of 3'-end of m-RNA is a distinguishing feature of eukaryotic transcription events. But it does not occur in

a. m-RNA for tumour cells

b. m-RNA for apolipoprotein-B

c. m-RNA for histone protein

d. m-RNA for interferon protein

59. Primary and secondary active transport both

a. Use ATP directly

b. Can move solutes against their concentration gradient

c. Include the passive movement of glucose molecule

d. Are based on passive movement of sodium ions

60. prokaryotes lack the membranous sub-cellular organelles characteristic of eukaryotes, but their plasma membrane may be enfolded to from

a. Plasmosome   b. Mesosome

c. Lysosome   d. Endo some

61. Proof reading activity is performed by

a. 3'–5' exonuclease activity of DNA polymerases

b. 5'–3' exonuclease activity of DNA polymerases

c. 3'–5' exonuclease activity of RNA polymerases

d. 5'–3' exonuclease activity of RNA polymerases

62. Protein present in coated pits involved in receptor mediated endocytosis is

a. Coatoamer   b. Diamine

c. Clathrin   d. Adopter

63. Protein cannot be synthesized in

a. Nerve fibers   b. Sieve tubes

c. WBCs   d. None of these above

64. Protein synthesized on ER-bound ribosome cannot be transported in to

a. Golgi complex   b. ER

c. Peroxisome   d. Lysosome

65. Pseudo dominance is caused by

a. Inversion   b. Deletion

c. Translocation   d. Duplication

66. Pseudo linkage is caused by

a. Translocation
b. Deletion
c. Duplication
d. Inversion

67. Pyrimidine dimmers are repaired by

a. DNA photolyase
b. DNA polymerase II
c. AP-endonuclease
d. Exconuclease

68. Quorum sensing in bacteria involves

a. Cell signalling cascading mediated by cGMP
b. Cell signalling cascading mediated by cAMP
c. Tyrosine phosphorylation
d. Histidine phosphorylation

69. Quorum sensing in gram positive bacteria occurs through

a. G-protein coupled signalling
b. Two component system
c. One component system
d. Stringent response

70. RBCs uptake glucose through

a. Symporter
b. Antiporter
c. Active porter
d. Passive porter

71. Receptors for neurotransmitters are located on the

a. Cytosol
b. Nucleoplasm
c. Nuclear membrane
d. Cell surface

72. Which one of the following statements is not correct?

a. Transport through symporter is fast than ion channels
b. Transport through channel is always passive
c. Oubain can inhibit Na+/K+ pump
d. None of these

73. Recombination is thought to be the primary source of variations which are spice of evolution because

a. It creates new alleles
b. It creates new gene
c. It creates new recombination of gene
d. It creates new recombination of alleles

74. Which one of the following statements is not correct?

a. Unsaturated fatty acids in the plasma membrane have cis-double bonds
b. Unsaturated fatty acids in the plasma membrane have trans-double bonds
c. Fatty acids in the plasma membrane are saturated and unsaturated
d. None of these

75. Recombination-dependent mechanism for DNA repairing is

a. Photo reactivation repair
b. Post-replication repair
c. SOS repair
d. Excision repair

76. Regarding gene expression in prokaryotes and eukaryotes, which statement is correct?

a. m-RNA and DNA are collinear
b. m-RNA and protein synthesis can occur simultaneously
c. RNA polymerase can bind to promoters situated upstream to gene
d. Processing of hn-RNA yield m-RNA

77. Replicate copies of each chromosome are called .... and are joined at the.....

a. Sister chromatids/centromere
b. Sister chromatids/kinetochore
c. Homologues/kinetochore
d. Homologous/centromere

78. Restriction endonucleases hydrolyze a polynucleotide from

a. From either terminal
b. Only the 5' end
c. At an internal phosphodiester bond
d. A phosphodiester bond within a specific sequence

79. Ribophorins proteins are found in the membrane of

a. ER
b. Golgi body
c. Chloroplast
d. Ribosome

80. Reverse transcriptase is a

a. DNA-dependent RNA polymerase
b. RNA-dependent DNA polymerase
c. DNA-dependent DNA polymerase
d. RNA dependent RNA polymerase

81. Ribosomal subunits are assembled in

a. Nucleolus
b. Nucleus
c. Cytoplasm
d. ER

82. Ribosome are attached to endoplasmic reticulum through

a. r-RNA
b. t-RNA

c. Hydrophobic interaction

d. Ribophorins

83. Which one of the following statements is not correct?

a. Tetrodotoxin blocks Na+ channels

b. DAG is a membrane derived second expression at

c. Rab protein are trimeric G-protein that are involved in vesicle fusion

d. Exocytosis and endocytosis are energy consuming process

84. Riboswitches can regulate gene expression at

a. Translation level

b. Transcription level

c. Post translation level

d. Both a and b

85. RNA interference is an extremely effective and widely used method for

a. Regulation of gene expression at the mRNA level

b. RNA processing in vitro

c. Interfering with transcription

d. Gene transfer

86. RNA is very much susceptible to hydrolysis in alkali because

a. Cleavage occurs in the glycosidic bonds of purine bases

b. Its 2'-OH group participate in intramolecular cleavage of phosphodiester backbone

c. Cleavage occurs in the glycosidic bond of pyrimidine bases

d. None of these

87. Secondary metabolites in plant cell accumulate in

a. Vacuoles

b. Oleosomes

c. Glyoxysomes

d. Lysosome

88. Secondary structures of protein are stabilized by

a. Hydrogen bonds between peptide bonds

b. Hydrogen bonds between R groups

c. Ionic bonds and hydrogen bonds between R groups

d. Disulphide bonds

89. Secretary proteins are mainly modified in

a. ER lumen

b. Golgi apparatus

c. Ribosome

d. Nucleus

90. Several staining technique yield characteristic patterns of alternating light and dark chromosome bands which results from the preferential binding of stains to

a. AG-rich versus CT-rich DNA

b. AT-rich versus GC-rich DNA

c. Exon-rich versus CT-rich DNA

d. Histone-rich versus non histone rich DNA

91. Sexual reproduction is called as "master piece of nature" because it involve gamete formation through meiosis. What property of the meiosis justifies the above saying?

a. Recombination of alleles during meiosis

b. Separation of homologous chromosomes during gamete formation

c. Independent assortment of alleles during anaphase I

d. Pairing of homologous chromosomes

92. Siderophores are

a. Magnesium binding protein

b. Calcium binding protein

c. Iron binding protein

d. Phosphorus binding protein

93. Signal hypothesis is associated with

a. Synthesis of secretary protein

b. Transport of mRNA from nucleus

c. Transport of ribosomes from nucleus

d. Anterograde transport

94. Signalling process mediated by insulin and epidermal growth factors occurs through

a. Cell adhesion molecule

b. Ion channel linked receptor

c. G-protein linked receptor

d. Tyrosine kinase linked receptor

95. Smooth ER is the site of synthesis and metabolism of

a. Carbohydrate

b. Proteins

c. Glycogen

d. Fatty acids and phospholipids

96. Somatic pairing is often seen in

a. Chromosomes of somatic cell

b. Polytene chromosome

c. Lampbrush chromosomes

d. During meiosis in germ cells

97. Some m-RNA of bacteria is polyadenylated. Here Polyadenylation

    a. Increases half life of m-RNA

    b. Increases rate of translation

    c. Provides polycistronic tendency

    d. Triggers degradation of m-RNA

98. Sometimes the presence of Introns allows the exons of a gene to be joined in different combinations resulting in the synthesis of different proteins from the same gene. Here Introns play role in

    a. Cis-splicing

    b. Alternative splicing

    c. Tans-splicing

    d. None of these

99. Spectrin is integral membrane protein of

    a. Macrophages

    b. Endosomes

    c. RBCs

    d. Epithelial cells

100. Spliceosome removes Introns from hn-RNA in

    a. Nucleus   b. Mitochondria

    c. Chloroplast   d. Archaebacteria

ANSWERS OF MODEL PAPER 4

1. b	2. a	3. a	4. b	5. a	6. d	7. b
8. b	9. c	10. d	11. b	12. c	13. a	14. c
15. b	16. d	17. d	18. a	19. c	20. d	21. c
22. a	23. b	24. a	25. c	26. b	27. a	28. c
29. b	30. c	31. c	32. b	33. b	34. b	35. d
36. b	37. a	38. a	39. a	40. b	41. c	42. c
43. c	44. a	45. c	46. c	47. b	48. d	49. b
50. a	51. c	52. a	53. b	54. c	55. d	56. c
57. c	58. c	59. b	60. b	61. a	62. c	63. b
64. c	65. b	66. a	67. a	68. d	69. b	70. d
71. d	72. a	73. b	74. b	75. b	76. c	77. a
78. d	79. a	80. b	81. c	82. d	83. c	84. d
85. a	86. b	87. a	88. a	89. a	90. b	91. a
92. c	93. a	94. d	95. d	96. b	97. d	98. b
99. c	100. a					

Model Test Paper 5

1. **The biologically active proteasome is**
   a. 20S
   b. 30S
   c. 26S
   d. 50S

2. **The biologically predominant form of DNA is**
   a. Left handed B-DNA
   b. Right handed A-DNA
   c. Left handed A-DNA
   d. Right handed B-DNA

3. **The concentration of glucose in the blood plasma is usually in the range of**
   a. 60–70 mg/100 ml
   b. 68–88 mg/100 ml
   c. 5–50 mg/100 ml
   d. 180–200mg/100 ml

4. **The conformational variation between B and z from of DNA is fartly due to**
   a. Lack of hydrophobic interaction
   b. Loss of H-bond
   c. Rotation of glycosidic bond
   d. Increase in humidity

5. **The curve for renaturation of denatured DNA is**
   a. Hyperbolic
   b. Direct
   c. Inverse
   d. Linear

6. **The cytoskeleton consist of**
   a. Intermediate filament, microtubules and cilia
   b. Intermediate filaments, microfilaments and microtubules
   c. Microfilament, cilia and flagella
   d. Microtubules, cilia and microfilament

7. **The DNA molecule having no grooves and left handed is known as**
   a. B-DNA
   b. Z-DNA
   c. A-DNA
   d. C-DNA

8. **The enzyme protein kinase–G is activated by**
   a. cGMP
   b. DAG
   c. IP3
   d. None of these

9. **The epithelial cells that line our intestine uptake glucose by**
   a. Na+/glucose symporter
   b. K+/glucose symporter
   c. Na+/glucose antiporter
   d. Facilitated diffusion

10. **The expression of genetic information can be regulated at the level of**
    a. Conjugation
    b. Transcription
    c. Replication
    d. Cell division

11. **The fastest known rate of any in vivo polymerization reaction is**
    a. Glycogen synthesis
    b. DNA synthesis
    c. Starch synthesis
    d. Protein synthesis

12. **The genetic event that result in Down's syndrome can be described as**
    a. Chromosomal duplication
    b. Uniparental disomy
    c. Non disjunction
    d. Non-reciprocal crossing over

13. **The golgi apparatus**
    a. Packages and modifies proteins
    b. Is found in prokaryotes
    c. Is found only in animals
    d. Is the appendage that moves a cell around in its environment

14. **The hormone testosterone is produced by**
    a. Sertoli cells
    b. Vas deferens
    c. Spermatocytes
    d. Leyding cells

15. **The hormone which is secreted by both hypothalamus and gastrointestine is**
    a. Somatostatin
    b. Cholecystokinin
    c. Secretin
    d. Gastrin

16. **The imidazole groups are parts of the active sites of many enzymes. This group is found in**

    a. Proline
    b. Histidine
    c. Glutamine
    d. Asparagines

17. **The inner side of plasma membrane is negatively charged. The reason behind it is**

    a. Facilitate diffusion
    b. Active transport
    c. Simple diffusion
    d. Donann equilibrium

18. **The internal system of protein fibres that contributes to a eukaryotic cell's structure and allows movement is called**

    a. Cytoskeleton
    b. Lysosomal system
    c. Extracellular matrix
    d. Endomembrane system

19. **The main force in membrane resealing of ruptured biomembrane in aqueous environment is**

    a. Covalent forces between membrane lipids
    b. Force between proteins and lipids
    c. Hydrophobic forces between membrane lipids
    d. Ionic interaction between membrane lipids

20. **The major constituent of the cell organelle centriole is**

    a. Actin
    b. Myosin
    c. Tubulin
    d. Intermediate filament

21. **The major function of nucleolus in a nucleus concern**

    a. Replication of DNA
    b. Synthesis of Ribosome
    c. Chromatids separation
    d. Organisation of chromosome

22. **The maximum frequency of recombination of genes at two loci is**

    a. 25%
    b. 50%
    c. 75%
    d. 100%

23. **The mechanism for transporting components of surrounding medium in to cytoplasm is:**

    a. Endocytosis
    b. Transduction
    c. Exocytosis
    d. Phagocytosis

24. **The melting temperature Tm of DNA depends upon**

    a. The purine content of DNA
    b. The length of DNA
    c. G-C content of DNA
    d. None of these

25. **The membrane protein of RBCs which are responsible for transport of glucose in to them functions as**

    a. Carrier
    b. Pump
    c. Ion channel
    d. Receptor

26. **The molecular motor that is involved in chromosome movement during cell division comprises**

    a. Kinesins and dyneins
    b. Kinesin and microtubules
    c. Microtubules and actin
    d. Troponin and dynein

27. **The most important point in the regulation of cell cycle occurs in the**

    a. G_1 phase
    b. S phase
    c. M phase
    d. G_0 phase

28. **The movement of material from the ER through the Golgi complex toward the plasma membrane is called**

    a. Anterograde transport
    b. Bulk flow
    c. Facilitated diffusion
    d. Retrograde transport

29. **The mutation which has no effect on the phenotype is called**

    a. Read through mutation
    b. Missense mutation
    c. Neutral mutation
    d. All of these

30. **The Na+/K+ pump is found in**

    a. Bacteria
    b. Animal
    c. Plant
    d. All of these

31. **The normal intracellular concentration of free Ca^{+2} is**

    a. $10^{-5}M$
    b. $10^{-6}M$
    c. $10^{-7}M$
    d. $10^{-8}M$

32. The operon consists of
    a. Regulator, structural and operator gene
    b. Structural, operator and promoter gene
    c. Regulator, structural and operator gene
    d. Regulator and repressor gene

33. The overall process of nitrogen fixation in bacteria involves
    a. Oxidation of NH_3 b. Reduction of N_2
    c. Oxidation of NO_2 d. Reduction of NO_2

34. Which one of the following is not a characteristic feature of cancer cells?
    a. They avoid programmed cell death
    b. Their cytoskeleton structure is changed
    c. Glycosyl transferases become more active
    d. Cell cycle check points are failed

35. The phenomenon of reverse transcription was discovered by
    a. Beadle and tatum   b. Lederberg and hays
    c. Temin and Baltimore   d. None of these

36. The primay cause of Aneuploidy in an organism
    a. Non-disjunction   b. Translocation
    c. Double fertilization   d. Pericentric inversion

37. The process by which a cell secretes macro-molecules by fusing a vesicle to the plasma membrane is called
    a. Pinocytosis   b. Exocytosis
    c. Phagocytosis   d. Endocytosis

38. Which one of the following is not a characteristic feature of cancerous cells?
    a. They have increased blood vessels
    b. Their cell surface markers remains unchanged
    c. Their monomeric G-protein rho is mutated
    d. They avoid programmed cell death

39. The protein complex 'dicer' is involved in
    a. Gene silencing
    b. Transcription
    c. Translation
    d. Protein sorting

40. The protein of Golgi complex which contain irregular cisternae and tubules is known as
    a. Intercisternal Golgi
    b. Cis Golgi
    c. Trans Golgi
    d. Medial Golgi

41. The region where RNA polymerase binds to promoter in prokaryotes is called
    a. Hogness box   b. Homeo box
    c. Pribnow box   d. Shine-dalgrano box

42. The shortening of eukaryotic chromosome during replication is prevented by
    a. Telomerase   b. Ligase
    c. Reverse transcriptase   d. RNA polymerase

43. Which one of the following hormones binds to intracellular receptor?
    a. Insulin   b. Estrogen
    c. Glucagon   d. Growth hormone

44. The Tm of DNA can be calculated using the formula: Tm = 69.1 + 0.41 (GC) where GC is the percent of guanine + cytosine. A double stranded DNA has 27% adenine. Its Tm is:
    a. 79°C   b. 80.73°C
    c. 95.50°C   d. 88°C

45. The type of intercellular signalling in which one cell can communicate with anoter over long distances is called
    a. Autocrine   b. Paracrine
    c. Juxtacrine   d. Endocrine

46. The uptake of cholesterol by mammalian cells can be explained by
    a. Pinocytosis
    b. Phagocytosis
    c. Transcytosis
    d. Receptor mediated endocytosis

47. The Z-DNA helix
    a. Tends to be found at the 3' end of genes
    b. Is favoured by an alternating GC sequence
    c. Has fewer base pair per turn than the B-DNA
    d. None of these

48. Thymine dimmers in eukaryotes are repaired by
    a. Mismatch repair mechanism
    b. Nucleotide excision repair mechanism
    c. Base excision repair mechanism
    d. Direct repair mechanism

49. To achieve active conformation calmodulin protein binds minimum
    a. Three Ca^{+2} ions   b. One Ca^{+2} ions
    c. Six Ca^{+2} ions   d. Four Ca^{+2} ions

50. which one of the following enzyme is involved in translation step in protein biosynthesis

a. RNA polymerase
b. Ribozyme
c. Reverse transcriptase
d. Aminoacyl –tRNA synthetase

51. Toll-like receptor play a central role in the signalling process which result is

a. Humoral immunity
b. Cell-mediated immunity
c. Innate immunity
d. Artificial passive immunity

52. Tonofilaments are the structural units of

a. Microfilaments
b. Intermediate filament
c. Micro tubules
d. Flagella

53. Transcription coupled DNA repair is an example of

a. Mismatch repair
b. Excision repair
c. SOS response
d. Direct repair

54. Which one of the following components of the plasma membrane of eukaryotic cells is not found in the membrane of prokaryotes?

a. Cholesterol
b. Glycoprotein
c. Sphingolipids
d. Glycerophospholipids

55. Transport of m-RNA from nucleus to Cytosol is

a. Simple diffusion
b. Facilitated diffusion
c. Secondary active process
d. Primary active process

56. Transport of molecules through channel protein present in the plasma membrane is?

a. Always passive
b. May be active or passive
c. Always active
d. None of the above

57. Transport of sodium ions from outer side to the inner side of an eukaryotic cells is

a. Primary active
b. Facilitated diffusion
c. Simple diffusion
d. Secondary active

58. Transport vesicles involved in retrograde transport are coated with

a. COP I
b. COP II
c. Clathrin
d. Caveolin

59. Transposons cause mutation in plants, animal and bacteria. These are

a. Retroviruses
b. Mutagenic viruses
c. Infective protein molecule
d. Mobile genetic element

60. Trehalose is found in the exoskeleton of insects, it is

a. Polysaccharide
b. Disaccharide
c. Trisaccharide
d. Oligosaccharide

61. Two sisters chromatids are separated at anaphase by the action of

a. Seprarin
b. Cohesion
c. APC
d. MAD2

62. Tyrosine kinase is activated by

a. Methylatioon
b. Acetylation
c. Dephosphorylation
d. Phosphorylation

63. Ubiquitinatiohn of proteins is marked for all of the following *except*:

a. Chromatin remodelling
b. Protein degradation
c. Correct folding of protein
d. Endocytosis

64. UGA is a stop codon, but in mitochondrial genome it codes for

a. Trp
b. Met
c. Try
d. Asp

65. Under what thermodynamic conditions will a reaction proceed spontaneously?

a. $\Delta H < 0$
b. $\Delta S < 0$
c. $\Delta G < 0$
d. $\Delta S = 0$

66. UV rays usually causes

a. Gene mutation
b. Genome mutation
c. Chromosome mutation
d. Both a and c

67. Vascular ATPases are

a. Ca+2 pumps
b. K+ pumps
c. H+ pumps
d. Na+ pumps

68. **Vertebrates achieved terrestrial habit due to presence of**

   a. Aminiotic egg
   b. Vivipary
   c. Thermoregulation
   d. Internal fertilization

69. **Viagra is used in the treatment of erectile dysfunction because**

   a. Inhibits NO synthase
   b. Inhibits diesterase
   c. Increase half-life of guanyly cyclase
   d. Stimulates nitric oxide synthesis

70. **Vibrio cholera causes diahorrea by**

   a. Destroys cells of intestinal lining
   b. Closing absorption of water from gut epithelium
   c. Constitutive expression of adenylate cyclase
   d. Opening ion channel

71. **Vinblastin is used as anticancerous drug because it**

   a. Causes cell death
   b. Blocks cell division and functions as antimitotic drug
   c. Promotes cell growth
   d. Stimulates DNA synthesis

72. **Vincristine is an anticancerious drug. It is obtained from**

   a. Atropa
   b. Colchicum
   c. Catharanthus roseus
   d. Taxus baccata

73. **Viral encoded 'ras' oncogene transforms normal mammalian cells in to cancer cells. Viral Ras protein differs from its normal counterpart by**

   a. Diminished ATPase activity
   b. Increased ATPase activity
   c. Increased GTPase activity
   d. Diminished GTPase activity

74. **Viruses can cross biological membranes with the help of**

   a. Integral membrane proteins
   b. Glycocalyx
   c. Pores
   d. Lipid bilayer

75. **What cellular connection is "leak-proof"?**

   a. Tight junction   b. Gap junction
   c. Plasmodesmata   d. Anchoring junction

76. **What happens to the Cdk-cycA complex at metaphase?**

   a. Only cyclin A is degraded
   b. Both cyclin A and Cdk remain under graded
   c. Both cyclin A and Cdk are degraded
   d. Only Cdk is degraded

77. **What is fate of most duplicated genes?**

   a. Gene activation
   b. They become orthologous
   c. They are transferred to a new organism using lateral gene transfer
   d. Gain of a novel function through subsequent mutation

78. **What is the maximum number of hydrogen bonds that can be formed by each molecule of water?**

   a. 3   b. 5
   c. 4   d. 2

79. **When a cell expands energy to move a solute across its membrane against a concentration gradient, the process is called**

   a. Active transport   b. Passive transport
   c. Facilitated duffusion   d. Osmosis

80. **When a mutation changes a termination codon in to codon specifying an amino acid, it is called**

   a. Read through mutation
   b. Synonymous mutation
   c. Reverse nonsense mutation
   d. Back mutation

81. **When bcl-2 gene is mutated it results in tumor, like chronic lymphoblastic leukemia (CLL). Normally this gene regulates**

   a. Cell differentiation
   b. Cell division
   c. Programmed cell death
   d. Synthesis of growth factor

82. **When one amino acid is replaced by another by another owing to a mutation, it is called**

   a. Silent mutation
   b. Missense mutation
   c. Frame shift mutation
   d. Synonymous mutation

83. **When release factor binds to stop codon on m-RNA during translation, the synthesized peptide chain is transferred to**

   a. H+   b. Water
   c. Amino acids   d. t-RNA

84. **When repressor protein binds to operator of an operon which of the following process is regulated?**
    a. Translation
    b. Transcription
    c. Replication
    d. None of the above

85. **When the forces arise from the electrostatic attraction between the positively charged nucleus of one atom and the negatively charged electrons of the other it is called**
    a. Hydrogen bonding
    b. Stacking force
    c. Vanderwaals force
    d. Ionic bonding

86. **Which element is present in diatoms**
    a. Si   b. Ca
    c. Mg   d. Na

87. **Which enzyme is exclusively involved in DNA repair mechanism**
    a. DNA polymerase
    b. Photolyase
    c. RNA polymerase
    d. Restriction endonuclease

88. **Which group of bacteria on sporulation show cell coordination and social behaviour?**
    a. Actino bacteria   b. Archaebacteria
    c. Myxobacteria   d. Bacillus species

89. **Which GTPases regulates intracellular transport in mammalian cells through vesicle fusion?**
    a. Rab   b. Ran
    c. Ras   d. Rho

90. **Which is crossing over suppressor?**
    a. Translocation   b. Deletion
    c. Duplication   d. Inversion

91. **Which is responsible for Cytoplasmic streaming?**
    a. Microtubules
    b. Endoplasmic reticulum
    c. Intermediate filament
    d. Microfilament

92. **Which is true for gap junction?**
    a. It is made of connexion protein
    b. Allows free movement of large molecules across cells
    c. Made up of two subunit of connexions
    d. None of these

93. **Which of the following amino acids can easily be ionized at cellular pH?**
    a. Histidine   b. Tryptophan
    c. Lysine   d. Arginine

94. **Which one of the following components of cytoskeleton plays a crucial role in vesicular transport?**
    a. Molecular motors
    b. Microtubules
    c. Intermediate filaments
    d. Microfilaments

95. **Which of the following antibiotics causes misincorportation of amino acid in synthesizing polypeptide?**
    a. Streptomycin
    b. Polymixin B
    c. Chloramphenicol
    d. Bacitracin

96. **Which of the following antibiotic occasionally cause death when administered to persons who are allergic to them?**
    a. Penicillin   b. Streptomycin
    c. Polymixin   d. Bacitracin

97. **Which of the following anticancerous drugs does not act on microtubules?**
    a. Taxol   b. Methotrexate
    c. Thiabendazole   d. Colchicines

98. **Which of the following are not true cells?**
    a. Lymphocytes   b. Basophils
    c. Platelets   d. Phagocytes

99. **Which of the following bio molecules crosses nuclear membrane?**
    a. Lipid
    b. Carbohydrate
    c. RNA
    d. Protein

100. **Which of the following can induce SOS response in bacteria?**
    a. Thymine dimmers
    b. 5-flurouracil
    c. 2-aminopurine
    d. Hydroxylamine

ANSWERS OF MODEL PAPER 5

1. c	2. d	3. a	4. c	5. a	6. b	7. b
8. a	9. a	10. b	11. b	12. c	13. a	14. d
15. a	16. b	17. b	18. a	19. c	20. c	21. b
22. b	23. a	24. c	25. a	26. a	27. a	28. a
29. d	30. c	31. c	32. b	33. b	34. c	35. c
36. a	37. b	38. b	39. a	40. d	41. c	42. a
43. b	44. d	45. d	46. d	47. b	48. b	49. b
50. a	51. c	52. a	53. b	54. a	55. d	56. a
57. b	58. a	59. d	60. b	61. a	62. d	63. c
64. a	65. a	66. d	67. c	68. a	69. b	70. c
71. b	72. c	73. d	74. b	75. a	76. a	77. d
78. c	79. a	80. a	81. c	82. b	83. b	84. b
85. c	86. a	87. b	88. d	89. a	90. b	91. a
92. a	93. d	94. b	95. a	96. a	97. b	98. c
99. c	100. a					

Model Test Paper 6

1. **In liposome mediated gene transfer DNA enters the protoplast due to**
   a. Osmosis
   b. Endocytosis
   c. Exocytosis
   d. Collision

2. **Which of the following is a green tissue specific promoter?**
   a. Pea vicilin
   b. Bean phyutahemaglutinin
   c. 35 s CaMV
   d. Arabidopsis small sub unit of Rubisco

3. **During Agrobacterium infections the plant cell begins to synthesize an arginine derivative is called as**
   a. Opines
   b. Acetobenzylpurine
   c. Hygromycin
   d. Acetosyringone

4. **Which of the following enzyme is used for making cDNA**
   a. Reverse transcriptase
   b. DNA ligase
   c. Restriction enzyme
   d. Polynucleotide transterase

5. **Replication of the DNA by rolling circle mechanism give rise to a**
   a. Blunt end DNA
   b. Theta structure
   c. Concatamer
   d. Single strand DNA with nick

6. **Cosmid have the Cos site of**
   a. Lambda
   b. Plasmid
   c. ML3
   d. YAC

7. **Relaxed plasmid**
   a. Can not be purified
   b. Have multiple copies per cell
   c. Does not exist in bacteria
   d. Have only single copy per cell

8. **Restriction enzyme that cuts straight across the DNA produces**
   a. Nicks
   b. Blunt ends
   c. Single stranded
   d. None

9. **In-vitro packging is required for which one of the following vector**
   a. BAC
   b. YAC
   c. PAC
   d. None

10. **Lambda has short single stranded 5′ projection of**
    a. 5-nucleotide length
    b. 10-nucleotide length
    c. 8- nucleotide length
    d. 12-nucleotide length

11. **Electrophoretic separations of DNA and RNA in agarose is based on**
    a. Charge
    b. Size
    c. Both a and b
    d. Base sequence

12. **Which of the following reagent is useful for visualizing DNA?**
    a. 14 C uracil
    b. Diphenylamine
    c. Ethidium bromide
    d. DNA polymerase

13. **Endochitinase can be used as an**
    a. Antibacterial
    b. Antiungal
    c. Antinematodal
    d. Antivirus

14. **If adenine makes up 35% of DNA, cytosine will make**
    a. 15%
    b. 25%
    c. 30%
    d. 35%

15. **Which of the following is an herbicide resistant gene?**
    a. Bar
    b. Hpt
    c. Cholesterol oxidase
    d. Chitinases

16. Cytoplasmic channels connecting adjacent cells are called
    a. Ionic channels
    b. Conjugation tube
    c. Protoplasmic channel
    d. Plasmodesmata

17. Homologous pairs line up along equatorial plane during
    a. Anaphase II
    b. Metaphase I
    c. Interphase
    d. Telophase

18. Thee browing of the culture medium induced by some explants can be prevented by addition of
    a. GA
    b. Polyvinylpyrrolidone
    c. 2,4-D
    d. IBA

19. The yolk of chicken egg serves a nutritive function for the developing embryo. A functionally comparable structure in plants is
    a. Lignin
    b. Cellulose
    c. Pectin
    d. Endosperm

20. Between mitotic divisions, the cell is in
    a. G_0
    b. G_1
    c. G_2
    d. S phase

21. In meosis, as in mmitosis, the chromosomal materials is replicated during
    a. G1 phase
    b. G_2 phase
    c. T phase
    d. S phase

22. Which of the following is not an antibiotic resistance gene?
    a. hpt
    b. neo
    c. gfp
    d. npt II

23. during Agrobacterium transformation the T-DNA coated by protein, which is the product of gene
    a. vir C
    b. Vir D
    c. Vir E
    d. Vir G

24. A general method to confirm expression of transgene at translation level is
    a. Sourthern blotting
    b. Western blotting
    c. Northern blotting
    d. Eastern blotting

25. The gene transferred from E. Coli to tobacco to increase the level of manitiole is
    a. Manitiol dehydrogenase
    b. Manitiol carboxylase
    c. Manitiol hydrolase
    d. Manitiol oxygenase

26. The T-DNA region of all the Ti and Ri plasmids are flanked by direct repeat sequence
    a. 25 bp
    b. 20 bp
    c. 15 bp
    d. 35 bp

27. The transgenic tomato plants showing delayed ripening due to suppression of ethylene was developed using methodology of
    a. Coat protein gene
    b. Antisense RNA
    c. Agrobacterium mediated gene transfer
    d. None

28. The direct DNA uptake by the protoplast is stimulated by the chemical
    a. Cellulose
    b. Sucrose
    c. Sodium chloride
    d. PEG

29. The chemical used as an inducer of the vir operons is
    a. Hygromycin
    b. Fanamycin
    c. Acetosyringone
    d. Kanamycin

30. Which of the following is not an insecticidal protein gene?
    a. Sunflower seed albumin
    b. Lectins
    c. Protease-inhibitor
    d. Alpha-amylase inhibitor

31. In Agrobacterium mediated plant transformation which one of the following is used to check the Agrobacterium growth
    a. Basta
    b. PPT
    c. Timentin
    d. Kanamycin

32. Most commonly used strategy to develop transgenic plant against any viral disease is to engineer a
    a. Liposome mediated transfer of viral RNA
    b. Anti-sense RNA for viral genome
    c. Coat or capsid protein gene
    d. Direct DNA transfer of viral gene

33. **The vir region is organied in to six operon viz., vir A, vir B, vir C, vir D, vir E and vir G, out of these which four operons are required for virulence**

    a. A, B, C, D
    b. A, B, C, G
    c. C, D, E, G
    d. None

34. **The large dark body in the nucleus is the nucleolus, which participates in the formation of**

    a. Ribosome
    b. RNA
    c. Protein
    d. DNA

35. **Nuclear envelop breaks down in**

    a. Telophase II
    b. Anaphase I
    c. Metaphase II
    d. Prophase I

36. **Most plant cells are surrounded by a rigid cell wall made primarily of**

    a. Triglycerides
    b. Polysaccharides
    c. Proteoglycans
    d. Pectins

37. **"9 + 2" describes the basic structure of which of the following one**

    a. Flagellum
    b. Lysosome
    c. Basal body
    d. Chloroplast

38. **Endoplasmic reticulum:**

    a. Is found only in animals
    b. In a site of ATP production
    c. Is called rough if mitochondria are attached to it.
    d. Is a system of membrane bound channels

39. **Scientist have postulated that small pores must exist in the cell membrane because**

    a. Of endocytosis
    b. Of turgor pressure
    c. CO and O moves freely through the membrane
    d. Water molecules move freely through the membrane

40. **The organelle that functions in the breakdown of cell and tissues is the**

    a. Episomes
    b. Mitochondrion
    c. Centrosomes
    d. Lysosmes

41. **Which of the following statements is not true?**

    a. Chloroplast are the sites of photosynthesis
    b. Chromoplast contain bright orange and yellow pigments
    c. Leucoplast is responsible for the bright colours of the fruits and leaves
    d. Leucoplast, Chromoplast, and chloromoplast are present only in the cells of plants and algae

42. **Which of the following statement is true**

    a. Facilitates diffusion can occur against conc. Gradient
    b. Diffusion requires an expenditure of energy by the cell
    c. The active transport requires protein complex in the cell
    d. Osmosis can occur against a concentration gradient

43. **The function of the nucleus includes**

    a. Cellular respiration
    b. Housing the hereditary information
    c. Synthesis of proteins
    d. Synthesis of carbon compounds

44. **Batch systems of culture are**

    a. Steady state process
    b. Non steady state process
    c. Completely mixed
    d. Plug flow system

45. **Which o the following is not used as measuring device in biosensor?**

    a. Whole organism
    b. Immunoelectrodes
    c. Biofilters
    d. Enzyme

46. **Thiobacillus thioxidans grows on**

    a. Iron
    b. Sulphur
    c. Pyrites
    d. Covellite

47. **Majority of bacculoviruses have been reported from species**

    a. Lepidoptera
    b. Dipteran
    c. Crustacean
    d. Both dipteral and Lepidoptera

48. **Bacculoviruses**

    a. RNA viruses
    b. DNA viruses
    c. Both a and b
    d. None

49. **Bacteria are preferred over yeast for production of single cell protein because**

    a. Of their fast growth
    b. They are small
    c. Of their lower content of methionine
    d. None

50. **Requefort cheese is ripened with the help of**
    a. Lactobacillus coxi
    b. Penicillum roquoforti
    c. Brevibacterium linens
    d. Propionibacterium shexmanii

51. **Production of biogas takes through the following sequential steps**
    a. Methanogenis-solubilization-Acidogenis
    b. Acidogenis- Solubilization-methanogenis
    c. Acidogenis- Methanogenis-solubilization
    d. Soluvilization-Acidogenis-Methanogenis

52. **White rot fungus phaneiochaete chrysasporium produces**
    a. Extra cellular enzymes
    b. Intra cellular
    c. Both a and b
    d. None

53. **Degradation of xenobiotics occurs rapidly in**
    a. Highly compressed soils
    b. Well aerated soil
    c. Heavily contaminated soils
    d. None of these

54. **Anthropogenic chemicals introduced in to the terrestrial carbon cycle is more recalcitrant when they contain**
    a. Unsaturated compounds
    b. Unbranched chain
    c. Aromatic ring substituted with halogens
    d. Chain length of less than 12 carbon atoms

55. **Which of the following reaction is not performed by lignin peroxidise?**
    a. Detoxification of toxic phenols
    b. Oxidative cleavage of aromatic ether bond
    c. Oxidation of phenyl alcohols to the respective aldehydes
    d. Hydroxylation of the aliphatic double bonds in

56. **If meiosis does not occur, the chromosome number would .... in each generation**
    a. Remain same
    b. Triple
    c. Reduce
    d. Double

57. **An example of naturally occurring Auxin is**
    a. BAP
    b. 2,4-D
    c. ABA
    d. IAA

58. **The shine-dalgarno sequence is known as**
    a. Ribosome binding site
    b. Initiation site
    c. Promoter binding site
    d. None

59. **Plant protoplast fusion can be achieved with**
    a. TZZ
    b. PEG
    c. PM
    d. Zeatin

60. **Amino acid fermentatioin employs**
    a. Unicells
    b. Filamentous organisms
    c. Both a and b
    d. None

61. **An example of commercially important primary metabolites is**
    a. Toxin
    b. Alkaloid
    c. Alcohol
    d. None

62. **In PCR, the ds DNA is generally denatured by**
    a. Acid treatment
    b. Alkali treatment
    c. Temperature
    d. None

63. **Secondary mmetabolites like antibiotics are not essential for**
    a. Log phase growth
    b. Exponential growth
    c. Both a and b
    d. None of these

64. **Anther culture provides a method for the production of**
    a. Pollyploid
    b. Apomictic line
    c. Homozygous line
    d. Heterozygous line

65. **Which of the following is not used as cryoprotectant?**
    a. Glycerol
    b. Dimethyl sulfoxide
    c. Polyclar
    d. Ethylene glycerol

66. **The shoot apical meristem is characterized buy**
    a. Trapezoidal shape
    b. Round shape
    c. Dome shape
    d. None

67. **Explantation is a process of**
    a. Planting of explants
    b. Dissection and culture of small organs or tissue section
    c. Choice of explants
    d. Culture of plants

68. Cryo-preservation involves

a. Cutting, application of cryo-protectant and storage at -196°C

b. Freezing and thawing

c. Specimen treatment, freezing storage at ultra low temperature

d. None

69. Germplasm preservation of meristem and shoot tip culture involves

a. Storage in dry ice

b. Storage in liquid nitrogen

c. Culturing under low temperature

d. Cry-preservation and slow growth

70. In commercial fermentation process, it is desirable to have

a. Minimal lag phase

b. Minimum stationary phase

c. Minimal death phase

d. Minimal log phase

71. The term somaclonal variation was termed by

a. Larken and scowhoft

b. Skirvin

c. Eyans

d. Murashige and skoog

72. Micropores contained within the anther gives rise to

a. Callus culture and gynogenesis

b. Anthogenesis and callus culture

c. Gynogenesis and androgenesis

d. None

73. Callus and suspension culture normally produce secondary metabolites when

a. Emit fragrance

b. The callus turn red with age

c. Show lightful tracheids

d. All of the above

74. Inclusion of osmoticum in both isolation and culture media

a. Facilitates formation of heterokaryotes

b. Facilitates fusion of protoplast

c. Prevent rupture of protoplast

d. None

75. Micro propagation involves

a. Thorough callusing

b. Adventitious bud transfer

c. Shoot culture, asceptic initiatioin transfer to pot and rooting

d. Initiation of asceptic culture, shoot multiplier, rooting and transplantation

76. Which one of the following does not regulate nitrogenise activity?

a. H_2 b. M_O

c. NH_4 d. Energy supply

77. Nodulin genes are found in

a. Cyanobacteria

b. Bradyrhizobium

c. Plant

d. Bacteria

78. During reduction of dinitrogen by nitrogenise, how many net electrons re required

a. Six   b. Two

c. Four   d. None

79. Which one of the following is the first stable product of photosynthesis?

a. RuBP   b. DAHP

c. Glucose   d. 3-PGA

80. Which one of the following amino acids is specified by single codon in genetic code?

a. G   b. K

c. W   d. D

81. Ferredoxin is reduced by

a. PS-II only   b. PS-I only

c. PS-I and II   d. Mitochondria

82. Leghaemoglobin is synthesized exclusively in

a. Nitrogen fixing nodules

b. Leg of ruminants

c. Klebsiella

d. Cyanobacteria

83. The *in-vitro* electron donor to PS-II is

a. Water   b. Ascorbate

c. PS-I   d. Plastoquinone

84. Cyclic phosphorylation involves

a. PS-II   b. PS-I

c. Mitochondria   d. Both a and b

85. The in-vitro electron donor to PS-I is

a. PS-II   b. Plastoquinone

c. Oxygen   d. Ascorbate

86. **Oxidation of water during photosynthesis involves**
    a. PS-II
    b. PS-I
    c. Both a and b
    d. Mitochondria

87. **Which o the following is commonly used as a protecting group during peptide synthesis?**
    a. Dicyclohexylurea
    b. Ten-butyloxylcarbonyl
    c. Hydrogen fluoride
    d. Dicyclohexylurea
    e. Carbodimide

88. **Cyanobacteria protect nitrogenise from oxygen by**
    a. Heterocyst
    b. Gum production
    c. Prossession of catalase
    d. Possession of superoxide dismutase

89. **Which one of the following is not a component of nitrogenise?**
    a. Mg^{+2}
    b. NADP
    c. MoFe-protein
    d. Fe-protein

90. **Fe -protein of nitrogenase is**
    a. Heteropolymer tetramer
    b. Homomeric dimmer
    c. Homomeric tetramer
    d. Heteromeric dimmer

91. **Which of the following statement is not true?**
    a. An acidic protein will give pl less than 7
    b. A basic protein will give a pl greater than 7
    c. At a pH value equal to its pl, a protein will not move in the electric field of an electrophoresis experiment
    d. The pl is the pH value at which a protein has no charge

92. **Which one of the following chemical causes frame shift mutation?**
    a. 2- bromo uracil
    b. Acridine orange
    c. 2-aminopurine
    d. Hydroxyglamine

93. **Which one of the following is not formed in calvin cycle?**
    a. RuBP
    b. DAHP
    c. Glucose
    d. 3-PGA

94. **Which one of the following amino acids residues are likely to be found on the inside of a water soluble protein?**
    a. H
    b. R
    c. E
    d. V

95. **Which one of the following amino acid may alter the direction of polypeptide chains and interrupt alpha helices?**
    a. Pro
    b. Cys
    c. Phe
    d. His

96. **Which one of the following radioisotope is used to elucidate carbon pathway in calvin cycle?**
    a. 14C
    b. 32P
    c. 35S
    d. 3H

97. **Which one of the following is not the basic requirement of biological nitrogen fixation?**
    a. Mg^{+2} and ATP
    b. Nitrogenase
    c. Glutamine
    d. Strong reducing agent

98. **The enzyme nitrogenise is composed of:**
    a. Four-oxygen sensitive non-haem iron protein
    b. Three oxygen sensitive non-haem iron protein
    c. Two oxygen sensitive non haem iron protein
    d. One oxygen sensitive non-haem iron protein

99. **The restriction enzyme useful to the molecular biologist belong to**
    a. Type-I
    b. Type-II
    c. Type-III
    d. Type-IV

100. **Which of the following vector is suitable for DNA sequencing?**
    a. HCl
    b. $CaCl_2$
    c. Glycine
    d. NaCl

1. b	2. d	3. a	4. a	5. c	6. a	7. b
8. b	9. c	10. d	11. c	12. c	13. b	14. a
15. a	16. d	17. b	18. b	19. d	20. b	21. b
22. c	23. c	24. c	25. a	26. a	27. b	28. d
29. c	30. a	31. c	32. c	33. b	34. b	35. d
36. b	37. c	38. d	39. d	40. d	41. c	42. c
43. b	44. b	45. c	46. c	47. d	48. b	49. a
50. b	51. d	52. a	53. b	54. c	55. a	56. d
57. d	58. a	59. b	60. c	61. c	62. c	63. c
64. c	65. b	66. c	67. b	68. a	69. d	70. a
71. a	72. b	73. d	74. c	75. d	76. a	77. c
78. a	79. d	80. d	81. c	82. a	83. a	84. a
85. b	86. a	87. b	88. a	89. b	90. b	91. d
92. b	93. c	94. d	95. a	96. a	97. c	98. c
99. b	100. b					

Model Test Paper 7

1. **The chemical used to prevent RNAase contamination during RNA isolation is**
   - a. DEEPP
   - b. DEPCE
   - c. DCPPE
   - d. DEPC

2. **Introduction of a gene or DNA fragment from one organism into another organism in such a form, so that it is maintained, replicated and expressed in the new host is known as**
   - a. DNA fingerprinting
   - b. DNA cloning
   - c. RNA fingerprinting
   - d. RNA cloning

3. **Adenine pairs with Thymine with**
   - a. Phosphodiester bond
   - b. Glycosidic bond
   - c. 4 hydrogen bond
   - d. 2 hydrogen bond

4. **Guanine pairs with thymine with**
   - a. Phosphodiester bond
   - b. Glycosidic bond
   - c. 3 hydrogen bond
   - d. 2 hydrogen bond

5. **The DNA sequence which appear to have no function is called as**
   - a. Satellite DNA
   - b. selfish DNA
   - c. Palindrome DNA
   - d. Ct DNA

6. **Each strand in a chain of nucleotides are held together by**
   - a. Phosphodiester bonds
   - b. 2 hydrogen bond
   - c. Glycosidic bond
   - d. 3 hydrogen bond

7. **The set of bases in a t-RNA that pairs with a codon of a m-RNA is know as**
   - a. Cistron
   - b. Codon
   - c. Exon
   - d. Anti-codon

8. **The technique that is generally used for the identification of crininals from blood strains. Semen etc., and for establishing parentage in case of dispute is called**
   - a. DNA fingerprinting
   - b. RNA fingerprinting
   - c. DNA cloning
   - d. RNA cloning

9. **Purine and pyramidines are joined with de oxyribose by**
   - a. 2 hydrogen bond
   - b. 4 hydrogen bond
   - c. Glycosidic bond
   - d. Phosphodiester bonds

10. **All the reaction in the translational process from the formation of the first peptide bond to that of the last peptide bond of the polypeptide chain is called as**
    - a. Deformation
    - b. Elongation
    - c. Transition
    - d. Transition

11. **The enzyme that calalyses the covalent joining of okazaki fragments is called**
    - a. DNA polymerase
    - b. DNA ligase
    - c. DNA helicase
    - d. DNA gyrase

12. **The coding region of split genes is divided in to few to several small segments; each segment which is having the expressed sequences are called as**
    - a. Recon
    - b. Anti-codon
    - c. Exons
    - d. Codon

13. **In eukaryotic transcription units, a conserved sequence located upstream of start point and recognized by a large group of transcriptional factors is called.**
    - a. TTAA box
    - b. TATA box
    - c. CAAT box
    - d. CCTT box

14. **The DNA in which the base pair sequence can be read same in both the directions is called.**
    - a. Satellite DNA
    - b. Selfish DNA
    - c. Ct DNA
    - d. Palindrome DNA

15. **Which of the following is a mode of replication?**
    - a. Semiconservative
    - b. Dispersive
    - c. Conservative
    - d. All of the above

16. **The semi-conservative mechanism of replication was demonstrated by**

    a. Watson and crick
    b. Mendel
    c. Hershey and chase
    d. Meselson and stahal

17. **In meselson and stahl experiment, the E.coli cells were labelled with isotope of**

    a. Nitrogen
    b. Sulphur
    c. Uranium
    d. Potassium

18. **The modification of RNA polymerase in such a way that it does not recognize specific terminator sequences and continues transcription beyond the regular terminators is know is**

    a. Termination
    b. Annotation
    c. Bioconversion
    d. Anti-termination

19. **The point at which separation of the strands and synthesis of new DNA takes place is known as**

    a. Initiation
    b. Replication fork
    c. Origin
    d. Template

20. **The enzyme that catalyses the formation of supercoils is**

    a. DNA ligase
    b. DNA polymerase
    c. DNA gyrase
    d. DNA helicase

21. **The initiation of DNA replication within a replicon always occurs at a fixed point called as**

    a. Initiation
    b. Origin
    c. Template
    d. Replication fork

22. **Among the following, the example for highly repetitive DNA is**

    a. Histone cluster
    b. Dispersed repetitive DNA
    c. DNA minisatelites
    d. DNA microsatellites

23. **The enzyme that can relieve super coiling in DNA by creating transitory breaks in sone or both strands of helicase backbone is called as**

    a. Topoisomerase
    b. Gyrase
    c. Helicase
    d. Ligase

24. **The concept of central dogma was given by**

    a. Watson
    b. Crick
    c. Jones
    d. Korenbeg

25. **The enzyme that is responsible for transcription is**

    a. Polynuclease
    b. RNA polymerase
    c. DNA polymerase
    d. Endonuclease

26. **The labelling of a gene by a marker gene or specific DNA sequence closely kinked with the gene in question is called**

    a. Genetic code
    b. Gene tagging
    c. Gene therapy
    d. Gene translation

27. **A part of an RNA transcription unit i.e., transcribed but discarded during maturation is called as**

    a. Transcribed spacer
    b. Transcriptional unit
    c. Terminator sequence
    d. None of these

28. **A group of gene that are related by sequence homologies usually are also related by their functions are called as**

    a. Multi-gene family
    b. Multiple-cloning site
    c. Multicistronic message
    d. Multi locus probe

29. **The codon, usually but not exclusively 5′ AUG 3′ which indicates the point at which translation of an mRNA should begin is**

    a. Initiation complex
    b. Initiation codon
    c. Termination factor
    d. Translation factor

30. **The transfer or movement of a gene or gene fragment from the chromosomal location to another location is called**

    a. Gene translocation
    b. Gene coding
    c. Gene tagging
    d. Gene therapy

31. **The protein molecule that play an ancillary role in the initiation stage of translocation is called as**

    a. Initiation factor
    b. Termination factor
    c. Transcription factor
    d. Translation factor

32. **The protein required to obtain release of the newly synthesized polypeptide chain from t-RNA is called as**

    a. Termination factor
    b. Initiation factor
    c. Initiation codon
    d. Initiation complex

33. **A region of DNA at one end of an operon that acts as a binding sire for a specific repressor protein and so controls the functioning of adjacent cistrons is termed as**

    a. Operon
    b. Promoter gene
    c. Operator gene
    d. Reporter gene

34. A group of structural genes whose transcription is regulated by the coordinated action of a regulator gene, promoter, and operator elements is known as

    a. Operon fusion
    b. Operator gene
    c. Operon
    d. Reporter gene

35. The largest element within a gene, which is a unit of function, is called

    a. Exon
    b. Recon
    c. Muton
    d. Cistron

36. In case of repressible operons, the repressor can bind DNA only when it is associated with the effector; in such cases, the effector is called

    a. Operator
    b. Reporter
    c. Co-repressor
    d. Terminator

37. The enzymes that produce internal cuts, called cleavage, in DNA molecules are called

    a. Endonucleases
    b. Kinases
    c. Ligase
    d. Galactase

38. When a single pre-mRNA molecule is processed in two or more ways to yield more than one type of mature m-RNA is called

    a. Direct splicing
    b. Alternative splicing
    c. Destructive splicing
    d. Alienation

39. Premature aging due to loss a DNA repair enzyme, perhaps a ligase in human beings are the symptoms of the disease is called

    a. Edward syndrome
    b. Patau's syndrome
    c. Progeria
    d. Klinfelter syndrome

40. Nick translation is useful in labelling of molecules like

    a. Protein sequence
    b. Nucleotide sequence
    c. ds-DNA molecules
    d. none of these

41. The chemical, which is used for breaking the plasma membrane during DNA isolation is known as

    a. DNAase
    b. Ligase
    c. CTAB/SDS
    d. Helicase

42. The absolute radical requirement for both RNA synthesis and DNA replication in the organisms is

    a. Free 3'-CH4
    b. Free 3'-OH
    c. Free 5'-OH
    d. Free 3'-H

43. A sequence of DNA nucleotide which codes for specific polypeptide chian is called as

    a. Genome
    b. Gene
    c. Genetic code
    d. Genetic marker

44. The bond between sugar and nitrogenous base in case of DNA is known as

    a. Hydrophobic bond
    b. Glycosidic bond
    c. Hydrogen bond
    d. Wander wall bond

45. Restriction site for cloning should be

    a. Palindromic in nature
    b. Repeated sequence
    c. Hexanucleotide
    d. Tandemly tepeated

46. GAATTC is restriction sequence of CTTAAG indicates

    a. Bam HI
    b. Sam I
    c. Eco RI
    d. Null

47. For cloning Eukaryotic gene in prokaryotic, genes should be isolated from

    a. Genomic library
    b. Eukaryotic host
    c. C-DNA library
    d. None of these

48. Which enzyme play important role in reverse transcription?

    a. Ribonuclease
    b. DNA polymerase
    c. RNA polymerase
    d. Reverse transciptase

49. A term used to describe the excess DNA which is present in the genome beyond that required to encode protein is called as

    a. Split gene
    b. Active DNA
    c. Junk DNA
    d. Dead DNA

50. Micro-satellite are also known as

    a. STRs
    b. RAPDs
    c. ISSR
    d. RFLP

51. An enzyme that separate the two strand of a DNA duplex, usually using the energy from hydrolysis of ATP, is called

    a. Ligase
    b. Helicase
    c. Gyrase
    d. Topoisomerase

52. The sequence that consists of self complementary regions which from a stem loop/hairpin structure in RNA product is

    a. Regulator
    b. Terminator
    c. CAAT box
    d. TATA box

53. The enzyme that is responsible of heterogeneous nuclear RNA, the precursor of m-RNA is
   a. DNA polymerase I
   b. RNA polymerase I
   c. RNA endonuclease
   d. All of the above

54. Remova of the topological strain by inducting the negative super coiling, which is carried out by
   a. DNA gyrase
   b. DNA polymerase
   c. RNA polymerase
   d. RNA gyrase

55. Genomic imprinting is a kind of epistasis which occurs due to
   a. DNA polyI
   b. DNA gyrase
   c. DNA methylation
   d. RNA polymerase

56. The strand that is used as a template to which ribonucleotides base pair for the synthesis of the RNA is called as
   a. Sense strand
   b. Antisense strand
   c. Template strand
   d. Both b & c

57. The scientist, who had worked out fine structure of gene through cis-trans complementation test is
   a. Fleming
   b. Benzer
   c. Jones
   d. Shull

58. The temperature at which of the E.coli RNA polymerase performs elongation reaction is
   a. 37°C
   b. 30°C
   c. 40°C
   d. 45°C

59. Reverse transcription enzyme was discovered by
   a. Fleming and shull
   b. Shull and jones
   c. Watson and crick
   d. Vilmorin and jones

60. A construct that joins the coding region of two open reading frames such that expression of the product results in a chimeric protein is called as
   a. Gene cloning
   b. Gene family
   c. Gene fusion
   d. Gene construct

61. The enzyme that can synthesize a new DNA strand on a template DNA strand is called
   a. DNA pol III
   b. DNA gyrase
   c. DNA polymerase
   d. All of the above

62. DNA replicating enzyme in bacteria is called is
   a. DNA gyrases
   b. DNA poly III
   c. DNA polymerase
   d. DNA methylation

63. How many type of RNA polymerase were found in prokaryotes?
   a. 4
   b. 3
   c. 2
   d. 6

64. The distance between sites of initiation and termination by RNA polymerase is called as
   a. Transcription unit
   b. Transition unit
   c. Transformation unit
   d. Transduction unit

65. The DNA strand that is used as template during transcription is called as
   a. Antisense RNA
   b. Antisense DNA
   c. CAT box
   d. CPT box

66. In eukaryotes, DNA methylation is mainly concerned with regulation of
   a. Gene pairing
   b. Gene amplification
   c. Gene Index
   d. Genetic imprinting

67. The attachment point for the catabolite activator protein is called as
   a. CAT box
   b. CAC box
   c. CAP box
   d. CATT box

68. A series of DNA sequence fixed as distinct spots on a suitable solid support, such as a glass chip is called as
   a. DNA array
   b. DNA foot printing
   c. DNA sequencing
   d. All of the above

69. An RNA copy of a gene is described as
   a. RNA replicase
   b. RNA polymerase
   c. RNA transcript
   d. RNA splicing

70. The presence of a gene in multiple copies due to polyploidy, polytenic chromosomes, gene amplification, or chromosomal duplication is called
   a. Gene redundancy
   b. Gene splicing
   c. Gene stacking
   d. All of the above

71. The removal of large non-coding sequence from the primary RNA transcript followed by rejoining of coding sequences to produce the functional m-RNA is called
   a. RNA polymerase
   b. RNA editing
   c. RNA splicing
   d. RNA transcript

72. A polymerase enzyme that catalyses self replication of single stranded RNA is called
   a. RNA replicase
   b. RNA ligase
   c. RNA polymerase
   d. DNA polymerase

73. The sequence 3'AAAAAAT5' in sense strand of DNA is called as

    a. Transcribed spacer
    b. Transcriptional unit
    c. Terminator sequence
    d. Translational unit

74. A genetic marker that is detected as differential mobility of a protein/DNA fragment is known as

    a. Molecular marker
    b. Molecular breeding
    c. Molecular genetics
    d. All of the above

75. The nucleotide sequence in DNA downstream of the of the termination codon of a gene which is transcribed and not translated is called as

    a. Antitrailer
    b. Transcribed spacer
    c. Terminator sequence
    d. Transcriptional unit

76. Mini-satellites are also known as

    a. RFLPs
    b. RAPD
    c. STS
    d. VNTRs

77. Protein involved for joining the DNA during replication is

    a. Topoisomerase
    b. Ligase
    c. Gyrase
    d. Helicase

78. The use of DNA marker for indirect selection of difficult to select traits like yield etc. Is known as

    a. Marker assisted selection
    b. Yield selection
    c. DNA selection
    d. RNA selection

79. The c-DNA libraries can be prepared by isolating

    a. m-RNA
    b. t-RNA
    c. r-RNA
    d. All of the above

80. Actinomycin-D, rifampicin and 5-bromouracil are inhibitors to the synthesis of

    a. t-RNA
    b. m-RNA
    c. r-RNA
    d. all of the above

81. A CsCl gradient will separate DNA molecule by

    a. Resorption
    b. Density
    c. Adhesion
    d. Absorption

82. Which of the following DNA structure forms left hand helix?

    a. DNA B
    b. DNA C
    c. DNA Z
    d. DNA A

83. m-RNA usually is being extracted using

    a. poly T resin
    b. RNase P
    c. Poly A resin
    d. None of the above

84. DNA is fit for making tools in case of nano-technology, which is due to

    a. Small size of DNA
    b. Flexibility in DNA conformation
    c. Branching nature of DNA
    d. All of the above

85. RFLP markers mapped in one species or genus can often be used to construct parallel gentic maps in related species or genera, which is called as

    a. Reverse mapping
    b. Parallel mapping
    c. Targeted mapping
    d. None of these

86. Transgenic expression study can be done by

    a. Transcription profiling
    b. RT-PCR
    c. Transcription profiling
    d. All of the above

87. The midpoint of -10 sequence is about 10 bp on the upstream of the start point and has the consensus sequence TATAAT; this sequence is commonly known as

    a. TATA box
    b. CATA box
    c. CAAT box
    d. Pribnow box

88. Removal of the topological strain by inducing the negative super coiling is carried out by

    a. Primases
    b. DNA gyrase
    c. DNA polymerase
    d. Topoisomerase

89. The process of modification, mainly through cleavage and /or spicing, of primary RNA transcripts so as to produce functional molecules is called

    a. DNA processing
    b. RNA processing
    c. Enzyme processing
    d. Protein processing

90. Virions are

    a. DNA virus
    b. RNA virus
    c. Naked DNA viruses
    d. Naked RNA viruses

91. In case of negative control of regulation of transcription, the binding of the regulator proteins to the operator DNA prevents transcription to take palce, such regulator protein are called

    a. Initiator
    b. Repressor
    c. Promoter
    d. Translator

92. **The protein needed for splicing out the particular intro from the pre-mRNA and to stabilize intron in that particular conformation, which is required for splicing is called**

   a. RNA maturase   b. DNA desaturase

   c. DNA maturase   d. RNA desaturase

93. **Ribosome are synthesiszed in**

   a. Nucleolus   b. Cytoplasm

   c. Nucleus   d. All of the above

94. **Virons are**

   a. RNA virus   b. Naked RNA virus

   c. Naked DNA virus   d. DNA virus

95. **Taq polymerase used in PCR is**

   a. Highly processive enzyme

   b. Thermotolerant

   c. Osmotolerant

   d. None of these

96. **When pyrimidine is substituted by purine and vice versa, this type of mutation is know as**

   a. Nonsense mutation   b. Transition

   c. Transversion   d. Missence mutation

97. **Some highly repetitive sequence differ in density from the rest of chromosomal DNA; and from a separate minor band in $CsCl_2$ desity gradient centrifugation and are called**

   a. Split gene   b. Smart gene

   c. Satellite DNA   d. None of these

98. **An artificially constructed genetic molecule composed of one or more gene encoding a protein to be expressed and a region that will only allow the protein to be expressed under specific condition is called**

   a. Satellite gene   b. Split gene

   c. Sequence tagged site   d. Smart gent

99. **The DNA sequence that suppresses the promoter activity are called**

   a. Transmitters   b. Repressor

   c. Silencers   d. None of these

100. **Singe base positions in genomic DNA at which different nucleotides occur in different individuals of a population are called**

   a. SNPs   b. STSs

   c. RAPDs   d. RFLPs

ANSWERS OF MODEL PAPER 7

1. d	2. b	3. d	4. c	5. b	6. a	7. d
8. a	9. c	10. b	11. b	12. c	13. c	14. d
15. d	16. d	17. a	18. d	19. b	20. c	21. b
22. c	23. a	24. a	25. b	26. b	27. b	28. c
29. a	30. c	31. d	32. c	33. a	34. c	35. c
36. c	37. b	38. b	39. a	40. b	41. a	42. c
43. a	44. c	45. a	46. c	47. a	48. c	49. a
50. a	51. b	52. a	53. c	54. b	55. a	56. a
57. a	58. c	59. c	60. d	61. c	62. a	63. b
64. c	65. a	66. c	67. b	68. b	69. b	70. d
71. c	72. c	73. d	74. c	75. a	76. d	77. b
78. a	79. a	80. b	81. b	82. c	83. a	84. d
85. b	86. d	87. d	88. b	89. b	90. d	91. b
92. a	93. a	94. b	95. b	96. c	97. c	98. d
99. c	100. a					

Model Test Paper 8

1. **Abnormal growth of a plant organ is**
   - a. Teratoma
   - b. Tumour
   - c. Witches broom
   - d. Callus

2. **Crown gall is caused by**
   - a. Aspergillus
   - b. Agrobacterium tumefaciens
   - c. Bacillus stolonifer
   - d. Rhizopus stolonifer

3. **TIP is**
   - a. Tuber inducing protein
   - b. Tuber inducing principle
   - c. Tumour inducing protein
   - d. Tumour inducing principle

4. **Root knots are generally due to**
   - a. Symbiotic bacteria
   - b. Symbiotic cyanobacteria
   - c. Nematodes
   - d. Insect larvae

5. **Teratoma is**
   - a. Abnormal swelling
   - b. Formation of a number of shoots from a tumour
   - c. Development of a number of close branches
   - d. Secretion of tumour inducing principle

6. **Witches broom is characterised by**
   - a. Hypertrophy
   - b. Typotrophy
   - c. Teratoma
   - d. A number of close branches

7. **Variation appearing suddenly in culture**
   - a. Somatic variation
   - b. Somaclonal variation
   - c. Mutation
   - d. Aberration

8. **Abnormal growth can be due to**
   - a. Infection
   - b. Injury
   - c. Hybridization
   - d. All of the above

9. **Virus free plants can be obtained through**
   - a. Shoot tip culture
   - b. Root tip culture
   - c. Haploid culture
   - d. Embryo culture

10. **What additional treatment is required by protoplast fusion in plant**
    - a. PEG and sodium nitrate
    - b. Coconut milk and glycine
    - c. Cellulose and pectinase
    - d. All of the above

11. **Protoplast fusion result in**
    - a. Genetic hybridization
    - b. Male sterility
    - c. Abundant seeds of rare plants
    - d. Parasexual/somatic hybridization

12. **Pollen culture produces**
    - a. Haploid plant where every gene can excess its effect
    - b. Homozygous diploid plant
    - c. Abundant seed of rare plant
    - d. Abundant pollen in male sterile plant

13. **An androgenic plant can be converted in to homozygous diploid plant through the application of**
    - a. Nitrogen mustard
    - b. Nitrous acid
    - c. Colchicines
    - d. Acridine orange

14. **The enzyme required to obtained wall free/naked protoplast are**
    - a. Cellulose and proteinase
    - b. Cellulose and pectinase
    - c. Cellulose and amylase
    - d. Amylase and pectinase

15. Which technique can be helpful in over coming hybridisation barrier

a. Shoot tip culture
b. Embryo rescue
c. Protoplast fusion
d. Both b and c

16. Two protoplast can be made to fuse through the application of

a. Electrofusion
b. PEG
c. Sodium nitrate
d. All of the above

17. Who developed the technique of nurse tissue to show cellular totipotency

a. Hilderbrandt
b. Steward
c. Muir
d. Konar

18. Pollen embryoids were discovered by

a. Konar and Nataraja
b. Guha and maheshwari
c. Skoog and miller
d. Heparin and wetherell

19. Which of the following can yield a completely haploid plant

a. Root tip
b. Anther
c. Carpel
d. Stem apical meristem

20. Cellular totipotency was demonstrated by

a. Theodore schwann
b. A.V. Leeuwenhoek
c. F.C. Steward
d. Robert hooke

21. A totipotency cell means

a. An undifferentiated cell capable of developing in to a system or entire plant
b. An undifferentiated cell capable of developing into an organ
c. An undifferentiated cell capable of developing in to complete embryo
d. Cell which lacks the capability to differentiate in to an organ or system

22. The smallest viable unit which can grow, multiply and from a plant in tissue culture

a. Chromosome
b. Cell
c. Tissue
d. Nucleus

23. Micropropagation is

a. Raising of plants from a small tissue in culture
b. Multiplication of small plant
c. Propagation of small parts of organisms
d. Indefinite maintenance of an organ or tissue

24. Tissue culture is

a. Growth and multiplication of cell on artificial medium
b. Growth of specific plant structure on artificial medium
c. Maintenance, growth and differentiation of cell, tissue and organs on artificial medium
d. None of the above

25. Part of plant used for culturing is called

a. Stock
b. Explants
c. Scion
d. Callus

26. Tissue culture technique was first attempted by

a. Nobecourt
b. Hanning
c. Haberlandt
d. Gautheret

27. Tissue culture technique was first performed successfully by

a. White
b. Harberlandt
c. Nobecourt
d. Gautheret

28. The structure employed by white for first successful tissue culture was

a. Root of carrot
b. Root of tomato
c. Leaf cells
d. Apical meristem

29. Calls is

a. Tissue that forms embryo
b. Tissue that grows to form embryoid
c. Unorganised actively dividing mass of cells maintained in culture
d. None of the above

30. Callus formation is promoted by

a. Proper light and subculturing
b. Excess of NAA
c. Absence of cell
d. Darkness and subculturing

31. Differentiation of callus into plant part is

a. Embryogenesis
b. Morphogenesis
c. Totipotency
d. Embryoid formation

32. Who discovered that morphogenesis in culture medium is controlled by hormones

a. Skoog and miller
b. Muir at al
c. Vasil and hilderbrandt
d. Helperin and wetherell

33. **Embryo culture technique was discovered by**
    a. Skoog and miller   b. Muir at al
    c. Vasil and hilderbrandt d. Steward

34. **Embryoid is**
    a. A miniature embryo
    b. Non-zygotic embryo formed in vitro culture
    c. Embryo raised in culture medium
    d. Cellular aggregate similar to embryo in appearance

35. **The concept of cellular totipotency was given by**
    a. Skoog and miller
    b. Steward
    c. Vasil and hilderbrandt
    d. Helperin and wetherell

36. **Ramet is**
    a. Clone   b. Cell aggregate
    c. Callus   d. Individual of clone

37. **Guha and Maheshwari are famous for**
    a. Protoplast culture   b. Pollen culture
    c. Shoot tip culture   d. None of the above

38. **The technique of protoplast fusion was developed by**
    a. Skoog and miller
    b. Muir at al
    c. Vasil and hilderbrandt
    d. Carlson et al

39. **Explants is required to be disinfectant before placing in culture. This done by**
    a. Autoclaving
    b. Ultraviolet rays
    c. Clorax or hyprochlorite
    d. X-rays

40. **Aseptic culture means**
    a. Presence of bacteria
    b. Absence of other organism like microbes
    c. Parthenogenetic development
    d. None of the above

41. **Micropropagation refer to**
    a. Mature stage of endosperm
    b. The phenomenon of manufacture of hormones
    c. Germination of seed where cotyledons come above the soil
    d. A technique to obtain new plants by culturing cell or tissue in culture medium

42. **A major use of embryo culture is in**
    a. Induction of Somaclonal variation
    b. Overcoming hybridisation barriers
    c. Production of alkaloids
    d. Clonal propagation

43. **On culturing the young anther of a plant a botanist got a few diploid plant along with haploid plants. Which of the following might have given the diploid plant?**
    a. Exine of pollen grain
    b. Vegetative cell of pollen
    c. Cells of anther wall
    d. Generative cell of pollen

44. **Which one produce androgenic haploids in anther cultures**
    a. Anther cell
    b. Tapetal layer of anther wall
    c. Connective tissue
    d. Young pollen grain

45. **In tobacco callus, which one shall induce shoot differentiation in combination of Auxin and cytokinin**
    a. Higher concentration cytokinin and lower concentration of Auxin
    b. Lower concentration cytokinin and higher concentration of Auxin
    c. Only cytokinin and no Auxin
    d. Only Auxin and no cytokinin

46. **In callus culture, roots can be induced by the supply of**
    a. Auxin and no cytokinin
    b. Higher concentration cytokinin and lower concentration of Auxin
    c. Lower concentration cytokinin and higher concentration of Auxin
    d. None of the above

47. **After demonstration of cellular totipotency, a botanist wishes to raise identical plants. The tissue or part likely to yield haploid embryo are**
    a. Stem apices   b. Root tips
    c. Young anther   d. Young leaves

48. **Who could grow tomato roots successfully and developed the technique of tissue culture for the first time**
    a. Hilderbrandt   b. P.R. white
    c. W.H. muir   d. F.C. Steward

49. Plant tumour/ crown gall/ abnormal growth is caused by

a. Agrobacterium   b. Azotobactor
c. Nostoc   d. E.coli

50. Which of the following plant cells will show totipotency

a. Sieve tubes   b. Xylem vessels
c. Meristem   d. Cork cell

51. Variations observing during tissue culture of some plant are known as

a. Clonal variation
b. Somaclonal variation
c. Somatic variation
d. Tissue culture variation

52. Virus free plants can be obtained by

a. Antibiotic treatment   b. Bordeaux mixture
c. Root tip culture   d. Shoot tip culture

53. Tissue culture technique can be produce in definite number of new plants from a small parental tissue. The economic importance of the technique is in raising

a. Variants through picking up Somaclonal variation
b. Genetically uniform population of an elites species
c. Homozygous diploid plants
d. Development of new species

54. Haploid plant culture are got from

a. Leaves   b. Root tip
c. Pollen grain   d. Buds

55. Somaclonal variation are the ones

a. Caused by mutagens
b. Produced during tissue culture
c. Induced during sexual embryogeny
d. Caused by gamma rays

56. Parasexual hydridisation means fusion of

a. Male gamete with female gametes
b. Male gamete with synergid
c. Somatic protoplasts
d. Male gamete with somatic cell

57. Application of embryo culture is in

a. Clonal propagation
b. Overcoming hybridization barrier
c. Production of alkaloids
d. Formation of Somaclonal variation

58. Plants developed *in vitro* culture from pollen grains are

a. Androgenic haploid   b. Pollen plant
c. Male plant   d. Sterile plant

59. In tissue/bacterial culture glassware and nutrients are sterilised through

a. Water bath at 200°C   b. Dry air oven at 200°C
c. Dehumidifier   d. Autoclave

60. Development of shoot and root in tissue culture is determined by

a. Cytokinin and Auxin ratio
b. Enzymes
c. Temperature
d. Plant nutrient

61. Plant raised from single germinating pollen grain under culture condition would be

a. Diploid   b. Haploid
c. Triploid   d. Tetraploid

62. Plant medium used widely in preparation of culture medium is got from

a. Cycas revolute   b. Cocus nucifera
c. Pinus roxburghii d. Borassus flabellifera

63. Clonal cell lines are got from

a. Tissue culture   b. Tissue fractionation
c. Tissue homogenisation d. Tissue system

64. Auxenic culture is

a. Culture of tissue
b. Culture of genes
c. Pure culture without contamination
d. Pure culture of microbes without any external nutrient

65. A cell from leaf is made to grow into complete plant under culture conditions. It shows cellular

a. Cloning   b. Totipotency
c. Hybridization   d. All of the above

66. The equation,

$$c(s) + \frac{1}{2}O_2(g) = CO(g); \ \Delta H = -26.4 \ kcal \ \text{shows that:}$$

a. Carbon monoxide is endothermic compound
b. Carbon monoxide is exothermic compound
c. Reaction is endothermic
d. Above reaction is not possible

67. If no heat is transferred to and from the system during a process, the process is called:

 a. Adiabatic
 b. Isothermal
 c. Isobaric
 d. Cyclic

68. If temperature is kept constant throughout a process, the process is called:

 a. Isobestic
 b. Isobaric
 c. Isothermal
 d. Adiabatic

69. The heat of combustion, "H, of hydrogen gas at 25°C is –68.4 kcal. The heat of formation of water liquid at 25°C

 a. – 68.4 kcal
 b. – 38.4 kcal
 c. – 92.4 kcal
 d. None of the above

70. The apparatus used from measuring the heat of reactions at constant volume is called:

 a. Colorimeter
 b. Pyrometer
 c. Calorimeter
 d. Pyknometer

71. The bond energy of C-H bond in CH_4 from thermo-chemical equation, $C(g) + 4H(g) \rightarrow CH_4(g)$; "H= –397.8 kcal is expected to be about:

 a. +99.45 kcal
 b. +379.8 kcal
 c. + 100 kcal
 d. +95.0 kcal

72. The heat of reaction does not depend upon:

 a. Physical state of reactants and products
 b. The method by which final products are obtained from reactants
 c. Temperature of the reaction
 d. Whether the reactions is carried out at constant pressure or at constant volume

73. The reaction, $N_2(g) + O_2(g) = 2NO(g)$; "H= +21.6 is:

 a. Isothermic
 b. Endothermic
 c. Explosive
 d. Exothermic

74. In the reaction, $H_2(g) + Cl_2(g) = 2HCl(g) + 44.0$ kcal:

 a. Enthalpy of products is equal to the enthalpy of reactant
 b. Enthalpy of products is twice the enthalpy of reactant
 c. Enthalpy of products is greater than the enthalpy of reactant
 d. None of these

75. Heat of formation of CO(g) and $CO_2(g)$ are –26.4 and –94.0 kcal respectively. The heat of combustion of carbon monoxide is:

 a. +120.0 kcal
 b. – 67.6 kcal
 c. + 35.4 kcal
 d. – 68.0 kcal

76. An endothermic reaction is one in which?

 a. Heat is converted into electricity
 b. Heat is absorbed
 c. Heat is given out
 d. Heat is converted into mechanical work

77. First law of thermodynamics deals with.

 a. Conservation of mass
 b. Conservation of both mass and energy
 c. Conservation of energy
 d. All of these

78. First law of thermodynamics may be stated as:

 a. $Q = \Delta E - W$
 b. $\Delta E = Q + W$
 c. $\Delta E = Q - W$
 d. $W = \Delta E + Q$

79. The heat of formation of carbon dioxide is -90.4 kcal. This shows that:

 a. CO_2 is isothermal compound
 b. CO_2 is exothermic compound
 c. CO_2 is endothermic compound
 d. All of the above

80. The sign of enthalpy change "H for an endothermic reaction reaction is:

 a. Positive
 b. Negative
 c. May be positive or negative
 d. None of the above

81. heat evolved is given:

 a. –ve sign
 b. +ve sing
 c. No sign
 d. None of the above

82. If total enthalpy of reactants and products are Hr and Hp respectively, then for an exothermic reaction:

 a. $H_R > H_P$
 b. $H_R < H_P$
 c. $H_R = H_P$
 d. None of the above

83. Select the correct relation:

 a. $Q_V = \Delta E$
 b. $Q_P = -\Delta H$
 c. $Q_P = QV$
 d. $Q_P = \Delta E$

84. The relation between heat of a reaction of constant pressure and at constant volume is:

 a. $Q_P = Q_V + \Delta n \times RT$
 b. $Q_P = Q_V - \Delta n \times RT$
 c. $Q_V = Q_P + \Delta n \times RT$
 d. $Q_V = Q_P - \Delta n \times RT$

85. ΔH is related to ΔE by the equation:

 a. $\Delta H = \Delta E + \Delta n \times RT$
 b. $\Delta H = \Delta E - \Delta n \times RT$
 c. $\Delta H = \Delta E \times PV$
 d. None the above

86. **Enthalpy H is defined as:**

    a. $H = E \times PV$
    b. $H = E + PV$
    c. $H = E - PV$
    d. None of the above

87. **By convention the enthalpy of an element in standard state is assumed to be:**

    a. 5
    b. 10
    c. 0
    d. 100

88. **Condition of standard state are:**

    a. 2°C and 1 atm
    b. 25°C and 1 atm
    c. 15°C and 1 atm
    d. 5°C and 1 atm

89. **The heat of formation of compounds:**

    a. May be positive or negative
    b. Is always negative
    c. Is always positive
    d. Is zero in standard state

90. **Select the correct order:**

    a. 1 erg > 1 joule > 1 cal
    b. 1 joule > 1 erg > 1 cal
    c. 1 erg > 1 cal > 1 joule
    d. 1 cal > 1 joule > 1 erg

91. **The heat of neutralization of a strong acid with a strong base:**

    a. Depends upon the nature of acid
    b. Is a constant value
    c. Depends upon the nature of base
    d. None of the above

92. **Heat of neutralization of acetic acid with sodium hydroxide is expected to be about:**

    a. – 13.7 kcal
    b. –14.7 kcal
    c. – 13.4 kcal
    d. – 15.5 kcal

93. **The quantity of heat which must be supplied to decompose a compound into its elements is equal to the heat evolved during the formation of that compound from the elements." This statement is called:**

    a. Le chatelier's principle
    b. Joule's principle
    c. Hess's law
    d. Lavoisier and Laplace law

94. **The resultant heat change in a chemical reaction is the same whether it takes place in one or several stage". This statement is called**

    a. Hess's law
    b. Le Chatelier's principle
    c. Joule Thomson principle
    d. None of the above

95. **Heat of combustion, DH, of methane, ethane, ethylene and acetylene gases are – 212.8, –373.0, – 337.0 and –310.5 kcal respectively at the same temperature. The best fuel among these gases is:**

    a. Ethylene
    b. Ethane
    c. Methane
    d. Acetylene

96. **3-D structure can be seen under**

    a. TEM
    b. SEM
    c. Phase-contrast microscope
    d. Light microscope

97. **5′ to 3′ exonuclease activity is found in**

    a. DNA polymerase I
    b. DNA polymerase III
    c. DNA polymerase II
    d. None of these

98. **A Barr body is**

    a. Inactive Y-chromosome
    b. Inactive X-chromosome
    c. A result of primary non-disjunction
    d. Gene that plays a key role in male development

99. **A cell has four DNA molecules. At metaphase stage it will have**

    a. Six DNA molecule
    b. Eight DNA molecule
    c. Five DNA molecule
    d. Two DNA molecule

100. **Diploid cells have 20 chromosome. What will be the number of DNA at metaphase?**

    a. 30
    b. 20
    c. 40
    d. 50

ANSWERS OF MODEL PAPER 8

1. b	2. b	3. d	4. c	5. b	6. d	7. b
8. d	9. a	10. c	11. d	12. a	13. c	14. b
15. d	16. d	17. c	18. b	19. b	20. c	21. a
22. b	23. a	24. c	25. b	26. c	27. a	28. b
29. c	30. d	31. b	32. a	33. d	34. b	35. b
36. d	37. b	38. c	39. c	40. b	41. d	42. b
43. c	44. d	45. a	46. c	47. c	48. b	49. a
50. c	51. b	52. d	53. b	54. c	55. b	56. c
57. b	58. a	59. d	60. a	61. b	62. b	63. a
64. c	65. b	66. b	67. a	68. c	69. a	70. c
71. a	72. b	73. b	74. c	75. b	76. b	77. c
78. c	79. b	80. a	81. a	82. a	83. a	84. a
85. a	86. b	87. c	88. b	89. a	90. d	91. b
92. c	93. d	94. a	95. c	96. b	97. a	98. b
99. b	100. c					

UNIT 3
Solved Examination Papers

Memory Based ARS/NET 2001

1. Nuclear envelop breaks down in:

   a. Telophase II   b. Anaphase I

   c. Metaphase II   d. Prophase I

Ans. (d) Prophase I

2. A good molecular marker must be:

   a. Polymorphic

   b. Heritable

   c. Both a and b

   d. None of the above

Ans. (c) Both a and b

3. Genetic improvement of crop plants through biotechnology needs conventional breeding due to:

   a. The elite cultivars developed by plant breeding will be parents of the next generation of transgenics

   b. Field testing across locations or cropping systems and over years will be needed to select the best transgenic event

   c. Breeding may be required to minimize pleitropic effects

   d. All of these

Ans. (d) All of these

4. Electrophoretic separations of DNA and RNA in agarose is based on:

   a. Charge   b. Size

   c. Both a and b   d. Base sequence

Ans. (c) Both a and b

5. Which of the following statement is not true?

   a. Chloroplast are the sites of photosynthesis

   b. Chromoplast contains bright orange and yellow pigments

   c. Leucoplast is responsible for the bright colours of the fruits and leaves

   d. Leucoplast chromoplast and chloromoplast are present only in the cells of plants and algae

Ans. (c) Leucoplast is responsible for the bright colours of the fruits and leaves

6. Degradation of xenobiotics occurs rapidly in:

   a. Highly compressed soils

   b. Well aerated soils

   c. Heavily contaminated soils

   d. None of these

Ans. (b) Well aerated soils

7. Which of the following is an herbicide resistant gene:

   a. Bar   b. Hpt

   c. Cholesterol oxidase   d. Chitinases

Ans. (a) Bar

8. Anthropogenic chemicals introduced into the terrestrial carbon cycle is more recalcitrant when they contain:

   a. Unsaturated compounds

   b. Unbranched chain

   c. Aromatic ring substituted with halogens

   d. Chain length of less than 12 carbon atoms

Ans. (c) Aromatic ring substituted with halogens

9. The yolk of a chicken egg serves a nutritive function for the developing embryo. A functionally comparable structure in plants is:

   a. Lignin   b. Cellulose

   c. Pectin   d. Endosperm

Ans. (d) Endosperm

10. "9 + 2" describe the basic structure of which of the following one:

   a. Flagellum   b. Lysosome

   c. Basal body   d. Chloroplast

Ans. (a) Flagellum

11. Between mitotic division, the cell is in:

   a. G   b. G1

   c. G2   d. S phase

Ans. (b) G1

12. **Most plant cell are surrounded by a rigid cell wall made primarily of:**
    a. Triglycerides
    b. Polysaccharides
    c. Proteoglycanes
    d. Pectin

Ans. (b) Polysaccharides

13. **Which is not correct about gamma-linolenic acid?**
    a. It is a non-essential fatty acid
    b. It is the first intermediate in the conversion of linoleic acid to arachidonic acid
    c. It is produced by desaturation of linoleic acid by the enzyme fatty acid desaturase
    d. It is beneficial in alleviation of may physiologica and pathological conditions such as hyper-cholestereremia, cancer and diabetes

Ans. (a) It is a non-essential fatty acid

14. **During Agrobacterium transformation the T-DNA is located by protein, which is the product of gene:**
    a. Vir C
    b. Vir D
    c. Vir E
    d. Vir G

Ans. (c) Vir E

15. **In liposome mediated gene transfer DNA enters the protoplast due to:**
    a. Osmosis
    b. Endocytosis
    c. Exocytosis
    d. Collision

Ans. (b) Endocytosis

16. **Endochitinase can be used as:**
    a. Antibacterial
    b. Antifungal
    c. Antinematodal
    d. Antivirus

Ans. (b) Antifungal

17. **The T-DNA region of all the Ti and Ri plasmids are flanked by direct repeat sequence:**
    a. 25 bp
    b. 20 bp
    c. 15 bp
    d. 35 bp

Ans. (a) 25 bp

18. **Bacteria are preferred over yeast for production of single cell protein because:**
    a. Of their fast growth
    b. They are small
    c. Of their lower content of methionine
    d. None of these

Ans. (a) Of their fast growth

19. **The transgenic tomato plant showing delayed ripening due to suppression of ethylene was developed using methodology of:**
    a. Coat protein gene
    b. Antisense RNA
    c. Agrobacterium mediated gene transfer
    d. None of these

Ans. (b) None of these

20. **Lambda has short single stranded 5 projection of:**
    a. 5-nucleotide length
    b. 10-nucleotide length
    c. 8-nucleotide length
    d. 12-nucleotide length

Ans. (d) 12-nucleotide length

21. **The direct DNA uptake by the protoplast is stimulated by the chemical**
    a. Cellulose
    b. Sucrose
    c. Sodium chloride
    d. PEG

Ans. (d) PEG

22. **The function of the nucleus includes:**
    a. Cellular respiration
    b. Housing the hereditary information
    c. Synthesis of protein
    d. Synthesis of carbon compounds

Ans. (b) Housing the hereditary information

23. **Which is not correct about virus cross protection?**
    a. The phenomenon of cross protection was first observed by McKinney in 1929 in case of tobacco mosaic virus
    b. Plants infected with a mild strain of virus resist the development of symptoms upon infection by a more severe strains of the same virus
    c. A mild protecting strain effective for one region may be serve for another region
    d. Selection of mild protecting strain is rather easy

Ans. (d) Selection of mild protecting strain is rather easy

24. **Which of the following reagent is useful for visualizing DNA?**
    a. 14 uracil
    b. Diphenylamine
    c. Ethidium bromide
    d. DNA polymerase

Ans. (c) Ethidium bromide

25. **Endoplasmic reticulum:**
    a. Is mound only in animals
    b. Is a site of ATP production
    c. Is called rough if mitochondria is attached to it
    d. Is a system of membrane bound channels

Ans. (d) Is a system of membrane bound channels

26. Which of the following is a green tissue specific promoter?

a. Pea vicilin
b. Bean phytahemaglutinin
c. 35 s CaMV
d. Arabidopsis small sub unit of Rubisco

Ans. (d) Arabidopsis small sub unit of Rubisco

27. Scientist have postulated that small pores must exist in the cell membrane because:

a. Of endocytosis
b. Of turgour pressur
c. CO and O move freely though the membrane
d. Water molecules move freely through the membrane

Ans. (d) Water molecules move freely through the membrane

28. If adenine makes up 5% of DNA, cytosine will make:

a. 15%   b. 25%
c. 35%   d. 45%

Ans. (a) 15%

29. A general method to confirm expression of transgene at translation level is:

a. Southern blotting   b. Western blotting
c. Northern blotting   d. Eastern blotting

Ans. (c) Northern blotting

30. The organelle that functions in the breakdown of ells and tissues is the

a. Episomes   b. Mitochondria
c. Centrosomes   d. Lysosomes

Ans. (d) Lysosomes

31. In vitro packaging is required for which one of the following vector:

a. BAC   b. YAC
c. PAC   d. None of these

Ans. (c) PAC

32. Which of the following statement is true?

a. Facilitates diffusion an our against concentration gradient
b. Diffusion requires an expenditure of energy by the cell
c. The active transport requires protein complex in the cell
d. Osmosis an our against a concentration gradient

Ans. (c) The active transport requires protein complex in the cell

33. Which is not about Scarlet?

a. It is a somaclonal variety of potato
b. It was selected from shoot tip culture derived plants
c. This variety is comparable to the parent cultivars in yield and disease resistant
d. It shows darker and more stable skin colour, which is a desirable quality trait

Ans. (a) It is a somaclonal variety of potato

34. Batch system of culture are:

a. Steady state process
b. Non steady state process
c. Completely mixed
d. Plug flow system

Ans. (b) Non steady state process

35. The browning of the culture medium induced by some explants can be prevented by addition of:

a. GA
b. Polyvinylpyrrolidone
c. 2,4,D
d. IBA

Ans. (b) Polyvinylpyrrolidone

36. The phosphofrutokinase an pyruvate kinage reaction are similar is that:

a. Both generate ATP
b. Both are essentially irreversible
c. Both involves a high energy: sugar derivative
d. Both involves three carbon compound

Ans. (b) Both are essentially irreversible

37. Which of the following is not used as measuring device in biosensor?

a. Whole organism   b. Immunonuclear
c. Enzyme   d. Biofilters

Ans. (c) Enzyme

38. Bacculoviruses:

a. RNA virus   b. DNA virus
c. Both a and b   d. None of these

Ans. (b) DNA virus

39. Bioreactor are used for:

a. Production of enzymes
b. Production of secondary metabolites
c. Production of cell structure
d. All of the above

Ans. (d) All of the above

40. **During agrobacterium infections the plant cell begins to synthesize an arginine derivative called as:**

    a. Opine
    b. Aetobenzylpurine
    c. Hygromycin
    d. Acetosyringone

Ans. (a) Opine

41. **Which of the following is not a general property of the enzyme?**

    a. Enzyme has great catalytic powers
    b. Enzyme bind specific substances
    c. Enzyme mostly use hydrophobic interactions to bind substrates
    d. Enzymes are almost exclusively proteins

Ans. (d) Enzymes are almost exclusively proteins

42. **Requefort cheese is ripened with the help of:**

    a. Lactobacillus coxi
    b. Penicillum reguoforti
    c. Brevibacterium linens
    d. Propionibacterium shexmanii

Ans. (b) Penicillum reguoforti

43. **Plant protoplast fusion and be achieved with:**

    a. TZZ
    b. PEG
    c. PM
    d. Zeatin

Ans. (b) PEG

44. **The gene transferred from *E. coli* to tobacco to increased the level of manitol is.**

    a. Manitol dehydrogenase
    b. Manitol carboxylase
    c. Manitol hydrolase
    d. Manitol oxygenase

Ans. (a) Manitol dehydrogenase

45. **Nick transition is directly involved in which of the following process:**

    a. RNA to DNA
    b. DNA to RNA
    c. DNA to DNA
    d. RNA to RNA

Ans. (c) DNA to DNA

46. **Production of biogas takes through the following sequential steps:**

    a. Methanogenis–Solubilization–Acidogenis
    b. Acidogenis–Solubilization–Methanogenis
    c. Acidogenis–Methanogenis–Solubilization
    d. Solubilization–Acidogenis–Methanogenis

Ans. (d) Solubilization–Acidogenis–Methanogenis

47. **Restriction enzyme cuts straight across the DNA produces:**

    a. Nicks
    b. Blunt ends
    c. Single stranded
    d. None of these

Ans. (b) Blunt ends

48. **White rot fungus *Phaneiochaete chrysasporium* produces:**

    a. Extra cellular enzymes
    b. Intra cellular
    c. Both a and b
    d. None of these

Ans. (a) Extra cellular enzymes

49. **During stress which of the following phytohormone is accumulated?**

    a. Auxin
    b. GA
    c. ABA
    d. Ethylene

Ans. (c) ABA

50. **In eukaryotes, DNA methylation is mainly concerned with:**

    a. Restriction
    b. Control of replication
    c. Regulation of gene pair
    d. DNA repair

Ans. (c) Regulation of gene pair

51. **Which of the following reactions is not performed by lignin peroxidise?**

    a. Detoxification of toxic phenols
    b. Oxidative cleavage of aromatic ether bonds
    c. Oxidative of phenyl alcohols to the respective aldehydes
    d. Hydrosylation of the aliphatic double bond in

Ans. (a) Detoxification of toxic phenols

52. **Cytoplasmic channels connecting adjacent cells are called:**

    a. Ionic channels
    b. Conjugation tube
    c. Protoplasmic channels
    d. Plasmodesmata

Ans. (d) Plasmodesmata

53. **If meiosis does not ours, the chromosome number would in each generation:**

    a. Remain same
    b. Triple
    c. Deduce
    d. Double

Ans. (d) Double

54. **Which of the following enzyme is used for making DNA:**

    a. Reverse transcriptase
    b. DNA ligase
    c. Restriction enzyme
    d. Polynucleotide trans sterase

Ans. (a) **Reverse transcriptase**

55. **An example of naturally occurring auxin is:**

    a. BAP
    b. 2,4-D
    c. ABA
    d. IAA

Ans. (d) **IAA**

56. **The in-vitro electron donor to PS-II is:**

    a. Water
    b. Ascorbate
    c. PS-I
    d. Plastoquinone

Ans. (a) **Water**

57. **Which of the following statements regarding simple Michaelis-Menten enzyme kinetics is not correct?**

    a. Km is expressed I terms of a reaction velocity
    b. Km is the concentration of substrates required to achieves one half of V_{max}
    c. Km is the concentration of substrates required to convert one half of the total enzyme into the enzyme substrates complex
    d. The maximum velocity, V_{max} is related to the maximal number of substrates molecules that and be turned over in unit time by a molecule of enzyme

Ans. (a) **Km is expressed I terms of a reaction velocity**

58. **Thiobacillus thioxidans grows on:**

    a. Iron
    b. Sulphur
    c. Pyrites
    d. Covellite

Ans. (c) **Pyrites**

59. **The Shine Dalgarno sequence is known as:**

    a. Ribosome binding site
    b. Initiation site
    c. Promoter binding site
    d. None of these

Ans. (a) **Ribosome binding site**

60. **In tissue culture regeneration of shoot and root occurs by manipulating the balance of:**

    a. Auxin and ABA
    b. Auxin and Cytokinin
    c. Cytokinin and ABA
    d. ABA and Etylene

Ans. (b)

61. **Relaxed plasmid:**

    a. Can not be purified
    b. Have multiple copies per cell
    c. Does not exist in bacteria
    d. Have only single copy per cell

Ans. (b) **Have multiple copies per cell**

62. **For mitochondrial structure and function mt-DNA species:**

    a. 20% protein
    b. 10% protein
    c. 100% protein
    d. 30% protein

Ans. (b) **10% protein**

63. **Amino acid fermentation employs:**

    a. Unicells
    b. Filamentous organisms
    c. Both a and b
    d. None of these

Ans. (c) **Both a and b**

64. **Homologous pairs line up along equatorial plane during:**

    a. Anaphase II
    b. Metaphase I
    c. Interphase
    d. Telophase

Ans. (b) **Metaphase I**

65. **An example of commercially important primary metabolites is:**

    a. Toxin
    b. Alkaloid
    c. Alcohol
    d. None of these

Ans. (c) **Alcohol**

66. **The chemical used as an inducer of the vir operons is:**

    a. Hygromycin
    b. Fanamycin
    c. Acetosyringone
    d. Kanamycin

Ans. (c) **Acetosyringone**

67. **The large dark body in the nucleus is the nucleolus, which participates in the formation of:**

    a. Ribosome
    b. RNA
    c. Protein
    d. DNA

Ans. (b) **RNA**

68. **State which of the following is not a desired characteristic of a vector?**

    a. Large size
    b. Autonomous replication
    c. Unique restriction site
    d. Genes that confer antibiotic resistance

Ans. (a) **Large size**

69. In meosis, as in mitosis, the chromosomal materials is replicated during:

a. G1 phase　　　　b. S phase

c. T phase　　　　d. G2 phase

Ans. (b) S phase

70. In PCR, the ds DNA is generally denatured by:

a. Acid treatment　　b. Alkali treatment

c. Temperature　　　d. None of these

Ans. (c) Temperature

71. Cyclic phosphorylation involves:

a. PS-II　　　　b. PS-I

c. Mitochondria　　d. Both a and b

Ans. (a) PS-II

72. Replication of chloroplast DNA is controlled by:

a. Nuclear DNA　　b. Mitochondrial DNA

c. Pollen grains　　d. Chloroplast

Ans. (a) Nuclear DNA

73. Which of the following is not used as cryoprotectant?

a. Glycerol　　　　b. Dimethyl sulfoxide

c. Polyclar　　　　d. Ethylene glycerol

Ans. (b) Dimethyl sulfoxide

74. The *in-vitro* electron donor to PS-I is:

a. PS-II　　　　b. Plastoquinone

c. Oxygen　　　d. Ascorbate

Ans. (b) Plastoquinone

75. Which one of the following controls gene expression in eukaryotes?

a. Effector　　　　b. Histones

c. Transcription factor　d. Transferase

Ans. (c) Transcription factor

76. The shoot apical meristem is characterized by:

a. Trapezoidal shape　b. Round shape

c. Dome shape　　　d. None of these

Ans. (c) Dome shape

77. Germplasm preservation of meristem and shoot tip culture involves:

a. Storage in dry ice

b. Storage in liquid nitrogen

c. Culturing under low temp

d. Cryo preservation and slow growth

Ans. (d) Cryo preservation and slow growth

78. Horizontal gene flow can be reduced by expressing genes in:

a. Nucleus

b. Chloroplast

c. Both a and b

d. None of these

Ans. (b) Chloroplast

79. The vir region is organized into six operons viz., virA, virB, vir C, vir D, vir E and vir G, out of these which four operons are required for virlence:

a. A,B,C,D　　　　b. A,B,D,G

c. C,D,E,G　　　　d. None of these

Ans. (b) A,B,D,G

80. Majority of bacculoviruses have been reported from species:

a. Lepidoptera　　b. Dipteral

c. Crustacean　　　d. Both a and b

Ans. (d) Both a and b

81. In commercial fermentation process, it is desirable to have:

a. Minimal lag phase

b. Minimum stationary phase

c. Minimal death phase

d. Minimal lag phase

Ans. (a) Minimal lag phase

82. Replication of the DNA by rolling circle mechanism give rise to a:

a. Blunt and DNA

b. Theta structure

c. Concatamer

d. Single strand DNA with nick

Ans. (c) Concatamer

83. Oxidation of water during photosynthesis involves:

a. PS-II

b. PS-I

c. Both a and b

d. Mitochondria

Ans. (a) PS-II

84. E.L. Tatum was a noble prize recipient, his work on:

a. Nurospora

b. *E. coli* gene expression

c. RNA polymerase

d. DNA polymerase

Ans. (a) Nurospora

85. **Shotgun approach is mainly used in:**
   a. Genomic library
   b. Gene mapping
   c. Gene transforming
   d. DNA sequencing

Ans. (a) Genomic library

86. **Which of the following is not an antibiotic resistance gene?**
   a. hpt   b. neo
   c. gfp   d. npt II

Ans. (c) gfp

87. **Callus and suspension culture normally produce secondary metabolites when:**
   a. Emit fragrance
   b. The callus turn red with age
   c. Show lightful tracheids
   d. All of these

Ans. (d) All of these

88. **Cosmid have the Cos site of:**
   a. Lambda   b. Plasmid
   c. ML 3   d. YAC

Ans. (a) Lambda

89. **Inclusion of osmoticum in both isolation and culture media:**
   a. Facilates formation of heterokaryotes
   b. Facilitates fusion of protoplast
   c. Prevent rupture of protoplast
   d. None of these

Ans. (c) Prevent rupture of protoplast

90. **Xeroderma pigmentation disese in man is due to defects in DNA repair system of:**
   a. Excision repair
   b. Mismatch repair
   c. Deletion repair
   d. Direct repair

Ans. (d) Direct repair

91. **Which of the following is not an insecticidal protein gene?**
   a. Sunflower seed albumin
   b. Lectins
   c. Protease-inhibitor
   d. Alphas amylase inhibitor

Ans. (a) Sunflower seed albumin

92. **Anther culture provides a method for the production of:**
   a. Pollyploid
   b. Apomictic line
   c. Homozygous line
   d. Heterozygous line

Ans. (c) Homozygous line

93. **The term somaclonal variation was termed by:**
   a. Larken and scowhoft
   b. skirvin
   c. Eyans
   d. Murashige ans skoog

Ans. (a) Larken and scowhoft

94. **Most commonly used organism in SCP is**
   a. Bacillus   b. E.coli
   c. Spirulina   d. Pseudomonas

Ans. (c) Spirulina

95. **In Agrobacterium mediated plant transformation which one of the following is used to check the Agrobacterium growth:**
   a. Basta   b. PPT
   c. Timentin   d. Kanamycin

Ans. (c) Timentin

96. **Which one of the following means transfer of genes in host without a biological agent?**
   a. Transduction
   b. Transformation
   c. Conjugation
   d. Perpetuation

Ans. (b) Transformation

97. **The sigma factor of RNA polymerase in *E. coli* involved :**
   a. DNA unwinding
   b. Binding with template DNA
   c. RNA synthesis
   d. Transcription initiation

Ans. (d) Transcription initiation

98. **Which of the following statements is not generally true about histones?**
   a. Present in nucleosome
   b. Homogenous in structure
   c. Always present in chromatin
   d. Heterogeneous in structure

Ans. (b) Homogenous in structure

99. Secondary metabolites like antibiotics are not essential for:

　a. Log phase growth
　b. Exponential growth
　c. Both a and b
　d. None of these

Ans. (c) Both a and b

100. Micro propagation involves:

　a. Thorough callusing
　b. Adventitious bud transfer
　c. Shoot culture, asceptic initiation transfer to pot and rooting
　d. Initiation of aseptic culture, shoot multiplier, rooting and transplantation

Ans. (d) Initiation of aseptic culture, shoot multiplier, rooting and transplantation

101. Nodulin genes are found in:

　a. Cyanobacteria
　b. Badyrhizobium
　c. Plant
　d. Bacteria

Ans. (c) Plant

102. Most commonly used strategy to develop transgenic plant against any viral disease is to engineer a:

　a. Liposome mediated transfer of viral RNA
　b. Anti sense RNA for viral genome
　c. Coat or capsid protein gene
　d. Direct DNA transfer of viral gene

Ans. (c) Coat or capsid protein gene

103. During isolation of protoplast:

　a. Cell membrane is removed
　b. Treated with pectinase
　c. Treated with proteases
　d. Cells are irradiated

Ans. (b) Treated with pectinase

104. Which one of the following is the first stable product of photosynthesis?

　a. RuBP
　b. DAHP
　c. Glucose
　d. 3-PGA

Ans. (c) Glucose

105. In replication of *E. coli* DNA, the protein complex involved is known as:

　a. Replisome
　b. Splisosome
　c. Endosomes
　d. Primososme

Ans. (a) Replisome

106. Which one of the following amino acids is specified by single codon in genetic code?

　a. G
　b. K
　c. W
　d. D

Ans. (c) W

107. The existence of mRNA was first indicated by:

　a. Palkade and Siekevitz
　b. H.G. Khurana
　c. Volkin and Astrachan
　d. Brahett and aspersson

Ans. (c) Volkin and Astrachan

108. Leghaemoglobin is synthesized elusively in :

　a. Nitrogen fixing nodules
　b. Leg of ruminants
　c. Klebsiella
　d. Cyanobacteria

Ans. (a) Nitrogen fixing nodules

109. Cyanobacteria protect nitrogenase from oxygen by:

　a. Heterocyst
　b. Gum production
　c. Possession of catalase
　d. Possession of superoxide dismutase

Ans. (a) Heterocyst

110. Which of the following does not regulate nitrogenease activity?

　a. H_2
　b. M_0
　c. NH_4
　d. Energy supply

Ans. (a) H_2

111. Which of the following enzymes is not involved in HMP pathway?

　a. Trasketolase
　b. Endolase
　c. Transaldolase
　d. 6-phosphogluonase

Ans. (b) Endolase

112. What is the role of SDS in case of SDS PAGE?

　a. It increases speed of proteins in gel
　b. It protects proteins from denaturation
　c. It provides negative charge to all the proteins so that separation can be done only on the basis of molecular weight
　d. SDS is detergent so is used to emulsify contaminating fats if any in sample

Ans. (c) It provides negative charge to all the proteins so that separation can be done only on the basis of molecular weight

113. Fe protein of nitrogenase is:

a. Heteropolymer tetramer

b. Homomeric dimmer

c. Homomeric tetramer

d. Heteromeric dimmer

Ans. (b) Homomeric dimmer

114. The length of okazaki fragments in *E.coli* are about:

a. 50–100 nucleotides

b. 100–200 nucleotides

c. 10000 nucleotides

d. 1000–2000 nucleotides

Ans. (d) 1000–2000 nucleotides

115. Ferrodoxin is reduced by:

a. PS-II only

b. PS-I only

c. PS-I and II

d. Mitochondria

Ans. (c) PS-I and II

116. Which of the following statements about conjugation are not true?

a. A recipient cell because of donor cell

b. As the chromosome replicates, the free and moves into the recipient cell

c. The recipient bacterium possess plasmids call F factor

d. Conjugation studies have produced maps of gene sequences on the bacterial chromosome

Ans. (c) The recipient bacterium possess plasmids call F factor

117. Which of the following statements is not true?

a. An acidic protein will give pI less than 7

b. A basic protein will give a pI greater than 7

c. At a pH value equal to its pI, a protein will not move in the electric field of an electrophoresis experiment

d. The pI is the pH value at which a protein has no charge

Ans. (d) The pI is the pH value at which a protein has no charge

118. Explanation is a process of:

a. Planting of explants

b. Dissection and culture of small organs or tissue section

c. Choice of explants

d. Culture of plants

Ans. (b) Dissection and culture of small organs or tissue section

119. During reduction of dinitrogen by nitrogenase, how many net electron are required

a. Six

b. Two

c. Four

d. None of these

Ans. (a) Six

120. In biotin labelling of probes, the detection method is:

a. Streptavidin labelling

b. Antibody labelling

c. Colorimetric

d. Fluorescene

Ans. (a) Streptavidin labelling

121. Micropores contained within the anther give rise to:

a. Callus culture and gynogenesis

b. Anthogenesis and callus culture

c. Gynogenesis and androgenesis

d. None of these

Ans. (b) Anthogenesis and callus culture

122. Operon comprise of:

a. Operator

b. Structural gene

c. Promoter

d. Repressor

e. All of these

Ans. (b) Structural gene

123. Which of the following is not a component of nitrogenase?

a. Mg^{++}

b. NADP

c. MoFe- protein

d. Fe protein

Ans. (b) NADP

124. Which one of the following is not formed in calvin cycle?

a. RuBP

b. DAHP

c. Glucose

d. 3′-PGA

Ans. (c) Glucose

125. The end product of transcription process in prokaryotes:

a. Monocistronic mRNA

b. Polycistronic mRNA

c. Both a and b

d. None of these

Ans. (b) Polycistronic mRNA

126. Which one of the following radioisotope is used to elucidate carbon pathway in calving cycle

a. 14C

b. 32P

c. 35S

d. 3H

Ans. (a) 14C

127. Pure plasmid DNA was isolated from a bacterium. Restriction enzyme digestion of this plasmid with either Bam HI or Eo RI resulted in two DNA fragments, A double digestion of the same plasmid with both these enzymes resulted in three DNA fragments. From this we an conclude that the isolated plasmid DNA is:

    a. Double stranded and linear
    b. Double stranded and circular
    c. Single stranded and linear
    d. Single stranded and circular

Ans. (a) Double stranded and linear

128. Which of the following is commonly used as a protecting group during peptide synthesis?

    a. Dicyclohexylurea
    b. Ten butyloxylcarbonyl
    c. Hydrogen fluoride
    d. Dicyclohexylurea carbodimide

Ans. (b) Ten butyloxylcarbonyl

129. Guanosine is:

    a. Pyrimidine base
    b. Purine nucleotide
    c. Purine base
    d. Pyrimidine nucleotide

Ans. (b) Purine nucleotide

130. The restriction enzyme useful to the molecular biologist belongs is:

    a. Type – I
    b. Type – II
    c. Type – III
    d. Type – IV

Ans. (b) Type – II

131. The number of consensus sequences in the promoter region of a gene in *E. coli* is generally:

    a. 2   b. 3
    c. 4   d. 6

Ans. (a) 2

132. Which category of microbes are used in retting process of jute?

    a. Microbes tolerant to high temperature
    b. Which process high amount of hydrolytic enzyme activity
    c. Anaerobic microbes
    d. Aerobic microbes only

Ans. (b) Which process high amount of hydrolytic enzyme activity

133. The proof reading function in DNA replication is done by:

    a. DNA helicase   b. 3′ exonuclease
    c. DNA gyrase   d. 5′ exonuclease

Ans. (b) 3′ exonuclease

134. When the PCR used to generate single stranded copies of DNA, that PCR reaction is called:

    a. Asymmetric PCR   b. RT-PCR
    c. Inverse PCR   d. All of these

Ans. (a) Asymmetric PCR

135. Which one of the following amino acids residues are likely to be formed on the inside of a water soluble protein?

    a. H   b. R
    c. E   d. V

Ans. (d) V

136. Which of the following chemical is used for preparation of competent cell?

    a. HCL   b. $CaCl_2$
    c. Glycine   d. NaCl

Ans. (b) $CaCl_2$

137. Cryo-preservation involves:

    a. Cutting, application of cryo-protectant and storage at 196°C
    b. Freezing and thawing
    c. Specimen treatment, freezing storage at ultra low temperature
    d. None of these

Ans. (a) Cutting, application of cryo-protectant and storage at 196°C

138. Which one of the following chemical causes frame shift mutation?

    a. 2-bromo uracil   b. Acridine orange
    c. 2-aminopurine   d. Hydroxyglamine

Ans. (b) Acridine orange

139. The conversion of IMP to AMP requires which of the following ?

    a. GTP   b. NAD
    c. ATP   d. Glutamine

Ans. (a) GTP

140. Up and down mutation occurs in:

    a. Promoter region   b. Intron
    c. Transcription start site d. Poly-A-region

Ans. (a) Promoter region

141. The hsd system of DNA methylationn in *E.coli* methylates:

    a. Guanine
    b. Thymine
    c. Cytosine
    d. Adenine

Ans. (d) Adenine

142. The existence of puffs in giant chromosome of the Brazilian guat support the concept that:

    a. Conjugation involves a transfer of genetic material
    b. DNA unwind for m-RNA transcription
    c. The sequence of gene on a chromosome can be determined on the basis of crossover frequencies
    d. Homologous chromatids exchange genetic material at meiosis

Ans. (b) Conjugation involves a transfer of genetic material

143. Transcription is directly involved in which of the following steps in the flow of genetic information:

    a. RNA to DNA
    b. RNA to Protein
    c. Protein to RNA
    d. DNA to RNA

Ans. (d) DNA to RNA

144. Which one of the following is not the basic requirement of biological nitrogen fixation?

    a. Mg^{++} and ATP
    b. Nitrogenase
    c. Glutamine
    d. Strong reducing agent

Ans. (c) Glutamine

145. DNA re-association kinetics provides information on the:

    a. Genomic size
    b. Presence of exon
    c. Presence of intron
    d. Existence of gene

Ans. (a) Genomic size

146. Which one of the following amino acids mat alters the direction of polypeptide chains and interrupt alpha helices?

    a. Pro
    b. Cys
    c. Phe
    d. His

Ans. (a) Pro

147. RNA molecules involve in splicing are:

    a. Sn rRNA
    b. 5s rRNA
    c. 16s RNA
    d. t RNA

Ans. (a) Sn rRNA

148. Substance, such as tryptophan, tha decreases the amount of enzyme produced by a cell is known as:

    a. Induces
    b. Repressor
    c. Promoter
    d. Corepressor

Ans. (d) Corepressor

149. In lambda phage the N, Cl and Cro gene are responsible for:

    a. Host lysis
    b. Gene regulation and immunity
    c. DNA synthesis
    d. Late function regulation

Ans. (d) Late function regulation

150. The sedimentary velocity of a protein sin a centrifuge does not depend on the:

    a. Density of the protein
    b. Charge on the protein
    c. Shape of the protein
    d. Density of the solution

Ans. (b) Charge on the protein

151. The evidence for semi-conservative replication of DNA was first given by:

    a. Meselson and Stahl
    b. Harshey and chase
    c. Avery and Malecode
    d. Watson and Crick

Ans. (a) Meselson and Stahl

152. The absolute requirement for both RNA synthesis and DNA replication is:

    a. UTP
    b. Free 3′ –OH
    c. Free 5′ –OH
    d. Primer

Ans. (b) Free 3′ –OH

153. The enzyme nitrogenase is composed of:

    a. Four – oxygen sensitive non haem iron protein
    b. Three – oxygen sensitive non haem iron protein
    c. Two– oxygen sensitive non haem iron protein
    d. One – oxygen sensitive non haem iron protein

Ans. (c) Two– oxygen sensitive non haem iron protein

154. Hybridization technology is used in production of:

    a. m-RNA
    b. Monoclonal serum
    c. Polyclonal antibodies
    d. Monoclonal antibodies

Ans. (d) Monoclonal antibodies

155. Which of the following enzyme is classified as hydrolases?

a. Aconitase   b. Catalase

c. Polynucleotide kinase   d. Pepsin

Ans. (d) Pepsin

156. Which of the following is the major metabolic product of glycolysis in higher organism?

a. Lactic acid   b. Acetone

c. Ethanol   d. Glycerol

Ans. (a) Lactic acid

157. Which of the following is true about the structure of ATP?

a. Has a free hemiacetal

b. Contains a ketose sugar

c. Contains a pyranose ring

d. Contains a beta N-glycosidic linkage

Ans. (d) Contains a beta N-glycosidic linkage

158. Which blotting technique is used for the detection of DNA that has been separated from a mixture of DNA restriction fragments by electrophoresis through an agrose gel and then transferred on to a nitrocellulose sheet?

a. Northern blotting

b. Southern blotting

c. Eastern blotting

d. Western blotting

Ans. (b) Southern blotting

159. During splicing of proteins which part is removed?

a. Exons   b. Introne

c. Exteins   d. Intein

Ans. (d) Intein

160. Which of the following pairs are anomers?

a. Glucose and mannose

b. Ribose and ribulose

c. Pyruvate lactate

d. Alpha D-glucose and beta D-glucose

Ans. (d) Alpha D-glucose and beta D-glucose

161. In the transcription process of eukaryotes, which of the following in not a true:

a. Translation occurs in cytoplasm

b. Translation is coupled with transcription

c. AUA is a coding sequence

d. 3′ end of m-RNA is polyadenylated

Ans. (b) Translation is coupled with transcription

162. If a polypeptide has 400 amino acid residue, what is the appropriate molecular weight of that polypeptide?

a. 11 kd   b. 44 kd

c. 22 md   d. 44 md

Ans. (b) 44 kd

163. Which of the following is not true for single stranded vector?

a. Replicate via RF intermediate

b. Has cohesive

c. Used for oligonucleotide directed mutagenesis

d. Used for dideoxy mediated DNA sequencing

Ans. (b) Has cohesive

164. The first product of purine nucleotide biosynthesis that contain a complete purine ring is:

a. GMP   b. IMP

c. AMP   d. XMP

Ans. (b) IMP

165. Physical maps of genome is based on:

a. Number of base pair

b. Recombination percentage

c. Both a and b

d. None of these

Ans. (a) Number of base pair

Memory Based Paper CSIR NET
June 2007

1. There are various types of bond in chemistry like metallic bond, ionic bond, wandervall and hydrogen bond. Among the following the weakest bond is

   a. Ionic bond
   b. Metallic bond
   c. Hydrogen bond
   d. Wandervalls bond

   Ans. (d) Wandervalls bond

2. Consider the following chemical reaction in which rate of forward reaction (K^+) is 1/sec and rate of backward reaction is 10^7/sec

   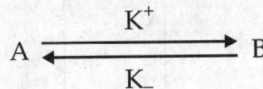

   If the reaction starts with one atom of substrate A, then what woud be the concentration of B at equilibrium?

   a. 1
   b. 10^7
   c. 10^{-7}
   d. 10^5

   Ans. (c) 10^{-7}

3. Find the oxidation state of Mn in $KMnO_4$

   a. −1
   b. −7
   c. +7
   d. −1

   Ans. (b) −7

4. In routine lab practice for dilution of concentrated sulphuric acid generally it is advised to drops of sulphuric acid in water instead of water in concentrated sulphuric acid because

   a. Pure sulphuric acid s very costly
   b. It is an endothermic reaction
   c. It is an exothermic reaction
   d. Latent heat of water is low

   Ans. (c) It is an exothermic reaction

5. If equal volumes of soild, liquid or vapour state of water is filled in thermos. Molecules of which state of matter will possess maximum mean kinetic energy

   a. Solid
   b. Liquid
   c. Vapour
   d. All will have same

   Ans. (c) Vapour

6. In plant water is transported from roots to shoots via

   a. Xylem
   b. Phloem
   c. Apoplast
   d. Symplast

   Ans. (a) Xylem

7. Among the following organelles where you will NOT find the process of transcription of genes

   a. Nucleolus
   b. Chloroplast
   c. Mitochondria
   d. Plasma membrane

   Ans. (d) Plasma membrane

8. Most common reason for genetic change from one generation to next generation among humans is

   a. Mutation
   b. Segregation
   c. Recombination
   d. Environmental

   Ans. (c) Recombination

9. In female which hormone is related with regulation of estrous cycle

   a. Cortisol
   b. Insulin
   c. Progesterone
   d. ACTH

   Ans. (c) Progesterone

10. The speed of nerve impulse in human is

    a. 10 μm/sec
    b. 10 mm/sec
    c. 10 m/sec
    d. 10 km/sec

    Ans. (c) 10 m/ sec

11. If a 0.5 Km asteroid from space hits the earth. Among the following in whch area of world would be least likely impact on life

    a. Sahara desert
    b. South east Asa
    c. North America
    d. Mid pacific ocean

Ans. (d) Mid pacific ocean

12. The major cause behind the damage of historica building like tajmahal is

    a. Atmospheric Ozone
    b. Presence of sulphuric acid in environment
    c. Increased CO_2 concentration
    d. Polluted water in rivers

Ans. (b) Presence of sulphuric acid in environment

13. Half life of Uranium-238 is 4.468×10^9 years. At present in any rock the concentration of ^{238}U is equal to concentration of Pb, then the age of rock will be

    a. 4.468×10^9
    b. 4.468×10^4
    c. 2.234×10^9
    d. 10117×10^9

Ans. (a) 4.468×10^9

14. The main reason behind earth's magnetic field

    a. Presence of Diamagnetic iron in earth core
    b. Matter present on earth curst
    c. Motion of iron in liquefied core
    d. Due to impact of asterioids

Ans. (c) Motion of iron in liquefied core

15. The main reason for presence of circum-pacific ocean seismic belt is

    a. Union of continent and oceanic pates
    b. Subduction of oceanic plates into contnental plates
    c. Sea floor spreading
    d. More human disturbance

Ans. (b) Subduction of oceanic plates into contnental plates

16. If p implies q and q implies r. It is given that q is true it means

    a. Both p and q are true
    b. Both p and q are false
    c. P is true and q false
    d. P is false and q is true

Ans. (a) Both p and q are true

17. On sudden power failure. Information of which memory will be NOT lost in computer

    a. RAM and CD
    b. Floppy and hardisk
    c. PRAM and ROM
    d. Floppy and EP-RAM

Ans. (b) Floppy and hardisk

18. How many values of integer with sign magnitude can be stored in 8 bits

    a. -511 to $+511$
    b. 255 to 0
    c. -127 to $+127$
    d. -128 to $+128$

Ans. (c) -127 to $+127$

19. Among the following which language is more near to one which is used by computer for execution of its programs

    a. C
    b. BASIC
    c. Assembly language
    d. SOL

Ans. (c) Assembly language

20. Half life of a radioactive element is one year. If at present there is one atom what is probability that it will not decay in next two years

    a. 1/2
    b. 1
    c. 1/4
    d. 0

Ans. (d) 0

21. Consider a weightless pulley, wire and spring as show in figure

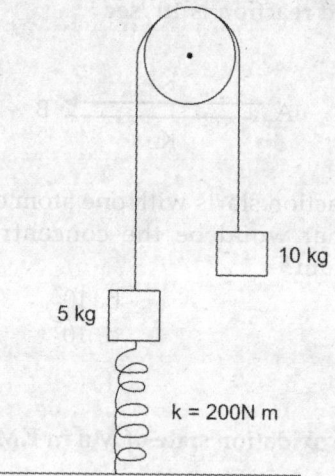

At balanced state what would be extensionb in spring

    a. 1 m
    b. 0.5 m
    c. 0.5 cm
    d. 0.1 cm

Ans. (b) 0.5 m

22. In the figure blow A and B are two point on wire. R is resistance and D is diode, wire is finally grounded at end

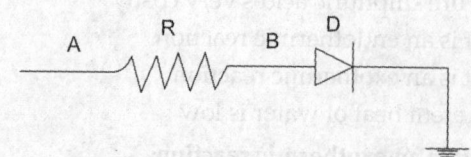

The effect of applied voltage V_A at point A on point $B(V_B)$ can be represented as-

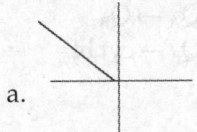 a.

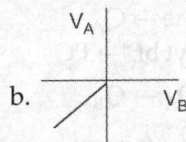 b.

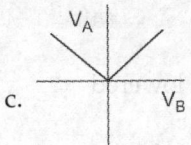 c.

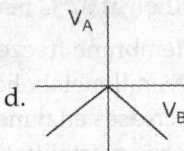 d.

23. An element was having 3×10^{29} atom at beginning of decay. At present it has 10^{20} atom, then ha fife of element is

a. Log 3/2
b. Log 2/3
c. Log 2
d. Log 3

Ans. (a) Log 3/2

24. If x is real integer, then the solution of equation will be

$F(x) = \log x (\log_e x)$ will be

a. 0
b. 1
c. Infinity
d. Cannot be predicted

Ans. (b) 1

25. Number of subsets in set of 'n' integer will be

a. n
b. 2^n
c. n+1/2
d. n(n+1)/2

Ans. (b) 2^n

SECTION B

1. Activity of Receptor tyros8ne kinase is regulated by

a. Phosphorylation
b. Dephosphorylation
c. Methylation
d. Acetylation

Ans. (b) dephosphorylation

2. Which of the following cell possess poly morphonucleus

a. B- cells
b. Neutrophils
c. Macrophage
d. Erythrocyte

Ans. (b) Neutrophils

3. DNA fragmentation is characteristic feature of

a. Cell death
b. Mutation
c. Cancer growth
d. Cell division

Ans. (a) Cell death

4. Complete photosynthetic apparatus of chloroplast necessary for photosynthyesis is coded by

a. Nuclear gene
b. Chloroplast gene
c. Nuclear and chloroplast gene
d. Chloroplast and mitochondrial genes

Ans. (c) Nuclear and chloroplast gene

5. Characterstc feature of k-selected species is

a. High intrinsic rate of groth
b. Small size and large number of offspring
c. Larger age at first reproduction
d. Short life span

Ans. (c) Larger age at first reproduction

6. Correct statement regarding the effect of ozone on biosphere is

a. Both atmospheric and stratospheric ozone is beneficial
b. Both atmospheric and stratospheric ozone s harmful
c. Atmospheric ozone s harmful but stratospheric ozone is beneficial
d. Atmospheric ozone s beneficial but stratospheric ozone s harmful

Ans. (c) Atmospheric ozone s harmful but stratospheric ozone is beneficial

7. During evolution if a single species give rise to may descendents of different phylogenetic taxons it is termed as

a. Clade
b. Cline
c. Cluster
d. Clone

Ans. (a) Clade

8. Biological species concept cannot be applied on

a. Parthenogenic species
b. Sympatric species
c. Species producing viable hybrids
d. Species of aquatic ecosystem

Ans. (c) Species producing viable hybrids

9. Increase in amount of the following is NOT a consequence of sewage effluents in river system

a. Microbial load
b. Phosphate level
c. Dissolved oxygen
d. Cynobacterial density

Ans. (c) Dissolved oxygen

10. In grasslands ergot feeds follows grazing cows. Cow during grazing exposes insects from grasses to ergots. This is an example of

a. Commensalisms

b. Parasitism

c. Ammensalism

d. Mutualism

Ans. (a) Commensalisms

11. The plant species which produces both oil and dye is

a. Sesannum indicum

b. Canavalia gladicosa

c. Carhamus tinctorinus

d. Riccinus cumminis

Ans. (c) Carhamus tinctorinus

12. Dfference at species and sub species level and gene flow between population is best illustrated by

a. Allozyme

b. Amino acid sequence

c. Double diffusion serology

d. Isoeletric

Ans. (a) Allozyme

13. Biodiversity hot spots are characterized on the basis of

a. Endemic fowering plants and threat perception

b. Endemic flowering plants

c. Species of flowering plants

d. Threat perception

Ans. (b) Endemic flowering plants

14. Sustainable harvesting for a fish population growing logistically is done by

a. Above carrying capacity

b. At carrying capacity

c. At half of the carrying capacity

d. At lowest level

Ans. (c) At half of the carrying capacity

15. Consider the following assumption

I. All known living organism is more then parasite

II. A single host species can harbour more then one type of parasites

III. Parasites are species specific

From above information it can be conclude that

a. Species of host oragansm is more then parasites

b. Species of parasites is more then host organisms

c. Number of parasite is equal to number of host

d. No valid conclusion can be drawn

Ans. (b) Species of parasites is more then host organisms

16. Dichloropheny dimethy urea inhibits photoshythesis at photosystem during

a. phe $\rightarrow Q_A$

b. $Q_A \rightarrow Q_B$

c. Cyt bf$_6$ $\rightarrow$ PC

d. $Q_B \rightarrow$ cyt bf$_6$

Ans. (b) $Q_A \rightarrow Q_B$

17. The bacteria can be best stored under starvation at 4°C then at 37°C because

a. Membrane freezes

b. Overall metabolic activity is lowered

c. Increases enzyme efficiency

d. Large mortality so low competition

Ans. (b) Overall metabolic activity is lowered

18. Which of the following index does not show relative abundance of species

a. Shanon weaver

b. Simpson

c. Brillion

d. Species richness

Ans. (d) Species richness

19. In caryophyllales the type of sieve tube plasmid is

a. Type-IIIP

b. TYPE- S

c. TYPE- C

d. TYPE- A

Ans. (a) Type-IIIP

20. Cardiac muscles can not be tetanised because

a. Resistant to tetanus toxin

b. Autorythmicity

c. Leng Refratory period

d. Highly evolved muscles

Ans. (c) Leng Refratory period

21. Correct order for increasing order of primary productivity is

a. Ocean-Desert-Tropical deciduous forest-tropical rain forest

b. Desert-Tropical deciduous- Ocean –Tropical rain forest

c. Tropical rain forest-Ocean-Tropical deciduous-Deserts

d. Tropical deciduous-desert-Ocean-tropical rain forest

Ans. (a) Ocean-Desert-Tropical deciduous forest-tropical rain forest

22. Silica cells are present in the member of family

a. Annonaceae

b. Poacaeae

c. Orchidaceae

d. Lamaceae

Ans. (b)

23. **Type III survivorship curve is shown by**

   a. Birds
   b. Pelagic fishes
   c. Humans
   d. Phytophagous insect

Ans. (b) Pelagic fishes

24. **The dwarfing gene which was responsible for green revolution is involved in signal transduction of over expression of**

   a. Gibberlic acid
   b. Cytokinin
   c. Absicic acid
   d. Ethylene

Ans. (a) Gibberlic acid

25. **Anemia due to lack of haemoglobin is associated with**

   a. Iron deficiency
   b. Calcium deficiency
   c. Vitamin B-6
   d. Vitamin B-12

Ans. (a) Iron deficiency

26. **Among the following hypothalum peptide hormone which is smallest**

   a. GnRH
   b. CRH
   c. TRH
   d. GH-RH

Ans. (c) TRH

27. **According to present concept the main cause of extinction of dinosaurs was**

   a. Competition
   b. Meteorite striking
   c. Environment change
   d. Unknown

Ans. (b) Meteorite striking

28. **Fat soluble vitamin involved in bone formation and blood clotting was**

   a. Vit D and Vit K
   b. Vit B and Vit D
   c. Vit D and Vit B
   d. Vit A and Vit K

Ans. (a) Vit D and Vit K

29. **In *E.coli* lac operon is positively as well as negatively regulated. It mean**

   a. *E.coli* depends only on glucose
   b. Depends only on lactose
   c. Can use both glucose and lactose simultaneously
   d. Use lactose only when glucose is absent

Ans. (c) Can use both glucose and lactose simultaneously

30. **Replcative transposons increases their copy number by relicating its copies and inserting into new position while keeping its copy at original place. The enzyme involved in this process are**

   a. Transposase
   b. Transposase and integrase

   c. Transosase and Resolvase
   d. Transosase, Resolvase and Integrase

Ans. (c) Transosase and Resolvase

31. **Generally limiting factor for primary productivity in aquatic ecosystem is**

   a. Nitrogen
   b. Phosphorus
   c. Sulphur
   d. Carbon

Ans. (b) Phosphorus

32. **During opening of stomata which ions are transported from neighbouring cells to guard cell**

   a. K^+ ion
   b. Cl^- ion
   c. Na^+ ion
   d. Ca^{++} ion

Ans. (a) K^+ ion

33. **Inhibitor of RNA polymerase during elongation of transcripton n both prokaryotes and eukaryotes is**

   a. Rifamcin
   b. á- aminitin
   c. streptomycin
   d. Actinomycin-D

Ans. (d) Actinomycin-D

34. **C-vlaue paradox suggest us about**

   a. Colinearity between genome size and complexity of organism
   b. Non- colinearity between genome size and complexity of organism
   c. Dosage compensation
   d. Number of chromosome

Ans. (b) Non- colinearity between genome size and complexity of organism

35. **Conctration of urine in mammls depends on**

   a. Glomerulus's
   b. Length of Henly's loop
   c. Osmotic pressure of blood
   d. Size of organism

Ans. (b) Length of Henly's loop

36. **If organism is triploid, then hardy-weinberg theorem applicable will be**

   a. $(p+q)^3$
   b. $(p+q)^2$
   c. $(p+q+r)^3$
   d. $(p+q+r)^2$

Ans. (d) $(p+q+r)^2$

37. **During the process of selection if number of individual are more in heterozygote state as compare to both homozygote, under such condition**

   a. Both alles well coexist in population
   b. Only dominant alleles will exist

c. Only recessive alleles will exist

d. Both the alleles will be lost

Ans. (a) Both alles well coexist in population

38. In honey bee queen and worker are diploid while male are haploid. It a queen honey bee is fertilized with equal number of sperms from two different males, then genetic relatedness in progeny

    a. 0.75
    b. 0.5
    c. 0.25
    d. 0.46

Ans. (d) 0.46

39. If mutation changes codon in such a way that there s no effect on functioning and overall structure of protein. This type of mutation is termed as

    a. Silent
    b. Mis-sense
    c. Transition
    d. Frameshift

Ans. (a) Silent

40. Which statement is true about nucleosome model of chromatin in eukaryotes

    a. It consist of one unit each of H2A, H2B, H3,H4 and 200 bp of DNA
    b. It consist of two unit each of H2A, H2B, H3, H4 and 200 bp of DNA
    c. It consist of H1 and 200 bp of DNA
    d. It consist of histone and non-histone protein

Ans. (b) It consist of two unit each of H2A, H2B, H3, H4 and 200 bp of DNA

41. Genetically identical nucleus are present in embryo sac of type

    a. Polygonum
    b. Adoxa
    c. Plumbago
    d. Fratillium

Ans. (a) Polygonum

42. YAC behaves similar t normal chromosomes because it possess

    a. Centromere
    b. Centromere and telomere
    c. Telomere and ARS
    d. Centromere, telomere and ARS

Ans. (d) Centromere, telomere and ARS

43. Angiosperms originated during

    a. Upper cretaceous
    b. Mid cretaceous
    c. Lower Jurassic
    d. Carboniferous

Ans. (b) Carboniferous

44. Paternal grandfather is haemophilic what is probability of his grandson to be hemohilic

    a. 1/2
    b. 1/4
    c. 1/8
    d. 0

Ans. (d) 0

45. Lipid phase transition and movement can be studies using

    a. ESR
    b. NMR
    c. Electron microscopy
    d. Phase contrast microscopy

Ans. (a) ESR

46. Split genes are present in

    a. All eukaryotes
    b. Most of eukaryotes and some Archaebacteria
    c. Most of eukaryotes and some eubacteria
    d. All organisms

Ans. (b) Most of eukaryotes and some Archaebacteria

47. Sucrose dose not occur in its anomeric from while its hydrolyzed products glucose and fructose have anomers. The reason is

    a. C1 of glucose and C1 of fructose are bounded in glycosidic linkage
    b. C2 of glucose and C2 of fructose are bounded in glycosidic linkage
    c. Sucrose is polysaccharide
    d. Sucrose is not soluble in water

Ans. (b) C2 of glucose and C2 of fructose are bounded in glycosidic linkage

48. Darwinian finches of three different size of beaks-large, intermediate and small feeds on seed. Size with bimodia distribution. Under such condition natural selection will favour finches having beak size

    a. Intermediate
    b. Large
    c. Large and small
    d. Large and intermediate

Ans. (c) Large and small

49. All of the mendelian alleles for different traits showed

    a. Epistasis
    b. Co dominance
    c. Incomplete dominance
    d. Dominance and recessiveness

Ans. (d) Dominance and recessiveness

50. UV-B induced damage of DNA by formation of pyridimine dimmer are repaired by photolyase on activation by

a. UV-C light

b. Green light

c. Blue light

d. IR light

Ans. (c) Blue light

51. If tow bacterial culture are growing exponentially with different in their intrinsic rate of growth. The difference in population of both will differ

a. Increased linearly

b. Decreased linearly

c. Increased exponentially

d. Decreased exponentially

Ans. (c) Increased exponentially

52. Translocation of photosynthatase in plant occurs through

a. Xylem

b. Phloem

c. Cambium

d. Endodermis

Ans. (b) Phloem

53. During evolution first multicellular organisms appeared during

a. 1 billion year ago

b. 2 billion

c. 600 million

d. 200 million

Ans. (a) 1 billion year ago

54. The amount of radiation hitting the retina per second is 2×10^6 Js of wavelength 600Å. The number of photon received per second by eye is

a. 6000

b. 4000

c. 2000

d. 3000

Ans. (a) 6000

55. The most probable amino acid occurring at bents and turns of polypeptide is

a. Proline

b. Leucine

c. Phenyl Alanine

d. Tryptophan

Ans. (a) Proline

56. Among the following which statement is correct regarding the promoter of the gene

a. It is always located upstreme of transcription start site

b. It is located downstream of translation start site

c. Different promoter elements are recognized by different RNA polymerase

d. None of these

Ans. (c) Different promoter elements are recognized by different RNA polymerase

57. Which of the following types of cells would you expect to contain a high density of Cytoplasmic intermediate filament?

a. Amoeba

b. Sperm

c. Epithelial cells

d. Plant cells

Ans. (c) Epithelial cells

58. Sodium laural sulphate disrupts protein by changing their

a. Primary structure

b. Primary and secondary structure

c. Secondary and tertiary structure

d. Secondary, tertiary and quarternary structure

Ans. (d) Secondary, tertiary and quarternary structure

59. Among the following which is responsible for nerve action potential

a. Influx of Na^+ and K^+

b. Out flux of Na^+ and K^+

c. Influx of Na^+ and out flux K^+

d. Out flux of Na^+ and influx K^+

Ans. (c) Influx of Na^+ and out flux K^+

60. Which molecule is continuously transported from nucleus to cytoplasm

a. DNA

b. RNA

c. Histone

d. Ribosome

Ans. (b) RNA

61. In severe combination immumodeficiency syndrome there is

a. Low number of Neutrophils

b. Low number of T or B cells

c. Low macrophages

d. Low amount of IgG

Ans. (b) Low number of T or B cells

62. In human somatic cell number of kenetochore at mitosis is

a. 23

b. 44

c. 46

d. 92

Ans. (c) 46

63. In meiosis crossing over occur during

a. Prophase-I

b. Prophase-II

c. Metaphase

d. Anaphase

Ans. (a) Prophase-I

64. The order of reaction catalyzed by enzyme at low substrate concentration

a. First order   b. Pseudo first order

c. Second order   d. Zero order

Ans. (a) First order

65. If the Km of enzyme for substrate A is 1×10^{-4} and for substrate B is 4×10^{-8}. It means

a. Enzyme has more affinity for substrate A then substrate B

b. Enzyme has more affinity for substrate B then substrate A

c. Enzyme has equal affinity for substrate A and substrate B

d. Enzyme is non-specific

Ans. (b) Enzyme has more affinity for substrate B then substrate A

66. In a sexuality responding organisms which is most important barrier for speciation

a. Geographical   b. Reproductive

c. Temporal   d. Ethological

Ans. (b) Reproductive

67. Source of energy for Urey and Miller experiment was

a. Electric spark

b. UV

c. Glycine

d. ATP

Ans. (a) Electric spark

68. Which national park is not correctly matched with its organism

a. Ranthambore Bengal Tiger

b. Rajaji Holleck gibbon

c. Kanchanjanga Rhinoceros

d. Bandipur Elephant

Ans. (b) Rajaji Holleck gibbon

69. Change in allele frequency at species or below species level is termed as

a. Microevolution

b. Macroevolution

c. Mega evolution

d. Silent evolution

Ans. (a) Microevolution

Memory Based Paper CSIR NET Dec 2007

1. The circuitis shown as follows with a true diode and circuit is finally earthed. The relationship between the V and I will be

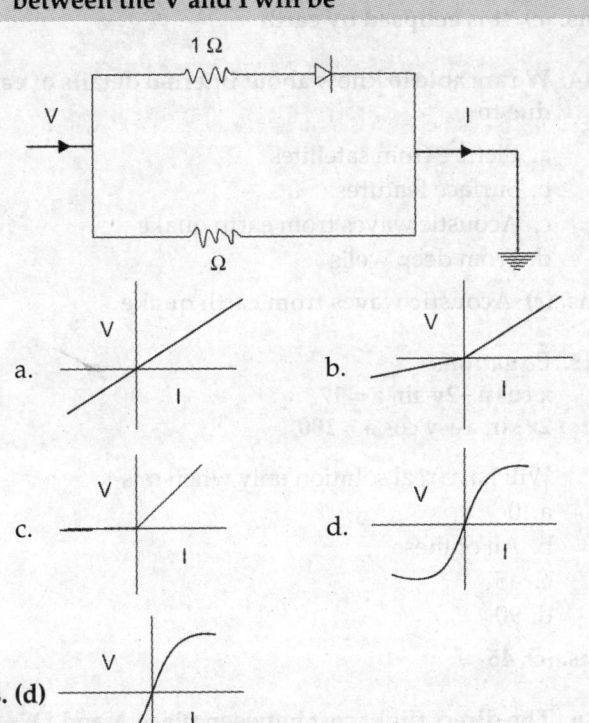

a.

b.

c.

d.

Ans. (d)

2. The pulley system is in equilibrium as shown in figure. Neglect mass of Pulley, what would be the mass of "M"

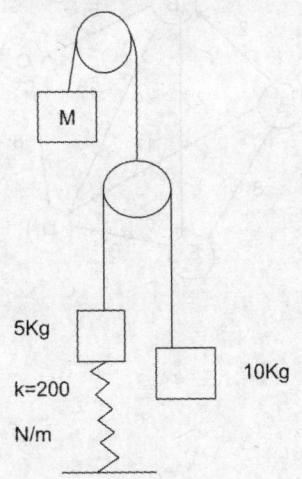

a. 10 kg
b. 5 kg
c. 2.5 kg
d. 20 kg

Ans. (d) 20 kg

3. If an beam of electron with velocity 4×10^8m/s enters along positive X axis in the magnet field 0.003 T aligned on positive Z axis. The change in path of electron will be

a. Curved along negative Z axis
b. Along positive Z axis
c. Along negative Y axis
d. Along Positive Y axis

Ans. (c) Along negative Y axis

4. Considering the earth as perfect black body. It is given that = 2900/T where T is 290K. The maximum radiation emitted by the earth will fall in which range of Electromagnetic spectrum

a. UV
b. Visible
c. X- rays
d. IR rays

Ans. (d) IR rays

5. A wire of length 'l' and cross section area 'A' has resistance 'R'. Another wire of length '2l' and Area of cross section 'A/2' will have resistance equal to

a. R
b. 2R
c. 4R
d. 8R

Ans. (c) 4R

6. When one gram ^{238}U is converted into Pb, eight a particles are emitted. The mass of Pb will be

a. 0 gm
b. Less than 1 gm
c. 1 gm
d. 206/208

Ans. (d) 206/208

7. A man along with a cylinder filled with Helium gas and a balloon was sitting in a boat. He fills some of gas from cylinder to the balloon as a result balloon swells. [Hint Do not neglect the density of air] What is effect on boat in water

a. Boat will rise in water
b. Boat will sink little in water

c. No effect on boat

d. Data are not sufficient to draw conclusion

Ans. (a) Boat will rise in water

8. Among the following which has highest boiling point

a. CH_3OH

b. CH_3CH_2OH

c.
$$CH_3 - \overset{\overset{\displaystyle CH_3}{|}}{\underset{\underset{\displaystyle CH_3}{|}}{C}} - OH$$

d. $CH_3CH_2CH_2CH_2OH$

Ans. (c)
$$CH_3 - \overset{\overset{\displaystyle CH_3}{|}}{\underset{\underset{\displaystyle CH_3}{|}}{C}} - OH$$

9. IUPAC name of given structure will be

$$CH_3 - \underset{\underset{\underset{\displaystyle CH_3}{|}}{\underset{\displaystyle CH_2}{|}}}{CH} - CH_2 - CH_2 - OH_3$$

a. 2-methyl pentane

b. 4 –methyl pentane

c. 3 methyl hexane

d. 4-methyl hexane

Ans. (c) 3 methyl hexane

10. If in a balloon air is filled, it was observed that it denies Boyles rule P a 1/V because as air is filled both the Pressure and volume inside the balloon increases. The explanation for this is

a. Air is not an real gas

b. Boyles law is applicable at low temperatures only

c. It is applicable at high temperatures only

d. Boyles law is applicable at all temp

Ans. (c) It is applicable at high temperatures only

11. If an substrate changes from X to Y and finally to Z by an first order reaction. The rate constant of X Y is 0.2 sec^{-1} and Y Z is 200 sec^{-1}. The overall rate of reaction from X Z will be

a. 0.2 sec^{-1}

b. 100 sec

c. 200 sec

d. 400 sec

Ans. (a) 0.2 sec^{-1}

12. Considering the isothermal condition, what would be change in the atmospheric pressure at height 0 Km, 8 Km and 16 Km .

a. No change

b. 1, 0.5, 0

c. 2, 1, 0

d. 4, 2, 0

Ans. (b) 1, 0.5, 0

13. Venus is visible only during the morning or evening because

a. It rotate very fast

b. It has very elliptical path

c. It is eclipsed by earth

d. It revolving path is smaller as compare to earth

Ans. (c) It is eclipsed by earth

14. We are able to know about internal details of earth due to

a. Picture from satellites

b. Surface features

c. Acoustic waves from earth quake

d. From deep wells

Ans. (c) Acoustic waves from earth quake

15. Equations

$x \cos a - 2y \sin a = 17$

$2x \sin a + y \cos a = 100$

Will have real solution only when α is

a. 0

b. All of these

c. 45

d. 90

Ans. (c) 45

16. The direct flight cost between place A and D is 17. What would be the minimum flight cost between A and D by any route?

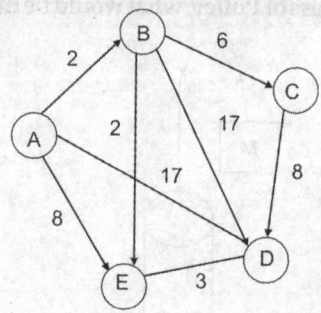

a. 7

b. 9

c. 14

d. 17

Ans. (a) 7

17. Peripheral devices are attached to computer to increase its basic functioning. Among the following which is not an peripheral device.

   a. USB flash drive   b. CPU

   c. Modem   d. Printer

Ans. (b) CPU

18. Floating number in computer has

   a. Indefinite range and indefinite precision

   b. Definite range and indefinite precision

   c. Definite range and definite precision

   d. Indefinite range and definite precision

Ans. (c) Definite range and definite precision

19. A is an array A[1], A[2].... A[10]

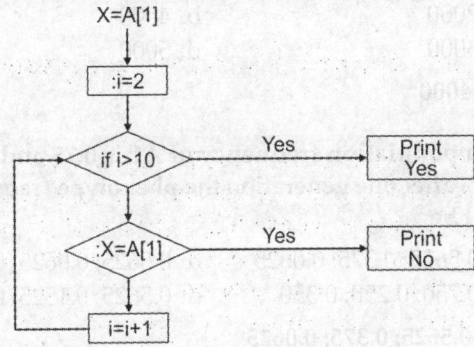

Programme will print " Yes" if the array A is

   a. Is sorted in increasing order

   b. Is sorted in decreasing order

   c. Has first element repeated

   d. Has a element less then 10

Ans. (c) Has first element repeated

20. First cell to be differentiated in developing embryo is

   a. Epithelial cells   b. Rods

   c. RBC   d. Nerves cells

Ans. (a) Epithelial cells

21. In plant if the sequence 5'-GATGGCACGAT-3' is transcribed, the corresponding m-RNA will be

   a. 5'-CUACCGUGCUA-3'

   b. 5'-GAUGGCACGAU- 3'

   c. 5-AUGUCCAUC-3'

   d. 5'-ATGTCCATC-3'

Ans. (c) 5-AUGUCCAUC-3'

22. Which of the following vaccine does not provide lifetime protection

   a. Typhoid

   b. Tetanus

   c. Polio

   d. Small pox

Ans. (b) Tetanus

23. The special roots termed as pneumatophores are visible at

   a. Oceans   b. Mangroves

   c. Epiphytes   d. Salt stress

Ans. (b) Mangroves

24. Efficiency of ATP synthesis is 40% and enthalpy of reaction ADP + iP → ATP is 8 K cal. If an individual consumes 2000 K cal, then the net ATP production from it would be

   a. 40   b. 100

   c. 200   d. 500

Ans. (b) 100

25. Pearl oysters are obtained from the genus

   a. Oysteria   b. Pinctada

   c. Mytillus   d. Pila

Ans. (b) Pinctada

26. Temperature sensitive mutation are important in molecular biology because it help in studying

   a. Genes for heat stress

   b. Genes for cold stress

   c. Genes necessary for survival of cell

   d. Genes required for development

Ans. (c) Genes necessary for survival of cell

27. In ecosystem the concept of entropy is used to explain

   a. Photosynthesis efficiency

   b. Energy flow in trophic level

   c. Population growth

   d. Competition

Ans. (b) Energy flow in trophic level

28. Rate of reaction for first order reaction for an radioisotope is 6.93×10^{-2} sec^{-1}. What is half life of radioisotope

   a. 10 sec   b. 100 sec

   c. 0 sec   d. 1000 sec

Ans. (a) 10 sec

29. Chlorinated hydrocarbons effects ecosystem by

   a. Biomagnifications   b. Bioconcentration

   c. Bioaccumulation   d. Bioremediation

Ans. (a) Biomagnifications

30. Morphologically similar species when interbreed produced viable fertile offspring. They are considered as single species according to

    a. Biological species concept
    b. Evolutionary species concept
    c. Genetic species concept
    d. Morphospecies concept

Ans. (a) Biological species concept

31. Natural selection against extreme phenotype is termed as

    a. Directional selection
    b. Diversifying selection
    c. Disruptive selection
    d. Stabilizing selection

Ans. (d) Stabilizing selection

32. At any OTU following dendrogram was obtained

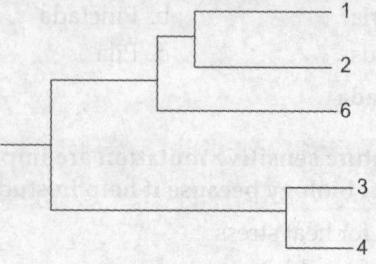

    Here species i, 2 and 6 represents
    a. Evolutionary relationship
    b. Phylogenetic relationship
    c. Overall smlarity
    d. Genetic similarity

Ans. (c) Evolutionary relationship

33. Extensive phyletic diversification of animals was obtained in

    a. Cambrian
    b. Silurian
    c. Devonian
    d. Mesozoic

Ans. (a) Cambrian

34. Which one of the following statement is not true for edge effect of two ecosystems

    a. T has its distinct physical environment differing from both side
    b. Moving corridors are always harmful
    c. It has different species composition as compare to both side
    d. It has high biodiversity

Ans. (b) Moving corridors are always harmful

35. In habitat A pike cichlid fishes preferentially feeds on large adult guppies, so guppies mature later and is of small size while in habitat B killer fish feeds on small, juvenile guppies so here guppies mature early and are large size. What will be effect if experimentally guppies for habitat A are transferred to habitat B.

    a. No change would be seen
    b. Mature late but small size adults
    c. Mature early but large size adults
    d. Mature late but large size adults

Ans. (c) Mature early but large size adults

36. If in a metabolic reaction at temperature 27°C increased in enthalpy is 1000 J and decreased in entropy is 10 J. Calculate the change in free energy

    a. 2000   b. 4000
    c. 3000   d. 5000

Ans. (b) 4000

37. In a population frequency of A1 is 0.75 and A2 is 0.25. after one generation the phenotype frequency will be

    a. 0.5625; 0.375; 0.0625   b. 0.5625; 0.0625; 0.375
    c. 0.750; 0.250; 0.350   d. 0.5625; 0.1525; 0.0625

Ans. (a) 0.5625; 0.375; 0.0625

38. The curve shown below shows a relationship between

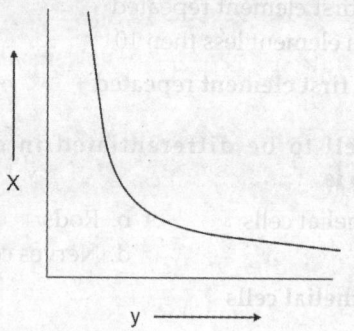

    a. Time (X) and population density (Y)
    b. Body size (X) and generation time (Y)
    c. Area (X) and number of species (Y)
    d. Fish length (X) and fish body weight (Y)

Ans. (b) Body size (X) and generation time (Y)

39. Phenotype A has selective advantage over B, B has over C and C has over A. The condition is like "paper-scissor-rock". Under such condition in nature

    a. All phenotype would be selected
    b. Only A and C would be selected

c. A and B together seleted

d. Only B would be selected

Ans. (a) All phenotype would be selected

---

40. Among the following which organelle is involved in apoptosis

a. Lysosome   b. ER

c. Golgi   d. Mitochondria

Ans. (d) Mitochondria

---

41. Tiger is not found in wild at

a. Punjab   b. Rajasthan

c. UP   d. Arunchal pradesh

Ans. (c) UP

---

42. Taxol, an anti-cancerous drug effects

a. Inhibiting polymerization of tubulin

b. Inhibiting depoymerization of tubulin

c. Polymerization of actin

d. Favouring depolymerisation of tubulin

Ans. (b) Inhibiting depoymerization of tubulin

---

43. Distance between gene A and B is 10 cM. If the F1 genotype $\dfrac{A \qquad B}{a \qquad b}$ was test crossed then what is probability of obtaining $\dfrac{A \qquad B}{a \qquad b}$ genotype

a. 40   b. 45

c. 50   d. 55

Ans. (b) 40

---

44. A spirin delays senescence in cut part of plant and keeps flower fresh for longer time . the effect of aspirin is

a. By increasing the synthesis of cytokinins

b. By decreasing the synthesis of absisic acid

c. By decreasing the synthesis of ethylene

d. By increasing the synthesis of gibberlic acid

Ans. (c) By decreasing the synthesis of ethylene

---

45. Gibberlic acid stimulates seed germination in monocots by activation of degradative enzyme by acting on

a. Endosperm   b. Embryo

c. Cotyledons   d. Aleurone layer

Ans. (d) Aleurone layer

---

46. Hemidesmosomes are structure found between

a. Two adjacent plant cells

b. Two adjacent animals cells

c. Between cell and extracellular matrix

d. Within a bacteria

Ans. (c) Between cell and extracellular matrix

---

47. Lymphatic system are mainly involved in

a. Innate immunity   b. Acquired immunity

c. Phagocytosis   d. Recycling lymph

Ans. (b) Acquired immunity

---

48. A zygote formed by a fusion of one normal gamete and another gamete where one of the chromosomes did not segregated at anaphase-II will lead into chromosomal aberration known as

a. Haploidy   b. Diploidy

c. Polyploidy   d. Aneuploidy

Ans. (d) Aneuploidy

---

49. The fluid mosaic model of plasma membrane given by singer and Nicolson is applicable to

a. Only prokaryotic membrane

b. Only eukaryotic membrane

c. Both prokaryotic and Eukaryotic membrane

d. Only to organelle membrane

Ans. (c) Both prokaryotic and Eukaryotic membrane

---

50. During which phase of infection cycle, the DNA polymerase of T_4-Phage is expressed maximally

a. Immediate early   b. Early

c. Late   d. Middle

Ans. (b) Early

---

51. In a chemical reaction catalyzed by enzyme following the Michales-menten equation what will be the concentration of substrate when the velocity of reaction s 90% of the maximum velocity

a. 5 Km   b. 6 Km

c. 8 Km   d. 9 Km

Ans. (d) 9 Km

---

52. Which of the following is involved in intermolecular hydrogen bonding with water

a. Urea   b. CH_4

c. CCl_4 d. $CHCl_3$

Ans. (a) Urea

---

53. If the length of one helix in DNA is 34 Å. The type of DNA is

a. A   b. B

c. C   d. D

Ans. (a) A

54. **Which statement is NOT correct regarding the genetic code**

    a. One Amino acid can have more then one codon

    b. In eukaryotes the start codon is AUG

    c. Genetic codes are not strictly universal

    d. Third base of anticodon in not necessary for specificity

Ans. (d) **Third base of anticodon in not necessary for specificity**

55. **In prokaryotes there is single multifunctional fatty acyl synthase sufficient for complete fatty acid synthesis where as in eukaryotes there are many different enzymes involved in fatty acid synthesis. The probable explanation for this difference is**

    a. Fatty acid synthesis is more stringent n eukaryotes

    b. Synthesis of fatty acid is by different mechanism in eukaryotes as compare to prokaryotes

    c. For better regulation of fatty acid synthesis in eukaryotes

    d. Fatty acids of eukaryotes are different from the prokaryotes

Ans. (c) **For better regulation of fatty acid synthesis in eukaryotes**

56. **Vitamin B complex is an essential for humans because**

    a. It is obtained only from plant sources

    b. It s obtained only from animal sources

    c. It act as cofactor for various metabolic reactions

    d. It s directly utilized in various metabolic reactions

Ans. (c) **It act as cofactor for various metabolic reactions**

57. **In submerged roots of mangrove plants the recycling of NAD+ is carried out by**

    a. Cellular oxidation

    b. Glycolysis

    c. Electron transport chain

    d. Fermentative metabolism

Ans. (d) **Fermentative metabolism**

58. **Electron acceptor in anaerobic condition in prokaryotes is**

    a. Glucose, fructose, maltose

    b. Fatty acids

    c. SO_4^{-2}, NO_3^{-2}

    d. Antioxidants such as vitamin K

Ans. (c) SO_4^{-2}, NO_3^{-2}

59. **The biggest disadvantage of sexual reproduction against the asexual reproduction is**

    a. Only half of genetic material is passed to offspring from each parent

    b. Lot of energy and time is consumed n locating mate

    c. At least two individual are required for sexual reproduction

    d. After fertilization in many cases zygote fails to develop

Ans. (a) **Only half of genetic material is passed to offspring from each parent**

60. **In test cross F1 progeny is crossed with**

    a. Either of the parent   b. Recessive parent

    c. Dominant parent   d. Heterozygous parent

Ans. (b) **Recessive parent**

61. **Polytene chromosome is generated due to**

    a. Failure of DNA replication

    b. Repeated DNA replication without segregation chromosomes

    c. Pairing of homologous chromosome

    d. Due to extensive transcription process

Ans. (b) **Repeated DNA replication without segregation chromosomes**

62. **An bacterial operon contains three structural genes A,B and C n the same order. If polar mutation occurs in gene B, then the effect in protein would be observed in**

    a. In all protein A, B and C

    b. Only in B and C

    c. Only in B

    d. Complete loss of all protein

Ans. (c) **Only in B**

63. **Among the following, which is sex linked disorder**

    a. Night blindness   b. Colour blindness

    c. Cretinism   d. Myxoderma

Ans. (b) **Colour blindness**

64. **Among the following which statement is not correct for X-linked recessive disorder**

    a. Females carrying the diseased allele are always diseased

    b. Males carrying the diseased allele are always diseased

    c. Females are diseased only when their mother is carrier and father is diseased

    d. Males always passes trait to all of his sons

Ans. (d) **Males always passes trait to all of his sons**

65. C-value measure

 a. Haploid content of genome
 b. Diploid content of genome
 c. Poly haploid genome content
 d. Anueploid genome content

Ans. (a) Haploid content of genome

66. The most ancient mode of energy generating metabolic reactions are

 a. Photosynthesis
 b. Oxidation of nitrate
 c. Reduction of sulphate
 d. Reduction of nitrate

Ans. (c) Reduction of sulphate

67. Chemolithotroph obtained their carbon from CO2 and energy from

 a. Sunlight
 b. Water
 c. Inorganic compound
 d. Organic compound

And. (c) Inorganic compound

68. Carrying capacity of a forest is 20 tones which increased 10% of its biomass annually. For sustainable forestry how much trees can be harvested for timber so that is has minimum effect on forest and can be harvested annually

 a. 2 tone
 b. 1 tone
 c. 0.5 tone
 d. 5 tone

Ans. (b) 1 tone

69. The characterstic of a population with low value of intrinsic growth (r = 0.2) is

 a. Later age at maturity and small clutch size
 b. Early age at maturity and small clutch size
 c. Late age at maturity and large clutch size
 d. Early age at maturity and large clutch size

Ans. (a) Later age at maturity and small clutch size

70. The characteristic survivorship curve III is shown by

 a. Fruit flies
 b. Pelagic fishes
 c. Birds
 d. Humans

Ans. (b) Pelagic fishes

71. Which statement is correct regarding arteries and veins

 a. Arteries has single valve while veins has two valves
 b. There is no difference
 c. Arteries carry deoxygenated blood and has thicker walls
 d. Veins contain deoxygenated blood and has thinner walls

Ans. (d) Veins contain deoxygenated blood and has thinner walls

72. Which statement is true regarding spore and seed

 a. Spore always generate diploid organisms
 b. Spore always give rise to sporophyte generation while gamete fuses with another haploid cells to give rise to zygote
 c. Spore and gametes are identical
 d. Spore are immotile and gametes are always motile

Ans. (b) Spore always give rise to sporophyte generation while gamete fuses with another haploid cells to give rise to zygote

73. Which is not considered as major threat to loss of species diversity

 a. Habitate destruction
 b. Overexploitation
 c. Alien invasion
 d. Pollution

Ans. (d) Pollution

74. The technique used for observing 3-D structure is

 a. Scanning electron microscopy
 b. Transmission electron microscopy
 c. Confocal microscopy
 d. UV microscopy

Ans. (a) Scanning electron microscopy

75. Pyrimidine dimmers formed due to UV rays can be repaired without removing any nucleotide by the repair mechanism known as

 a. Mismatch repair mechanism
 b. Photoactvation
 c. Base excision repair mechanism,
 d. SOS repair mechanism

Ans. (b) Photoactvation

76. Pentadactylity is a dominant trait, yet many individual having single dominant alleles does not show any sign of polydacylity. This is known as

 a. Incomplete penetrance
 b. Variable expressivity
 c. Co dominance
 d. Incomplete dominance

Ans. (a) Incomplete penetrance

77. Among the following which is not an correct explosion for high biodiversity at tropical rain forest

 a. Long evolutionary time
 b. More surface area
 c. High productivity
 d. Minimum competition

Ans. (d) Minimum competition

78. **Ribose-5-phosphate is precursor for ribose sugar in DNA and RNA and is obtained from**

    a. PPP
    b. Kerb cycle
    c. Glycolysis
    d. Aminoacids

Ans. (a) PPP

79. **First fossils were discovered**

    a. Prior to both Lamarck and Darwin
    b. Prior to Lamarck but after Darwin
    c. After Lamarck but prior to Darwin
    d. None of the above

Ans. (c) After Lamarck but prior to Darwin

80. **Prebiotic environment was different from present environment and was devoid of**

    a. CO_2
    b. O_2
    c. Atmosphere
    d. N_2

Ans. (b) O_2

81. **Type of biome in california and coastal regions of Mediterranean sea is**

    a. Taiga
    b. Savannah
    c. Chaparrals
    d. Tropical deciduous forests

Ans. (c) Chaparrals

82. **Biodiesel is obtained from**

    a. Caotropis
    b. Jatropa curcus
    c. Prosopis
    d. Catharanthus

Ans. (b) Jatropa curcus

83. **Homeotic genes are responsible for**

    a. Development
    b. Homeostasis
    c. Cell cycle
    d. Gene regulation

Ans. (a) Development

84. **An object of 1.5 m height s placed 8.5 m away from the human eye and image s formed on retina which is 1.7 cm away from the lense. The size of image will be**

    a. 3 cm
    b. 0.3 cm
    c. 3 mm
    d. 3m

Ans. (b) 0.3 cm

85. **The sign of cross between spatina X townsendaii represents**

    a. Cultivars
    b. Intergeneric hybridization
    c. Interspecific hybridization
    d. Grafts

Ans. (c) Interspecific hybridization

86. **The equation 1-Σ Pi^2 represents**

    a. Shannon weaver index
    b. Simposon index
    c. Bronaulli index
    d. Hills equation

Ans. (b) Simposon index

87. **Gram positive bacteria are further classified at generic and species level by analysis of**

    a. DNA
    b. Cell wall
    c. Protein
    d. Cell membranes

Ans. (c) Protein

88. **In E. Coli the complementation test is done by**

    a. Transformation
    b. Merozygotes
    c. Heterokaryons
    d. Making them diploid

Ans. (b) Merozygotes

89. **Absisisic acid can be degraded by**

    a. Oxidation and reduction
    b. Reduction and conjugation
    c. Oxidation and conjugation
    d. Light and oxidation

Ans. (c) Oxidation and conjugation

90. **Honey bee keep variations among the worker by**

    a. Matting with males many times
    b. Parthenogenesis
    c. Specialization of functional role
    d. Exensive recombination during oogenesis

Ans. (d) Exensive recombination during oogenesis

91. **Haematopoetic stem cells are found in**

    a. Bone marrow
    b. Skin
    c. Lymphoid organ
    d. Spleen

Ans. (a) Bone marrow

92. **Among the following which is not an density ndependent factor effecting population**

    a. Competition
    b. Food
    c. Temperature
    d. Nutrients

Ans. (c) Temperature

93. Under which condition of natural selection no allele would be lost

    a. Any one homozygote s favoured

    b. Both homozygote are favoured

    c. Heterozygote are favoured

    d. Heterozygote is not favoured

Ans. (c) Heterozygote are favoured

94. The properties of water include:

    a. Being a dipole, with the negative end at the oxygen atom

    b. A low dielectric constant

    c. A disordered structure in the liquid state

    d. The ability to form hydrophobic bonds with itself

Ans. (a) Being a dipole, with the negative end at the oxygen atom

95. A double stranded DNA has 30% thymine. The percentage of cytosine is:

    a. 70%   b. 30%

    c. 20%   d. 15%

Ans. (c) 20%

96. The isomerization of which chromophore by light is the first event in visual excitation:

    a. All- trans retinal   b. 11- cis retinal

    c. Retinol   d. Retinoic acid

Ans. (b) 11- cis retinal

97. Food web is:

    a. A matrix of food chain

    b. A series of produces

    c. A series of consumers

    d. A collection of producers and decomposers

Ans. (a) A matrix of food chain

98. An amino-acyl synthetase is responsible for:

    a. Formation of a peptide bond

    b. Binding of m-RNA to ribosomes

    c. Attaching an amino acid to an organic acid

    d. Joining to amino acid to t-RNA

Ans. (d) Joining to amino acid to t-RNA

99. Which of the following seed is used for commercial crop production:

    a. Foundation seed

    b. Registered seed

    c. Certified seed

    d. Breeders seed

Ans. (c) Certified seed

100. A mechanism that can cause a gene to move from one linkage group to another is:

    a. Translocation   b. Duplication

    c. Inversion   d. Deletion

Ans. (a) Translocation

Memory Based Paper CSIR NET June 2008

1. Among the following which process do not occur n nucleus

a. Replication
b. Transcription
c. Translation
d. Repair

Ans. (c) Translation

2. Consider the following algorithm

$n \geq 0$

f(n)

if n=0

then return 0

Else 2+ f (n-2)

Consider the initial valve of n=11, then the value returned after execution of program will be

a. 9
b. 11
c. 13
d. Program will no terminate

Ans. (d) Program will no terminate

3. Consider a series is n certain geometrical progression with exact difference 'd' between successive number. If series starts with 10 and consist 100 integers. Their sum can be represented by the equation

a. 100 (100 + 99d)
b. 100 (90 + 100d)
c. 20(50 + 99d)
d. 50(20 + 99d)

Ans. (d) 50(20 + 99d)

4. It is expected that around 2100 AD all ice in polar glaciers will melt and level of sea will increase as a consequence of global warming. What would effect of it on rotation speed of earth?

a. Increase
b. Decrease
c. No change
d. Stop

Ans. (b) Decrease

5. If a bar magnet is allowed to fall through solenoid connected to the closed circuit. Its acceleration will be

a. Equal to g
b. Greater than g
c. Smaller than g
d. It will not fall

Ans. (c) Smaller than g

6. Mumbai and Chennai are more humid cities as compare to Delhi because they are

a. Near to tropics
b. Near to equator
c. Coastal cities
d. Lies in low pressure

Ans. (c) Coastal cities

7. If accelerated charged particles with similar velocity are allowed to pass through the magnetic field which is perpendicular to their direction. It was observed that all have same radius of curvature. Thus we can conclude that

a. They have same mass
b. Have same mass: charge ration
c. Mass is directly proportional to square of charge
d. Charge is directly proportional to square of mass

Ans. (b) Have same mass: charge ration

8. Electron microscopes have comparatively better resolution as compare to light microsope because

a. They are costly
b. Uses more lenses
c. Carried out in vacuum
d. Wavelength used s lesser then visible light

Ans. (d) Wavelength used s lesser then visible light

9. If a ball of mass "m" was dropped from certain height "h". The distance covered by t after 2 sec will be

a. 4.9 m
b. 9.8 m
c. 19.6 m
d. 28 m

Ans. (c) 19.6 m

10. Elevation level altitude for a glacier is constant height when deposition of ice at top is equal to melting of ice from its base. It is estimated that height of Himalayan glaciers has reduced 500 m since ice age, considering that temperature change per km rise in height is 6°C. the global temperature during ice age as compare to present was

    a. 6° higher
    b. 3° higher
    c. 6° lower
    d. 3° lower

Ans. (d) 3° lower

11. At present half life of C^{14} is 5730 years. Its half life 11460 year ago was

    a. 5730
    b. 11460
    c. 2680
    d. 1680

Ans. (b) 11460

12. It is observed that tail of revolving comet is always directed away from sun. The probable reason is

    a. Due to gravitational pull of Saturn and Jupiter
    b. Due to repulsive force from sun
    c. Due to high seed
    d. Due to lesser evaporation at sunlight side

Ans. (b) Due to repulsive force from sun

13. Consider the following statements, where, := stands for implies to

    X:= x+y
    y:=x-y
    X:= x-y
    If x=2 and y=3, then b out put (x,y) will be
    a. 3,4
    b. 3,2
    c. 1,2
    d. 1,1

Ans. (b) 3,2

14. The order of stability in given structure would be

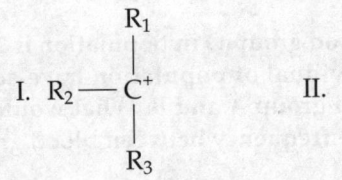

    III. $R_1 — C^+$
    a. I>II>III
    b. I<II<III
    c. II>III>I
    d. I>III>II

Ans. (a) I>II>III

15. The light falling on oil is split in to several colour due to phenomenon of

    a. Dispersion
    b. Refreaction
    c. Diffraction
    d. Interference

Ans. (d) Interference

16. Possible combination of gamete which can be formed by genotype AaBbCcDdEeFrGg are

    a. 16
    b. 32
    c. 64
    d. 128

Ans. (d) 128

17. If $f(x)=3^x$, such that f(x)=1, then value x will be

    a. 0
    b. 1
    c. 2
    d. 3

Ans. (a) 0

18. For an equation , the sum of root will be

    $X^5 +15 X^4 +10X +5X^2 +1 =0$
    a. 10
    b. 15
    c. -10
    d. -15

Ans. (d) -15

19. According to chares law a real gas at 1 atm pressure and temperature 't' was kept at absolute 0 degree. Its volume at this temperature will be

    a. 1
    b. 0
    c. V/273
    d. V/273+t

Ans. (a) 1

20. Volume of a person of 50 kg will be

    a. 50 ml
    b. 500 ml
    c. 5 lit
    d. 50 lit

Ans. (d) 50 lit

21. Which statement is correct regarding the meiosis

    a. There is two round of replication and two round of cell division
    b. There is one round of replication and one round of cell division
    c. There is one round of replication and two round of cell division
    d. There is two round of replication and one round of cell division

Ans. (c) There is one round of replication and two round of cell division

22. Which of the following monochromatic lights are more suitable for growth and development of plants

    a. Red, far red
    b. Red, blue, far red
    c. Red, green
    d. Blue, far red

Ans. (b) Red, blue, far red

23. Consider the following DNA sequence 5'-ATGGGCATAGACGATATGGTAG-3' IF DUE TO FRAME shift mutation there is insertion of G between 3rd and 4th position. Consider a reverse mutation occur n same mutated sequence. Which reverse mutation will have minimum effect in protein change

   a. Insertion of nucleotide between 5th and 6th position
   b. Insertion of three nucleotide between 5th and 6th position
   c. Deletion of a nucleotide between 5th and 6th position
   d. Deletion of a nucleotide between 11th and 12th position

Ans. (c) Deletion of a nucleotide between 5th and 6th position

24. A tryptophan auxotroph in corn showed 50 time more accumulation of IAA then the normal. Probable explanation for this is

   a. There may be some other precursor for IAA synthesis
   b. IAA is probably not inhibited by feed back mechanism
   c. IAA was not oxidized
   d. De-conjugation of ester linked IAA does not take place

Ans. (a) There may be some other precursor for IAA synthesis

25. Pitcher plant nepenthes alata would be expected to have

   a. NO$_3$- specific ion channel
   b. H$^+$-NO$_3$- symporter
   c. NH$_3$ tranporter
   d. ATP powered pump for NO$_3$-

Ans. (c) NH$_3$ tranporter

26. With time molecular distance between organisims increases during evolution due to

   a. Natural selection   b. Neutral selection
   c. Random drift   d. Point mutation

Ans. (b) Neutral selection

27. During gametohytic self incompatibility the primary response is

   a. Deposition of callose
   b. Pollen tube lysis
   c. Formation of concentric ring from golgi
   d. Self incompatibility triggers a Ca+2 dependent signaling cascade in incompatible pollen

Ans. (d) Self incompatibility triggers a Ca+2 dependent signaling cascade in incompatible pollen

28. Major cause of evolution of genes and protein is

   a. Point mutation
   b. Chromosomal aberration
   c. Sexual reproduction
   d. Gene duplication and divergence

Ans. (d) Gene duplication and divergence

29. Blood vessel A has thick wall, narrow lumen and no valves while blood vessel B has thin wall, wide lumen and have valves. Here A and B are

   a. A is artery and B is vein
   b. A is vein and B is artery
   c. A is vein and B is capillary
   d. A is capillary and B is artery

Ans. (a) A is artery and B is vein

30. Bacteria propels with the help of

   a. Actin like mreB protein
   b. Myosin
   c. Flagella made of protein flagelln
   d. Cytoskeleton

Ans. (c) Flagella made of protein flagelln

31. Photoperiodic stimulus from leaves to shoot apical meristem/ floral meristem is transported through

   a. Xylem   b. Phloem
   c. Plasmodesmata   d. Apoplast

Ans. (b) Phloem

32. Primary carnivores consume 40% production of herbivore and assimilate 70% of energy. What % of energy thee carnivores assimilates the energy available from herbivores

   a. 30   b. 28
   c. 10   d. 40

Ans. (b) 28

33. Frequency of blood group O in population is 25%. Remaining individual of population have equal number of blood group A and B. What would be the ratio of allele frequency between blood group O, A and B

   a. 1:1:1   b. 2:2:1
   c. 1:1:2   d. 3:3:1

Ans. (b) 2:2:1

34. The adaptation related to high altitude is

   a. Increase in RBC count
   b. Decrease in RBC count
   c. Increase affinity for oxygen by haemoglobin
   d. Decrease affinity for oxygen by haemoglobin

Ans. (a) Increase in RBC count

35. Natural selection is primarily based on fitness which is dependent on maximum number of offspring laid for next generation but at present new concept is added where organism help in reproduction of relatives to increase the overall fitness. This concept is termed as

    a. Evolutionary fitness
    b. Inclusive fitness
    c. Relative fitness
    d. Kin selection

Ans. (b) Inclusive fitness

36. Goucher disease where glucocerebrocde are not degraded is related to

    a. Mitochondria
    b. Lysosome
    c. Peroxisomes
    d. Golgi

Ans. (b) Lysosome

37. The genes for improving rice cultivars have been taken from the Indian rice variety

    a. Oriyza sativa
    b. O. Indica
    c. O. Nivara
    d. O. Rhyzae

Ans. (c) O. Nivara

38. Temperature of body is regulated by

    a. Hypothalamus
    b. Suprachaismatic
    c. Cerebellum
    d. Cerebrum

Ans. (c) Cerebellum

39. Which statement s Not correct for vitamin D

    a. it helps in bone formation
    b. It is produced by skin in presence of UV light
    c. It is water insoluble
    d. It helps in bone resorption

Ans. (d) It helps in bone resorption

40. Polar head group in membrane cholesterol is due to

    a. Hydroxyl group
    b. Long alkyl chain
    c. Benzene ring
    d. Carboxylic group

Ans. (a) Hydroxyl group

41. Which statement is Not true regarding genetic drift as an evolutionary force

    a. Small population size
    b. Reproductive variance
    c. Effective population
    d. Change in allele frequency

Ans. (b) Reproductive variance

42. Among the following which in endangered animal

    a. Indian tiger
    b. Indian lion
    c. Lion tailed macaque
    d. Indian wild ass

Ans. (c) Lion tailed macaque

43. Among the following critically endangered plant species is

    a. Dipterocarpus nilgirinsensis
    b. Suraca indica
    c. Cupressus cashmeriana
    d. Terminalia arjuna

Ans. (c) Cupressus cashmeriana

44. A pathogen is capable of transvarial transmission in it vector. During evolution host with become

    a. Resistance
    b. Susceptible
    c. Kill pathogen
    d. Cannot be predicted

Ans. (b) Susceptible

45. Calculate the pH of acid with $Ka=10^{-6}$ and 0.01 M

    a. 0
    b. 2
    c. 4
    d. 6

Ans. (c) 4

46. Consider that two population are growing exponentially with initial difference in growth rate of 10%. After 10 generation the difference between population size would be

    a. 1:1
    b. 4:1
    c. 2:1
    d. 10:1

Ans. (d) 10:1

47. Among the following which microorganism is involved in nitrogen fixation with woody trees?

    a. Frankia
    b. Rhyzobium
    c. Azotobactor
    d. Azospirillium

Ans. (a) Frankia

48. Genes between related organism exhibits high variation. The variations would maximally occur in

    a. Exons
    b. Intron
    c. Promoters
    d. Polyadenylation site

Ans. (b) Intron

49. Ecological adaptation in which some organism are favoured due to more energy investment on their reproductive rate while other on basis of channelizing energy for homeostasis. Such a selection strategies are termed as

    a. K selection and r selection
    b. Logistic and exponential selection
    c. Directional and disruptive selection
    d. Kin and group selection

Ans. (a) K selection and r selection

50. The possible type of gametes formed from genotype AABbCCDdEe will be

a. 4   b. 8
c. 16   d. 32

Ans. (b) 8

51. After meiosis the 20% gametes are recombinant for two genes. The distance between two genes will be

a. 5 cM   b. 10 cM
c. 20 cM   d. 40 cM

Ans. (c) 20 cM

52. If in a operon repressor binds to operator it will lead to

a. Switch on transcription
b. Switch off transcription
c. Enhanced transcription
d. Differential gene expression

Ans. (b) Switch off transcription

53. If activator binds to repressor, it will prevent

a. Transcription
b. Binding of RNA polymerase to promoter
c. Binding of repressor to operator
d. Binding of repressor to promoter

Ans. (b) Binding of RNA polymerase to promoter

54. In signal transduction trimeric G protein with α, β and ? is involved. Which subunit will activate adenylate cyclase.

a. α-subunit   b. β- subunit
c. ?-subunit   d. All of these

Ans. (a) α-subunit

55. Receptors for signaling for steroid hormones are located at

a. Plasma membrane
b. Organelle membrane
c. Intracellular
d. No receptor

Ans. (c) Intracellular

56. Among closely lying cells signal are communicated by

a. Neurotransmitter
b. Hormone
c. Gap junction
d. Cell membrane protein

Ans. (c) Gap junction

57. For an enzyme catalyzed reations exhibiting Michelis Menten equation what would be increase in substrate concentration to increase the rate of reation from 10% of V max to 90% of Vmax

a. 80 fold   b. 8 fold
c. 4 fold   d. 20 fold

Ans. (a) 80 fold

58. In TCA cycle malonate is competitive inhibitor structurally similar to

a. Succinate   b. Fumarate
c. Oxaloacetate   d. α-ketoglutrate

Ans. (a) Succinate

59. which mineral ion play important role in functioning of photosystem II

a. manganese   b. magnesium
c. iron   d. molybdenum,

Ans. (a) manganese

60. Primary acceptor of CO_2 in photosynthesis

a. ribose
b. Ribulose 5-P
c. Ribulose 1,5 bis phosphate
d. 3-phosphaoglycerate

Ans. (c) Ribulose 1,5 bis phosphate

61. During cell cycle sister chromatid are pulled apart during

a. Metaphase   b. Anaphase
c. Prophase   d. Interphase

Ans. (b) Anaphase

62. In chromosome 30 nm fiber during metaphase attached to

a. Scaffold   b. Centromere
c. Nuclear matrix d. Nuclear lamina

Ans. (a) Scaffold

63. Which of the following DO NOT bring variation in population

a. Random drift   b. Non- random matting
c. Recombination   d. Natural selection

Ans. (c) Recombination

64. In Drosophila XO are male and XXY are female while in humans XX are female and XY are female. On the bass of given information which statement is NOT true

a. Y chromosome do not play any role in sex determination of drosophila

b. Y chromosome is sex determination in human

c. N humans sex determination is based on number of X chromosome to sets of autosomes

d. In drosophila sex determination is based on number o X chromosome to sets of autosomes.

Ans. (c) N humans sex determination is based on number of X chromosome to sets of autosomes

65. **During transposition Transposon are exicised by**

a. Transposase   b. Nuclease

c. Topoisomerase   d. Exonuclease

Ans. (a) Transposase

66. **Which of the following statement regarding plasma cell is correct**

a. They are produce during secondary immune response

b. They are mature antibody secreting cell

c. They are involved in removal of intercellular viruses

d. Involved in inflammatory responses

Ans. (b) They are mature antibody secreting cell

67. **Immunological diversity in antibody is generated by**

a. Rearrangement of immunoglobulin genes

b. Alternative RNA processing

c. Post transcriptional modification

d. Post translation modification

Ans. (a) Rearrangement of immunoglobulin genes

68. **In honey bee males are developed parthenogenetically while workers are developed as sexual reproduction. The workers exhbts more similarity among them selves as compare to queen. If workers starts giving organisms parthenogenetically then offspring would most likely resembles to**

a. Among themselves and with mother

b. Among themselves and slightly differ from mother

c. Among themselves and with queen

d. Among themselves and with father

Ans. (b) Among themselves and slightly differ from mother

69. **Negative potential across plasma membrane is maintained by**

a. Active transport   b. Passive transport

c. Ion channels   d. Transporters

Ans. (a) Active transport

70. **Receptor mediated endocytosis is carried from specific portions of membrane termed as**

a. Coated vesicle

b. Coated pits

c. Endocytosis

d. Exocytosis

Ans. (b) Coated pits

71. **Which of the following statement is correct with reference to replication in eukaryotes**

a. Single origin and continuous replication

b. Multiple origin and continuous and discontinuous replication

c. Multiple origin and continuous replication

d. Single origin and continuous and discontinuous replication

Ans. (b) Multiple origin and continuous and discontinuous replication

72. **Gene for fungal resistance is found cytoplasm. If a susceptible female and resistant male are crossed then progeny will exhibit**

a. All resistance

b. All susceptible

c. Half resistance and half susceptible

d. Can not be predicted

Ans. (b) All susceptible

73. **Renaturation of human genome has reveled that it contain both repetitive and non repetitive sequence. Which statement is incorrect**

a. Human have more unique sequence

b. Repetitive sequence are located only to centromere

c. Repetitive sequences renaturate fast

d. Unique sequence renaturate fast

Ans. (c) Repetitive sequences renaturate fast

74. **In india which conservation program is related with protection of entire "tropic ladder".**

a. Project tiger

b. Project elephant

c. Ramsar sites

d. Biosphere reserve

Ans. (d) Biosphere reserve

75. **Area under forest cover in india as per estimates of 2001**

a. 7.9   b. 12.7

c. 20.6   d. 16.3

Ans. (c) 20.6

76. **Among the following which data alone are capable for ppreparing dendograme from given operational taxonomic unit**

    a. Mean of similarity
    b. Similarity matrix
    c. Characters taken in to account
    d. Criteria for classification

    Ans. (b) Similarity matrix

77. **Shannon weaver index for biodiversity characterization can be represented as**

    a. $H=\Sigma Pi \log Pi$
    b. $D= H/\log Pi$
    c. $D=\Sigma(n/N^2)$
    d. $H=\log(N)-\Sigma\log(n)$

    Ans. (a) $H=\Sigma Pi \log Pi$

78. **In which of the following condition realized niche exceed over fundamental niche**

    a. Competition
    b. Commensalisms
    c. Ammensalism
    d. Mutualism

    Ans. (d) Mutualism

79. **Which of the following is characterstic feature of climax community**

    a. Simple food chain
    b. High resilience
    c. High roductivity
    d. Narrow niche specialization

    Ans. (d) Narrow niche specialization

80. **Cattle are known to be responsible for green house effect due to**

    a. High respiration rate
    b. More consumption of plant
    c. Fermentation in rumen
    d. High reproductive rate

    Ans. (c) Fermentation in rumen

81. **Gases used by Urey and Miller for experimentation of origin of life by Oparin and Hadane hypothesis**

    a. Hydrogen, methane and Ammonia
    b. Hydrogen, methane and CO_2
    c. Hydrogen, ammonia, methane and CO_2
    d. Hydrogen, Carboxylic acid and Amino acids

    Ans. (a) Hydrogen, methane and Ammonia

82. **Highest extinction during history of earth was observed during**

    a. End of Permian
    b. End of cretaceous
    c. End of Devonian
    d. End of carboniferous

    Ans. (a) End of Permian

83. **Bacteria cannot be classified as species by the biological species concept because they**

    a. Asexually reproduction organisms
    b. High growth rate
    c. Exhibits little morphological variation
    d. Do not have nucleus

    Ans. (a) Asexually reproduction organisms

84. **In eukaryotes shortening of chromosome from ends s prevented by**

    a. DNA polymerase
    b. RNA polymerase
    c. Telomerase
    d. Transposase

    Ans. (c) Telomerase

85. **Organisms with high growth and production are**

    a. Ectotherm
    b. Endotherm
    c. Carnivore insects
    d. Detrivores

    Ans. (a) Ectotherm

86. **On molar basis if DNA has 20% cytosine, then percentage of Adenine would be**

    a. 20%
    b. 30%
    c. 40%
    d. 60%

    Ans. (b) 30%

87. **The maximum BOD and minimum DO for pure drinking water should be**

    a. 25, 5
    b. 2, 5
    c. 3, 9
    d. 0, 6

    Ans. (b) 2, 5

Memory Based Paper CSIR NET Dec 2008

1. Which of the following pair is isotones?

a. ^3H, ^4He

b. ^{15}N, $^{14}N1$

c. ^{140}Ba, ^{140}Th

d. ^1H, ^3H

Ans. (a) ^3H, ^4He

2. What would be energy released on breaking H–H covalent bond (generally energy of covalent bond lies in between 100–200 Kcal/mol)

a. 4.36×105 l/mol

b. 1×10^{-19} l/mol

c. 5×10^{-19} l/mol

d. 8×10^{19} l/mol

Ans. (a) 4.36×105 l/mol

3. The mode of sex determination in humans is

a. Haploidy-diploidy

b. XX–XY

c. ZZ–ZW

d. Genic balance

Ans. (b) XX–XY

4. The region of visible light which is most useful for photosynthesis is

a. Blue, red

b. Green, red

c. Violet, blue

d. Green, blue

Ans. (a) Blue, red

5. Why the inner plant's surface are made up of rocky denser metals, where as the outer planets are made of mainly light gases which is lesser denser then the outer planets

a. Inner planets are formed earlier

b. Sun rays pushes gases far apart

c. Centrifugal force attract denser planet near sun

d. Inner planets are near to sun, thus high temperature has blown most of lighter gases

Ans. (d) Inner planets are near to sun, thus high temperature has blown most of lighter gases

6. The following algorithm loops how many times internal loops will be executed

```
i = 0
j = 0
while i = 1 to 100
    i = 1,100, 2
    j = 1,100, 2
    stop
```

a. 100

b. 501

c. 151

d. Infinity

Ans. (d) Infinity

7. Correct graphical representation for frequency of Indian population according to their annual income is

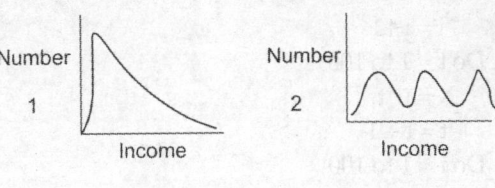

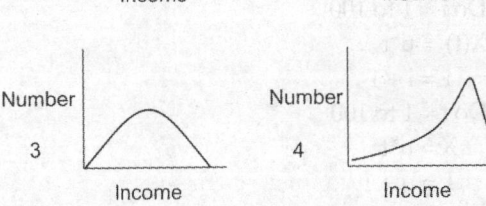

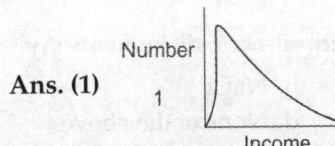

Ans. (1)

8. Among the following maximim reflectance s(albedo effect) will be observed at

a. Ice covered land

b. Ocean

c. Vegetation land

d. Deserts

Ans. (a) Ice covered land

9. A charged partical having mass 'm' and charged 'q' is moving through constant eletric field 'E' the time to cover given path will depends on

a. $m^{-1/2}$

b. $q^{-1/2}$

c. $E^{-1/2}$

d. $M^{-1/2} q^{-1/2} E^{-1/2}$

Ans. (d) $M^{-1/2} q^{-1/2} E^{-1/2}$

10. A cureent (I) carrying solenoid of length 'I', radius 'a', the charge in magnetic field along axis of solenoid 'r' will be

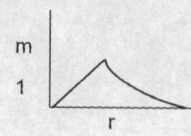
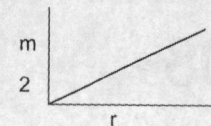
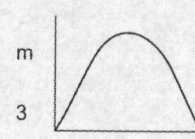
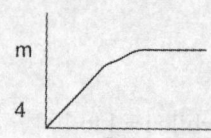

Ans. (1)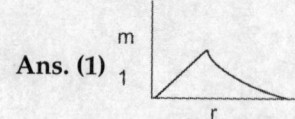

11. Correct algorthims for comuting distance (X = u*t) for time 1 to 100 sec. Will be (considering constnat speed).

   a. Do i = 1 to 100
      X(t) = x*i
      i = i +1
   b. Do t = 1 to 100
      X = u*t
      t = t + 1
   c. Do i = 1 to 100
      X(t) = u*t
      i = i +1
   d. Do t = 1 to 100
      X = u*t
      T = u + 1

Ans. (a) Do i = 1 to 100   X(t) = x*i   i = i +1

12. Among the following which salt occurs in human body

   a. KCl
   b. NaCl
   c. HCN
   d. None of the above

Ans. (b) NaCl

13. Rock 'A' is layered on rock 'B' and rock 'C' is intrusion through A and B as shown in diagram the correct explanation for diagram is

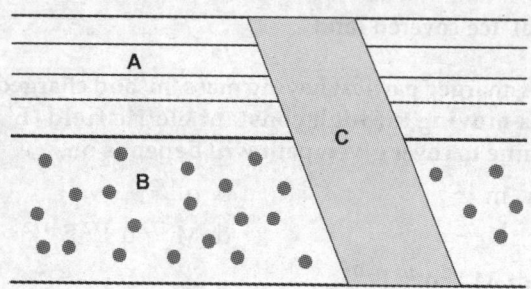

   a. 'A' is younger than B and C younger than A
   b. 'B' is younger than A and C younger than B
   c. 'C' is younger than B and C younger than A
   d. 'A' is younger than B and C younger than A

Ans. (a) 'A' is younger than B and C younger than A

14. Current passing through A–B n amperes as shown in diagram will be

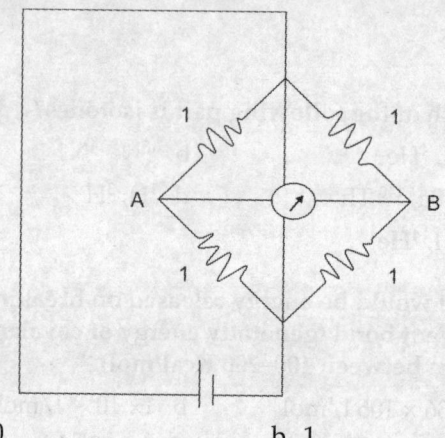

   a. 0
   b. 1
   c. 2
   d. 0.5

Ans. (a) 0

15. If 7g of NaOH is dissolved in 350 ml water the molarity of resultant solution will be

   a. 0.5 M
   b. 2.5 M
   c. 50 M
   d. 25 M

Ans. (a) 0.5 M

16. A race was held between Hare and tortoise. Hare rus fast and took rest in middle and then completed race while tortose moved at constant speed and completed race earlier then hare. The correct representation of this story is

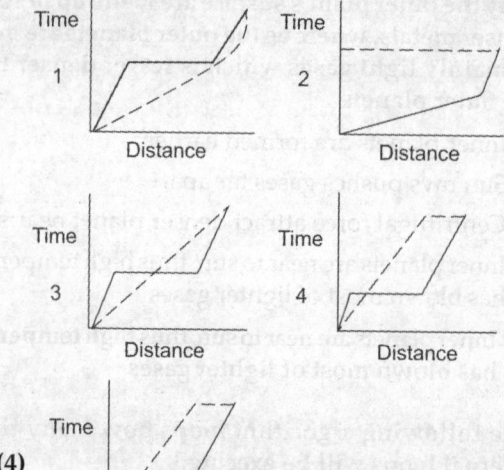

Ans. (4)

17. A bacterial population become half after one minute the reduction n population depends on population at time 't' what would the remaining population after 2 min of original population

a. ¼   b. ½
c. 1/8   d. 1/16

Ans. (a) ¼

18. Fog, which s commonly observed during winter and causes problem to flight take off mainly seen at

a. Low altitude with pollution
b. High altitude with no pollution
c. High latitude with pollution
d. Low latitude without pollution

Ans. (d) Low latitude without pollution

19. The algorithm comuters

X = 0, N = 0, T = 0
For
i = 1 to N
sum (X) = x + 1
STOP

a. Computer sum for array 'N'
b. Computer product for array 'N'
c. Computer factorial for array 'N'
d. Calculate sum of any integers

Ans. (a) Computer sum for array 'N'

20. An apple falls from a tree, to hit apple from a bullet gun fired (distance between apple and gun is 100 m both are at height 5 m).

a. Exactly at apple
b. Silightly above the apple
c. Slightly beneath the apple
d. 1m below orignal position to apple

Ans. (a) Exactly at apple

21. Minimum daily variation in temp. wil be observed at

a. Bangalore
b. Shimla
c. Coachin
d. Nagpur

Ans. (c) Coachin

22. Correct graphical representation for function x + sinx (x >0)

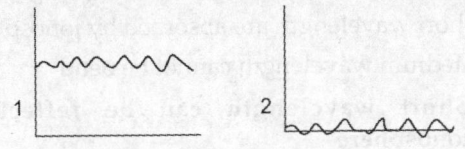

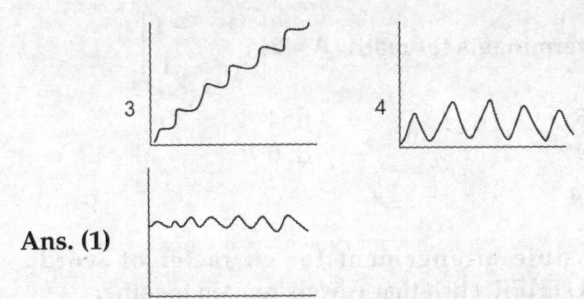

Ans. (1)

23. In equation sin 2x, value of x cannot be

a. 0   b. –1
c. 1   d. 2

Ans. (d) 2

24. What would be effect of increasing humidity on rate of transpiration?

a. Rate of transpiration will decreased
b. Rate of transpiration will increased
c. Initially low then it will be high
d. It will be unaffected

Ans. (a) Rate of transpiration will decreased

25. Maximum evaporation in ocean will occur at

a. Poles
b. Equators
c. Wetlands
d. Evenly at all places

Ans. (b) Equators

26. Graphical representation for rate kinetics for enzyme catalysed reaction will be

Time (sec) 0 30 60 90 120
K (rate)   8.00 5.35 3.5 2.15 1.15

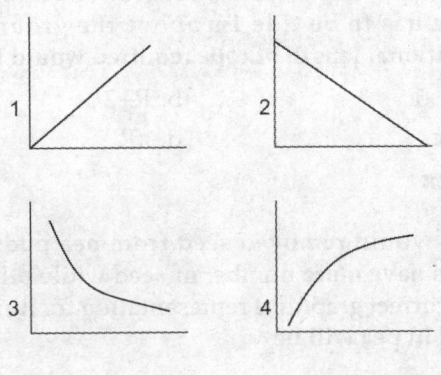

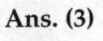
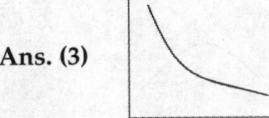

Ans. (3)

27. Determinants for matrix $A = 2 \begin{bmatrix} 1 & -1 \\ +i & 1 \end{bmatrix}$

    a. 5   b. 4
    c. 9   d. 0

Ans. (b) 4

28. Possible arrangement for character of word 'MOTHER' such that vowels remain together

    a. 120   b. 140
    c. 240   d. 280

Ans. (a) 120

29. A racer conplete 100m in very small time, another racer who runs 200m covers distance in time slightly greater than double of 100m race. Both achieve their maximum velocity at 50m the correct graphical for above situation will be

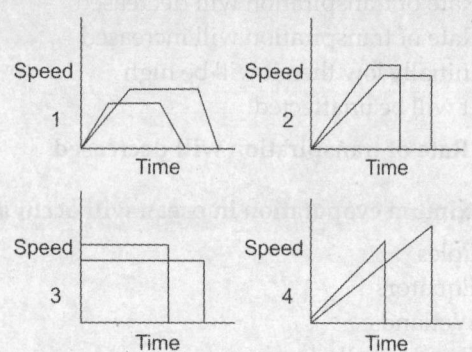

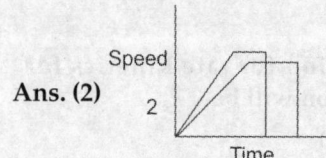

Ans. (2)

30. If a rope is tide around the radius 'R' of earth if the rope has to be tide 1m above the ground then additional length of rope required would be

    a. R+1   b. R+2
    c. 2π d. πR

Ans. (c) 2π

31. You would removed seed from pea pods; some pods have more number of seed while other less, the correct graphical representation for number of seed in pea will be

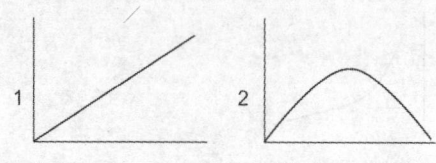

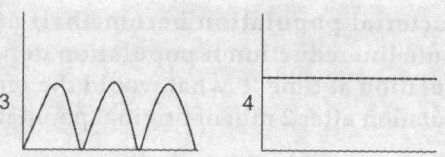

Ans. (2)

32. In graph line reprecenting y=ax-c [value of x and c are +ve]

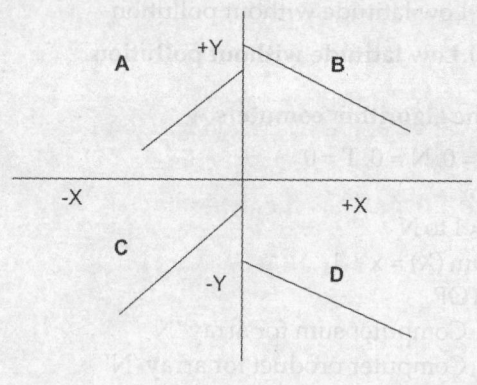

    a. A   b. B
    c. C   d. D

Ans. (d) D

33. The data of Rainfall for five cosequentive days in Hyderabaqd is given below

    2008 0, 0, 0, 0, 100
    2007 0, 20, 20, 40, 0

    Which statement is correct?
    a. Lesser variation in rainfall was observed in 2007 as compare 2008 at Hyderabad
    b. In 2008 Hyderabad experienced more rainfall
    c. In 2007 Hyderabad experienced more rainfall
    d. Variation in rainfall in 2007 and 2008 was equal

Ans. (a) Lesser variation in rainfall was observed in 2007 as compare 2008 at Hyderabad

34. Short wave can be received at longer distance during radio transition as compare to medium wave because

    a. Short wavelength can be reflected by ionosphere
    b. Medium waves are transmitted across space
    c. Short wavelength are absorbed by ionosphere
    d. Medium wavelength cannot be bend

Ans. (a) Short wavelength can be reflected by ionosphere

35. If $\delta_{ij}=1$ when i=j and o when i≠j . Then sum of δ_{ij} if it takes value of i and j from 1,2 and 3 respectively

a. 1
b. 2
c. 3
d. 4

Ans. (c) 3

36. Currently among the following which is used as a fuel for nuclear reactor

a. ^{232}Th
b. ^{238}Pu
c. ^{233}U
d. ^{235}Th

Ans. (a) ^{232}Th

37. NaCl can be electrolyzed on electrode. But ethanol cannot because

a. Ethanol has covalent bond
b. Ethanol is polar
c. Ethanol has hydrogen bonding
d. Ethanol is eclectically neutral

Ans. (a) Ethanol has covalent bond

38. Which of the following which s most orous:

a. Clay
b. Sand
c. Loamy soil
d. Granite

Ans. (b) Sand

39. Which graph represents the endothermic reaction with minimum activation energy? (A substrate → B product)

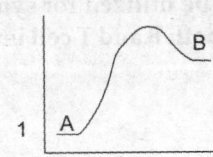
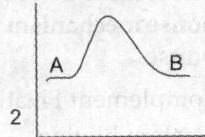
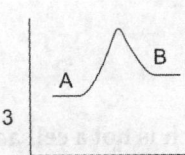
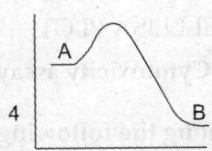
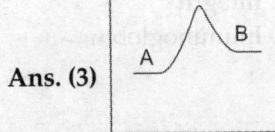

Ans. (3)

40. The process of photosynthesis which ieads to formation of glucose is a type of

a. Oxidation
b. Reduction
c. Condensation
d. Fixation

Ans. (b) Reduction

41. A perfuse kindey isolated from organism. What would be the effect of applying increasing arterial pressure on renal filtration rate?

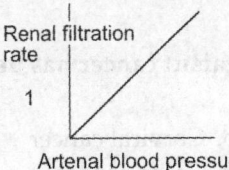
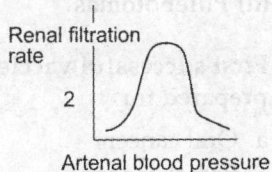
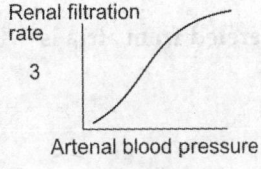
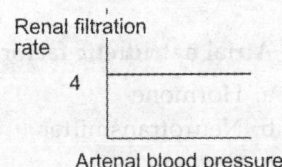
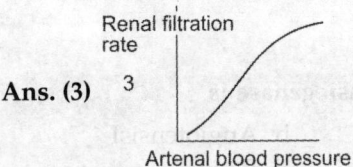

Ans. (3)

42. For 99% confidence interval the value of Y^ can be represented as

a. $\bar{Y}\pm1.53\ SD$
b. $\bar{Y}\pm2.58\ SD$
c. $\bar{Y}\pm2.56\ SE$
d. $\bar{Y}\pm1.53\ SE$

Ans. (b) $\bar{Y}\pm2.58\ SD$

43. The statistical test which can be utilized to validate he statement "people having high cholesterol suffer more from hypertension"

a. Student 't'
b. Regression Y
c. Pearson correlation coefficient
d. ANOVA

Ans. (c) Pearson correlation coefficient

44. Among the following which palnt family has been extensively used for phyto remediation

a. Poaceae
b. Brassicaceae
c. Malvaceae
d. Anonaceae

Ans. (b) Brassicaceae

45. Defective gene in Amyotropic lateral sclerosis is

a. Rb
b. P53
c. bCl2
d. TFG

Ans. (c) bCl2

46. Vector for transmission of disease Kalazar is

   a. Ades   b. Anoheles

   c. Glossina   d. Phlebotomas

Ans. (d) Phlebotomas

47. First successful vaccien agaisnt cancer has been prepared for

   a. Oral cancer   b. Cervical cancer

   c. Breast cancer   d. Colon cancer

Ans. (b) Cervical cancer

48. Atrial natriuretic factor sereted from atria is

   a. Hormone

   b. Neurotransmitter

   c. Enzyme

   d. Growth factor

Ans. (a) Hormone

49. Substrate for angitensiogenase is

   a. Angiotensinogen   b. AngiotensisI

   c. Angiotensin II   d. Renn

Ans. (a) Angiotensinogen

50. Among the following which mutant lines, λ lysogen phages will form clear bacterail plaques

   a. cI-   b. cII-

   c. INT-   d. XIS-

Ans. (a) cI-

51. Among the following which is not involved in plant defense signaling pathway

   a. Gibberlic acid   b. Ethylene

   c. Salisylic acid   d. jasmonic acid

Ans. (a) Gibberlic acid

52. Factor responsible for formation of early embryonic axis during early development pathway of palant is

   a. Auxin gradient

   b. Morhogens

   c. Orientation of embryo sac

   d. Plane of cell division

Ans. (a) Auxin gradient

53. During germination of barley enzymes for mobilization of reverse material to development embryo are secreted from

   a. Endosperm   b. Embryo

   c. Aleurone layer   d. Embryonic leaves

Ans. (c) Aleurone layer

54. Which statement is correct for given compound?

   a. It is always optically active

   b. It is always optically inactive

   c. It will be optically active if N is protonated

   d. It will be always optically neutral

Ans. (c) It will be optically active if N is protonated

55. Electrical activity of brain during brain mapping can be recorded by

   a. FMRI   b. ECG

   c. EEG   d. Polygraph

Ans. (c) EEG

56. Recently gene therapy for mutated gene has been experimentally proven in mouse utilizing

   a. Winged P element

   b. Cre-Lox system

   c. Non-homologous recombination

   d. Ac-Ds Element

Ans. (b) Cre-Lox system

57. Which technique can not be utilized for syudying response mechanism for both B and T cell immune response

   a. Complement Fixation

   b. Western bloting

   c. Cytotoxicity assay

   d. ELLLISA PLOT

Ans. (c) Cytotoxicity assay

58. Among the following which is not a cell adhesion rotein

   a. Adherin   b. Integrn

   c. Selection   d. Immunoglobin

Ans. (d) Immunoglobin

59. Which of following is not coded by MHC gene?

   a. Comonents of comlement pathway

   b. Immunoglobulin

   c. Glycoproteins

   d. Antigen presenting protein

Ans. (b) Immunoglobulin

60. Which is least likely to occur for removal of cancer cells?

a. T-cell based cytotoxicity

b. Complement fixation

c. Autophagy

d. Phagocytosis

Ans. (c) Autophagy

61. Leukemia inhibiting factor has been utilized in animal cell culture for

a. Stimulating growth of cell

b. Differentiation

c. Mrphogenesis

d. Arrest cells at mitosis

Ans. (b) Differentiation

62. Dorsal lip of amphibian is equivalent to chick

a. Hensen node

b. Primitive grove

c. Animal pole

d. Vegetal pole

Ans. (a) Hensen node

63. Homeotic enes are responsible for

a. Maintaining gaps in segments

b. Provide radient in developing embryo

c. Codes morphogenesis

d. Mutation result in formation of organ at unusual location

Ans. (d) Mutation result in formation of organ at unusual location

64. Mosaic developmental pattern is always

a. Autonomous

b. Non autonomous

c. Conditional

d. Regulative

Ans. (a) Autonomous

65. The specialzed structure pectin for clear eye sight s characteristic feature are

a. Birds

b. Amphibian

c. Nacturanal mammals

d. Aquatic mammals

Ans. (a) Birds

66. Which of the following is not correctly matched

a. Chanocyes-porifera

b. Malphigian tubes-Arthropods

c. Citellum-annelids

d. Cnidocytes-mollusc

Ans. (d) Cnidocytes-mollusc

67. Cytoplasmic streaming results into mobility of substance and organalles inovlves interaction of

a. Tubulin, kinesin

b. Tubulin, myosine

c. Actin, kinesin

d. Actin, myosin

Ans. (d) Actin, myosin

68. The main force in membrane resealing of ruptured biomembrane in aqueous environment is

a. Hydrophobic forces between membrane lipids

b. Covalent forces between membrane lipids

c. Force between protein and lipids

d. Ionic interaction between membrane lipids

Ans. (a) Hydrophobic forces between membrane lipids

69. What would happen if lysozyme membrane leaks its digestive enzyeme in cytosol

a. Acid hydrolases will be inactivated

b. Acid hydrolases will digest the cellular components

c. pH of cell will increase

d. It will causes I-cell disease

Ans. (a) Acid hydrolases will be inactivated

70. The maximum ionic interaction would be observed

a. In presence of polar solvant

b. In presence of mixture of water and alcohol

c. Almost equal in all kind of solvant

d. When ionic compound is out of the solvent

Ans. (d) When ionic compound is out of the solvent

71. Regulation of trp operon by binding of tryptophan to ryp repressor is termed as

a. Repression

b. Induction

c. Anti termination

d. Atteneution

Ans. (a) Repression

72. In salt tolerance plant the excess salt s transported to vacoule by

a. Na-H+ antiporter

b. Na-K+ pump

c. Na-Ca- symporter

d. Na-H+ ppase

Ans. (a) Na-H+ antiporter

73. Post translational modification takes place in

a. Nucleus

b. Mitochondria

c. Ribosome

d. ER

Ans. (d) ER

74. Which technique can not be utilized for detection of microdeletion on Y chromosome

a. Karyotyping

b. PCR

c. Microarray

d. Hybridization

Ans. (c) Microarray

75. **Individual having X chromosome and short arm of Y chromosome are Y is male while individuals having X chromosome and long arm of Y chromosome are female. This shows that**

    a. Genes for maleness are located on short arm of Y chromosome
    b. Genes for maleness are located on long arm of X chromosme
    c. Genes for malness are located on X chromosome
    d. Male determining genes are not located on Y chromosome

Ans. (a) Genes for maleness are located on short arm of Y chromosome

76. **If a cell has 'C' as the DNA content of cell and 'n' as the number of chromosme, then just immediately before the cell division in case of mitosis what would be value of 'c' and 'n'**

    a. 2c and 4n
    b. 4c and 2n
    c. 4c and 4n
    d. 2c and 2n

Ans. (b) 4c and 2n

77. **Which equation best describes the bacterial population growth**

    a. $\dfrac{dN}{dt} = KN$ b. $\dfrac{dN}{dt} = N$

    b. $\dfrac{dt}{dN} = KN$ c. $\dfrac{dN}{dt} = K$

Ans. (a) $\dfrac{dN}{dt} = KN$

78. **Genetic disorder xeroderma pigmentosum is due to error is**

    a. Base exicision repair mechanism
    b. Nucleotide excision repair mechanism
    c. Direct repair mechanism
    d. DNA replication mechanism

Ans. (b) Nucleotide excision repair mechanism

79. **In Lederbergs experiment which one of the following option they have used to prove their historical experiment**

    a. One auxotroph and one prototroph
    b. Two auxotroph and two prototroph
    c. Two auxotrophs
    d. Two prototroph

Ans. (c) Two auxotrophs

80. **Among the following which inhibitor of 80S ribosome**

    a. Tetracycline   b. Streptomycin
    c. Cyclohexamide   d. Chloromphenicol

Ans. (c) Cyclohexamide

81. **Diphtheria toxin causes**

    a. ADP ribosylation of EF-2
    b. ADP ribosylation EF-α
    c. Biocking activity of RNA polymerase
    d. Blocking DNA replication

Ans. (a) ADP ribosylation of EF-2

82. **Effect of release of IP3 during signal transduction pathway is**

    a. Closure of Ca+2 channel in ER
    b. Increase n intraellular Ca+2 level
    c. Increase of extracellular Ca+2 level
    d. Inactivation of calmodulin protein

Ans. (b) Increase n intraellular Ca+2 level

83. **Dorsal mutant in drosophila will result in**

    a. Dorsalization of ventral side
    b. Ventralzation of dorsal side
    c. There would be no effect
    d. Anterior posterior pattern formation will be effective

Ans. (a) Dorsalization of ventral side

84. **Intracelluar negative potential and extracelluar positive potential occurs in**

    a. In all cell
    b. In neurons
    c. In kidney cells
    d. In liver cells

Ans. (a) In all cell

85. **A major functional difference between the succinyl Co-A synthetase of plant and animal cell mitochondria is that it**

    a. Does not produce ATP in plant cell
    b. Produce UTP in plant cell
    c. Produces ATP in plants and GTP in animal cell
    d. Produces GTP in plant and ATP in animals.

Ans. (c) Produces ATP in plants and GTP in animal cell

86. **Among the following which is not monitered as daily potential pollutnat**

    a. CO   b. CO_2
    c. SO_2 d. NO_3

Ans. (b) CO_2

87. In plant lateral root initiates from

a. Pith
b. Pericycle
c. Cortex
d. Endoderm

Ans. (b) Pericycle

88. Oxygenase activity of RUBISCO generates

a. Two molecules of PGA
b. Two molecules f phosphoglycolate
c. One molecules each of PGA and hosphoglycolate
d. Tw molecule each of PGA and phoshoglycolate

Ans. (c) One molecules each of PGA and hosphoglycolate

89. Plant family having characteristic umbel nflorescence is

a. Asteraceae
b. Acanthaceae
c. Apiaceae
d. Poaceae

Ans. (c) Apiaceae

90. Dendrogram in numerical taxonomy represent

a. Phenetic similarites
b. Phlogenetic similarity
c. Evolutionary similarities
d. No similarities

Ans. (a) Phenetic similarites

91. A plant with genotype r+h+/r-h- was test crossed. Out of total 280 progeny 260 are r+h+/r-h- and r-h-/r-h-. The recombination frequency will be

a. 92.8
b. 46.4
c. 7.2
d. 3.6

Ans. (c) 7.2

92. Genetic mapping reveals that distance between two genes 'A' and 'B' is 10 cM. What is chance of getting Aabb progeny if AaBb is test crossed?

a. 5%
b. 10%
c. 45%
d. 90%

Ans. (a) 5%

93. The regulattors of circadyn rythms in plants is

a. Phycobillins
b. Phytochromes
c. Phototropins
d. Cryotophores

Ans. (c) Phototropins

94. The following pedgree reresents the inheritance of a rare disorder.

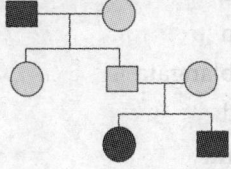

Based on the above pedigree, what is the most likely mode of inheritance?

a. Autosomal dominant
b. X-linked recessive
c. X-linked dominant
d. Autosomal recessive

Ans. (d) Autosomal recessive

95. Quantitative inheritance defines

a. Variation in phenotype
b. Variation in genotype
c. Variation in environment
d. Variation in gene

Ans. (b) Variation in genotype

96. Which of the following which is not intrensic flour

a. Tryptophan
b. Phenyl alanine
c. Tyrosine
d. Histidine

Ans. (d) Histidine

97. Among the following which group has maximum number of endangered an critically endangered species as per HJCN red data list?

a. Amphibian
b. Reptile
c. Mammals
d. Aves

Ans. (a) Amphibian

98. Germination of moth beat in dark is an example of

a. Photomorphogenesis
b. Skotomorphogenesis
c. De-etiolation
d. Shadding effect

Ans. (b) Skotomorphogenesis

99. Birds besides lungs have highly branched air sacs. The major function of air sac is to

a. Increase surface area for air sac is to
b. Help in ventilation during inhalation
c. Help in ventilation during exhalation
d. Help in ventilation during both iinhalation and exhalation

Ans. (d) Help in ventilation during both iinhalation and exhalation

100. Which is correct hierchical sequence in taxonomy?

a. Phylum-class-order-family-genus
b. genus-class-order-family-phylum
c. Phylum-genus-order-family-class
d. Phylum-class-order-genus-family

Ans. (a) Phylum-class-order-family-genus

101. Among the following which moleucle has been frequently used for molecular systematic

a. Insulin   b. Cytochrome C

c. Globin   d. Collagen

Ans. (b) Cytochrome C

102. Rate of molecular evolution would be least in

a. Non-synonymous change in codon

b. Synonymous change in codon

c. Flanking region of gene

d. Introns of gene

Ans. (a) Non-synonymous change in codon

103. The most probable place where life would have originated

a. Outer space

b. Barren rocks

c. In oceans

d. Deep hydrotheral vents

Ans. (d) Deep hydrotheral vents

104. In population of 10 million individual birth rate is 19 per 100 and death rate is 14 per 1000. Annual rise in population would be

a. 50000   b. 5000

c. 14000   d. 500000

Ans. (a) 50000

105. Which of the following curves represents the general relationship between population size (N) and growth rate (dN/dt) for logistically growing population

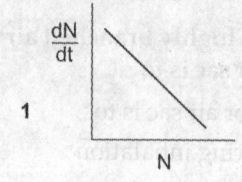
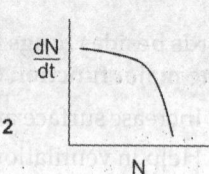
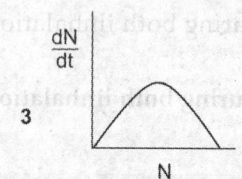
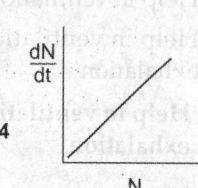

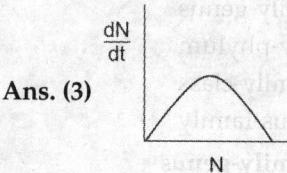

Ans. (3)

106. Which factor is least responsible for genetle drift?

a. Migration

b. Founder effect

c. Bottleneck

d. Restriction of resources

Ans. (d) Restriction of resources

107. In spite of the revalence of herbivory the earth continues to be largely green because

a. The number of herbivors species is low

b. Herbivors are very inefficient feeders

c. Herbivors numbers are kept low by their predator

d. Herbivory promotes plant growth

Ans. (d) Herbivory promotes plant growth

108. Biomass turnover time is the ration between biomass and productivity of an ecosystem. Which of the following forests shoud have highest bomass turnover time?

a. Tropical dry forest

b. Tropical wet forest

c. Temperate deciduous forest

d. Boreal forest

Ans. (b) Tropical wet forest

109. Smoth movement of bacteria during chemitaxis is due to

a. Due to tumbling

b. Phosphorylation of CheY

c. Movement of H+ across plasma membrane

d. Phoshorylation of Che A

Ans. (c) Movement of H+ across plasma membrane

110. Which statement is least likely to be observed amongst the animals showing extensive parental care

a. Male polyamous

b. Sexual dmorphism

c. Difference in body size of male and female

d. No investment in selection of mates by female

Ans. (d) No investment in selection of mates by female

111. Maximum density of dopamine and nor adregenic receptor occurs at

a. Cerebellum

b. Cerebellem

c. Medulla oblangata

d. Spinal cord

Ans. (a) Cerebellum

112. **Chitin occurs in cell wall of**
   a. Bacteria
   b. Arthropods
   c. Fungus
   d. Mollusck

Ans. (c) Fungus

113. **The emergence of polarity of an embryo is the result of**
   a. Positive and negative charges nteracting in early development
   b. Cytoplasmic differences between cells
   c. Cytoplasmic determinant within cells.
   d. All of the above

Ans. (c) Cytoplasmic determinant within cells.

114. **Which anti cancerous drug is obtained from catharanthus roseus**
   a. Taxol
   b. Vincristine
   c. Colchicine
   d. Serpentine

Ans. (b) Vincristine

115. **Which technique is used to study de novo RNA SYNTHESIS?**
   a. Southern blotting
   b. Northern blotting
   c. Microarray
   d. RT-PCR

Ans. (d) RT-PCR

Memory Based Paper CSIR NET June 2009

1. Electrical charge is stored in

   a. Battery   b. Capacitor

   c. Voltmeter   d. Wire

Ans. (b) Capacitor

2. Which of them will have minimum resistance to flow of electric current?

   a. Glass   b. Saline aquifer

   c. Granite   d. Lime stone

Ans. (b) Saline aquifer

3. What would be effect on shape of cupper metallic tube carrying electric current due to nerate magnetic field

   a. No effect

   b. It will swell from middle

   c. It will shrink from middle

   d. Will be eclipse shape

Ans. (b) It will swell from middle

4. The main reason for release of energy from sun is

   a. Fusion of hydrogen   b. Fission of hydrogen

   c. Fusion of helium   d. Fission of helium

Ans. (a) Fusion of hydrogen

5. What would be effect on time period of endulum one laced on equator and other on pole

   a. No effect

   b. Time period would be greater at pole

   c. Time period would be greater at equator

   d. Pendulum will stop at poles

Ans. (c) Time period would be greater at equator

6. At ground state of hydrogen atom its Bohr radius is 5.3×10^{-11}m and mean velocity is 2.1×10^6m/s. What would be value of fundamental time unit?

   a. 2.52×10^{-27} b. 2.52×10^{-5}

   c. 1.2×10^{-17} d. 1.52×10^{-27}

Ans. (a) 2.52×10^{-27}

7. Angle between two vector 2i+3j and 3i-2j will be

   a. 30°   b. 45°

   c. 60°   d. 90°

Ans. (d) 90°

8. Relative mean kinetic energy for He atom and Ar would be

   a. 1:10   b. 1:4

   c. 1:100   d. 1:16

Ans. (a) 1:10

9. During combustion of carbon in presence of oxygen CO_2 is formed. What will be effect on release of CO_2 if availability of O_2 is doubled?

   a. No change

   b. Will double

   c. Will half

   d. Will increase four times

Ans. (a) No change

10. If iodine stored in a closed chamber is slowly evacuated to sublime. What would be effect on sublimation rate and mean free path?

   a. Both will increase

   b. Both will decrease

   c. Sublimation rate will increase while free path decrease

   d. Sublimation rate decrease and free path increase

Ans. (a) Both will increase

11. Assuming equal density through out different layers of the earth, if radius 'r' of selected part is gradually increased from centre of earth (where $r < r_e$) what would be correct graphical representation for change in mass?

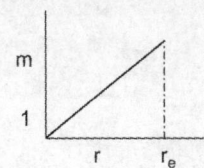 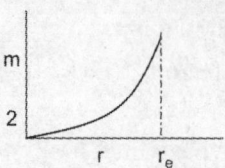

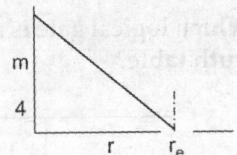

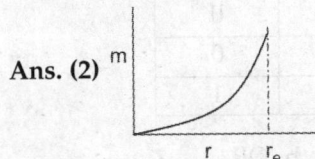

Ans. (2)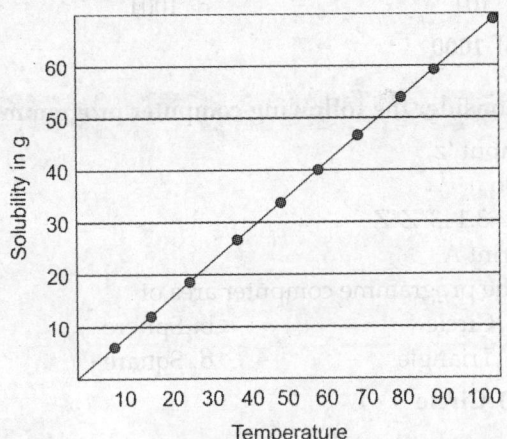

12. As shown in graph solubility of $CuSO_4$ increase as the temp. of solution is increased. Suppose under saturated condition temp. of solution is dropped from 60° to 30°, amount of $CuSO_4$ deposited will be

a. 24 g   b. 44 g
c. 20 g   d. 100 g

Ans. (a) 24 g

13. Which of the following is not a major green house gas n stratosphere?

a. CO_2 b. Methane
c. Ozone   d. Water vapour

Ans. (d) Water vapour

14. Boiling point of water at sea level is 100°C what would be its boiling point at top of mount Everest?

a. 100°C   b. 104°C
c. 114°C   d. 74°C

Ans. (d) 74°C

15. Atmospheric pressure decline with altitude as shown in table

Height	0 Km	2 Km	4 Km	6 Km	8 Km
Pressure	900	800	650	450	200

What would be atm. Pressure at height of 5 Km?

a. 720   b. 550
c. 640   d. 420

Ans. (b) 550

16. Mostly inner material of earth remains in solid state. Seldom has it melted and do not remain inside and expelled to the surface of earth because

a. It is just beneath the earth crust
b. Due to buoyancy
c. Due to high pressure
d. More density of surrounding rocks

Ans. (b) Due to buoyancy

17. Among the following which ocean receives maximum sediments?

a. Arabian ocean
b. Indian ocean
c. Bay of Bengal
d. Dead sea

Ans. (c) Bay of Bengal

18. The amount of rainfall in summer at any receives maximum sediments?

Jan	March	June	Dec
550	30	10	450

The probable place would be
a. India
b. North America
c. Australia
d. Sri Lanka

Ans. (c) Australia

19. Half life of any radioactive material is 50 days. How many half life it will take to become 12.5 % of the original amount?

a. 1   b. 2
c. 3   d. 4

Ans. (c) 3

20. What is probability of getting first three female pus out of a little of 7?

a. 1/8   b. 7/8
c. 3/27   d. 37/64

Ans. (a) 1/8

21. If two sides of isosceles triangle are 7 cm and 16 cm respectively. What would be length of its third side?

a. 7 cm   b. 16 cm
c. 23 cm   d. 10 cm

Ans. (b) 16 cm

22. A crystalline sphere of radius 1 cm is broken into pieces of 0.01 cm radius each. What would be change in surface area?

a. 0
b. 10
c. 100
d. 1000

Ans. (c) 100

23. Graphical representation for function e^{-ixi} will be

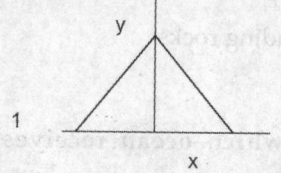
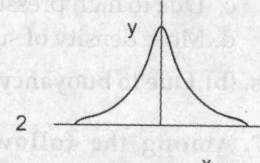
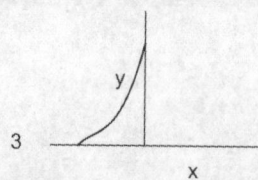
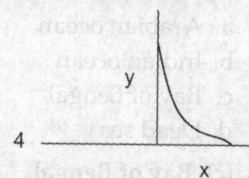

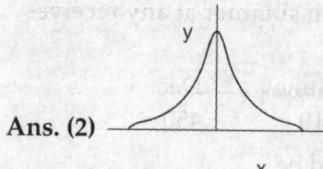

Ans. (2)

24. If value of Φ is 360°, then as per equation $r=a\Phi$, shape of object would be (where r is distance from origin and a is constant)

a. Spiral
b. Circle
c. Sphere
d. Eclipse

Ans. (a) Spiral

25. A non-malignant tumor with radius 'r' shrinks at constant rate with time 't'. It can be reprewented by equation

a. $r = r_0 + k/t$
b. $r = r_0 - k/t$
c. $r = r_0 - kt$
d. $r = r_0 + kt$

Ans. (c) $r = r_0 - kt$

26. A committee of two member has to be selected out of 3 men and 2 women. In how many possible ways it can be done

a. 10
b. 25
c. 100
d. 120

Ans. (a) 10

27. Which logical gate is represented by the following truth table?

P	Q	RESULT
0	0	0
0	1	0
1	0	0
1	1	1

a. AND
b. OR
c. NOR
d. XOR

Ans. (a) AND

28. Sum of two binary number 101 and 011 would be

a. 1000
b. 100
c. 101
d. 1001

Ans. (a) 1000

29. Consider the following computer programme

Input 'z'
Do
A=3.143*Z*Z
Print A
The programme computer area of

a. Circle
b. Sphere
c. Triangle
d. Square

Ans. (a) Circle

30. Among the following which s a object oriented language

a. PASCAL
b. FORTRAN
c. C++
d. COBAL

Ans. (c) C++

31. If five flower have nectar amount 10, 20, 30 40, 50 µl respectively. If a bee consumes all the nectar from flower, then at the end bee is rewarded with how much mean amount of nectar

a. 10
b. 20
c. 30
d. 150

Ans. (d) 150

32. Starch on treatment with dilute H_2SO_4 yields free glucose but cellulose not because

a. Cellulose is linear
b. Cellulose is branched
c. Starch is carbohydrate
d. Starch is linear

Ans. (a) Cellulose is linear

33. **Major weight of human body is due to**

a. C

b. P

c. N

d. O

Ans. (a) C

34. **If all parameters related with cockroach are doubled such as height, width and length, it will not survive because of**

a. Low surface area to volume ration

b. High surface area to volume ratio

c. Exchange of gases

d. Problem is excretion

Ans. (a) Low surface area to volume ration

35. **The graph represents**

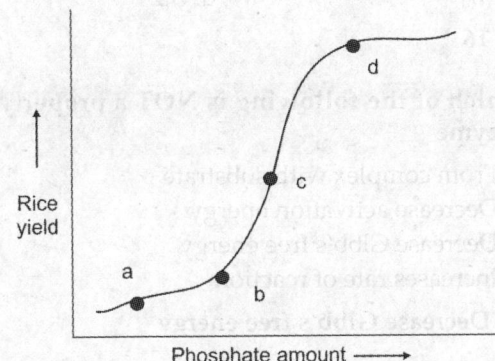

a. Exothermic reaction

b. Isolated reaction

c. Endothermic reaction

d. Physiological reaction

Ans. (d) Physiological reaction

36. **Corollas force is due to rotation of earth on moving object. The direction of corollas force is**

a. Along the axis rotation of the moving object

b. Against the axis of rotation of the moving effect

c. Perpendicular to the of rotation of the moving object

d. Tangential to the axis of rotation of the moving object

Ans. (a) Along the axis rotation of the moving object

37. **area required to store fats in seed as compare to carbohydrate would be**

a. equal

b. more

c. less

d. slightly more

Ans. (c) less

38. **Terminal electron acceptor for metabolic reaction in organism would be**

a. CO_2

b. H_2

c. O_2

d. H_2O

Ans. (c) O_2

39. **If parents with genotype AABBcddeeFF and aabbCCDDEEff are crossed, the genotype of resulting progeny will be**

a. AABBccDDeeFf

b. AaBbCcDdEeFf

c. aaBBccDDeeFF

d. AaBbCCddEeFf

Ans. (b) AaBbCcDdEeFf

40. **The effect of input of any fertilizer on rice yield is shown in graph. The optimum utilization of nutrient is at point?**

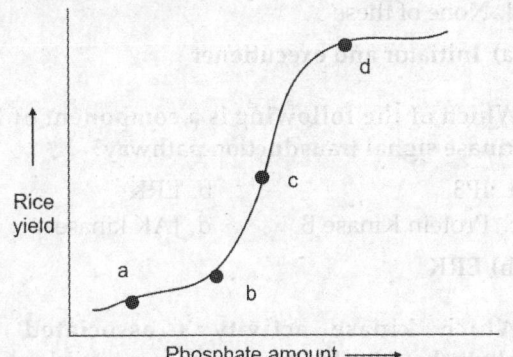

a. A

b. B

c. C

d. D

Ans. (c) C

41. **Transduction has been used extensively for genome mapping for bacteria. Which of the following process is useful for gene mapping?**

a. Generalized transduction

b. Specialized transaction

c. Site specific recombination

d. Bacterial lysis

Ans. (a) Generalized transduction

42. **Molecular marker can not be utilized for**

a. Mapping of gene

b. Identifying the clones

c. Identifying the locus of gene on chromosome

d. Identifying the expressed product

Ans. (d) Identifying the expressed product

43. **Sxi genes of Drosophila regulate expression at**

a. Transcriptional level

b. Post trnascriptional level

c. Translational level

d. Post translational level

Ans. (b) Post trnascriptional level

44. Which function is not related with Th1 cells

a. Secretion of IL-2
b. Promoting antibody binding to soluble antigens
c. IFN-?
d. Induce phagocytosis

Ans. (b) Promoting antibody binding to soluble antigens

45. Cysteine Aspartate protein kinases involved in process of apoptosis function as

a. Initiator and executioner
b. Initiator and inflammatory
c. Initiator, inflammatory and executioner
d. None of these

Ans. (a) Initiator and executioner

46. Which of the following is a component of MAP kinase signal transduction pathway?

a. IP3
b. ERK
c. Protein Kinase B
d. JAK kinase

Ans. (b) ERK

47. Which kinase activity s associated with phytochrome photoreceptors responsible of Red/far red response?

a. Histidine
b. Tyrosine
c. Aspartate
d. Ser/thr kinase

Ans. (d) Ser/thr kinase

48. Fas protein involved in cell mediated immune response

a. Have death domain
b. Act as inducer
c. Generates G Protein
d. Inhibits apoptosis

Ans. (a) Have death domain

49. Bubonic plaque caused by Yersinia pestis cannot be eradicated completely because

a. Casual organism cannot be culture in vitro
b. Antibodies are not generated by causal organism
c. Causal organism do not express surface antigens
d. Y. pestis have broad host range

Ans. (d)

50. Mycobacteria tuberculosis is able to cause disease because as it enters host cell it donor allow endosome to mature into

a. Lysosomes
b. Peroxisomes
c. Er
d. Golgibody

Ans. (a) Lysosomes

51. Sendai virus enters host cell by

a. Endocytosis
b. Phagocytosis
c. Cell fusion
d. Receptor mediated endocytosis

Ans. (c) Cell fusion

52. Red wine and red grapes are important source of which anti-tumor agent

a. Taxol
b. Vincristine
c. Resveratol
d. Bradystanin

Ans. (c) Resveratol

53. Maximum possible isomer for glucose are

a. 4
b. 8
c. 16
d. 32

Ans. (c) 16

54. Which of the following is NOT a property of a enzyme

a. From complex with substrate
b. Decrease activation energy
c. Decrease Gibb's free energy
d. Increases rate of reaction

Ans. (c) Decrease Gibb's free energy

55. Which era is characterized by dramatic diversification among eukaryotes?

a. Cambrian
b. Devonian
c. Carboniferous
d. Triassic

Ans. (a) Cambrian

56. An organism influence the evolutionary pace of the other organism in

a. Co-evolution
b. Parallel evolution
c. Convergent evolution
d. Divergent evolution

Ans. (a) Co-evolution

57. A population of 200 is in Hardy – Weinberg equilibrium with allele frequency of 'A'=0.7 and 'a'=0.3. the number of carrier in population will be

a. 18
b. 42
c. 84
d. 98

Ans. (c) 84

58. Air inhaled during breathing contains rincipal gases in order N2>O2>CO2>H2. The gases n exhaled air would be in order

a. $H_2>O_2>CO_2>N_2$
b. $N_2>O_2>CO_2>H_2$
c. $N_2>CO_2>O_2>H_2$
d. $N_2>O_2>H_2>CO_2$

Ans. (b) $N_2>O_2>CO_2>H_2$

59. Distance between the tow linked genes A and B is 20 cM. On test cross of $\dfrac{A \quad b}{a \quad B}$ with recessive parent how many offspring will have genotype $\dfrac{A \quad B}{a \quad b}$

a. 10
b. 20
c. 30
d. 40

Ans. (a) 10

60. In Neurospora crassa tetrad analysis showed following result + : m :: 6 : 2. The phenomenon involved for above result would be

a. Branch migration
b. Strand exchange
c. Holiday junction
d. DNA replication

Ans. (b) Strand exchange

61. A poky Neurospora was crossed with normal Neurospora and following results were obtained

✳Poky   X   ✳Normal → all poky

✳Normal X   ✳poky → all normal

The mode of inheritance is

a. Maternal inheritance
b. Maternal effect
c. X-Linked
d. Sex influenced

Ans. (a) Maternal inheritance

62. The mendelian law of independent assortment is due to arrangement of chromosome during

a. Anaphase-I
b. Anaphase-II
c. S-phase
d. Cytokinesis

Ans. (a) Anaphase-I

63. Among the following most variable stage of cell cycle is

a. G1
b. S
c. G2
d. M

Ans. (a) G1

64. It has been observed that during prolong animal cel culture and differentiation cell tends to stop dividing. They are said to be in

a. Apoptosis
b. Quiescent
c. Senescence
d. G1

Ans. (c) Senescence

65. Type of mutation which is most suitable for study of regulation of cell like DNA replication is

a. Gain of function
b. Loss of function
c. Suppressor mutation
d. Conditional mutation

Ans. (d) Conditional mutation

66. The glycocalyx around cell membrande can be determined by

a. Methylene blue
b. Iodine
c. Saffranin
d. Lectins

Ans. (d) Lectins

67. Small amount of lethal mutation always tend to remain in population is due to

a. Mutation selection balance
b. Frequency dependent selection
c. Positive selection
d. Negative selection

Ans. (a) Mutation selection balance

68. During evolution increased ornamentation in male is a result of

a. Directional selection
b. Co-evolution
c. Sexual selection
d. Natural selection

Ans. (c) Sexual selection

69. The harmone responsible for regulating spermatogenesis in human is

a. Testosterone
b. FSH
c. LH
d. Estrogen

Ans. (b) FSH

70. Exponential growth in bacteria would be expected during

a. Lag phase
b. Log phase
c. Stationary phase
d. Deceleration phase

Ans. (b) Log phase

71. Thylokoid membrane has lateral asymmetrical positioning of photosystem in chloroplast. Which statement is correct?

a. PS-I in non appressed portion and PS-II in appressed portion
b. PS-II in non appressed portion and PS-I in appressed portion
c. Both PS-I and PS-II in appressed portion
d. Both PS-I and PS-II in non appressed portion of thylakoid

Ans. (a) PS-I in non appressed portion and PS-II in appressed portion

72. Which organelle required intact membrane system for ATP synthesis

a. Chloroplast
b. Mitochondria
c. Both a and b
d. ER

Ans. (d) ER

73. The movement of chloroplast is mediated by

   a. Dynein   b. Kinesin

   c. Actin   d. Myosin

Ans. (d) Myosin

74. The flagellin protein is associated with

   a. Bacteria   b. Protest

   c. Virus   d. EK cell

Ans. (a) Bacteria

75. Starch filled plastids are responsible for geotropism in columella cel beneath the root cap. They are termed as

   a. Amyloplast   b. Elioplast

   c. Chloroplast   d. Proplastid

Ans. (a) Amyloplast

76. ABC transporter in plant which are responsible for detoxification of senobiotics and revent oxidative damage are located at

   a. Tonoplast

   b. Peroxisome

   c. ER

   d. Plasma membrane

Ans. (a) Tonoplast

77. Which technique is most suitable to study transcription factor and its binding site

   a. DNAse I foot printing

   b. Western blotting

   c. Northern botting

   d. Microarray

Ans. (a) DNAse I foot printing

78. Which of them is not utilized for comparison of operational taxonomic unit in numerical taxonomy

   a. Unweighted pair group method

   b. Percentage similarity

   c. Jaccard coefficient

   d. Genetic similarity

Ans. (d) Genetic similarity

79. Which statement is correct regarding c-oncogenes

   a. They are viral genes

   b. They mutated from of genes controlling cell division

   c. They are mutated viral enes

   d. They suppresses tumors

Ans. (b) They mutated from of genes controlling cell division

80. A sample is in normal distribution ranging from $(\mu - 1\sigma)$ to $(\mu + 2\sigma)$. The data in range would be

   a. 17   b. 50

   c. 67   d. 98

Ans. (c) 67

81. Among the following which graph represent correct relationship between intrinsic rate of growth 'r' and generation time 't'

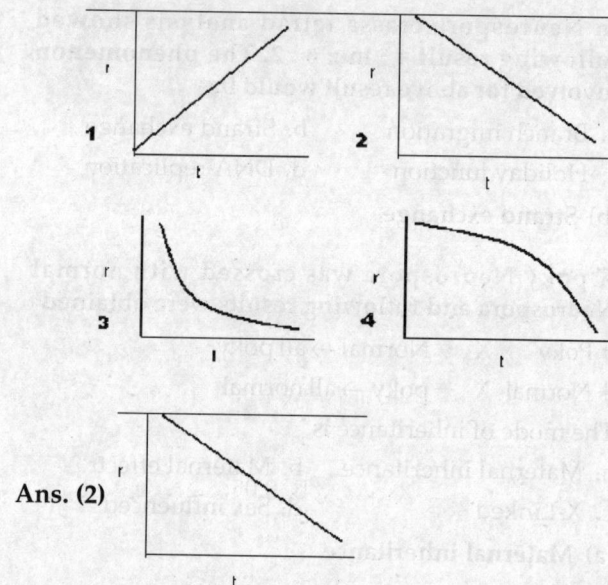

Ans. (2)

82. Among the following which is not a result of acid rain

   a. Low amount of phosphate availability

   b. Low amount of aluminium availability

   c. Low availability of nutrient to plant

   d. Increased acidity of soil

Ans. (b) Low amount of aluminium availability

83. Organ identity genes are responsible for correct positioning of floral organ on floral meristem, mutation in them will lead to

   a. Loss of organs from certain whorls

   b. More number of organs in certain whorls

   c. Appearance of organs at incorrect positions

   d. No flower

Ans. (c) Appearance of organs at incorrect positions

84. In hydra if any part is lost remaining portion re-pattern itself and given rise to complete organism. Such a pattern of development is termed as

   a. Epimorphosis   b. Morphallaxis

   c. Regeneration   d. Healing

Ans. (b) Morphallaxis

85. Generally organism ends to remain in realized niche. Under what condition realized niche can be greater than fundamental niche

   a. Abundance of resources
   b. Heterogeneity of resources
   c. One species helping other in utilization of resources
   d. Moving of organism from source to new sink area

Ans. (d) Moving of organism from source to new sink area

86. According to survival of fittest concept of natural selection one species out compete other species. Under such condition no two species tan co-exist in same niche but more than one species can live in same niche under condition

   a. Abundant resources
   b. High competition
   c. Marginal overlapping
   d. Utilization of different resources

Ans. (a) Abundant resources

87. The inbreeding coefficient of offspring on marriage between brother and sister sibling will be

   a. 0.5   b. 0.05
   c. 0.25   d. 0.75

Ans. (c) 0.25

88. Which would be suitable fr constructing the genomic library of 70 kb of DNA

   a. YAC   b. BAC
   c. P1 based vector   d. Cosmid

Ans. (c) P1 based vector

89. If we want to obtained glycosylated protein from microbe, suitable choice will be

   a. Bacteria   b. Yeast
   c. Mycoplasma   d. Animal cell

Ans. (b) Yeast

90. Glycosylation of protein occurs n

   a. ER   b. Golgi
   c. Mitochondria d. Nucleus

Ans. (b) Golgi

91. Among the following which antibiotic will inhibit protein synthesis in chloroplast?

   a. Cyclohexamide
   b. Chloromphenicol
   c. Riifamcin
   d. Ricin

Ans. (b) Chloromphenicol

92. Worldwide maximum cultivated transgenic crop is

   a. Insect resistance cotton
   b. Herbicide resistance soybeans
   c. Growing plant for desired molecule
   d. Edible vaccine

Ans. (b) Herbicide resistance soybeans

93. Elevated level of RBC and low affinity of haemoglobin for oxygen is an adaptation for

   a. High altitude   b. Poles
   c. Low altitudes   d. marine

Ans. (a) High altitude

94. perennial habit among trees would be more preferred under conditions

   a. low survival during sapling stage and high during adult
   b. high survival during sapling stage and low during adult
   c. low survival during sapling stage and low during adult
   d. High survival during sapling stage and low during adult

Ans. (a) low survival during sapling stage and high during adult

95. Most of trees of India in tropical forest belongs to family

   a. Arecacea
   b. Fabaceae
   c. Dipterocarpaceae
   d. Bromeliacae

Ans. (c) Dipterocarpaceae

96. Scientific names of bacteria, fungi plant and animals are given by

   a. International union of biological nomenclature
   b. There is different organization for naming plants and fungus
   c. There are three different ograniztion for naming bacteria, plant and animals
   d. Names of plants and animals are given by same organization

Ans. (c) There are three different ograniztion for naming bacteria, plant and animals

97. Among the following imino acid is

   a. Proline
   b. Arginine
   c. Typtophan
   d. Lysine

Ans. (a) Proline

98. pI for hypothetical protein consisting of only apolar amino acids will be

a. Independent on charge over N and C terminus

b. Depend on number of amino acids

c. Depend on mass of amino acids

d. Independent of type of amino acids

Ans. (d) Independent of type of amino acids

99. What would be effect on photosynthesis in C3 and C4 plants on elevating the concentration of CO_2 under light saturated condition?

a. No effect on both type plants

b. C3 plants will saturates fast and C4 plant remain unaffected

c. C4 plants saturate fast and C3 plants remain unaffected

d. Both type plants will saturate fast

Ans. (b) C3 plants will saturates fast and C4 plant remain unaffected

100. Common metabolites in nucleotide biosynthesis from glucose by pentose phosphate pathway is

a. PRPP

b. Glyceraldehydes-3-phosphate

c. Di Hydroxy Acetone Phosphate

d. Fructose -6-P

Ans. (a) PRPP

Memory Based Paper CSIR NET Dec 2009

1. Correct arrangement from smallest to largest is

- a. Nucleus < Cell < Tissue < Organ < System< organism
- b. Cell <Nucleus < Tissue < Organ < System< organism
- c. Nucleus < Cell < Tissue < system <organ< organism
- d. Nucleus < Cell < organ < tissue < System< organism

Ans. (a) Nucleus < Cell < Tissue < Organ < System< organism

2. If complete atmospheric gases are removed than what would be effect on global temperature of earth

- a. It will fall
- b. It will increase
- c. No effect
- d. Unstable temperature

Ans. (a) It will fall

3. Which of the following are not utilized in photosynthesis?

- a. CO_2, N_2, Chlorophyll, sunlight
- b. CO_2, N_2, Chlorophyll, sunlight
- c. CO_2, N_2, Chlorophyll, sunlight, NADP
- d. CO_2, N_2, Chlorophyll, sunlight, carbohydrates

Ans. (a) CO_2, N_2, Chlorophyll, sunlight

4. There are two Ecosystems, A with high species diversity and B with low species diversity. Which statement is not correct for above ecosystem?

- a. Ecosystem A would be more stable
- b. Ecosystem B would be more stable
- c. More extinction rate at ecosystem A
- d. There will be more competition in ecosystem A

Ans. (b) Ecosystem B would be more stable

5. The following graph shows population growth curve for rabbit n certain ecosystem. The point x on graph after which population become stable represents

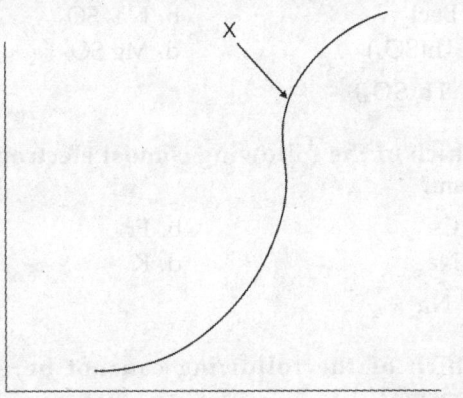

- a. Carrying capacity
- b. More mortality
- c. Scarcity of food
- d. Natural selection

Ans. (a) Carrying capacity

6. Which of the following is not a function of blood?

- a. Provide immunity
- b. Production of hormones like insulin
- c. Repair of damage parts
- d. Gaseous transport

Ans. (b) Production of hormones like insulin

7. Among the following which is biopolymer

- a. Nucleic acid
- b. Polystyrene
- c. Latex
- d. Nylon

Ans. (a) Nucleic acid

8. Among the following which will be basic in nature

- a. Lemon juice
- b. Baking soda in water
- c. Ammonium chloride in water
- d. Vinegar in water

Ans. (b) Baking soda in water

9. **Among the following which s optically active**

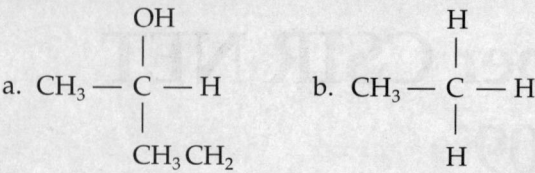

a. $CH_3 — \overset{\overset{\displaystyle OH}{|}}{\underset{\underset{\displaystyle CH_3\,CH_2}{|}}{C}} — H$ b. $CH_3 — \overset{\overset{\displaystyle H}{|}}{\underset{\underset{\displaystyle H}{|}}{C}} — H$

c. $CH_3 — \overset{\overset{\displaystyle CH_3}{|}}{\underset{\underset{\displaystyle H}{|}}{C}} — H$ d. $CH_3 — \overset{\overset{\displaystyle CH_3}{|}}{\underset{\underset{\displaystyle CH_3\,CH_2}{|}}{C}} — H$

Ans. (a)

10. **Which of the following is radioactive substance?**

    a. $Becl_2$ b. $Na_2\,SO_3$
    c. $Th(SO_4)$ d. $Mg\,SO_4$

Ans. (c) $Th(SO_4)$

11. **Which of the following is most electropositive atom?**

    a. Cs   b. Fr
    c. Na   d. K

Ans. (c) Na

12. **Which of the following can not be used as abrasive?**

    a. Diamond   b. Calcite
    c. Granite   d. Topaz

Ans. (c) Granite

13. **Which is correct about spectra for H atom and He+ ion**

    a. Similar
    b. Similar but He+ ion having one/fourth frequency
    c. Similar but He+ ion having four time more frequency
    d. Similar but He+ ion having four times more frequency

Ans. (c) Similar but He+ ion having four time more frequency

14. **Mean half life of a radioisotope is $\left\{\dfrac{1}{0.693}\right\}$ second. The time required for decay of 10 mg radioactive substance in to 2.5 mg will be**

    a. $\left\{\dfrac{1}{0.693}\right\}$ sec   b. $\left\{\dfrac{2}{0.693}\right\}$ sec
    c. 1 sec   d. 2 sec

Ans. (d) 2 sec

15. **Path of a comet entering into our solar system cannot be**

    a. Circle   b. Parabola
    c. Eclipse   d. Straight line

Ans. (d) Straight line

16. **Correct representation of a graph for a pebble falling from a certain height would be**

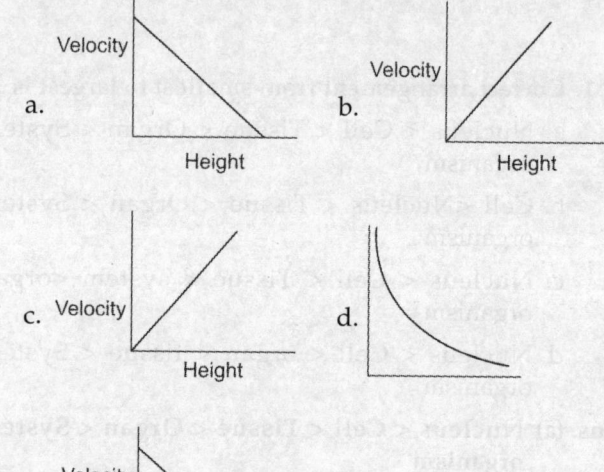

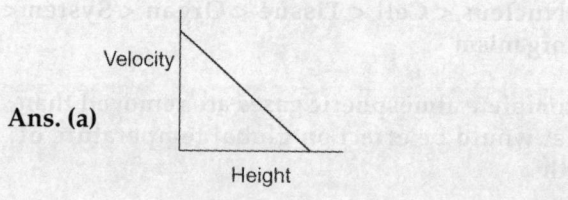

Ans. (a)

17. **Various rectangles can be drawn in circle of radius 'r'. The rectangle with maximum area will be**

    a. $2r^2$
    b. $V2r^2$
    c. $2r$
    d. None of these

Ans. (a) $2r^2$

18. **A metallic solid sphere is fully charged. The charge on sphere will be**

    a. Only at surface
    b. Concentrated at centre
    c. Evenly distributed
    d. Unevenly distributed

Ans. (a) Only at surface

19. **Why air is cooler at high altitude such as mountain than at lowlands**

    a. Higher pressure at high altitude
    b. Low density of air at high altitude
    c. Heat of air is due to reflected radiation from earth
    d. Lesser oxygen

Ans. (b) Low density of air at high altitude

20. The undisturbed layers of sedimentary rocks are deposited down from west to east as shown in figure. The order of layers from oldest to youngest will be

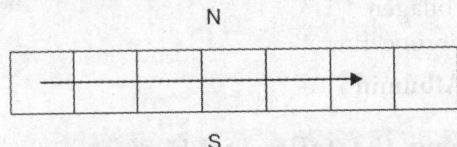

a. North to south
b. East to west
c. West to east
d. South to North

Ans. (b) East to west

21. An object is placed 100 cm from a lens of focal length 50 cm. The image is formed at 'x' and magnification is 'm'. The value of x and m will be

a. 100, 100
b. 50, 100
c. 100, 50
d. 100, 1

Ans. (d) 100, 1

22. Sum of two binary number 1101 and 1011 will be

a. 10111
b. 11001
c. 11111
d. 10001

Ans. (a) 10111

23. Time required for downloading a file of 2.4 Mb from a broadband connection having speed of 256 kbps will be

a. Lesser than 5 minutes
b. 30 minutes
c. 3 minutes
d. Lesser than 30 second

Ans. (d) Lesser than 30 second

24. The programme first to run on starting computer is

a. Operating system
b. Checking keyboard
c. Checking power on
d. Bios booting

Ans. (d) Bios booting

25. The function of heat sink in PC is

a. To heat up CPU
b. To cool CPU
c. To cool memory
d. To dissipate heat from RAM

Ans. (b) To cool CPU

26. Vinblastin has been extensively used for treating cancer. This is an example of

a. Radiotherapy
b. Chemotherapy
c. Heat therapy
d. Surgery

Ans. (b) Chemotherapy

27. When tryptophan in excess most of times RNA polymerase dismount after transcription of first 150 nt in trp operon. This is termed as

a. Antitermination
b. Attenuation
c. Catabolite repression
d. Feed back inhibition

Ans. (b) Attenuation

28. Under which phase of bacterial growth bacteria increased is size but do not divide

a. Lag
b. Log
c. Stationary
d. Death phase

Ans. (a) Lag

29. Which of the following can be regarded as programmed cell death?

a. Death induced by toxin
b. Death by inflammation
c. Death of cell during normal development
d. Death due phagocytosis

Ans. (c) Death of cell during normal development

30. Which of the following is necessary for transport of m-RNA from nucleus

a. RNA editing
b. 5' capping
c. 3' polyadenylation
d. Secondary structure

Ans. (d) Secondary structure

31. Among the following which is not a function of hydrogen peroxide release during plant stress response

a. Crosslinking glycans in cell wall
b. Lignin deposition
c. Production of ethylene and salicyclic acid
d. Production of jasmonic acid

Ans. (d) Production of jasmonic acid

32. Promoters for RNA polymerase III are located at

a. +1 to +10
b. Downstream after termination
c. – 35 to – 10
d. With in transcribed sequence

Ans. (b) Downstream after termination

33. Transport of ions across membrane depends on

a. Concentration gradient
b. Membrane potential
c. Concentration gradient and membrane potential both
d. Independent of both

Ans. (c) Concentration gradient and membrane potential both

34. **Among the following which amino acid do not absorbs wavelength of 250 to 300 nm**

    a. Cystine   b. Phenylalanine
    c. Tryptophane   d. Histidine

Ans. (a)

35. **The efficient conversion of fructose to fructose-6 phosphate occurs in**

    a. Liver   b. Muscles
    c. Adipose   d. Intestine

Ans. (a) Liver

36. **Which statement is not true about E.coli DNA ligase**

    a. Links double stranded blunt ends
    b. NAD is source of AMP as cofactor
    c. Requires ATP as energy source
    d. Do not link single stranded DNA

Ans. (d) Do not link single stranded DNA

37. **Which statement is correct regarding edge effect**

    a. They are poor in diversity
    b. They are rich in diversity
    c. Low completion
    d. High predation pressure

Ans. (b) They are rich in diversity

38. **In Sickle cell anemia the RBC are sickle shaped due to**

    a. Change in shape of haemoglobin before binding of oxygen
    b. Change in shape of haemoglobin after binding with oxygen
    c. Loss of spectrin cytoskeleton protein
    d. Plasma membrane of RBC is sickle shaped

Ans. (a) Change in shape of haemoglobin before binding of oxygen

39. **If organism is at very high risk of extinction according to IUCN, then it is kept in category of**

    a. Critically endangered   b. Endangered
    c. Rare   d. Vulnerable

Ans. (a) Critically endangered

40. **Activity of single channel on neuron can be studied using**

    a. Single neuron recording
    b. Patch clamp technique
    c. ECG
    d. EEG

Ans. (b) Patch clamp technique

41. **Which of the following is not an extracellular matrix protein**

    a. Albumin
    b. Lamin
    c. Collagen
    d. Fibronectin

Ans. (a) Albumin

42. **Among the following highest assimilation efficiency is observed in**

    a. Herbivores
    b. Carnivores
    c. Microbivores
    d. Omnivores

Ans. (a) Herbivores

43. **To focus image the accommodation in lens of eye is mainly at**

    a. Due to change surface of front of lens
    b. Due to change surface of back of lens
    c. Due to sphincter muscles which vary the curvature the both surface of lens
    d. Due to type of ciliary muscles and fiber

Ans. (d) Due to type of ciliary muscles and fiber

44. **Cell with rigid lignified cell wall and dead protoplasm is**

    a. Collenchymas
    b. Sclerenchyma
    c. Cholrenchyma
    d. Companion cell

Ans. (b) Sclerenchyma

45. **Which of the following is not a co-dominant marker**

    a. RFLP   b. SNP
    c. RAPD   d. ISSR

Ans. (c) RAPD

46. **The best technique for analyzing total m-RNA**

    a. Northern analysis
    b. Southern analysis
    c. DNA hybridization
    d. RNA in situ hybridization

Ans. (d) RNA in situ hybridization

47. **Among the following which radioisotope is not a emitter**

    a. C^{14} b. I^{125}
    c. P^{32} d. H^3

Ans. (b) I^{125}

48. In sandwich ELISA the molecule capture is

a. Antibody

b. Antigen

c. Enzyme

d. Antgen-antibody complex

Ans. (b) Antigen

49. Taq enzyme utilized in PCR is a

a. RNA polymerase

b. Reverse transcriptase

c. DNA polymerase

d. Ligase

Ans. (c) DNA polymerase

50. Maximum diversity of reptiles was during

a. Cretaceous

b. Jurassic

c. Ordovician

d. Triassic

Ans. (b) Jurassic

51. Among the following which is not an assumption of Hardy-Weinberg rule

a. Small population size

b. Random mating

c. No natural selection

d. No mutation

Ans. (a) Small population size

52. Wings of insect and birds have be come flat, large and stream lined. This is an example of

a. Convergent evolution

b. Parallel evolution

c. Divergent evolution

d. Co-evolution

Ans. (a) Convergent evolution

53. The correct expression of Hamilton rule for the evaluation of altruism is [C= the cost of a behavioural act to the act, b= the benefit of that act to a beneficiary, and r= the genetic relatedness between the actor and the beneficiary] where C is 0.5 and r=0.5

a. C>r.b

b. C<b.r

c. C must be more than 0.5 and r lesser than 0.5

d. Benefits must be more than genetic relationship

Ans. (b) C<b.r

54. Phonetic classification is based on

a. Over all similarity of characters and gaps between variation

b. Phylogenetic relationship

c. Genetic relationship

d. Anatomical and embryological characters

Ans. (a) Over all similarity of characters and gaps between variation

55. Among the following which group of animals do not belongs to deutrostomes

a. Brachypoda

b. Chordates

c. Nematodes

d. Echinodermates

Ans. (c) Nematodes

56. Which of the following molecule can be utilized for establishing early evolutionary process

a. Mitochondrial DNA

b. Ribosomal RNA

c. Chloroplalst DNA

d. Nuclear DNA

Ans. (b) Ribosomal RNA

57. The family Dipterocarpacae occurs in

a. Temp. deciduous forest

b. Tropical deciduous forest

c. Semi arid forest

d. Tropical forest

Ans. (d) Tropical forest

58. Certain species of birds shown variation n beak size only when they are sympatric. This is example of

a. Character displacement

b. Natural selection

c. Ecological variation

d. Mutation

Ans. (a) Character displacement

59. Maximum growth rate s observed in logistic equation when the organism are at

a. N excess than K+

b. K/2

c. N = K

d. N is greater than K

Ans. (b) K/2

60. Which of the following are abiotic factor?

a. Temperature, rainfall, pH, parasites

b. Temperature, rainfall, pH, soil

c. Temperature, rainfall, pathogens

d. Temperature, rainfall, pH, viruses

Ans. (b) Temperature, rainfall, pH, soil

61. During the process of succession arrival of late successional stage depends on environment modified by earlier succession stage. The process is referred as

a. Co-evolution

b. Facilitation

c. Tolerance

d. Inhibition

Ans. (b) Facilitation

62. The ecosystem having longest energy transfer time is

a. Tropical rain forest

b. Open Ocean

c. desert

d. temperate deciduous forest

Ans. (a) Tropical rain forest

63. the term used for bubble like structure generated during early process of origin of life by Oparin is

a. micelles   b. protobionts

c. probiont   d. coacervates

Ans. (b) protobionts

64. which gas was absent during pre-biotic environment?

a. CO_2 b. CH_4

c. O_2 d. SO_2

Ans. (c) O_2

65. Toll like receptors are a type of pattern recognition receptor and recognize molecules that are broadly shared by pathogens but distinguishable from host molecules, collectively referred to as pathogen associated molecular pattern. They are

a. Present only in mouse

b. Present on membrane of ER

c. Are transmembrane protein

d. Present on cytosolic face of plasma membrane

Ans. (c) Are transmembrane protein

66. Function of CD+4 T-lymphocyte is

a. Secretion of cytokinin

b. Secretion of complement proteins

c. Production of antibodies

d. Destroys antigen

Ans. (a) Secretion of cytokinin

67. In regulative development , the prospective potency of cells

a. Equal to prosective fate

b. More than prospective fate

c. Lesser than prospective fate

d. Not determined

Ans. (b) More than prospective fate

68. For translation process besides eIF2, Met-t-RNA eukaryotic 80-S ribosome also requires

a. GTP   b. ATP

c. CTP   d. UTP

Ans. (a) GTP

69. T4 bacteriophage after infecting E. Coli generally hacks host machinery for transcrton of its own genes. It is done by

a. Degrading host RNA polymerase

b. Synthesis of own RNA polymerase

c. Degradation of host genome

d. Modifying host RNA polymerase

Ans. (d) Modifying host RNA polymerase

70. Influenza virus enters host cell by

a. Cell fusion   b. Exocytosis

c. Endocytosis   d. Transcytosis

Ans. (c) Endocytosis

71. The vector responsible for Japanese encephalitis is

a. Culex tritaeniorhynchus

b. C. jenseni

c. C.pipiens

d. C. pusillus

Ans. (a) Culex tritaeniorhynchus

72. Which lipid is found exclusively on one face of membrane

a. Cholestrole

b. Phosphyatidyl choline

c. Phophatidy inisitol

d. Phosphatidy lethanolamine

Ans. (b) Phosphyatidyl choline

73. Chaperons (Hsp 70) are absent in

a. Mitochondria

b. Chloroplast

c. Endoplasmic reticulum

d. Golgi bodies

Ans. (d) Golgi bodies

74. Prolamellar body are present in

a. Leucoplast

b. Chloroplast

c. Chromoplast

d. Eiloplast

Ans. (d) Eiloplast

75. Uptake of mineral like zinc, Mg and Fe across membrane in plant is by

a. ABC transporter

b. H+- co-transporter

c. ZIP transporter

d. ATP dependent transporter

Ans. (c) ZIP transporter

76. During development homing of cell is mediated by

    a. Laminin   b. Integrin

    c. Cadherin   d. Selection

Ans. (a) Laminin

77. Which of the following vaccine will not pose any problems n immune-compromised person

    a. Measles   b. Mumps

    c. BCG   d. Pneumonococcal

Ans. (d) Pneumonococcal

78. Morphylaxis can be defined as

    a. Reinitiation of cell division in existing cells, followed by repatterning of those cells

    b. Production of lost organ by division in remaining cell

    c. Production of complete organism by single cell

    d. Movement of organism toward stimulus

Ans. (a) Reinitiation of cell division in existing cells, followed by repatterning of those cells

79. The grafting of the dorsal lip of the blastopore from an early Xenopus astrula onto the ectopic ventral side of an early embryo will result in two complete embryos. Thus dorsal can be designated as

    a. Primary organizer

    b. Cytoplasmic determinant

    c. Morphogen

    d. Primitive

Ans. (a) Primary organizer

80. Three classed of gene A,B and C regulates the development of flowers in Arabidopsis. If a loss-of-function mutation occurs in the B-type genes, what will be the compostion of the flower whorls?

    a. Sepals-petals-stamens-carpels

    b. Sepals-sepals-stamens-carpels

    c. Sepals-sepals-carpels-carpels

    d. Petals-petals-stamens-stamens

Ans. (c) Sepals-sepals-carpels-carpels

81. Plant dissipate excess excitation energy as heat so as to protect rom hto-oxidative damage. The mechanism is known as

    a. Photo chemical quenching

    b. Non-photo chemical quenching

    c. Photonhibition

    d. Merven effect

Ans. (b) Non-photo chemical quenching

82. Major transport of nitrogen n xylem sap is in form of

    a. Glutamate   b. Allantoin

    c. Glutamine   d. Ammonia

Ans. (b) Allantoin

83. According to the polymer trap hypothesis small sugars such as sucrose are converted t raffinose and other larger oligosaccharides is loaded in phloem. Major site of synthesis if raffinose is

    a. Sieve tube   b. Companion cell

    c. Intermediate cell   d. Transfer cells

Ans. (c) Intermediate cell

84. E.coli based Humulin is a

    a. Insulin   b. Interferon

    c. Growth factor   d. Disaccharide

Ans. (a) Insulin

85. Agrobacterium tumefaciens causes crown gall seases in dicot plants. Which phytohormone genes are present in T-DNA

    a. Auxin and cytokinin

    b. Auxin only

    c. Cytokinin

    d. Cytokinin and brassicosteroids

Ans. (a) Auxin and cytokinin

86. In formaldehyde the pure orbitals involves n bonding between C and O is

    a. Only C   b. Both C and O

    c. Only O   d. H, C &O

Ans. (b) Both C and O

87. Retinoblastoma is one of the important protein involved in cancer. The function of Rb is to hold the protein involved in

    a. G1 arrest

    b. G2 arrest

    c. DNA repair

    d. Replication initiation

Ans. (d) Replication initiation

88. The major function of type-III secretion by pathogenic bacteria is

    a. Efflux of drug

    b. Release signal for quorum sensing

    c. Release virulence factors

    d. Release of competence factor

Ans. (c) Release virulence factors

89. **Under what condition reaction will always occurs**
   a. $\Delta H<0$ and $\Delta S<0$
   b. $\Delta H<0$ and $\Delta S>0$
   c. $\Delta H>0$ and $\Delta S>0$
   d. $\Delta H>0$ and $\Delta S<0$

   Ans. (b) "H<0 and " S>0

90. **Which thermodynamics property cannot be directly measured in cell**
   a. Free energy
   b. Enthalpy
   c. Entropy
   d. Temperature

   Ans. (a) Free energy

91. **Which statement is correct for globular proteins**
   a. Always contain α helix
   b. Contain β sheet
   c. Contain β pleated sheet
   d. Turns

   Ans. (a) Always contain á helix

92. **Which organelles have characterstic galactolipids in its membrane**
   a. Mitochondria
   b. Chloroplast
   c. ER
   d. Golgibody

   Ans. (b) Chloroplast

93. **If cell is not dividing which repair mechanism will not occurs**
   a. Recombination repair mechanism
   b. Excision repair mechanism
   c. Transcriptional coupled repair mechanism
   d. DNA synthesis annealing repair

   Ans. (a) Recombination repair mechanism

94. **The virus inserted in genome can be recognised by**
   a. FISH
   b. Microarray
   c. Northern blot
   d. Southern blot

   Ans. (a) FISH

95. **Different strains of virus can be identified by**
   a. Fluorescence Microscopy
   b. Electron Microscopy
   c. PCR
   d. Observing symptoms of disease in patient

   Ans. (c) PCR

96. **Bacterial two component system includes**
   a. Sensory kinase and response regulator
   b. Sensory kinase and hoshotransferase
   c. Signal and receptor
   d. Stimulus and response

   Ans. (a) Sensory kinase and response regulator

97. **Which of the following represent the gametophyte generation in plant**
   a. Ovule
   b. Megaspore
   c. Embryo sac
   d. Egg

   Ans. (c) Embryo sac

98. **The major function of cortical granules in cytoplasm of egg is to**
   a. Fast block to polyspermy
   b. Slow block to polyspermy
   c. Allowing meiosis to complete
   d. Helping in reorganization of sperm

   Ans. (a) Fast block to polyspermy

99. **Among the following which plant removes heavy metal from water**
   a. Chlorophyll
   b. Lycopene
   c. Xanthophylls
   d. Coumarin

   Ans. (b) Lycopene

100. **Among the following which plant removes heavy metal from water**
   a. Eichornia crassipes
   b. Nymhia vishin
   c. Pistia stratiotes
   d. Salvia officinalis

   Ans. (a) Eichornia crassipes

Memory Based Paper CSIR NET June 2010

1. Cupper sulphate in presence of excess or ammonia gives blue colour. The blue is due to
   a. Complex ligand formation
   b. Cuperic ion
   c. Cuperous ions
   d. Ammonium sulphate

Ans. (a) Complex ligand formation

2. $NH_3 + H_2O \rightarrow NH_4OH$

   What would be weight of ammonia used for complete utilization of one liter of water for formation of ammonium hydroxide
   a. 1000 g
   b. 943.5 g
   c. 17.7 g
   d. 35 g

Ans. (b) 943.5 g

3. Moon centre do not show movement in its core, so it will result in
   a. No gravitational force on moon
   b. Moon will not have its magnetism
   c. It will lack atmosphere
   d. It will be heavily bombarded with meteors

Ans. (b) Moon will not have its magnetism

4. $H_2O \rightarrow H^+ + OH^-$. If $[H+] [OH] = 1 \times 10^{-14}$ M^2 and H_2O = 55 M. Then ratio of non ionized water to ionized water will be
   a. $1 : 1.8 \times 10^{-7}$
   b. $1 : 1.8 \times 10^{-6}$
   c. $1 : 1.8 \times 10^{-13}$
   d. $1 : 1.8 \times 10^{-16}$

Ans. (d) $1 : 1.8 \times 10^{-16}$

5. A myopic person is also suffering from astigmatism, to correct his vision which lenses must be used
   a. Plane concave lens
   b. Plane convex lens
   c. Combination of concave and cylindrical
   d. Combination of convex and cylindrical

Ans. (c) Combination of concave and cylindrical

6. Four times the square of an integer is one greater than three times of an integer: the value of integer is
   a. +4
   b. –4
   c. +1
   d. –1

Ans. (c) +1

7. Oxidation of cupper occurs in
   1. $CuSO_4 + Zn \rightarrow ZnSO_4 + Cu$
   2. $Cu + AgNO_3 \rightarrow CuNO_3 + Ag$
   3. $Fe + CuSO4 \rightarrow Fe_2(SO4)_3 + Cu$
   4. $Cu + AuCl_3 \rightarrow 3CuCl + Au$

   a. 1 and 2
   b. 2 and 3
   c. 2 and 4
   d. 1 and 4

Ans. (c) 2 and 4

8. Two dice are thrown having number 1 to 6. maximum probability for getting sum of two dice will be
   a. 4
   b. 6
   c. 7
   d. 8

Ans. (c) 7

9. Blue color of sky is due to
   a. Scattering only
   b. Due to composition of sunlight
   c. Both
   d. Crompton scattering

Ans. (a) Scattering only

10. Three balloons are filled with hydrogen (A), Helium (B) and CO_2 (C) respectively and then dipped in water, so order of buoyancy force operating on them will be
    a. F1 > F2 > F3
    b. F3 > F2 > F1
    c. F1 = F2 > F3
    d. F1 = F2 < F3

Ans. (a) F1 > F2 > F3

11. **Duration of day length n summer(southern) hemisphere will**

   a. Decrease with increase n ongitudes
   b. Increase with increase in longitudes
   c. Increase with increase in latitudes
   d. Decrease with increase n latitude

Ans. (c) Increase with increase in latitudes

12. **Which statement is correct regarding ratio of half life of radioactive material to its mean life?**

   a. Will remain constant
   b. Will be always greater than one
   c. Will increase with increase n duration of half life
   d. Will depends on amount of radioactive

Ans. (a) Will remain constant

13. **An object is dropped from certain height. Among the following which graph correctly explain change in magnitude of acceleration and velocity before hitting the ground**

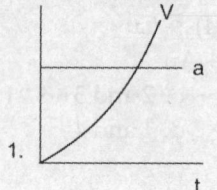 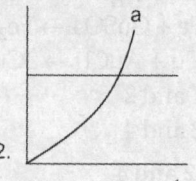

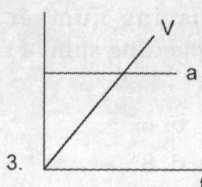 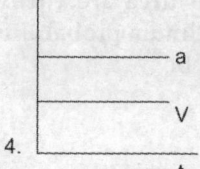

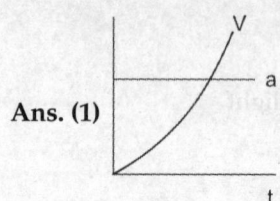

Ans. (1)

14. **Frequency of incident light on hotovoltaic material is 1.5 times of requried threshold frequency fr generation of electrons. If the frequency s haved and ntensity is doubled what will happen**

   a. Electron emission will remain same
   b. No emission of electrone
   c. Electron emission will reduce to half
   d. Electron emission will be double

Ans. (b) No emission of electrone

15. **A plane flying at certain altitude completes a complete turn around the earth at equator n 24 hours. What would be time taken to complete revolution around 60° N of earth flying at same speed and altitude**

   a. 24 hrs
   b. 18 hours
   c. 12 hours
   d. 6 hours

Ans. (b) 18 hours

16. **A plane is flying at height 10 km with speed of 1000 Km/hour. What would be angular velocity of plane when it is observed by person standing on earth**

   a. 1 rad/sec
   b. 36 rad/ sec
   c. π rad/ sec
   d. $\pi/2$ rad/sec

Ans. (b) 36 rad/ sec

17. **$a^2 + b^2 + c^2 < 10$, where a, b and c are integers. The maximum possible ways of arrangement of ntegers such that statement is satisfide**

   a. 3   b. 4
   c. 5   d. 6

Ans. (c) 5

18. **For the equation $x^5 + x^4 + 2x^3 + 3x^3 + 4x + 5 = 0$, product of root will be**

   a. 0   b. 16
   c. 15   d. 12

Ans. (b) 16

19. **The value of given matrix will be**

$$\begin{bmatrix} 1 & 2 & 0 & 1 \\ 0 & 2 & 2 & 1 \\ 0 & 0 & 2 & 1 \\ 0 & 0 & 0 & 1 \end{bmatrix}$$

   a. 0   b. 1
   c. 2   d. 5

Ans. (a) 0

20. **A string of length six characters is to be arranged using codes R, G and B such as RRRRRR, RRGBBRR etc. In how many ways it can be done**

   a. 150   b. 650
   c. 729   d. 216

Ans. (c) 729

21. Consider the following flow chart. F string starts from A than what be position at end of reading string 00111000111100000

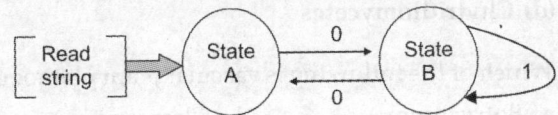

a. State A
b. State B
c. 1/3 chance state A and 2/3 chance of state B
d. 2/3 chance of state A and 1/3 chance of state B

Ans. (a) State A

22. Fossil gives better idea for age of rocks because

a. Organic evolution is irreversible
b. Rocks are formed after fossil deposition
c. Rocks with fossils are stable
d. Fossils do not allow weathering of rocks

Ans. (a) Organic evolution is irreversible

23. In atmosphere lowest concentration of CO_2 is measured durng September. The major causes is

a. High utilization of CO_2 by plants during summer
b. CO_2 is more soluble n warm oceanic water
c. CO_2 sinks below earth
d. Pollution is lesser in September

Ans. (a) High utilization of CO_2 by plants during summer

24. Genome of virus is made up of

a. DNA
b. RNA
c. DNA and RNA
d. Protein

Ans. (c) DNA and RNA

25. Which element is present in least amount by weight in human body?

a. H   b. C
c. N   d. P

Ans. (d) P

26. The characteristic of organisms reaching first to barren island are

a. Slow growth and small generation time
b. Slow growth and large generation time
c. Fast growth and small generation time
d. Fast growth and large generation time

Ans. (c) Fast growth and small generation time

27. Among the following which would be absent in the insects flying in night?

a. Color vision   b. Vibration sensation
c. Rods   d. Black and white vision

Ans. (a) Color vision

28. Sucrose is composed of

a. Glucose and galactose
b. Fructose and galactose
c. Glucose and fructose
d. Mannose and fructose

Ans. (c) Glucose and fructose

29. During replication of DNA during S phase of cell cycle DNA is duplicated, what happens to chromosome number

a. They also doubles
b. Remains same
c. Reduced to half
d. Reduced to one fourth

Ans. (b) Remains same

30. On selfing urple plants out of 100 plants in next generation 79 plants were purple and 21 plants were white. The conclusion which can be drawn is

a. One gene is involved
b. Two independent genes are involved
c. Two genes showing epistasis
d. Three gene are involved

Ans. (a) One gene is involved

31. Green house effect is observed due to absorption of

a. Primary radiation from sun
b. Secondary radiation coming from earth
c. CO_2
d. Water vapour

Ans. (b) Secondary radiation coming from earth

32. The out come following equation would be

$n \to \infty (1 + 2/n)^n$

a. e^2 b. e
c. $e^2 + 1$ d. $e^2 - 1$

Ans. (a) e^2

33. Temperature decreases at the rate of 6°C per Km with altitudes. At hat height there is least likeliness of water vapours to exist

a. 0.1 km   b. 1 Km
c. 2 Km   d. 10 Km

Ans. (d) 10 Km

34. The perimeter of right angle isosceles triangle with unit area will be

    a. 2
    b. $\sqrt{2}$
    c. $2\sqrt{2}$
    d. $2+\sqrt{2}$

Ans. (d) $2+\sqrt{2}$

35. Among the following which is not a polymer?

    a. Polysterene
    b. Vinyl alcohol
    c. Polyethylene
    d. Rubber

Ans. (b) Vinyl alcohol

36. Which is isomer of C_2H_5OH is

    a. CH_2CH_2CHO
    b. $CH_3CH_2OCH_3$
    c. CH_3OCH_3
    d. CH_3CH_2COOH

Ans. (c) CH_3OCH_3

37. Humans have originated in Africa is supported by the fact that

    a. Less variation in DNA of African population
    b. More variation in DNA of African population
    c. More evidences of human fossil in African population
    d. Conserved fossils in Africa

Ans. (a) Less variation in DNA of African population

38. In a lake low nutrients occur in upper strata due to consumption by algae while high nutrients are present at bottom due to activity of decomposer, which is correct graphical representation of nutrients with depth for such lakes under steady state?

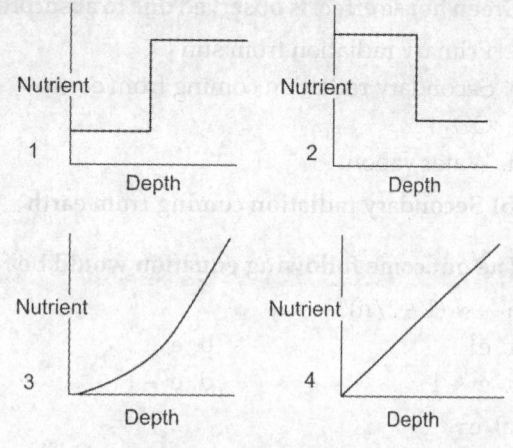

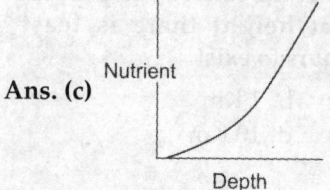

Ans. (c)

39. Motile zoospore occur in

    a. Basidiomycetes
    b. Ascomycetes
    c. Zygomycetes
    d. Chytridiomycetes

Ans. (d) Chytridiomycetes

40. Which of the following is vascular plant plathogen?

    a. Botrychium
    b. Claviceps
    c. Fusarium
    d. Verebarium

Ans. (c) Fusarium

41. Origin of tropical weed Eupatorium odoratum is

    a. Ethopia
    b. Peru
    c. Mexico
    d. Brazil

Ans. (c) Mexico

42. Which statement is correct for $\Delta G = 0$

    a. Reaction is in equilibrium
    b. Operates only under constant P and V
    c. Follows PdV equation
    d. All of the above

Ans. (d) All of the above

43. Among the following maximum gross productivity is observed at

    a. Boreal forests
    b. Temperate deciduous
    c. Temperate confer
    d. Cold deciduous

Ans. (b) Temperate deciduous

44. Which biogeographical region covers maximum part of India?

    a. Semi arid
    b. Deccan peninsular
    c. Gangatic plains
    d. Himalaya

Ans. (b) Deccan peninsular

45. Tigers do not occurs in Srilanka while they are seen India. While the leopards areseen in both India and srilanka. The main reason is

    a. Tigers are not swimmers
    b. Srilankans have removed tiger due to excessive hunting
    c. India care more for tigers
    d. Leopard originated before separation of India and srilanka due to plate shifting

Ans. (d) Leopard originated before separation of India and srilanka due to plate shifting

46. Chromatids appear in form of dyads during

    a. Metaphase of Mitosis
    b. Metaphase of Meiosis
    c. Prophase of Mitosis
    d. Anaphase of Mitosis

Ans. (b) Metaphase of Meiosis

47. Meiosis produces n, n + 1 and n − 1 gametes. The probable reason is

a. Non-disjunction during metaphase I

b. Non-disjunction during metaphase II

c. Non-disjunction during metaphase I and II

d. Non-disjunction during anaphase I

Ans. (b) Non-disjunction during metaphase II

48. A cross between hens with different comb shape was carried as show in figure.

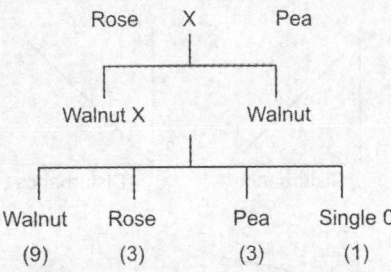

This conclusion which can be drawn is

a. Single gene is involved for comb shape

b. Two independent segregating genesare involved

c. Two genes are showing epistasis

d. Four independent segregating alleles are involves

Ans. (c) Two genes are showing epistasis

49. Mendel during his experiment on garden pea observed F2 ratio of 3:1 on selfing round seed plants where 3 were round and 1 was wrinkled. If all round seed plant are selfed to raise the F3 generation the observed ratio will be

a. Half of plants with round seed and rest with wrinkled seed

b. 3/4 of plants with round seed and 1/4 with wrinkled seeds

c. All plants with round seeds

d. 1/3 of plants with round seeds and 2/3 of plants bearing round and wrinkled seeds

Ans. (d) 1/3 of plants with round seeds and 2/3 of plants bearing round and wrinkled seeds

50. Darwinian evolutionary fitness is measured in turn of

a. Good health

b. Ability to fight with others

c. Reproductive success

d. Lesser mutation

Ans. (c) Reproductive success

51. Hardy-weinberg law will NOT operate under condition, when

a. 3 alleles are involved

b. Weak selection on one of the allele

c. Skewed sex ration

d. Mutated allele is not involved in sexual selection

Ans. (b) Weak selection on one of the allele

52. Reversal of sexual dimorphism is observed under condition

a. Strong female choice

b. Skewed sex ration

c. Number of males are very low

d. Male and females changes their roles

Ans. (b) Skewed sex ration

53. The donor and acceptor of electron for cytb/f6 are

a. PQ and UQ   b. UQ and Cyt C

c. UQ and PC   d. PQ and PC

Ans. (d) PQ and PC

54. The chemical salicyl hyrooxamic acid inhibits

a. Cytochrome oxidase

b. Alternate oxidase

c. ATP synthese

d. NADH- dehyrogenase

Ans. (b) Alternate oxidase

55. Phytochromes involved in red/far red response are dimeric chromoproteins. The two sub-units of phytochromes are linked with

a. PAS domain

b. PTB domain

c. Hinge region

d. Kinase domain

Ans. (c) Hinge region

56. Which of the following DONOT occur during seed development?

a. Accumulation of storage proteins

b. Synthesis of LEA proteins

c. Desiccation

d. Synthesis of Gibberlic acid

Ans. (d) Synthesis of Gibberlic acid

57. In signal transduction pathway of which plant hormones genes 'rht', spy', 'gay' are associated

a. Auxin   b. Gibberlic acid

c. Absiccic acid   d. Ethylene

Ans. (b) Gibberlic acid

58. Most of DNA binding proteins binds to DNA by particular motif to modulate gene expression. Gene which are under regulation of gibberllic acid have GRE where, GREB binds. The motif in GREB is

    a. Leucine Zipper

    b. b ZIP

    c. Zinc finger

    d. Homeodomain

Ans. (a) Leucine Zipper

59. In plants gene 'sepallata' is NOT involved in formation of organ

    a. Sepals   b. Petals

    c. Stamens   d. Carpels

Ans. (a) Sepals

60. The lateral separation of amphibian embryo at two celled stage will result in

    a. Identical twins

    b. Two embryos joined at bell region

    c. Single embryo

    d. Two embryos missing various organs

Ans. (a) Identical twins

61. If hydra is fragmented into various parts, separates group of cell repattern themselves into various small hydras. Such an mode of developments termed as

    a. Regeneratioin

    b. Morphlaxis

    c. Epimorphogenesis

    d. Morphylaxis and epimorphogenesis

Ans. (b) Morphlaxis

62. An embryo lacking biocoid is injected with biocoid m-RNA at middle portion. It will result

    a. Two heads and no tarsons

    b. Head in middle and tarsons at both end

    c. No head and tarson at both ends

    d. Normal phenotype

Ans. (b) Head in middle and tarsons at both end

63. Which of the following is a species specific protein in sea urchin which play an important role in recognization during acrosomal reaction

    a. Bindin

    b. Avidine

    c. Fertiline

    d. Cortical granules

Ans. (a) Bindin

64. In an experimental population birth rate is 18 per 1000 and death rayte is 14 per 1000. Size of population is 10,000 at times , 't' , then what will be the size of population at time 't+1'

    a. 10,000   b. 10,040

    c. 10,140   d. 11,040

Ans. (b) 10,040

65. Whichis correct graphical representation of effect of disturbance on species diversity as per island biogeography ?

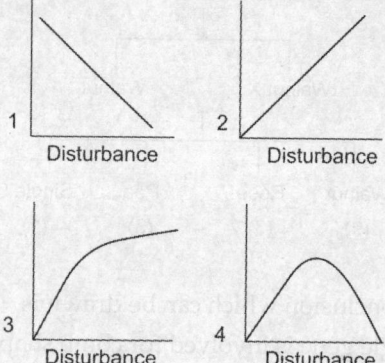

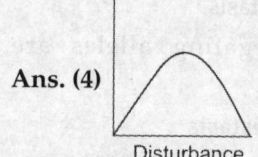

Ans. (4)

66. Which statement is correct for r selection species ?

    a. Large number of progeny with large size

    b. Small number of progeny with large size

    c. Large number of progeny with small size

    d. Small number of progeny with large size

Ans. (c) Large number of progeny with small size

67. To explain origin of life the first biomolecule generated under lab condition were

    a. Amino acid

    b. Nucleic acid

    c. Carbohydrate

    d. Lipid

Ans. (a) Amino acid

68. Dinasaurs becomes extinict during

    a. 1.6 billion year ago

    b. 6.5 billion year ago

    c. 6.5 million year ago

    d. 65 million year ago

Ans. (d) 65 million year ago

69. When a new sapling is transferred to soil, roots have very loose contact with soil particles and its suffer from water stress because of

a. Cavitation
b. Positive hydrolic pressure
c. Capiilary action
d. Loss of water from root to soil

Ans. (a) Cavitation

70. Km for enzyme is equal to where

a. $V_0 = Vmax$
b. $2V_0 = Vmax$
c. $4V_0 = Vmax$
d. $V_0 = 2 max$

Ans. (b) $2V_0 = Vmax$

71. During regulation of trp operon by attenuation there is

a. Immature termination of translation
b. Immature termination of transcription
c. Termination of replication
d. Ribosome fails to read transcript

Ans. (b) Immature termination of transcription

72. In an experimental approach trp operon and lac operon were fused. Under what condition there would be expression of β galactosidase?

a. Low lactose and glucose
b. High lactose and glucose
c. Low tryptophan
d. High tryptophan

Ans. (c) Low tryptophan

73. Which selectablemarker gene is routinely rused for selection of transgenic plant?

a. Amphicillin
b. Tetracycline
c. Hygromycin
d. Carbenicillin

Ans. (c) Hygromycin

74. Which microbe has been used against insect plant pathogens?

a. Agrobacterium tumefaciens
b. Agrobacterium rhizogenes
c. Bacillus thuringennesis
d. Fusarium nudum

Ans. (c) Bacillus thuringennesis

75. Which instrument is used to measure electrical activity of heart?

a. Electrocardiograph
b. Electrocardiogram
c. Sphygmomanometer
d. Electroencephalogram

Ans. (b) Electrocardiogram

76. Flow cytometer is used to measure the number of

a. Cells
b. DNA
c. RNA
d. Protein

Ans. (a) Cells

77. In bioinformatics for structural proteomics, the structure of protein can be spectrum

a. PDB
b. EMBL
c. NIH
d. Gene bank

Ans. (a) PDB

78. How many H atoms would be replaced CCl4 in presence of ethanol during NMR spectrum

a. 1
b. 2
c. 3
d. 4

Ans. (c) 3

79. polygalacatournidase antsense RNA is use in reference to which phenomenon

a. Seed setting
b. Herbicide resistance
c. Viral resistance
d. Fruit Ripening

Ans. (d) fruit Ripening

80. which of the following diseases or pathogen have been completely eradicated from India?

a. Small pox, polio
b. Yellow fever, Plaque
c. Small pox, Guinea worm
d. Sleeping sickness, yellow fever

Ans. (c) Small pox, Guinea worm

81. A person suffering from gucose-6-phosphate dehydrogenase deficiency are found to be resistance to

a. Plasmodium
b. Fungus
c. Leishmania
d. Bacteria

Ans. (a) Plasmodium

82. Which of the following cell has been proved in elucidation of lipid bilayer of plasma membrane?

a. Bacterial cell
b. Virus
c. RBC
d. Kidney cell

Ans. (c) RBC

83. In HIV diagnosis technique based on western blotting, the patient sample is screened for

a. Antigen
b. Antibody
c. Virus outer coat protein
d. Virus

Ans. (b) Antibody

84. In which cancer treatment erb-B antibodies are used

a. Breast

b. Oral

c. Prostrate

d. Lung

Ans. (a) Breast

85. Bcl-2 and Bax proteins involved in apoptosis are

a. Proapoptic and anti apoptic

b. Both proapoptic

c. Both anti-apoptic

d. Anti-apoptic and pro-apoptic

Ans. (d) Anti-apoptic and pro-apoptic

86. Vif gene is one of the important regulatory gene in lifecycle of HIV virus. It was observed that HIV virus with mutated vif gene fails to culture of normal T-helper cells. The main reason is

a. Vif gene helps in reverse transcription process

b. Vif gene helps in transport of HIV genome to nucleus

c. Vif gene helps in insertion of viral genome into host genome

d. Vif product targets the enzyme responsible for hypermutation to ubiquitination and cellular degradation

Ans. (d) Vif product targets the enzyme responsible for hypermutation to ubiquitination and cellular degradation

87. Nick translation means

a. Translation by cytosolic ribosome

b. Translation of protein from stalled site

c. Replication by DNA polymerase I after removing RNA primers

d. Replication of DNA by DNA polymerase I from nick produced by DNase treatment

Ans. (d) Replication of DNA by DNA polymerase I from nick produced by DNase treatment

88. According to Holiday model if markers are present outside of crossover point, then recombinant molecules would be generated when

a. There is no resolution

b. Always recombinant would be produced

c. Nick is on outer strand during resolution

d. Nick is on inner strand during resolution

Ans. (c) Nick is on outer strand during resolution

89. E. coli cells were transformed with plasmid carrying tetracycline resistance gene and later on plated on LB medium and various colonies were observed but same number of colonies were observed for control non transformed E. coli cells. The probable reason is

a. No transformation has occurred

b. Bacteria are plated just after heat shock and incubation with plasmid

c. E. coli cells were already resistance to tetracycline

d. Wrong plasmid was used

Ans. (c) E. coli cells were already resistance to tetracycline

90. Which antibiotic is responsible for premature termination of translation n bacteria?

a. Tetracycline

b. Choloramphenicol

c. Penicillin

d. Puromycin

Ans. (d) Puromycin

91. Among the following which DNA polymerase lacks proof reading activity

a. DNA polymerase α

b. DNA polymerase δ

c. DNA polymerase ε

d. DNA polymerase α and ε

Ans. (a) DNA polymerase α

92. Which statement is correct for archaebacteria?

a. Lacks histone protein

b. Have 9 + 2 arrangement in flagella

c. Lacks introns in genes

d. Cell wall is made up of peptidogycan

Ans. (a) Lacks histone protein

93. In a m-RNA mmature termination occurs from codon UAA, which of the following transition mutation will lead to its reversal

a. Change at first U

b. Change at first A

c. Change at second A

d. All of these

Ans. (a) Change at first U

94. The major function of surfactant protein secreted by lungs is

a. Do not allow growth of bacteria

b. Stops entry of dust particles into lungs

c. Keeps alveolies inflated

d. Helps in absorption of oxygen

Ans. (c) Keeps alveolies inflated

95. In brain meninges are absent at

a. Dura matter

b. Pia mater

c. Grey mater

d. Arachnoid mater

Ans. (c) Grey mater

96. Which phylum is characterized by absence of body symmetry, no tissue or organs and lack of nervous system?

a. Porifera

b. Cnidaria

c. Pteniphora

d. Rhyzopoda

Ans. (d) Rhyzopoda

97. Secondary structure of RNA is stabilized by hydrogen bonding between

a. GC and AU

b. GC and AT

c. GC, AU and GU

d. GC only

Ans. (c) GC, AU and GU

98. Which of the following enzyme of nitrogen metabolism is located in plastid?

a. Nitrate reductase

b. Nitrite reductase

c. Aspartate synthetase

d. Nitrogenase

Ans. (b) Nitrite reductase

99. ABC transporter are NOT involved in

a. Transport of chloroplast content for degradation in vacuole

b. Accumulation of pigment in plant vacuole

c. Secretion of matting factor in yeast

d. Uptake f phosphorus

Ans. (a) Transport of chloroplast content for degradation in vacuole

100. Which plant has been used in phyto-remediation for uptake of cadmium from contaminated soil?

a. Helianthus annus

b. Brassica juncea

c. Silene vulgaris

d. Oscimum basalcum

Ans. (b) Brassica juncea

Memory Based Paper CSIR NET Dec 2010

1. The correct configuration for given structure is

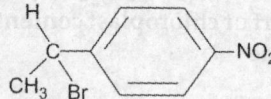

a. L configuration   b. D configuration
c. R configuration   d. S configuration

Ans. (c) R configuration

2. Pumice is the name of the most common volcanic rocks that floats. It has various air bubbles and capillaries which trap air. Which statement is correct for this rock

a. Air cavities are interconnected
b. Air cavities are not connected
c. Density of rock is more than water
d. Rock is very older

Ans. (b) Air cavities are not connected

3. Fr a reaction A→B, the rate of reaction can be represented is

$$\frac{dx}{dt} = K(a-x)$$

Where a and (a-x) are concentration of reactant at time 0 and t, then the unit of K will be
a. $Mol^{-1}L^{-2}$
b. $Mol^{-2}L^{-1}$
c. $L.mol^{-1}s^{-1}$
d. Sec^{-1}

Ans. (d) Sec^{-1}

4. Identify the graph of the logarithmic function $f(x)=xe^2$

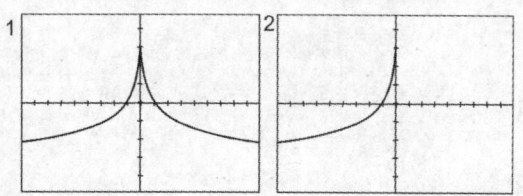

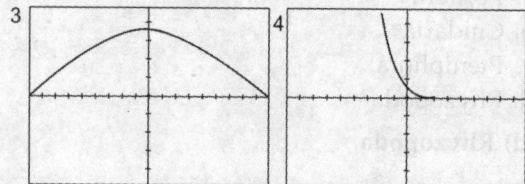

Ans. (1)

5. What amount has to be taken from 11 N HCl to make 50 ml of 2N HCl

a. 11.0 ml
b. 9.09 ml
c. 6.03 ml
d. 2.0 ml

Ans. (b) 9.09 ml

6. High biological oxygen demand in water body indicates

a. Chemical pollution
b. Organic pollutant
c. High photo-autograph
d. Pressure of heterotrophs

Ans. (b) Organic pollutant

7. If standard enthalpies of formation for $H_2O(g)$-242, CH_4 (g) -75 and CO_2 (g) is -111 Kjmol-1 respectively. Determine the heat of reaction of the following reaction.

$$CH_4(g)+2H_2O (g) \rightarrow CO_2 (g)+ 4H_2$$

a. $- 206\ Kj\ mol^{-1}$
b. $+ 206\ Kj\ mol^{-1}$
c. $- 448\ Kj\ mol^{-1}$
d. $- 670\ Kj\ mol^{-1}$

Ans. (c) $- 448\ Kj\ mol^{-1}$

8. Slope of line in given plot will be

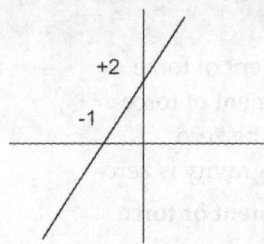

  a. −1   b. −½

  c. +1/2   d. 2

Ans. (d) 2

9. If period of f(x) = sin x s 2π, then the period of g(x) = sin (2X) will be

  a. π b. 2π

  c. $\pi/2$ d. 4π

Ans. (a) π

10. It is predicted that due to global warming there would be rise in level of oceans. If radius of earth is R and rise in level of water is 'h'. Then the volume of water will be

  a. $\Pi r^2 h$ b. $\frac{3}{4}\pi r^2 h$

  c. $2\pi r^2 h$ d. $4\pi r^2 h$

Ans. (d) $4\pi r^2 h$

11. If a rectangle is inscribed in circle of diameter 'D'. Then the area of rectangle will be

  a. Independent of length and breadth

  b. Will be always smaller than $D^2/2$

  c. Will be always smaller than $D^2/4$

  d. Will be always greater than $\pi D^2/4$

Ans. (b) Will be always smaller than $D^2/2$

12. An aero plane flies with a ground speed of 800 km/h and velocity of wind is constant 50 km/h. If this aero pane flies one hour upstream an one hour downstream of wind. Then total distance covered and average speed will be

  a. 1600 km and 800 km/h

  b. 1650 km and 825 km/h

  c. 1550 km and 775 km/h

  d. 1700 km and 850 km/h

Ans. (a) 1600 km and 800 km/h

13. Which of the following element is required for production of thyroxin?

  a. Nacl   b. Iodine

  c. Bromine   d. Fluorine

Ans. (b) Iodine

14. Temperature above which gas cannot be liquefied even by applying pressure is termed as

  a. Critical temperature

  b. Boyle temperature

  c. Curie temperature

  d. Charles temperature

Ans. (a) Critical temperature

15. If a nail is hammered in the bark of tree at height 4m, after ten year the height of tree is doubled. Then the height of nail will be

  a. 4 m

  b. 8 m

  c. 16 m

  d. 10 m

Ans. (a) 4 m

16. Let f:[0,1] → (0, ∞) be a continuous function. Suppose f(0) =1 and f(1)=7. Then

  a. F s uniformly contimuous and is not onto

  b. F is increasing and f([0,1])= [1,7]

  c. F is not uniformly continuous

  d. F is not bounded

Ans. (c) F is not uniformly continuous

17. The net direction of force on charge placed at origin as shown in diagram will be in

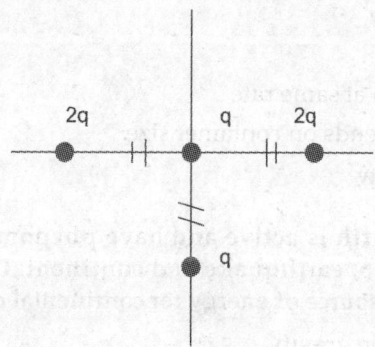

  a. +Y   b. −Y

  c. +X   d. −X

Ans. (a) +Y

18. Zinc oxide is thermochromic, changing from white to yellow when heated to high temperature. This color change s caused due to

  a. Stoichiometric property of metal

  b. Non-stoichiometric property of metal

  c. Burning of oxygen

  d. Fluorescence at high temperature

Ans. (b) Non-stoichiometric property of metal

19. **A wild from animal gives one egg and mutant from gives three egg per year respectively. If all parents and progenies survive, then what would be ratio of number of wild to mutant after four years.**

    a. 4
    b. 2×4
    c. $2 \times 3 \times 4$
    d. $2 \times 2 \times 2 \times 2$

Ans. (d) $2 \times 2 \times 2 \times 2$

20. **If a certain place shown stable population distribution. If means maximum number of individual will be**

    a. Healthy
    b. Youngest
    c. Oldest
    d. Reproductively more active

Ans. (b) Youngest

21. **Which of the following is responsible for ozone hole?**

    a. CO_2
    b. CH_4
    c. Chlorine
    d. NO

Ans. (c) Chlorine

22. **At 35°C ambient room temperature any liquid in two container are allowed to cool from 100°C to 70°C and 80 to 50°C respectively. If we compare rate cooling in we find that rate of cooling in later will be**

    a. Slow
    b. Fast
    c. Both at same rate
    d. Depends on container size

Ans. (a) Slow

23. **The earth is active and have phenomenon like volcano, earthquake and continental drift. The major source of energy for continental drift is**

    a. Moon gravity
    b. Earth gravity
    c. Radioactivity in core of earth
    d. Energy from sun

Ans. (c) Radioactivity in core of earth

24. **The mean salinity of sea 35 g per liter. The main cause of this observed salinity is**

    a. Evaporation and rainfall
    b. Photosynthesis
    c. Crust erosion and surface run off
    d. Rivers drainage

Ans. (a) Evaporation and rainfall

25. **If the handle of a door placed at hinges is displaced toward centre, more force is required to open it because**

    a. Less moment of force
    b. More moment of force
    c. Force will be zero
    d. Centre of gravity is zero

Ans. (a) Less moment of force

26. **If a gas is released from pressurized bottle, then which statement will be true for release gas?**

    a. It will gain energy
    b. It will have same temperature as in bottle
    c. It will gain temperature
    d. It will cool as compare to gas in container

Ans. (d) It will cool as compare to gas in container

27. **Among the following which cell can divide by binary fission**

    a. Muscle cell
    b. Nerve cell
    c. RBC
    d. Bone marrow cell

Ans. (d) Bone marrow cell

28. **Which statement is not correct for all mammals?**

    a. Absence of scales
    b. Absence of laying egg
    c. Absence of segmentation
    d. Presence of asexual reproduction

Ans. (d) Presence of asexual reproduction

29. **Smog is due to**

    a. Air pollution derived from smoke and vehicles
    b. More moisture in environment
    c. Increased in CO_2
    d. Low temperature of earth surface

Ans. (a) Air pollution derived from smoke and vehicles

30. **Cell with large round size has more chance to survive as compare to thin cell under desiccation because**

    a. Low surface to volume ration
    b. High surface to volume ratio
    c. Thin membrane
    d. Thick membrane

Ans. (a) Low surface to volume ration

31. **Which of the following is not a direct consequence of green house effect?**

    a. Increase in sea level
    b. Rainfall
    c. Tsunami
    d. Global warming

Ans. (c) Tsunami

32. NaCl has ionic because

    a. Both Na and Cl has same number of valence electron

    b. Both Na and Cl belongs to same group

    c. Na losses one electron and chlorine receive one electron

    d. Due to difference in their electronegativity

Ans. (c) Na losses one electron and chlorine receive one

33. Brown ring test is confirmatory test for which anionic species

    a. Nitrate   b. Bromide

    c. Chloride   d. Fluoride

Ans. (a) Nitrate

34. The graph below shows frequency distribution of different sizes of cell during different stages of cell culture

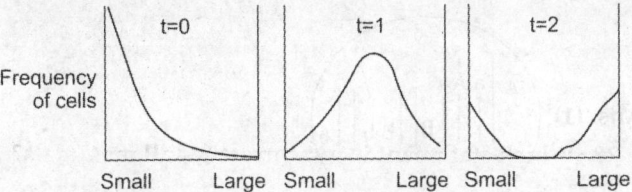

From this pattern of growth we can draw conclusion that

    a. Most of the cell divides at same time

    b. Rate of cell division is constant

    c. Cell does not divide

    d. All of cell divides at same time

Ans. (a) Most of the cell divides at same time

35. The computer codes for decimal number 99 will be

    a. 1100011   b. 1110111

    c. 1000011   d. 011000111

Ans. (d) 011000111

36. Parts per billion can be represented as

    a. ng/ kg   b. µg/kg

    c. µl/kg   d. µg/g

Ans. (b) µg/kg

37. Which of the following is not possible in biological systems?

    a. DNA → RNA → protein

    b. Protein → RNA → DNA

    c. Glucose → amino acid → protein

    d. RNA → DNA → Protein

Ans. (b) Protein → RNA → DNA

38. The liquid is following in tube as shown in diagram.

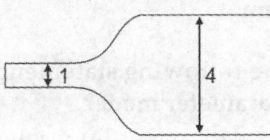

The rate of flow at position A as compare to B will be

    a. Four times

    b. Sixteen times

    c. Half

    d. One fourth

Ans. (b) Sixteen times

39. In given circuit voltage drop at diode is 0.9 V.

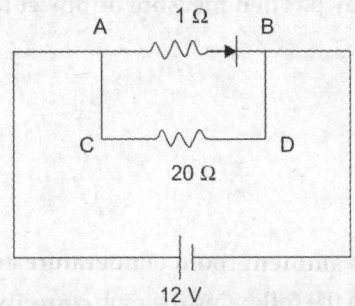

Then which statement is correct

    a. More current is flowing through path AB

    b. More current is flowing through path CD

    c. Equal current is flowing from both routes

    d. Resistance is not influencing flow of current

Ans. (a) More current is flowing through path AB

40. Which is not a structural alignment tool?

    a. SSAP

    b. TM-align

    c. T-coffee

    d. DALI

Ans. (c) T-coffee

41. Which of the following is major radioactive indoor air pollutant in home air conditioner?

    a. Cs

    b. U

    c. Sr

    d. Rn

Ans. (d) Rn

42. Variation in two characters in two or more species can be best represented by

    a. Histogram

    b. Scattered diagram

c. Triangular box

d. Linear curve

Ans. (a) Histogram

43. Which of the following statement correctly refer statistical parameter mode?

    a. Most of insect mature on third day of development

    b. Major part of population fails to advance their education above 10+2

    c. The average number of seeds by plant is 3.5

    d. The height of plant range from 5 to 10

Ans. (a) Most of insect mature on third day of development

44. In statistical error type-I is represented by α and type-II by β. Then measure of power of error will be

    a. 1-α

    b. 1-β

    c. α-β

    d. β-α

Ans. (b) 1-β

45. Which of the following diagram correctly represents co-existance of two species even during niche overlapping?

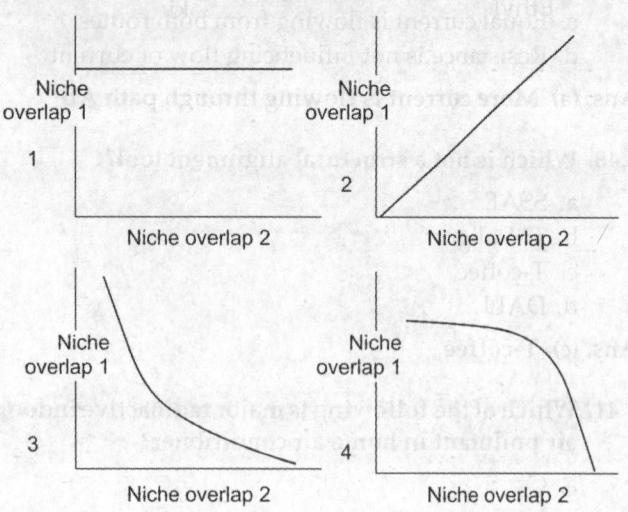

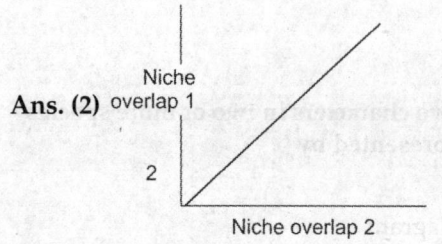

Ans. (2)

46. If all four gametes AB, aB, Ab and ab formed in equal probability. Then arrangement of chromosomes at metaphase-I of meiosis will be

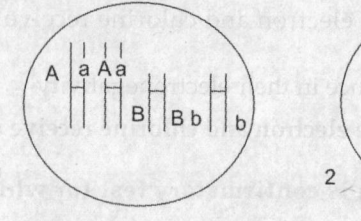 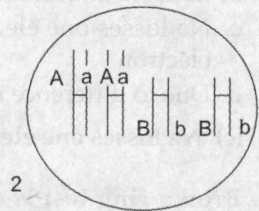

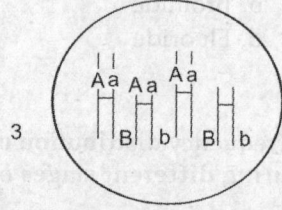 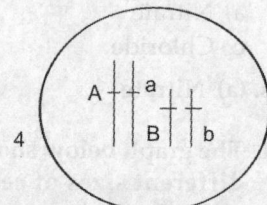

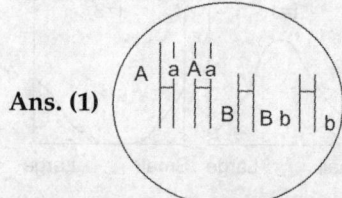

Ans. (1)

47. The distance between gene A and B is 10 cM. If a genotype $\dfrac{A \quad\quad b}{b \quad\quad B}$ is selfed, the percentage of progeny with genotype aabb will be

    a. 10%

    b. 25%

    c. 0.25%

    d. 0.01%

Ans. (c) 0.25%

48. Male parental care is expected to observed during

    a. Polygynous species

    b. Small population

    c. Life long bond pairing

    d. Reverse sexual dimorphism

Ans. (d) Reverse sexual dimorphism

49. Which of the following is the major environmental cue for migration of birds during winter?

    a. Duration of day length

    b. Instinct

    c. Falling temp.

    d. Learning

Ans. (a) Duration of day length

50. **Which cyclin is involved in formation of per transcriptional enhancer binding protein?**

   a. Cyclin D
   b. Cyclin k
   c. Cyclin E
   d. Cyclin T

Ans. (b) Cyclin k

51. **Binding of erythroprotin to its EPO receptor leads to activation enhancer binding protein?**

   a. JAK-STAT pathway
   b. NF-kβ pathway
   c. Apaf-smad pathway
   d. Tyrosine kinase pathway

Ans. (a) JAK-STAT pathway

52. **Receptors for FSH is present on**

   a. Leyding cell
   b. Sertoli cell
   c. Peritubular cells
   d. Spertogonium germ cell

Ans. (b) Sertoli cell

53. **During gametogenesis in male, cell during development are termed as primary spermatocytes when they are**

   a. Before meiosis-I
   b. After meiosis-I
   c. After meiosis-II
   d. Mature sperms

Ans. (a) Before meiosis-I

54. **Which statement is true about progenitor cells?**

   a. They are same as stem cells
   b. They are totipotent cell
   c. They can divide but do not remain differentiated as stem cell
   d. They can not divide

Ans. (c) They can divide but do not remain differentiated as stem cell

55. **Neuropeptides and neurotransmitters are molecules secreted by neuron. Which statement is correct statement about neuropeptide as compare to neurotransmitter?**

   a. Less potent and short acting
   b. More potent but short acting
   c. Less potent but long acting
   d. More potent and longer acting

Ans. (d) More potent and longer acting

56. **There is small gap between two neuron at synapses. The purpose of gap s**

   a. Unidirectional flow of information
   b. Reabsorbtion of neurotransmitter
   c. Coupling of charge over membrane
   d. Slow down speed of propagation

Ans. (a) Unidirectional flow of information

57. **Most abundant intracellular ion in plants is**

   a. Iron
   b. Calcium
   c. Potassium
   d. Zinc

Ans. (c) Potassium

58. **Na^+-K^+ pump operates under intracellular concentration of**

   a. High Na and low K
   b. High Na and High K
   c. Low Na and low K
   d. Low Na and high K

Ans. (d) Low Na and high K

59. **Precursor for amino acid proline is**

   a. Pyruvate
   b. 3-phosphoglycerate
   c. Oxalo acetate
   d. α-keto glutarate

Ans. (d) α-keto glutarate

60. **S-adenosyl methionine is a precursor of which plant hormone?**

   a. Absicic acid
   b. Auxin
   c. Ethylene
   d. Cytokinin

Ans. (c) Ethylene

61. **Under certain conditions pyruvate can be allowed to decarboxylation into acetyl CoA and CO_2. For evolution of ^{14}C labelled carbon in CO_2, which carbon atom must be radolbelled in glucose prior to glycosis?**

   a. C1 or C6
   b. C3 OR C4
   c. C3 OR C3
   d. C5 OR C2

Ans. (b) C3 OR C4

62. **Which cycle has been used in hetero lactic fermentation?**

   a. Entner-Doudroff pathway
   b. Phosphoketolase pathway
   c. Pentose phosphate pathway
   d. Glycoate pathway

Ans. (b) Phosphoketolase pathway

63. **The characteristic of mitochondrial genome is?**

   a. Intron free DNA
   b. Repetitive DNA
   c. Polycistronic RNA
   d. Satellite DNA

Ans. (a) Intron free DNA

64. In scanning simple sequence repeats primer are used against

a. Random sequence
b. Repetitive sequence
c. Flanking region of repetitive sequence
d. Conserved region of exon of gene

Ans. (c) Flanking region of repetitive sequence

65. Integrity of introduced transene in mouse can be validate by

a. Male pronuclei insertion
b. Fusion of enucleated eg with somatic cells
c. Transfer into competent embryogenic cell
d. Sourthern blot analysis

Ans. (d) Sourthern blot analysis

66. Techniques used to assess HIV-I seroconversion are

a. Immunoblot and ELISA
b. Immuno precipitation and PCR
c. PCR and immunofluroscence
d. PCR and ELISA

Ans. (b) Immuno precipitation and PCR

67. Which of the following cancerous transformation if due to retero virus?

a. Human T-cell leukemia b. Burkitt Lymphoma
c. Oral epithelial cancer   d. Colon cancer

Ans. (a) Human T-cell leukemia

68. Among the following which is termed as proof reading activity of DNA polymerase?

a. $5' \rightarrow 3'$ polymerase activity
b. $3' \rightarrow 5'$ polymerase activity
c. $5' \rightarrow 3'$ exonuclease activity
d. $3' \rightarrow 5'$ exonuclease activity

Ans. (d) $3' \rightarrow 5'$ exonuclease activity

69. The carboxy-terminal domain of RNA polymerase II consists of hepta-peptide repeats. Other protein often binds the C-terminal doman of RNA polymerase in order to activate polymerase activity. Which of the following is not a function associated with CTD of RNA polymerase?

a. Promoter recognition   b. Promoter clearance
c. 5' capping   d. Splicing

Ans. (a) Promoter recognition

70. Which of the following is reactive centre for splicing of exons during processing of m-RNA

a. U1 and U5
b. Branch point, U2 and U6

c. Branch point, U4 and U6
d. U2 and U4

Ans. (b) Branch point, U2 and U6

71. Which of the following is the first step in translational proof reading?

a. Aminoacylation of t-RNA by amino acyl t-RNA synthetase
b. Peptide bond formation
c. Entry into A site
d. Formation of amino acyl t-RNA 40 S ribosome and m-RNA ternary complex

Ans. (b) Peptide bond formation

72. Puromycin blocks translation. Mode of action of drug puromycin is

a. Binds to A site and stop elongation
b. Stops peptidyl trenasferase activity
c. Binds EF-TU-GTP and prevent initiation
d. Donot allow termination of translation

Ans. (a) Binds to A site and stop elongation

73. Etracyclines are a group of broad spectrum anti-biotics against bacterial resistance. Tetracycline antibiotics are protein synthesis inhibitor and exerts ts effect by binding to

a. 30S subunit of ribosome
b. 50 S subunit of ribosome
c. A site of ribosome
d. Peptidyl transferase

Ans. (a) 30S subunit of ribosome

74. Ciprofloxacin is a synthetic chemotherapeutic antibiotic of the fluoroquinlone drug class. The target of antibiotic ciprofloxacin is

a. Replication   b. Protein synthesis
c. Cell wall synthesis   d. Membrane structure

Ans. (a) Replication

75. The one of the most widely used herbicides methyl viologens interfere photosynthesis of higher plants. They are responsible for

a. Evolution of more oxygen
b. Dissipation of proton gradient across thylakoid membrane
c. Inhibition of flow of electron from PS II to PS I
d. Transfer of electrons from PS I to molecular oxygen

Ans. (d) Transfer of electrons from PS I to molecular oxygen

76. **Which would be the result of mutation in genes responsible for radial patterning in roots of higher plants?**

    a. No apical root formation
    b. Root hair will fail to develop
    c. Variation in number and position of cell in vascular system
    d. Roots will be positively geotropic

Ans. (c) Variation in number and position of cell in vascular system

77. **In Arabidoposis gene responsible for formation shoot meristem is**

    a. Leafy   b. Agamous
    c. Clavata   d. Wus

Ans. (c) Clavata

78. **Among the following which gene product migrates from leaves to shoot meristem during transition of shoot meristem into floral meristem?**

    a. Flowering locus T   b. Flowering locus D
    c. Leafy   d. Apetala 1

Ans. (a) Flowering locus T

79. **The position of collagen triple helix in Ramachandran plot is at:**

    a. Top left   b. Top right
    c. Bottom right   d. Bottom left

Ans. (a) Top left

80. **One of the most important gene, involved in dorsal-ventral axis determination in Drosophila is dorsal. It codes Dorsal protein which**

    a. Is taken up into the nuclei of cells and this side will become the ventral side
    b. Remains in the cytoplasm of cell and this side will become ventral side
    c. Is taken up into the nuclei of cells and this side will become the dorsal side
    d. Degraded in one side and that will become dorsal side

Ans. (a) Is taken up into the nuclei of cells and this side will become the ventral side

81. **Which is true for amount of yolk and cleavage in egg of amphibian?**

    a. Mesolecithal and holoblastic cleavage
    b. Isolecithal and holoblastic cleavage
    c. Mesolecithal and meroblastic cleavage
    d. Microlecithal and meroblastic cleavage

Ans. (a) Mesolecithal and holoblastic cleavage

82. **Among the following which enzyme used NAD as cofactor?**

    a. Histone acetyl transferase
    b. Histone methyl transferase
    c. Histone deacetylase
    d. Histone demethylase

Ans. (c) Histone deacetylase

83. **Which of the following system can be utilized for glycosylation of peptides expressed using RDT?**

    a. Large bacterial fermenters
    b. Small bacterial fermentors
    c. Normal bacterial bioreactors
    d. Mammalian cell line

Ans. (d) Mammalian cell line

84. **Among the following which is not responsible for producing near UV signal in circular dichorasim for secondary structure determination of proteins**

    a. Tyrosine   b. Tryptophan
    c. Disulphide bond   d. Peptide bond

Ans. (d) Peptide bond

85. **β-α-β structure in protein structure are known for**

    a. Ligand binding
    b. Stereological hindrance in binding of ligand
    c. Catalytic centre
    d. Transmembrane domain

Ans. (a) Ligand binding

86. **Which of the following is most unstable condition in protein folding?**

    a. Non-polar side chain exposed to outside
    b. Polar side chain present in core of protein
    c. Non polar side chains in core of protein
    d. Polar amino acids exposed to outside

Ans. (a) Non-polar side chain exposed to outside

87. **Most effective protein denaturant from of guanidinium when used in equimolar concentration is**

    a. Iodide   b. Chloride
    c. Bromide   d. Sulphate

Ans. (b) Chloride

88. **The melting temperature (Tm) is defined as the temperature at which half of the DNA strand are in the double-helical state and half are in the random coil states. Tm of DNA does not depends on**

    a. Length of DNA   b. % GC content
    c. Presence of cations   d. Presence of anions

Ans. (d) Presence of anions

89. In a heterozygous two recessive mutation at different site will give mutant phenotype when genes involved are
    a. Allelic and placed in cis
    b. Allelic and placed in trans
    c. Non-allelic and placed in cis
    d. Non allelic and placed in trans

Ans. (a) Allelic and placed in cis

90. Allele frequency of a particular allele was found to be 0.6 in three different populations. It is probably due to is
    a. Neutral allele
    b. Stable polymorphism
    c. Heterozygote advantage
    d. Natural selection

Ans. (a) Neutral allele

91. Molecular evolution do not reflects
    a. Species divergence
    b. Convergent evolution
    c. Natural selection
    d. Neutral mutation

Ans. (c) Natural selection

92. Somatic hypermutation in immunoglobulin genes is responsible for
    a. Class switching
    b. Affinity maturation
    c. Clonal selection
    d. VDJ Recombination

Ans. (b) Affinity maturation

93. To assess the mutation in bacteria, bacteria were inoculated in various aliquots and later on shifted on screening media for selection of mutants. The most important for assessing mutation would be
    a. Total number of mutant
    b. Average number of mutant per aliquot
    c. Petri plates with single mutant colony
    d. Petri plates without any mutant colony

Ans. (b) Average number of mutant per aliquot

94. Interaction of antibody with antigen is like lick and key. The major force responsible for antigen antibody interactions is
    a. Hydrogen bond
    b. Vander wall interaction
    c. Disulphide bond
    d. Peptide bond

Ans. (a) Hydrogen bond

95. Which is common cytokine secreted by both T_{H1} and T_{H2} cells
    a. IL-2   b. IL-4
    c. INF-   d. IL-5

Ans. (a) IL-2

96. Major Histocompatibility complex I (MHC I) is present at
    a. All nucleated cells
    b. Only on antigen presenting cells
    c. Only on B and T lymphocytes
    d. Macrophages and Dendritic cells

Ans. (a) All nucleated cells

97. Major reason for evolution for diversity in immune system is
    a. Natural selection   b. Neutral mutations
    c. Directed evolution   d. Co-evolution

Ans. (d) Co-evolution

98. At any place if more diversity and variation is observed in any species of domestic animal, then it can be concluded that
    a. Place is natural centre of origin of species
    b. Animal has been introduced once and is invasive
    c. Animal has been introduced more than once
    d. People take more care of animals

Ans. (c) Animal has been introduced more than once

99. Among the following which is typical tree of Indian desert ecosystem?
    a. Prosopis cineraria
    b. Avicennia officinalis
    c. Mangifera indica
    d. Acer negundo

Ans. (a) Prosopis cineraria

100. Which of the following is not an invasive plant species in India?
    a. Parthenium hysterophorus
    b. Salvinia molesta
    c. Lantana camara
    d. Myristica fica

Ans. (d) Myristica fica

101. The causal organism for blast of rice is
    a. Pyricularia grisea
    b. Ustilago tritici
    c. Erwinia chrysanthemi
    d. *Cercospora janseana*

Ans. (a) Pyricularia grisea

102. **Which group of algae is believed to be most closely related to higher plants?**

    a. Charophyceae
    b. Chlorophyceae
    c. Rhodophyceae
    d. Pheophyceae

Ans. (a) Charophyceae

103. **Following cladogram represent changes in annelids during evolution**

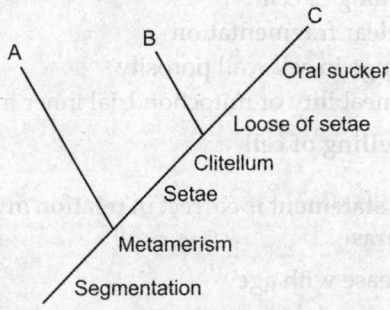

    The group 'C' in cladogram represents

    a. Hirudinea
    b. Echiura
    c. Polychaetes
    d. Oligochaeta

Ans. (a) Hirudinea

104. **Characteristic feature of Cnidaria is**

    a. No tissue or organ system
    b. Diploblastic or bilayered
    c. Triploblastic or three layered
    d. Segementation

Ans. (a) No tissue or organ system

105. **Nilgiri Tahr is restricted only to upper heights (1200 to 2600 metres) of western ghat. The major reason is**

    a. Habitat preferences
    b. Habitat shrinkage
    c. Urbanization in other part of habitat
    d. Pressure of tiger predation at lower height

Ans. (a) Habitat preferences

106. **Which of the following is not a characteristic of climax community?**

    a. Wide niche
    b. Complex food web
    c. Low resilience
    d. Inter biotic nutrients dependence

Ans. (a) Wide niche

107. **In an abandoned area first nitrogen fixing communities arrives and carry out nitrogen fixation with non-nitrogen fixers, later on this community is nitrogen fixers are lost and it is dominated by non nitrogen fixing species. In the mechanism of succession this is in general agreement according to**

    a. Facilitating   b. Tolerance
    c. Inhibition   d. Adaptation

Ans. (a) Facilitating

108. **Under what thermodynamically condition reaction would be spontaneous?**

    a. $\Delta H > 0$ and $\Delta S > 0$
    b. $\Delta H < 0$ and $\Delta S > 0$
    c. $\Delta H < 0$ and $\Delta S < 0$
    d. $\Delta H > T \Delta S$

Ans. (b) $\Delta H < 0$ and $\Delta S > 0$

109. **Which is most favourable for maximum sustainable harvesting of resources?**

    a. Major part of population is near of around the carrying capacity
    b. Population is half of the carrying capacity
    c. Population is one fourth below the carrying capacity
    d. Population has slow doubling time

Ans. (a) Major part of population is near of around the carrying capacity

110. **Which statement is not correct for blood?**

    a. Mature RBC is of larger size as compare to its precursor cells
    b. Platelets play important role in blood clotting
    c. Neutrophils are major phagocytotic cells
    d. Basophils are present in least amount

Ans. (a) Mature RBC is of larger size as compare to its precursor cells

111. **Mammalian jaw has evolved from**

    a. Pharyngeal arches
    b. Temporal bone
    c. Frontal bone
    d. Dentary and squamosal bones

Ans. (d) Dentary and squamosal bones

112. **Which eukaryotic RNA polymerase transcribes t-RNA genes?**

    a. RNA polymerase I
    b. RNA polymerase II
    c. RNA polymerase III
    d. DNA polymerase I

Ans. (c) RNA polymerase III

113. An insertion of single nucleotide in coding region of gene leads to frame shift mutation and result is formation of non functional protein. Under certain condition second suppressor mutation in another gene may result into formation of functional protein.

How suppressor mutation can do this

a. There is insertional mutation in gene of t-RNA anticodon such that it is able to interact with four nucleotide codon

b. Mutation in gene of ribosome leading to frameshift over transcript

c. Mutation in gene whose product buldge out extra nucleotide

d. Another mutation reverses the original insertion

Ans. (a) There is insertional mutation in gene of t-RNA anticodon such that it is able to interact with four nucleotide codon

114. Which statement is correct regarding ABC transporters?

a. Consist of the transmembrane domain as well as the nucleotide binding domain

b. All are P glycoprotein

c. Preset in only eukaryotes

d. Makes membrane porous

Ans. (a) Consist of the transmembrane domain as well as the nucleotide binding domain

115. The organelle of C_3 plants, where glyoxylate is formed is

a. Chloroplast

b. Peroxisome

c. Mitochondria

d. Cytosol

Ans. (b) Peroxisome

116. In prokaryotes during replication, the lagging strand is synthesized in a series of short fragments known as okazaki fragment, consequently requiring many primers, the RNA primers of Okazaki fragments are subsequently degraded by DNA polymerase I and the gap are filled. How DNA polymerse I fills the gap once the primer have been removed from lagging stands?

a. DNA polymerase I has its own primer

b. DNA polymerase I do not require Primer

c. DNA from leading stand serves as primer

d. Ends of existing Okazaki fragments on lagging stand serves as primer

Ans. (d) Ends of existing Okazaki fragments on lagging stand serves as primer

117. Which of the following small G-protein is involved in nuclear transport and targeting?

a. Ras

b. Ran

c. Rab

d. Rho

Ans. (b) Ran

118. Which of the following is not a characteristic feature of Apoptosis?

a. Swelling of cell

b. Nuclear fragmentation

c. Change in cell wall porosity

d. Permeability of mitochondrial inner membrane

Ans. (a) Swelling of cell

119. Which statement is correct in relation of activity of telomerase?

a. Increase with age

b. Observed in all cancers and responsible for immortality

c. Responsible for apoptosis but not for ageing

d. Re-synthesize telomeres

Ans. (b) Observed in all cancers and responsible for immortality

120. In an organism if number of linkage group is 12 then, number of haploid set of chromosome is

a. 12

b. 6

c. 24

d. 4

Ans. (a) 12

121. Chromopore associated with phytochrome of plants is

a. Phycobillin

b. β-carotene

c. Pterin

d. Flavin adenine dinucleotide

Ans. (a) Phycobillin

122. During the early origin of earth oxygen was absent in environment. Later on the oxygen increased and reached to present level. The main source of oxygen was

a. Photosynthesis

b. Released from $CaCO_3$

c. Escape of CO_2 to environment

d. Escape of oxygen from internal sources

Ans. (a) Photosynthesis

123. Which of the following is produced in phenyl propanoid pathway?

a. Phenolics   b. Carotenes

c. Alkaloids   d. Terpenes

Ans. (a) Phenolics

124. Which of the following helps in osmoprotection in plant?

a. Proline   b. Tryptophan

c. Glycine   d. Levulinic acid

Ans. (a) Proline

125. Frog A has length "I" and weight "w". Another frog "B" has double length and four times weight. It means

a. Frog A is more cylindrical

b. Frog B is more cylindrical

c. Both frogs have same surface to volume ratio

d. Frog B is overweight

Ans. (a) Frog A is more cylindrical

126. In a certain genetic cross, 1/16 proportion of progeny shows mutant phenotype. It means

a. Two independent assorting genes are involved for trait

b. Two independently assorting duplicate genes are involved

c. Two linked genes are involved for trait

d. Two independent segregating alleles are responsible for trait

Ans. (b) Two independently assorting duplicate genes are involved

127. Which statement is correct for membrane receptors for signal transduction?

a. Contain single or multiple membranes spanning domain

b. Always coupled with trimeric G protein

c. Always results in production of secondary messanger

d. Recognized non polar signaling molecules

Ans. (a) Contain single or multiple membranes spanning domain

128. Spontaneity of mutation means

a. Mutation in absence of exogenous mutagen

b. Mutation directly proportion to presence of mutagen

c. Mutation inversely proportion to presence of mutagen

d. Mutation at in appropriate time

Ans. (a) Mutation in absence of exogenous mutagen

129. Plasmid copy number achieved by plasmid encoded control elements that regulate the initiation of the replication step. For example in stringent plasmid protein Rep A dimerize and binds to origin of replication and do not allow replication more than once. What mutation may convert this stringent mode of replication in plasmid into relaxed one?

a. Over expression in rep A protein

b. Mutation in rep A gene in dimerization domain

c. Mutation in rep A other than dimerization domain

d. Gain of function in recognization domaon of rep A

Ans. (b) Mutation in rep A gene in dimerization domain

130. Ants and bees social structure include queen, sterile female workers and soldier drones, this best example of

a. Eusociality

b. Sub social

c. Group selection

d. Altruism

Ans. (a) Eusociality

131. Among the following which is insulin dependent glucose transporter?

a. GLUT1   b. GLUT2

c. GLUT4   d. GLUT5

Ans. (c) GLUT4

132. What would be effect on serum concentration of TSh if a bolus of thyroxine is injected to a person?

a. Remain unchanged

b. First increase and then come to normal

c. Initially decrease but after short time will be normal

d. Remain high for prolonged period of time

Ans. (c) Initially decrease but after short time will be normal

133. Substrate for DNA synthesis is?

a. Nucleotide tri phosphate

b. Nucleoside tri phosphate

c. Nucleoside pyrophosphate

d. Ribonucleotide tri phosphate

Ans. (b) Nucleoside tri phosphate

134. Optimum temperature for growth of extemo thermophiles is

a. 0°C   b. 20°C

c. 50°C   d. Over 80°C

Ans. (d) Over 80°C

135. Treatment of acetosyringone is given during transfer of transgene using Agrobacterium as vector. The rationale behind this is that acetosyringone

    a. Helps in anchorage of bacteria to plant cell was

    b. Activates vir operon of bacteria

    c. Helps in integration of T-DNA in plant genome

    d. Promotes bacterial growth by activating genes in plant

Ans. (b) Activates vir operon of bacteria

136. When a person enters a dark room from bright sunlight he cannot see anything for a few seconds because

    a. Rhodoposin pigment of rod cells is inactivated in bright light which takes time and is activated in dark and associate with opsin protein

    b. Scotopsin proteins of rods are denatured

    c. All scotopsin are bound with retinal in rod cells

    d. All Scotopsin becomes non-functional in bright light

Ans. (a) Rhodoposin pigment of rod cells is inactivated in bright light which takes time and is activated in dark and associate with opsin protein

137. Largest reservoir of carbon is

    a. Atmosphere

    b. Ocean sediments

    c. Carbonate and silicate Rocks

    d. Inorganic carbon in earth mantle

Ans. (b) Ocean sediments

Memory Based Paper CSIR NET June 2011

1. The cumulative profits of a company since its inception are shown in the diagram. If the net worth of the company at the end of the 4th year is 99 crores, the principal it had started with

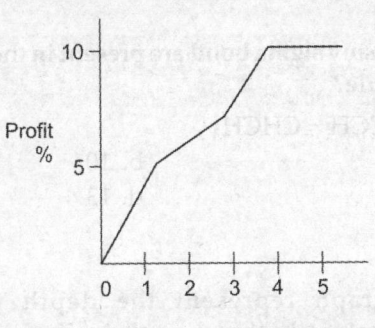

   a. 9.0 Crore   b. 99 Crore

   c. 90 Crore   d. 9.9 Crore

Ans. (c) 90 Crore

2. Popular use of which of the following fertilizers increase the acidity of soil?

   a. Potassium nitrate   b. Ammonium sulphate

   c. Urea   d. Superphosphate of lime

Ans. (b) Ammonium sulphate

3. Exposing an organism to a certain chemical can change nucleotide bases in a gene, causing mutation. In one such mutated organism if a protein had only 70% of the primary amino acid sequence, which of the following is likely?

   a. Mutation broke the protein

   b. The organism could not make amino acid

   c. Mutation created a terminator codon

   d. The gene was not transcribed

Ans. (c) Mutation created a terminator codon

4. A reference material is required to be prepared with 4 ppm calcium. The amount of $CaCO_3$ required to prepare 1000 g of such a reference material is

   a. 10 µg   b. 4 µg

   c. 4 mg   d. 10 mg

Ans. (d) 10 mg

5. Identify the figure which depicts a first order reaction.

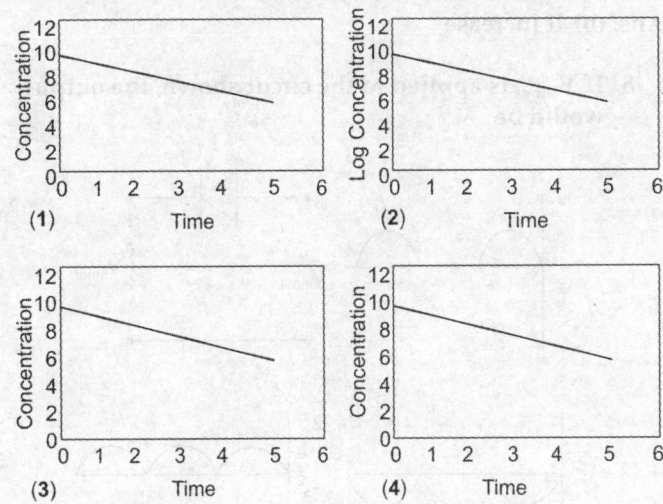

Ans. (2)

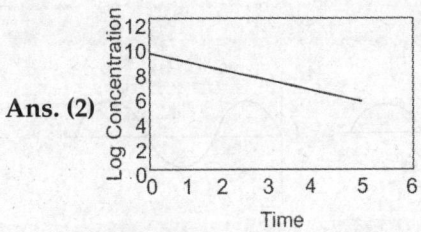

6. The speed of a car increase every minute as shown in the following table. The speed at the end of the 19th minute would be

Time (minute)	Speed (m/sec)
1	1.5
2	3.0
3	4.5
.	.
.	.
24	36.0
25	37.5

a. 26.5   b. 28.0

c. 27.0   d. 28.5

Ans. (d) 28.5

7. If the atmospheric concentration of carbon di oxide is doubled and there are favourable condition of water, nutrient, light and temp., what would happen to water requirement of plants?

   a. It decrease initially for short time and then return to original value

   b. It increase

   c. It decrease

   d. It increase initially for short time and then return to original value

Ans. (b) It increase

8. If V_{input} is applied to the circut shown, the output would be

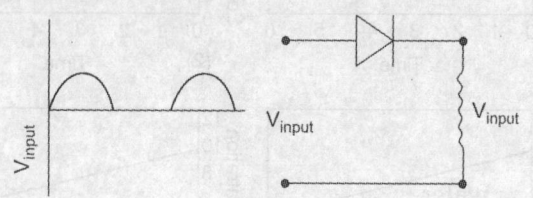

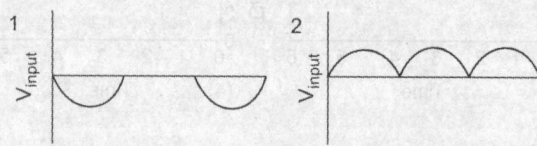

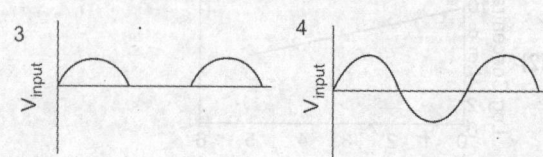

Ans. (3)

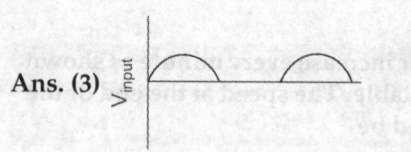

9. A physiological disorder X always leads to the disorder Y. however, disorder Y may occur by itself. A population shows 4% incidence of disorder Y. which of the following inferences is valid?

   a. 4% of the population suffers from both X & Y

   b. Less than 4% of the population suffers from X

   c. At least 4% of the population suffers from X

   d. There is no incidence of X in the given population

Ans. (b) Less than 4% of the population suffers from X

10. Water is dripping out of a tiny hole at the bottom of three flasks whose base diameter is the same, and are initially filled to the same height, as shown

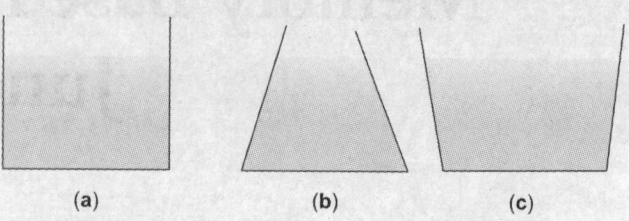

Which is the correct comparison of the rate of fall of the volume of water in the three flasks?

   a. A fastest, B slowest   b. B fastest, A slowest

   c. B fastest, C slowest   d. C fastest, B slowest

Ans. (d) C fastest, B slowest

11. How many sigma bond are present in the following molecule?

$$HC \equiv CCH = CHCH_3$$

   a. 4   b. 10

   c. 6   d. 13

Ans. (b) 10

12. The graph represent the depth profile of temperature in the open ocean; in which region this is likely to be prevalent?

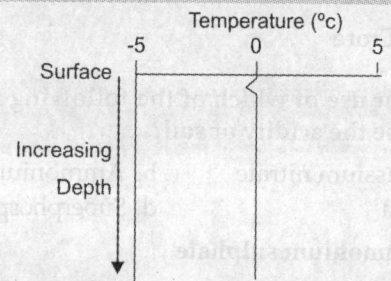

   a. Tropical region   b. Equatorial region

   c. Polar region   d. Sub tropical region

Ans. (c) Polar region

13. The normal boiling point of a solvent (whose vapour pressure curve is shown in the figure) on a planet whose normal atmosphere pressure is 3 bar, is about

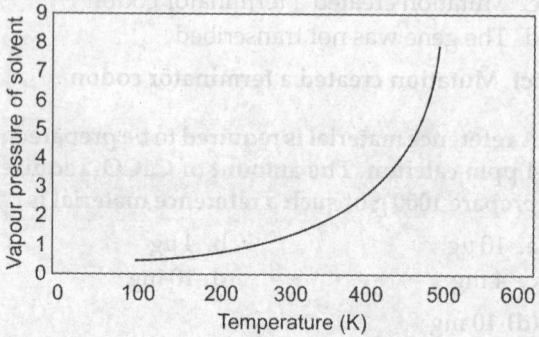

a. 400 K
b. 273 K
c. 100 K
d. 500 K

Ans. (a) 400 K

14. **Diabetic patients are advised a low gycaemic index diet. The reason for this is**

    a. They require less carbohydrate than healthy individual
    b. They can not assimilate ordinary carbohydrates
    c. They need to have slow, but sustained release of glucose in their blood stream
    d. They can tolerate lower, but not higher than normal blood sugar levels

Ans. (c) They need to have slow, but sustained release of glucose in their blood stream

15. **Glucose molecule diffuse across a cell of diameter d in time τ. If the cell diameter is tripled, the diffusion time would**

    a. Increase to 9 τ
    b. Decrease to τ/3
    c. Increase to 3r
    d. Decrease to τ/9

Ans. (d) Decrease to τ/9

16. **The reason for the hardness of diamond is**

    a. Extended covalent bonding
    b. Layered structure
    c. Formation of cage structure
    d. Formation of tubular structure

Ans. (a) Extended covalent bonding

17. **Which f the following particle has the largest range in a given medium if their initial energies are the same?**

    a. Alpha   b. Gamma
    c. Positron   d. Electron

Ans. (b) Gamma

18. **A ball is dropped from a height h above the surface of the earth. Lgnoring air drag, the curve that best represent its variation of acceleration is**

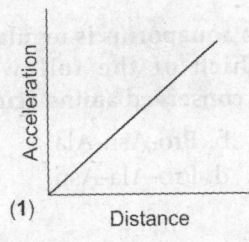
(1)

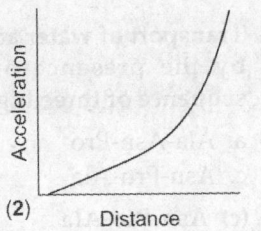
(2)

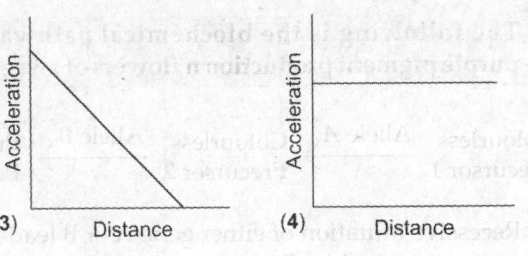
(3)   (4)

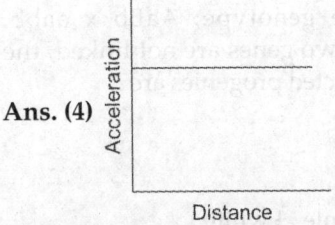

Ans. (4)

19. **Standing on a polished stone floor one feels colder than on a rough floor of the same stone. This is because**

    a. Thermal conductivity of the stone depends on the surface smoothness
    b. Specific heat of the stone changes by polishing it
    c. The temperature of the polished floor is lower than that of the rough floor
    d. There is greater heat loss from the soles of the feet when in contact with the polished floor than with the rough floor

Ans. (d) There is greater heat loss from the soles of the feet when in contact with the polished floor than with the rough floor

20. **The acidity or normal rain water is due to**

    a. SO_2 b. CO_2
    c. NO_2 d. NO

Ans. (b) CO_2

21. **Recent studies on Archaea suggest that life could have originated**

    a. Extraterrestially and seeded through meteorite impact
    b. In shallow coastal areas
    c. In deep hydrothermal vents
    d. In hot, terrestrial habitats

Ans. (a) Extraterrestially and seeded through meteorite impact

22. **If the ratio of the number of non synonymous to snynonymous substitutions per site in protein coding gene is greater than one, it is an evidence of selection that is**

    a. Positive   b. Negative
    c. Neutral   d. Random

Ans. (a) Positive

23. The following is the biochemical pathway for purple pigment production n flowers of sweet pea:

Colourless Precursor 1 $\xrightarrow{\text{Allele } A}$ Colourless Precursor 2 $\xrightarrow{\text{Allele } B}$ Purple Pigment

Recessive mutation of either gene A or B leads to the formation of white flower. A cross is made between two parent with the genotype; AaBb x aabb. Considering that the two genes are not linked, the phenotypes of the expected progenies are

a. 9 purple : 7 white
b. 3 white : 1 purple
c. 1 purple : 1 white
d. 9 purple : 6 light purple : 1 white

Ans. (b) 3 white : 1 purple

24. The frequency of alleles 'A' and 'a' in a population at hardy-weinburg equilibrium are 0.7 an 0.3, respectively. In a random sample of 250 individual taken from the population, how many are expected to be heterozygous?

a. 112   b. 81
c. 105   d. 145

Ans. (c) 105

25. The transition to flowering in plant requires

a. Growth of plant under long-day condition
b. Growth of plants under short-day condition
c. Reprogreamming of the shoot apical meristem
d. Synthesis of the flowering hormone florigen

Ans. (c) Reprogreamming of the shoot apical meristem

26. In an altruistic act, if a donor sacrifices 'C' offspring which helps the recipients to gain 'B' offspring and the donor is related to the recipient by a coefficient ~, under which condition would kin selection favour this altruistic trait?

a. B > C
b. B > ~C
c. ~B – C = 0
d. ~B – C > 0

Ans. (d) ~B – C > 0

27. Aneuploid females with only one X chromosome is a characteristic of individual with

a. Cri du chat syndrome
b. Klinefelter syndrome
c. Down syndrome
d. Turner syndrome

Ans. (d) Turner syndrome

28. Which of the following food crops has recently been genetically engineered to obtain edible vaccine to develop immunity against hepatitis B?

a. Banana   b. Maize
c. Potato   d. Tomato

Ans. (c) Potato

29. The most commonly used method of estimating primary productivity of a pond involves measurement of the amount

a. CO_2 utilized   b. Autotroph biomass
c. Oxygen released   d. Organic carbon

Ans. (c) Oxygen released

30. The area of allowed regions in the Ramachandran map will be least for

a. Gly   b. L-Ala
c. L-prol   d. α-methyl-L-valine

Ans. (c) L-prol

31. Small RNAs with internally complementary sequences that form hairpin-like structure, synthesized as percursor RNAs and cleaved by endonucleases to form short duplexes are called

a. snRNA   b. mRNA
c. tRNA   d. miRNA

Ans. (d) miRNA

32. A much greater proportion of energy fixed by autotrophs is transferred to the herbivore level in the open ocean ecosystem than in a forest ecosystem because

a. Aquatic autotrophs are small
b. Aquatic herbivores are more efficient feeders
c. Terrestrial autotrophs are less efficient feeders
d. Terrestrial autotrophs have more indigestible tissues

Ans. (d) Terrestrial autotrophs have more indigestible tissues

33. Polar bears maintain their body temperature because they have more of

a. Transducin protein   b. Uncoupling protein
c. Myoglobin protein   d. FoF1 ATPase

Ans. (b) Uncoupling protein.

34. Transport of water across aquaporins is regulated by the presence of which of the following sequence of three highly conserved amino acids?

a. Ala-Asn-Pro   b. Pro-Asn-Ala
c. Asn-Pro-Ala   d. Pro-Ala-Asn

Ans. (c) Asn-Pro-Ala

35. Which of the cyclins have/has essential functions in S phase of cell cycle?

    a. A-type   b. B-type

    c. D-type   d. Both B- and D-types

Ans. (a) A-type

36. During generation of an action potential, depolarization is due to

    a. K + efflux   b. Na + efflux

    c. Na + influx   d. K + influx

Ans. (c) Na + influx

37. G protein-linked receptors are trans-membrane proteins of

    a. Single-pass   b. Three-pass

    c. Five-pass   d. Seven-pass

Ans. (d) Seven-pass

38. Release of nutrients, oxidants or electron donors into the environment to stimulate naturally occurring microorganisms to degrade a contaminant, is referred to as

    a. Biostimulation

    b. Phytoremediation

    c. Bioaugmentation

    d. Bioremediation

Ans. (a) biostimulation

39. A mechanism that can cause a gene to move from one linkage group to another is

    a. Crossing over   b. Inversion

    c. Translocation   d. Duplication

Ans. (c) Translocation

40. Th2 response is generated and maintained mainly by which of the following pair of cytokines?

    a. IL-4 and IL-10

    b. IL-12 and IFN-γ

    c. IFN-γ and TNF-α

    d. IL-2 and IL-12

Ans. (a) IL-4 and IL-10

41. Cytoplasmic determinants coding for anterior structure of Drosophila embryo if injected elsewhere in the recipient embryo, would lead to

    a. Normal development

    b. Formation of additional ectopic head

    c. Degeneration

    d. A phenotype with two heads and two tails

Ans. (b) Formation of additional ectopic head

42. The dwarf pea mutant (*le*) used by Mendel was defective in which of the following enzyme involved in gibberellins biosynthesis?

    a. Ent-Kaurene synthase

    b. GA 3 β-hydroxylase

    c. GA 20-oxidase

    d. Ent-Kaurenoic acid hydroxylase

Ans. (b) GA 3 β-hydroxylase

43. ELISA assay uses

    a. An enzyme which can react with secondary antibody

    b. An enzyme which can react with the antigen

    c. A substrate which gets converted into a coloured product

    d. A radiolabelled secondary antibody

Ans. (c) A substrate which gets converted into a coloured product

44. Which of the following molecules is involved in Ca2 + -dependent cell-cell adhesion?

    a. Calmodulin

    b. Cadherin

    c. N-CAM

    d. Calpain

Ans. (b) Cadherin

45. The 5' Cap of RNA is required for the

    a. Stability of RNA only

    b. Stability and transport of RNA

    c. Transport of RNA only

    d. Methylation of RNA

Ans. (b) Stability and transport of RNA

46. Yeast artificial chromosome (YAC) vectors contain selectable markers. Loss of which marker at the cloning site distinguishes the religated YACs from the original vector marker?

    a. TRP1   b. SUP4

    c. URA3   d. CEN

Ans. (b) SUP4

47. In amphibian oocyte, the germplasm which gets segregated during cleavage to give rise to primordial germ cells (PGC's) is normally

    a. Distributed evenly throughout the oocyte

    b. Localized at animal pole

    c. Localized at vegetal pole

    d. Aggregated in central part of oocyte

Ans. (c) localized at vegetal pole

48. **Which of the following statements with respect to alternate oxidase activity in cyanide-resistant respiration in plants, is not correct?**

    a. Alternate oxidase accepts electrons directly from cytochrome C

    b. Some plants exhibit thermogenesis during inflorescence development

    c. Transcription of alternate oxidase gene is often induced by various abiotic stresses

    d. When electrons pass to alternate oxidase, two sites of proton pumping are bypassed

Ans. (a) Alternate oxidase accepts electrons directly from cytochrome C

49. **In mature Arabidopsis embryo, root apical meristem consists of cells derived from**

    a. Embryo and apical suspensor cells

    b. Embryo only

    c. Suspensor only

    d. Hypophysis only

Ans. (a) Embryo and apical suspensor cells

50. **Na + -K + ATPase is a tetramer of 2α and 2β subunits. On which of the following subunits are the Na + and K + binding sites present?**

    a. Both on α

    b. Both on β

    c. Na + on α and K + on β

    d. Na + on β and K + on α

Ans. (a) Both on α

51. **A mother of blood group 0 has a group a child. The father could be of blood type**

    a. A or B or O   b. A only

    c. A or B   d. AB only

Ans. (a) A or B or O

52. **Following figure shows McArthur and Wilson's equilibrium model of biota on a single island.**

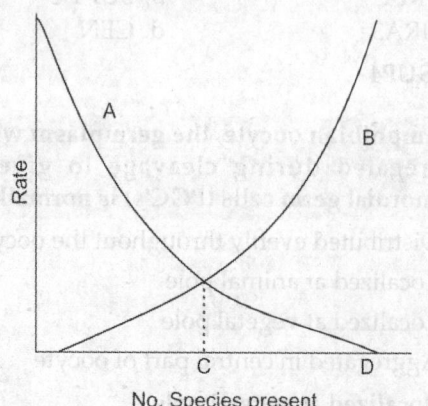

No. Species present

In this figure, terms A, B, C and D in order are

    a. Extinction. immigration, equilibrium number of species size of species pool

    b. Immigration. extinction, equilibrium number of species, size of species pool

    c. Extinction. immigration, size of species pool, equilibrium number of species

    d. Immigration, extinction, size of species pool, equilibrium number of species

Ans. (b) Immigration. extinction, equilibrium number of species, size of species pool

53. **Routinely used glucose biosensor estimates blood glucose level by sensing the concentration of**

    a. Glucose   b. Oxygen

    c. δ-gluconolactone   d. H_2O_2

Ans. (b) Oxygen

54. **Name the ectothermic animal that can thermo-regulate by behavioural means rather than by physiological means.**

    a. Bumble bee in an orchard

    b. Tuna fish in the ocean

    c. Lizard in a desert

    d. Flatworm in a pond

Ans. (c) Lizard in a desert

55. **Which of the following methods of plant transformation can be used to introduce a gene into chloroplast genome?**

    a. Agrobacterium-mediated transformation

    b. Particle delivery system

    c. Permeabilization

    d. Electroporation

Ans. (b) Particle delivery system

56. **The μ and σ of wing length (a normally distributed parameter) in a population of fruitflies are 4 and 0.2 mm. respectively. In a random sample of 400 fruitflies, how many individuals are expected to have wing lengths greater than 4.4 mm?**

    a. 20   b. 64

    c. 10   d. 336

Ans. (c) 10

57. **Which of the following characteristic of an early community?**

    a. Narrow niche specialization

    b. High species diversity

    c. Community production

    d. Open mineral cycling

Ans. (c) Community production

58. A culture of an E. coli strain that is lysogenic for phage lambda is grown at 32°C. Induction of the prophage from the host chromosome will occur when the culture is exposed to

a. 40°C

b. Ultra violet radiation

c. Infra red radiation

d. Wild type *E. coli* culture

Ans. (b) Ultra violet radiation

59. During urine formation the filtration of blood at the glomerulus is

a. An active process

b. An osmotic process

c. Is a pressure-dependent physical process

d. A non energy- mediated transport process

Ans. (c) Is a pressure-dependent physical process

60. If the core body temperature of a human rises above normal, which of the following processes would be initiated sequentially for Thermo-regulation?

a. Peripheral vasodilation, increased rate of respiration, tachycardia

b. Peripheral vasoconstriction, increased rate of respiration, bradycardia

c. Peripheral vasodilation, decreased rate of respiration, tachycardia

d. Peripheral vasodilation, decreased rate of respiration, bradycardia

Ans. (a) Peripheral vasodilation, increased rate of respiration, tachycardia

61. With which protein of *Yersinia* would integrin proteins of mammalian cells interact for internalization?

a. Pilin

b. Fimbrin

c. Lnvasin

d. Adherin

Ans. (c) Lnvasin

62. Graves disease is associated with

a. Insufficiency of thyroid hormones

b. Excess of thyroid hormones

c. Insufficiency of corticosteroids

d. Excess of growth hormones

Ans. (b) Excess of thyroid hormones

63. The fidelity of replicative base selection can be reduced by a factor of 102 when the repair of DNA synthesis involves

a. AP endonuclease

b. ABC exinuclease

c. DNA photolyase

d. TLS DNA polymerase

Ans. (d) TLS DNA polymerase

64. What is the minimum number of NTPs required for the formation of one peptide bond during protein synthesis?

a. One

b. Two

c. Four

d. Six

Ans. (b) Two

65. 'Imperfect fungi' is a group represented by fungal species which have

a. Simple mycelia

b. No known mechanisms of sexual reproduction

c. Unkown phylogenetic relationship

d. Lost its survival mechanism against harsh environments

Ans. (b) No known mechanisms of sexual reproduction

66. The photoreceptor commonly involved In light entrainment of the biological clock in flies, moulds and plants is

a. Phytochrome

b. Rhodopsin

c. Carotenoid

d. Cryptochrome

Ans. (d) Cryptochrome

67. The free energy ΔG of a dissolved solute

a. Increases with solute concentration

b. Decreases with solute concentration

c. Is independent of solute concentration

d. Depends only on temperature

Ans. (a) Increases with solute concentration

68. Which of the following is not a characteristic of phylum Chordata?

a. Pharyngeal slits

b. Amniotic egg

c. Post anal tail

d. Notochord

Ans. (b) Amniotic egg

69. In India, brown antlered deer (sangai) is found only in the floating landmasses of

a. Wular lake

b. Sasthamkotta lake

c. Dal lake

d. Lok Tak lake

Ans. (d) Lok Tak lake

70. Both halophytes and glycophytes compartmentalize cytotoxic ions into the intracellular compartment or actively pump them out of the cell to the apoplasts with the help of membrane transport proteins. Among these, the Na + -H + antiporter, NHX1, is localized in

    a. The plasma membrane
    b. Chloroplast (inner envelope)
    c. Mitochondria (outer membrane)
    d. Tonoplast

Ans. (d) Tonoplast

71. You are studying the binding of proteins to the cytoplasmic face of cultured liver cells and have found a method that gives a good yield of inside-out vesicles from the plasma membrane. Unfortunately, your preparations are contaminated with variable amounts of right-side-out vesicles. Nothing you have tried avoids this contamination. Somebody suggests that you pass the vesicles over an affinity column made of lectin coupled to Sepharose beads. What is the rational of this suggestion?

    a. Right-side-out-vesicles wIll be lysed by lectin coupled to Sepharose beads
    b. Right-side-out-vesicles will simply bind to the lectin coupled Sepharose beads
    c. Lectin will bind to the carbohydrate residues present only on the inside out vesicles
    d. Lectin will bind to only glycoproteins and glycolipids present on the inside-out vesicles

Ans. (b) Right-side-out-vesicles will simply bind to the lectin coupled Sepharose beads

72. The overall length of the cell cycle can be measured from the doubling time of a population of exponentially proliferating cells. The doubling time of a population of mouse L cells was determined by counting the number of cells in samples of culture at various times. What is the overall length of the cell cycle in mouse L cells?

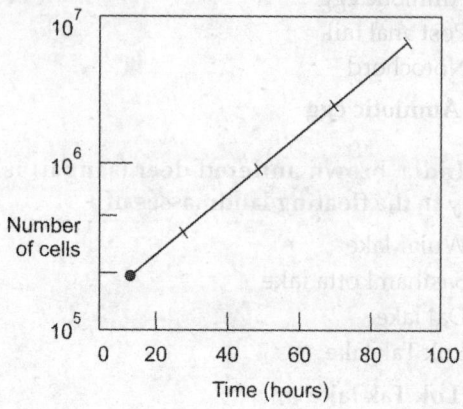

    a. 30 h   b. 20 h
    c. 10 h   d. 40 h

Ans. (b) 20 h

73. Using molecular clock, it was estimated that two species A and B must have diverged from their common ancestor about 9×10^6 years ago. If the rate of divergence per base pair is estimated to be 0.0015 per million years, what is the proportion of base pairs that differ between the two species now?

    a. 0.0270   b. 0.0135
    c. 0.00017   d. 0.0035

Ans. (a) 0.0270

74. A protein in 100 mM KCl solution was heated and the observed Tm (midpoint of unfolding) was 60°C. When the same protein solution in 500 mM KCl was heated, the observed Tm was 65°C. What is the most probable reason for this increase in Tm?

    a. Hydrophobic interaction is increased and electrostatic repulsion is decreased
    b. Hydrophobic interaction is decreased and electrostatic repulsion is increased
    c. Hydrogen-bonding is increased
    d. van der Waals interaction is increased

Ans. (a) Hydrophobic interaction is increased and electrostatic repulsion is decreased

75. During receptor-mediated endocytosis, apolipo-protein B on the surface of a LDL particle binds to the LDL-receptor present in coated pits containing clathrin. The receptor-LDL complex is internalized by endocytosis, trafficked to lysosomes and the LDL-receptor is finally recycled. A patient reports with familial hypercholesterolemia. This could be due to

    a. Mutation in the LDL molecule
    b. Defect in LDL-receptor recycling
    c. Mutation in the LDL-receptor
    d. Defect in cholesterol binding with its receptor

Ans. (c) Mutation in the LDL-receptor

76. Budding yeast cells that are deficient for Mad2, a component of the spindle-attachment-check point, are killed by treatment with benomyl, which causes microtubles to depolymerise. In the absence of benomyl, however, the cells are perfectly viable. Which explanation out of the following is able to justify this observation?

    a. In the absence of be no my I, the majority of spindles forms normally and the spindle-attachment checkpoint (Mad2) plays no role
    b. In the presence of be no my I, the majority of spindles form normally and Mad2 plays critical role in cell survival

c. Other than the role in cell survival, microtubule depolymerization affects oxidative phosphorylation in the absence of Mad2

d. Benomyl also affects protein synthesis in the absence of Mad2

Ans. (a) In the absence of be no my I, the majority of spindles forms normally and the spindle-attachment checkpoint (Mad2) plays no role

77. Eukaryotic genomes are organized into chromosomes and can be visualized at mitosis by staining with specific dyes. Heat denaturation followed by staining with Giemsa produced alternate dark and light bands. The dark bands obtained by this process are mainly

a. AT -rich and gene rich regions
b. AT -rich and gene desert regions
c. GC-rich and gene rich regions
d. GC-rich and gene desert regions

Ans. (c) GC-rich and gene rich regions

78. An amino acid contains no ionizable group in its side chain (R). It is titrated from pH 0 to 14. Which of the following ionizable state is not observed during the entire titration in the pH range 0 - 14?

Ans. (d) $H_2N-\underset{\underset{H}{|}}{\overset{\overset{R}{|}}{C}}-COOH$

79. A researcher has isolated a restriction endonuclease that cleaves at only one specific 10 base pair site.

a. Would this enzyme be useful in protecting cells from viral infections, given that a typical viral genome is 5×10^4 base pairs long?

b. Restriction endonucleases are slow enzymes with turnover number of $1\ s^{-1}$. Suppose the isolated endonuclease was faster with turnover numbers similar to those for carbonic anhydrase ($10^6\ s^{-1}$), would this increased rate be beneficial to host cells, assuming that the fast enzymes have similar levels of specificity?

The correct combination of answer is
a. (A) : No (B) : Yes
b. (A) : No (B) : No
c. (A) : Yes (B) : No
d. (A) : Yes (B) : Yes

Ans. (b) (A) : No (B) : No

80. Lac repressor inhibits expression of genes in *lac*-operon whereas purine biosynthesis is repressed by the *Pur* repressor. The two proteins have 31% identical sequences and have similar three-dimensional structures. The gene regulatory properties of these proteins differ in relation to

a. Binding of small molecules to the repressor.
b. Presence of recognition sites on the genome.
c. Oligomeric nature of the repressor.
d. DNA binding property.

The correct statements are
a. A and B
b. A, B and C
c. A and C
d. B, C and D

Ans. (a) A and B

81. An α-helix in a peptide or protein is characterized by hydrogen bonds and characteristic dihedral angles. Choose the right combination.

a. Hydrogen bonding between the amide CO of residue i and amide NH of residue i + 4. Dihedral angles in the region ~ = –50°, ψ = –60°

b. Hydrogen bonding between the amide NH of residue i and amide CO of residue i + 4. Dihedral angles in the region of ~ = –50°, ψ = –60

c. Hydrogen bonding between the amide CO of residue i and amide NH of residue i + 4. Dihedral angles in the region of ~ = –50°, ψ = + 60

d. Hydrogen bonding between the amide CO of residue i and amide NH of residue 1 + 3. Dihedral angles in the region of ~ = –50°, ψ = –60

Ans. (a) Hydrogen bonding between the amide CO of residue i and amide NH of residue i + 4. Dihedral angles in the region ~ = –50°, ψ = –60°

82. Mouse bone marrow cells were fractionated to derive stem cell antigen-1 + (Sca-1 +) cells. These cells were cultured with interleukin-3, or granulocyte-macrophage colony stimulating factor, or macrophage-colony stimulating factor, or granulocyte colony stimulating factor. Most numerous and varied colonies were obtained in the culture stimulated with

a. Interleukin-3
b. Granulocyte-macrophage colony stimulating factor
c. Macrophage-colony stimulating factor
d. Granulocyte-colony stimulating factor

Ans. (b) Granulocyte-macrophage colony stimulating factor

83. Precursors of the atoms in the purine skeleton are

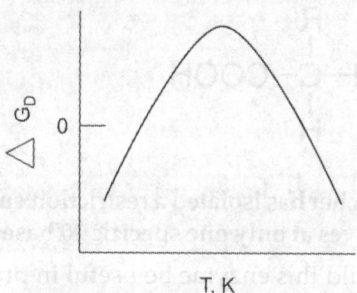

a. N1, Asp; C2 and C8, formate; N3 and N9 guanidine C4, C5 and N7, Gly; C6, CO_2

b. N1, Asp; C2 and C8, citrate; N3 and N9, amide nitrogen of Gln, C4,,C5 and N7; Gly; C6, CO_2

c. N1, Asp; C2 and C8, formate; N3 and N9 amide nitrogen of Gln, C4, C5 and N7, Gly; C6, CO_2

d. N1, Glu; C2 and C8, acetate; N3 and N9, amide nitrogen of Asn; C4, C5 and N7, Gly; C6, CO_2

Ans. (c) N1, Asp; C2 and C8, formate; N3 and N9 amide nitrogen of Gln, C4, C5 and N7, Gly; C6, CO_2

84. Two *E. coli* cultures A and B are taken. Culture A was earlier grown in the presence of optimum concentration of gratuitous inducer IPTG. Both the cultures are now used to inoculate fresh medium containing sub-optimal concentration of gratuitous inducer. It was observed that culture B was unable to utilize lactose, whereas culture A did so efficiently. The reason behind this is

a. Pretreatment with IPTG has resulted in a mutation as a result of which lac operon is constitutively expressed

b. IPTG has made the cell membrane more porous to small molecules and so lactose is taken up more efficiently by A as compared to B

c. In culture A, lactose permease was induced to a high level, during pretreatment with IPTG, which allowed the preferential uptake of lactose

d. In culture A, IPTG activated a receptor which bound lactose more efficiently, thereby triggering a signal

Ans. (c) In culture A, lactose permease was induced to a high level, during pretreatment with IPTG, which allowed the preferential uptake of lactose

85. Cancer causing genes can be functionally classified into mainly three types: (i) genes that induce cellular proliferation, (ii) tumor suppressor genes, (iii) genes that regulate apoptotic pathway. Epstein-Barr virus that causes cancer by modulating apoptotic pathway, contains a gene having sequence homology with which of the following genes?

a. Bax
b. Bcl-2
c. P53
d. Caspase-3

Ans. (b) Bcl-2

86. It has been observed that in 5-10% of the eukaryotic mRNAs with multiple AUGs, the first AUG is not the initiation site. In such cases, the ribosome skips over one or more AUGs before encountering the favourable one and initiating translation. This is postulated to be due to the presence of the following consensus sequence (s):

a. CCA CC AUG G
b. CCG CC AUG G
c. CCG CC AUG C
d. AAC GG AUG A

Which of the following sequence sets related to the above postulations is correct?

a. A and B
b. A and C
c. C and D
d. B and D

Ans. (a) A and B

87. Values of Tm (midpoint of denaturation), DHm (enthalpy change at Tm) and DCp (constant-pressure heat capacity change) of a protein are measured in a differential scanning calorimeter. DGD(T), the Gibbs free energy change at any temperature T(K) can be estimated using the following form of the Gibbs-Helmholtz equation with the values obtained from these measurements:

$$\Delta G_D(T) = \Delta H_m \left(\frac{T_m - T}{T_m} \right) - \Delta Cp[T_m - TIn(T/T_m)]$$

The stability curve for the protein simulated using the observed thermodynamic values is given below:

The shape of the stability curve is due to

a. Hydrogen-bonding and electrostatic interactions only

b. Van der Waals and electrostatic interactions only

c. Only electrostatic interactions

d. Only hydrophobic interaction

Ans. (c) Only electrostatic interactions

88. Toll-like receptor 4 is associated with responsiveness to LPS, an endotoxin that causes lethal endotoxic shock. The mice deficient In Toll-like receptor 4 and BALB/c mice were injected with Escherichia coli. In addition, some BALB/b mice were also injected with the same bacteria alone or with anti-interleukin-10 (IL-10) antibody. The mice resistant to the lethal effect of the bacteria were:

a. BALB/b mice receiving the bacteria
b. BALB/b mice receiving the bacteria and the anti-IL-10 antibody
c. Mice deficient In Toll-like receptor
d. BALB/c mice receiving the bacteria

Ans. (c) Mice deficient In Toll-like receptor

89. Presence of circular mRNAs for a specific protein in an eukaryotic cell reflects a rapid rate of synthesis of that protein. Following mechanisms are suggested:

A eIF-4G and PABP promote this process through 5'-3' interaction of mRNA.
B Ribosomes are less active in recognizing circular mRNA.
C PABP and eIF-4A promote this process.
D Ribosomes can reinitiate translation without being disassembled.
Which of the following is correct?

a. A and D
b. B and D
c. A and C
d. B and C

Ans. (c) A and C

90. siRNAs and miRNAs are used for achieving gene silencing. Although, major steps are similar there are distinct differences in the key players of the two processing pathways. Following statements relate to some characteristic features of gene silencing.

a. Both siRNAs and miRNAs are processed by cytoplasmic endonuclease Dicer.
b. 'Drosha' is needed for processing miRNAs and precursor siRNAs.
c. Both siRNAs and miRNAs show association with Argonaute protein.
d. Both the processing pathways involve RISe complex.
Which of the following combinations is NOT correct?

a. A and C   b. C and D
c. A and B   d. D and A

Ans. (b) C and D

91. Glucose is mobilized in muscle when epinephrine activates Gαs. In an experiment in which muscle cells were stimulated with epinephrine, glucose mobilization was observed even after withdrawal of epinephrine. This could be

a. Due to the presence of a cAMP phosphodiesterase inhibitor
b. Very low rates of cyclic AMP formation
c. Due to the presence of a cAMP phosphodiesterase activator
d. Due to the absence of protein kinase A

Ans. (a) Due to the presence of a cAMP phosphodiesterase inhibitor

92. In eukaryotic chromatin, 30 nm fiber (solenoid) can open up to give rise to two kinds of chromatin. In one type (A), the promoter of a gene within the open chromatin is occupied by a nucleosome whereas in the other (B), the promoter is occupied by histone H1. The following possibilities are suggested.

A The gene in (A) is repressed.
B The gene in (B) is repressed.
C The gene in (A) is active.
D The gene in (B) is active.
Which of the following sets is correct?

a. A and D   b. A and B
c. Band D   d. C and D

Ans. (a) A and D

93. Intracellular pathogens like *Mycobacteria, Salmonella, Leishmania* and *Listeria* survive in macrophages by modulating host cellular machinery. In order to study the fate of these intracellular pathogens in macrophages, cells were labelled with lysotracker Red arid infected with GFP-Iabelled organisms. After 2 hours at 37°C, cells were fixed, stained with anti-transferrin receptor antibody and probed with secondary antibody conjugated-blue dyes. Cells were viewed under confocal microscope.

Observation: GFP-labelled *Mycobacteria, Salmonella* and *Listeria* were localized in the same compartment labelled with blue dyes; whereas GFP-*Leishmania* colocalize with red labelled compartment.

Which of the following statement is true based on these observations?

a. *Mycobacteria, Salmonella* and *Listeria* reside in the lysosomes
b. *Leishmania* reside in lysosome like compartment
c. *Leishmania* reside in a compartment which bears characteristics of early endocytic compartment
d. *Mycobacteria, Salmonella* and *Listeria* lyse the phagosomal membrane and reside in cytosol

Ans. (b) *Leishmania* reside in lysosome like compartment

94. Macrophages were collected from BALB/c mice, CD40- deficient mice, CD86- deficient mice and ICAM-1-deficient mice. These macrophages were co-cultured with LCMV peptidespecific T cells in presence of the LCMV peptide for three days. The cells were recovered and co-cultured with BALB/c-derived macrophages in presence of the peptide. During the last twelve hour of the co-culture, 3H-thymidine was added to the cultures. The cells were harvested and 3H- thymidine incorporation was assessed. The highest incorporation was observed in

   a. BALB/c macrophage-T cell co-culture
   b. CD40-deficient macrophage-T cell co-culture
   c. CD86-deficient macrophage-T cell co-culture
   d. ICAM-1-deficient macrophage-T cell co-culture

Ans. (c) CD86-deficient macrophage-T cell co-culture

95. Genetic studies demonstrated that TBP mutant cell extracts are deficient in transcription of genes from all three promoters viz. class I, II and III. Following statements describe characteristic features of TBP.

   (A) TBP is considered as an universal basal transcription factor
   (B) TBP is not required for transcription of archaeal genes
   (C) TBP is involved in recognizing TATA box
   (D) TBP operates at all promoters regardless of their TATA content

   Which of the following combinations is NOT correct?
   a. A and D   b. C and D
   c. B and D   d. A and C

Ans. (c) B and D

96. cAMP signalling plays a very important role in the development and differentiation of *Dictyostelium discoideum*. This morphogen' is synthesized by different adenyl cyclises expressed at different stages of its life cycle. The following statements (AD) refer to the effect of mutations in different adenyl cyclase genes:

   (A) *aca* deficient cells can be a1l0wedto aggregate by exposing them to pulses of cAMP.
   (B) *acb* deficient cells would lorm normal fruiting bodies and the spores can germinate when exposed to favourable conditions.
   (C) *acg* deficient cells develop normally and the spores germinate in the spore head itself.
   (D) spores formed from the *acg* deficient cells will germinate irrespective of the osmotic conditions.
   Which of the above statements are correct?
   a. A and D
   b. A only

   c. A and B
   d. C and D

Ans. (a) A and D

97. Fill in the blanks (a, b, c and d) in the following statements with a proper combination of m, n, 0 and p. Where in m represents – longer n represents – shorter o represents –prevents p represents – induces Short day (SD) plants flower when night lengths are _____a____ than a critical dark period. Interruption of the dark period by a brief light treatment _____b_____ flowering in SD plants. Long day (LD) plants flower when night length is _____c_____ than a critical period. Shortening of the night with a brief light treatment _____d_____ flowering in LD plants. a b c d

   a. m o n p
   b. n p m o
   c. n o m p
   d. m p n o

Ans. (a) m o n p

98. The total variance in a phenotypic character can be split into two components - genetic (VG) and environmental (VE). The heritability of a phenotypic trait can be expressed quantitatively as heritability coefficient (h2) which is calculated as h2 =

   a. VG-VE
   b. VE/VG
   c. VG/VG + VE
   d. VG/VG-VE

Ans. (a) VG-VE

99. Mutations in *CONSTANS* (CO) of *Arabidopsis thaliana* results in late flowering phenotype. Transcript levels of CO were determined in long day and short day seedlings. Which of the following would likely represent the transcript profile of CO?

Ans. (1) ▬▬▬▬ ──────

100. **Following are some statements for synthesis of secondary metabolites in plants.**

(A) Terpenes are synthesized by shikimic acid pathway and mevalonic acid pathway.

(B) Alkaloids are nitrogen containing compounds and are synthesized by shikimic acid pathway.

(C) Phenolic compounds are synthesized by shikimic acid pathway and mevalonic acid pathway.

(D) Both alkaloids and terpenes are synthesized by mevalonic acid pathway and MEP pathway. Which one of the following combinations of the above statement is true?

a. A and D
b. A and C
c. B and C
d. B and D

Ans. (b) A and C

101. **During early cleavage of *Caenorabditis elegans* embryos, each asymmetrical division produces one founder cell which produces differentiated descendants and one stem cell. The very first cell division produces one anterior founder cell, namely AB and one posterior stem cell, namely P1. When these blastomeres are experimentally separated and allowed to proceed further with development, one could get the following possible outcomes:**

a. P1 cell would develop autonomously while the AB would show conditional development

b. P1 cells would show conditional development while AB would show autonomous development

c. Both would show autonomous specification and result in mosaic development

d. Both would show conditional specification and result in regulative development

Ans. (a) P1 cell would develop autonomously while the AB would show conditional development

102. **In case of sea urchin, which of the following is the correct sequence of events taking place during the interaction of sperm and egg?**

a. Chemoattraction of sperm to the egg by soluble molecules secreted by the egg? exocytosis of the sperm acrosomal vesicle to release its enzymes? binding of the sperm to the extracellular matrix of the egg? passage of sperm through this extracellular matrix? fusion of egg and sperm cell membranes

b. Chemoattraction of sperm to the egg by soluble molecules secreted by the egg? binding of the sperm to the extracellular matrix of the egg? exocytosis of the sperm acrosomal vesicle to release its enzymes? passage of sperm through this extracellular matrix? fusion of egg and sperm cell membranes

c. Chemoattraction of sperm to the egg by soluble molecules secreted by the egg? binding of the sperm to the extracellular matrix of the egg? passage of sperm through this extracellular matrix? exocytosis of the sperm acrosomal vesicle to release its enzymes? fusion of egg and sperm cell membranes

d. Chemoattraction of sperm to the egg by soluble molecules secreted by the egg? passage of sperm through this extracellular matrix? binding of the sperm to the extracellular matrix of the egg? exocytosis of the sperm acrosomal vesicle to release its enzymes? fusion of egg and sperm cell membranes

Ans. (b) Chemoattraction of sperm to the egg by soluble molecules secreted by the egg? binding of the sperm to the extracellular matrix of the egg? exocytosis of the sperm acrosomal vesicle to release its enzymes? passage of sperm through this extracellular matrix? fusion of egg and sperm cell membranes

103. **The time taken for atrial systole and diastole in a normal heart are tas and tad seconds, respectively. If ventricular systole takes tvs seconds, calculate the ventricular diastolic time (seconds)**

a. (tas + tad) - tvs
b. (tas- tad) + tvs
c. (tad- tas) - tvs
d. (tas + tad) x tvs

Ans. (a) (tas + tad) - tvs

104. **A patient undergoes liver transplantation and during the course of post-operative treatment, becomes susceptible to infection. The patient can be treated in two different modes and can have alternative outcomes. Which of the following statements is correct?**

a. Treatment with immunostimulatory drugs reducing the infection but rejecting the transplant

b. Treatment with immunostimulatory drugs reducing the infection and retaining the transplant

c. Treatment with antibiotics reducing the infection but retaining the transplant

d. Treatment with antibiotics reducing the infection but rejecting the transplant

Ans. (c) Treatment with antibiotics reducing the infection but retaining the transplant

105. **The dependence of the rate of sucrose uptake with respect to sucrose concentration in plant cell was studied and data are shown in the following graph. From the above data it can be inferred that**

a. The sucrose uptake is energy independent and no special carrier is involved

b. The sucrose uptake is energy dependent and a special carrier is involved

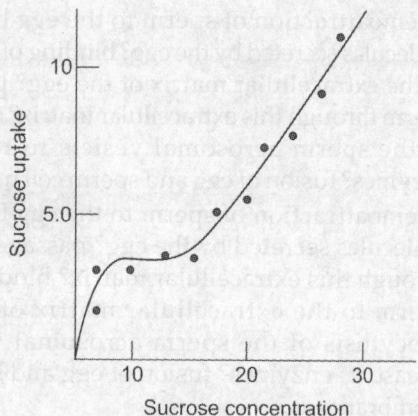

c. At lower concentration of sucrose the uptake of sucrose is energy dependent and carrier mediated

d. At higher concentration of sucrose the uptake is energy dependent and carrier mediated

Ans. (c) At lower concentration of sucrose the uptake of sucrose is energy dependent and carrier mediated

106. **During episodes of anoxia in plants, pyruvate produced in glycolysis is initially fermented to lactate. During later stage, there is an increase in the fermentation to ethanol and decrease in the fermentation to lactate, a phenomena which helps plants survive anoxia. Which of the following statements is correct about this change of fermentation flux from lactate towards ethanol?**

a. The cytosolic pH increases, thus activating both lactate dehydrogenase and pyruvate decarboxylase activity

b. The cytosolic pH increases, thus inhibiting lactate dehydrogenase activity and activating pyruvate decarboxylase activity

c. The cytosolic pH decreases, thus activating both lactate dehydrogenase and pyruvate decarboxylase activity

d. The cytosolic pH decreases, thus inhibiting lactate dehydrogenase and activating pyruvate decarboxylase activity

Ans. (d) The cytosolic pH decreases, thus inhibiting lactate dehydrogenase and activating pyruvate decarboxylase activity

107. **Bacteria often acquire genes by the process of lateral or horizontal transfer. Such 'foreign' genes, if acquired in recent past, may be identified by their atypical GC content, as compared to 'native' genes. Suppose the genomic GC content of a bacterium is 40%. Gene A of this organism contains 1000 bases with 225 G and 215 C. Another gene B of length 800 bases contains 160 G and**

140 C. **Which one of the following would be the most acceptable hypothesis (given that x2 = 3.841 at 0.05 significance level)?**

a. A: native, B: Foreign

b. A: Foreign, B: Native

c. A: Foreign, B: Foreign

d. A: Native, B: Native

Ans. (b) A: Foreign, B: Native

108. **Injection of *noggin* mRNA into a 1-cell, UV-irradiated embryos of frog completely rescues dorsal development and allows the fonnation of a complete embryo. Some of the following statements (A-D) could possibly explain this observation.**

(A) Noggin is a secreted protein which induces dorsal ectoderm to form neural tissue and it dorsalizes the mesoderm cells which would otherwise contribute to ventral mesoderm.

(B) Noggin binds directly to BMP4 and BMP2 thus preventing complex formation with their receptors.

(C) Noggin along with other molecules prevent BMP from binding to and inducing ectodenn and mesoderm cells near the organizer.

(D) Noggin is a secreted protein which induces the dorsal ectoderm to form the epidermis and it ventralizes the mesoderm cells which would otherwise contribute to dorsal mesoderm.

Which of the above statements are correct?

a. A, B and C   b. A and B

c. B and C   d. A and D

Ans. (d) A and D

109. **Atmospheric CO_2 contains the naturally occurring stable carbon isotopes 12C and 13C in the proportion of 98.9% and 1.1%, respectively. Following are some of the statements regarding CO_2 assimilation:**

(A) Both C3 and C4 plants assimilate less $13CO_2$ than $12CO_2$.

(B) Both C3 and C4 plants assimilate less $12CO_2$ than $13CO_2$.

(C) C3 plants assimilate lesser $13CO_2$ than $12CO_2$ as compared to C4 plants.

(D) C4 plants assimilate lesser $13CO_2$ than $12CO_2$ as compared to C3 plants.

Which one of the following combinations of above statements is true?

a. A and B   b. A and C

c. C and D   d. A and D

Ans. (d) A and D

110. Spinal cord of an animal was transected at C1/C2 level. The respiration of the animal stopped and it needed artificial respiration. However, the heart continued to beat although at a slower rate. Some of the explanations given were:

   (A) Respiration regulatory centre is located in the medulla.
   (B) Respiration regulatory centre is located above the C1/C2 cut.
   (C) Heart regulatory centre is above the C1/C2 cut.
   (D) Heart has autoregulation.
   Which one of the following is most appropriate?

   a. A only
   b. B and C only
   c. A, B and D only
   d. B, C and D only

Ans. (c) A, B and D only

111. An organism having heart for circulation, excretes through green glands. It has several ganglia and tactile organs on its body and its larval form is very different than its adult form. This organism is most likely to respire by:

   (A) Exchanging oxygen and carbon dioxide through an extensive tracheal system.
   (B) Gaseous exchange over thinner areas of cuticle or by gills
   (C) An efficient tracheal system that delivers oxygen directly to the tissues
   (D) A double transport system, where the circulating fluid contains a dissolved respiratory pigment.

   Choose the correct option.

   a. A and C
   b. Only D
   c. Only B
   d. B and D

Ans. (c) Only B

112. The MALDI spectrum of a peptide shows a peak at m/z corresponding to 3600. When the ESI spectrum is recorded, peaks at m/z corresponding to 721,904 and 1801 were obtained. When the MALDI MS/MS spectrum was recorded, large number of peaks with m/z less than 3600 were observed. The spectral data indicate that the peptide is

   a. Highly impure
   b. Pure with molecular mass of 3600 and partial sequence of the peptide can be determined
   c. Highly unstable and degrades rapidly
   d. Degraded under condition employed for recording ESI spectrum

Ans. (b) Pure with molecular mass of 3600 and partial sequence of the peptide can be determined

113. In a stressful condition, ACTH secretion was increased and as a result glucocorticoid concentration was elevated in blood. One or a combination of the following changes most likely taking place in this condition:

   (A) Decreased circulating eosinophils and basophils.
   (B) Reduced IL2 release.
   (C) Potentiated inflammatory response to tissue injury.
   (D) Increased mitotic activity of lymphocytes in lymph nodes.

   The correct answer is

   a. B and C　　　　　b. A and B
   c. B and D　　　　　d. C and D

Ans. (b) A and B

114. In one study, a group of 5 day rat pups were fed for 3 weeks a diet A and the pups gained weight by 300%. In a second study, when the same diet fed for 3 weeks to rats of 350 gms, they did not gain weight significantly. In a third study, a diet B was fed to 250-350 gms rats and it was observed that they delivered normal pups after five weeks. Based on these observations which of the following statements is correct?

   a. Diet A facilitates weight gain than diet B
   b. Diet B facilitates pregnancy and child-bearing
   c. More control experiments are to be conducted for definitive conclusion
   d. Diet A is more energy containing that diet 'B'. Hence, its quantity should be reduced

Ans. (c) More control experiments are to be conducted for definitive conclusion

115. In *Neurospora* a cross between the genotypes 'A' and 'a' results in an ascus with ascospores of genotypes as shown below. Statements A to D are events that could have occurred during meiosis.

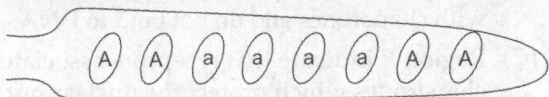

   (A) Crossing over between the centromere and the gene.
   (B) Segregation of alleles 'A' and 'a' in meiosis I.
   (C) Segregation of alleles 'A' and 'a' in meiosis II.
   (D) Assortment of alleles 'A' and 'a'.
   Which of the above events could correctly explain the observation shown in the figure?

   a. A followed by C　　　b. C alone
   c. A followed by B　　　d. D alone

Ans. (a) A followed by C

116. Which of the following graph represents normal sexual cycle in a normal human female?

— Estrogen - - Progestrone

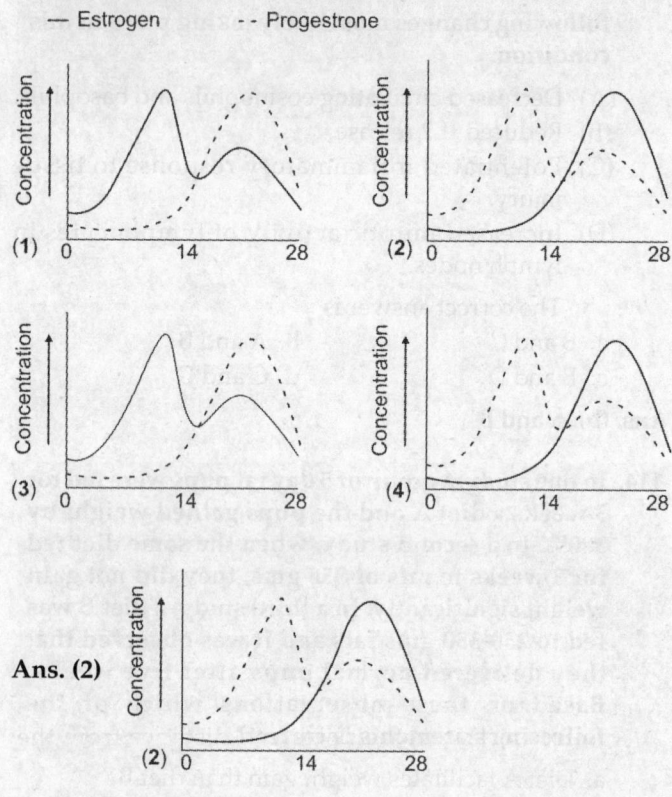

(1)   (2)   (3)   (4)

Ans. (2)

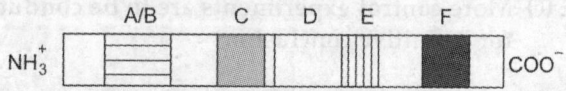

(2)

117. Based on the structural regions of a nuclear receptor shown in the diagram, the following predictions were made.

NH_3^+ A/B C D E F COO^-

(A) Region F is responsible for binding to ligands and contains two zinc finger-like binding motifs

(B) Receptors with A/B domains generally associate with chaperones and do not bind to DNA.

(C) Region E indicate that receptors associate with chaperones which protect the nuclear hormone receptors.

(D) Region C contains the P-box and the D-box required for dimerization of the receptor and creates contact with DNA phosphate backbone.

Which one of the following is true?

a. A and B
b. B and C
c. B and D
d. C and D

Ans. (c) B and D

118. When F1 female *Drosophila* of the genotype $a + a$ $b + b$ $c + c$ is test crossed, the following progenies were obtained:

Progeny classes*	No. of progenies
$a^+ b^+ c^+$	22
$a^+ b^+ c$	28
$a\, b\, c^+$	26
$a\, b\, c$	24
$a^+ b\, c^+$	230
$a^+ b\, c$	220
$a\, b^+ c^+$	225
$a\, b^+ c$	225
Total	1000

*The progeny has been shown as classes derived from the female gamete. Statements A to F as given below are conclusions derived from the above result.

(A) Genes a and b are linked in *cis*.

(B) Genes a and b are linked in *trans*.

(C) Genes a and b are linked in *cis* while b and c are linked in*trans*.

(D) The genotype of the parents are $a + a + b + b +$ and *aabb*

(E) The genotype of the parents are $a + a + bb$ and *aab* $+ b +$.

(F) Genes a and b are 10cM apart.

Which of the above statements are correct?

a. C alone
b. A, E and F
c. B, E and F
d. A, D and F

Ans. (c) B, E and F

119. Monoclonal antibodies (mAb) can be potentially used as therapeutic agents. The major advantage is that they can specifically target aberrant cells. However, there is a practical difficulty. Monoclonals are raised in mouse and therefore it is expected that an immune reaction will develop if these are injected into humans. It is therefore necessary to 'humanize' monoclonal antibody by

a. Expressing the genes for the mAb in cultured human cells and isolating the mAb from these cells

b. Replacing the Fv region of a mAb with one derived from a human IgG

c. Replacing CL and CH regions of the Mab with that obtained from a human IgG

d. Taking a human IgG and replacing the CDRs by those derived from the mouse mAb

Ans. (a) Expressing the genes for the mAb in cultured human cells and isolating the mAb from these cells

120. The following is a hypothetical pathway for the development of wild type (red) eye colour in an insect: Enzymes A and B are encoded by the genes *a +* and *b +*, respectively.

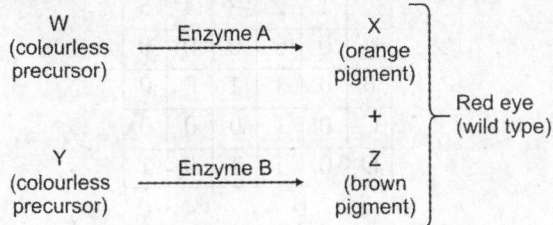

The following statements are made regarding inheritance of the genes involved in the development of eye colour:

(A) When two heterozygous individuals of the genotype *a + ab + b* are mated, progenies with red, orange, brown and white eye colour will be observed irrespective of whether the genes are independently assorting or showing incomplete linkage.

(B) When two heterozygous individuals of the genotype *a + ab + b* are mated, progenies with red, orange, brown and white eye colour will be observed in a ratio of 9:3:3:1, when the genes are independently assorting.

(C) When an heterozygous individual of the genotype *a + b/ a b +* is test crossed, progenies with red and white eye colour will be more in number.

(D) When an heterozygous individual of the genotype *a + b/ a b +* is test crossed, progenies with orange and brown eye colour will be more in number.

Which of the above statements is TRUE?

a. A and C
b. B and C
c. A, B and C
d. A, B and D

Ans. (d) A, B and D

121. Mendel crossed tall pea plants with dwarf ones. The F1 plants were all tall. When these F1 plants were selfed to produce F2 generation, he got a 3: 1 tall to dwarf ratio in the offspring. What is the probability that out of three plants (of F2 generation) picked up at random two would be dwarf and one would be tall?

a. 3/4
b. 3/8
c. 9/64
d. 9/32

Ans. (c) 9/64

122. Two new plant species, A and B, were described in 1872. Subsequently it was found that the type for species A was never designated and for species B there was one specimen designated as type but missing. As per International Code of Botanical Nomenclature (ICBN), typification should be

a. Neotype for A only
b. Neotype for A and lectotype for B
c. Neotypes for both A and B
d. Lectotype for both A and B.

Ans. (c) Neotypes for both A and B

123. According to MacArthur and Wilson's equilibrium theory, which of the following is true?

a. Larger islands and islands closer to continent are expected to have more species than smaller and isolated islands

b. Smaller islands and islands far from the continent are expected to have more species than larger and isolated islands

c. Smaller islands and islands closer to the continent are expected to have more species than far away smaller and isolated islands

d. More species are expected on all islands irrespective of their size and distance from the continent

Ans. (a) Larger islands and islands closer to continent are expected to have more species than smaller and isolated islands

124. Proteins in cells can be visualized by the following methods:

(A) Express the gene (coding for the said protein) as a fusion with the green fluorescence protein (GFP) and directly visualize under a fluorescence microscope.

(D) Express the gene (coding for the said protein) as a fusion with the β-galactosidase gene (*lac Z*) and directly visualize under a phase contrast bright field microscope.

(C) A fluorescence tagged antibody raised against the said protein could be used for visualization in a fluorescence microscope.

(D) Over express the protein and directly visualize it under a scanning electron microscope.

Which of the following methods you would choose to visualize a protein in a living cell?

a. A only
b. A and C only
c. A and B only
d. D only

Ans. (c) A and B only

125. Affected individuals from the pedigree given below are suffering from albinism, an autosomal recessive disease.

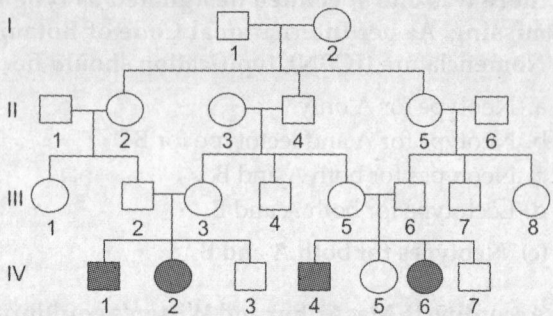

Identify the confirmed carrier individuals in this pedigree assuming that the members coming from outside the family are homozygous for the dominant allele.

a. III-2, 1II-3, III-5, 1II-6, II-I, II-3 and II-6

b. III-2, III-3, III-5, 1II-6, II-2, II-4, II-5 and I-2

c. III-2, 1II-3, III-5, III-6, 1I-2, II-4 and II-5

d. III-I, III-4, III-7, II-2, II-4 and II-5

Ans. (c) III-2, 1II-3, III-5, III-6, 1I-2, II-4 and II-5

126. Assume a new subspecies *Ficus callosa* subsp. *Microcarpa* has been published by Jacobs. The nomenclature of the resulting entities would be

a. *F callosa* and *F. callosa* subsp. *microcarpa* Jacobs

b. *F. callosa* subsp. *microcarpa* Jacobs and other yet to be named subspecies of *F. callosa*

c. *F. callosa* subsp. *callosa* Jacobs and *F.callosa* subsp. *microcarpa* Jacobs

d. *F. callosa* subsp. *callosa* and *F.callosa* subsp. *Microcarpa* Jacobs

Ans. (d) *F. callosa* subsp. *callosa* and *F.callosa* subsp. *Microcarpa* Jacobs

127. Primary production in aquatic ecosystem is measured using Light-and-Dark-Bottle technique. In this method, as an indirect measure of photosynthetic production, dissolved oxygen concentration of the pond water enclosed in a BOD bottle is measured initially (I) and after a fixed duration of incubation in a light bottle (L) and a dark bottle (D). Then, the gross and net primary productions are estimated is

a. (L-D) and (L-I), respectively

b. (L-I) and (L—D), respectively

c. (L-I) and (I-D), respectively

d. (L-D) and (I-D), respectively

Ans. (a) (L-D) and (L-I), respectively

128. Identify the most appropriate cladogram that can be constructed using the data matrix given below, assuming '0's are pleisomorphic and '1's are apomorphic characters.

	1	2	3	4	5
A	0	0	0	0	0
B	0	1	1	0	0
C	0	1	0	0	0
D	0	1	1	0	1

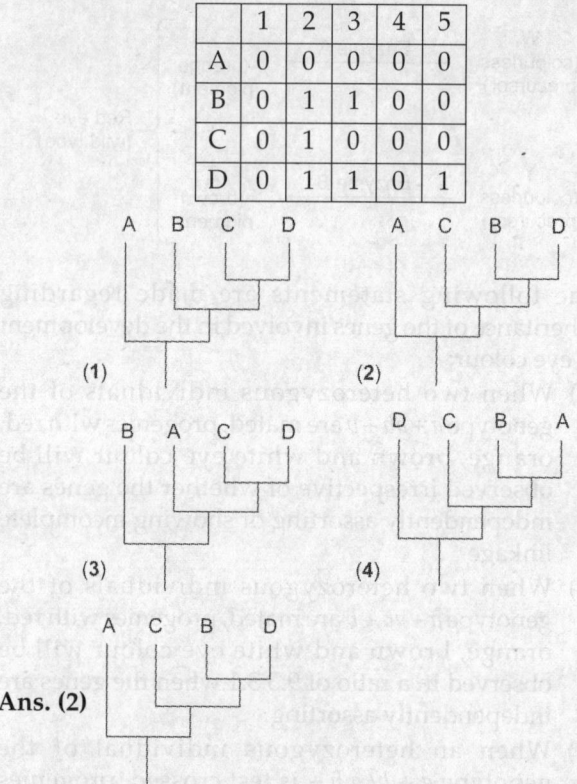

Ans. (2)

129. Gause's 'Competitive exclusion' principle states that two species with identical niches cannot coexist indefinitely. Which of the following statements is the most appropriate regarding the validity of the principle?

a. It depends on how one defines niche

b. There are in nature many instances of continued coexistence of closely related species

c. The principle is universally true

d. It does not predict the outcome where, both the species are equally strong competitors

Ans. (a) It depends on how one defines niche

130. In a lake ecosystem, bottom-up effects (B) refers to control of a lower trophic level by the higher trophic levels and top down effects (T) refer to the opposite. In a lake with three trophic levels - Phytoplankton (P), Zooplankton (Z) and Carnivore (C)

a. P and C are controlled by B, and Z is controlled by T

b. P, Z and C are all controlled by T

c. P is controlled by B, Z is controlled by T and C is controlled by B

d. P is controlled by T, Z is controlled by B and C is controlled by T

Ans. (a) P and C are controlled by B, and Z is controlled by T

Memory Based Paper CSIR NET Dec 2011

1. What is the angle θ in the quadrant of a circle shown below?

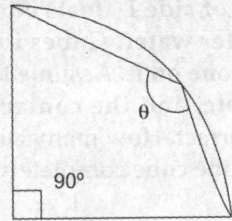

a. 135°
b. 90°
c. 120°
d. May have any value between 90° and 120°

Ans. (a) 135°

2. In ΔABC, angle A is larger than angle C and smaller than angle B by the small amount. if angle B is 67°, angle C is

a. 67°   b. 53°
c. 60°   d. 57°

Ans. (b) 53°

3. See the following mathematical manipulation.

   I. Let x =5
   II. Then $x^2-25 = x-5$
   III. $\{x-5\}\{x+5\}=x-5$
   IV. X+5 =1 [cancelling (x-5) from both sides]
   V. 10=1 [putting x=5]
Which of the above is wrong statement?
   a. I to II   b. II to III
   c. III to IV   d. IV to V

Ans. (d) IV to V

4. Inner plannet of the solar system are rocky, where as outer plannet are gaseous. One of the reason for this is that

a. Solar heat drove away the gases to the outer region f the solar system
b. Gravitational pull of the sun pulled all rocky material to the inner solar system

c. Outer planet are larger than the inner planet
d. Comets delivered the gaseous materials to the outer planet

Ans. (c) Outer planet are larger than the inner planet

5. The number f craters observed due to meteoritic impacts during the early stages of the formation, is less on the earth than that of Moon because

a. Formation of craters on the earth was difficults due to the presences of hard rocks
b. Impacting bodies on the Earth were smaller in size
c. Craters on the Earth are now covered by ocean water
d. Earlier craters are not preserved due to continuous modification of Earth's surface by geological process

Ans. (d) Earlier craters are not preserved due to continuous modification of Earth's surface by geological process

6. During a total solar eclipse occurring at noon, it becomes dark enough for few minute for star to become visible. The stars that are seen are those which will be seen from same location

a. On the following night only
b. On the night one month later
c. On the night three month later
d. On the night six months later

Ans. (d) On the night six months later

7. The variation of solublities of two compound X and Y in water with temperature is depicted below. Which of the following statement is true?

a. Solubility of Y is less than that of X
b. Solubility of X varies with temperature
c. Solubilities of X and Y are the same at 75°C
d. Solubilities of X and Y are independent of temp.

Ans. (c) Solubilities of X and Y are the same at 75°C

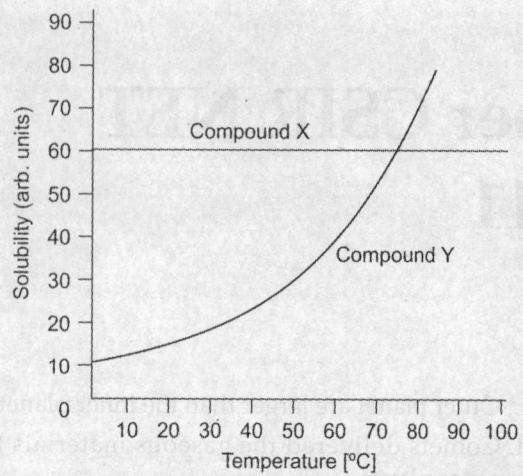

8. **Living being get energy frm foo through the process of aerobic respiration. One of the reactants is**

   a. Carbon dioxide   b. Water vapour
   c. Oxygen   d. Phosphorus

Ans. (c) Oxygen

9. **Restriction endonuclease cleaves DNA molecules at specific 'recognition sites'. One such enzyme has four recognition sites on a circular DNA molecule. After complete digestion, how many fragments would be produced upon reaction with this enzyme?**

   a. 4   b. 5
   c. 3   d. 6

Ans. (a) 4

10. **Which f the following statements about the concentration of CO_2 in the earth's atmosphere are true?**

    a. It was the highest n the very early atmosphere of the Earth
    b. It has steadily decreased since the formation of the Earth's atmosphere
    c. It has steadily increase since the formation of the Earth's atmosphere
    d. Its levels today are the highest n the Earth's history

Ans. (a) It was the highest n the very early atmosphere of the Earth

11. **Magnesium powder, placed in an air-tight glass container 1.0 bar, is burnt by focusing sunlight. Part of the magnesium burns off, and some is left behind. The pressure of the air in the container after it has returned to room temperature is approximately**

    a. 1.0 bar   b. 0.2 bar
    c. 1.2 bar   d. 0.8 bar

Ans. (d) 0.8 bar

12. **When a magnet is made to fall free in air, it falls with an acceleration of 9.8 ms^{-2}. But when it is made to fall through a long aluminium cylinder, its acceleration decreases, because**

    a. A part of the gravitational potential energy is lost in heating the magnet
    b. A part of the gravitational potential energy s lost in heating the cylinder
    c. The said experiment was one in the magnetic northern hemisphere
    d. The cylinder shields the gravitational force

Ans. (b) A part of the gravitational potential energy s lost in heating the cylinder

13. **A solid cube of side L floats on water 20% of its volumes under water. Cubes identical to ts are piled one by one on it. Assume that cubes do not slips or topple, and the contact between their surfaces is perfect. How many cubes are required to submerge one cube completely?**

    a. 4   b. 5
    c. 6   d. Infinite

Ans. (a) 4

14. **An overweight person runs 4 km everyday as an exercise. After losing 20% of his body weight, if he has t run the same distance in the same time, the energy expenditure would be**

    a. 20% more
    b. The same as earlier
    c. 20% less
    d. 40% less

Ans. (c) 20% less

15. **On exposure to desiccation, which of the following bacteria are least likely to experience rapid water loss?**

    a. Isolated rods
    b. Rods in chain
    c. Cocci in chain
    d. Cocci in clusters

Ans. (d) Cocci in clusters

16. **A cupboard is filled with a large number of bass of 6 different colours. You already have one ball of each colour. You already have one ball of each colour. If you are blindfolded, how many balls do you need to draw to be sure of having 3 colour matched pair of balls?**

    a. 3   b. 4
    c. 5   d. 6

Ans. (c) 5

17. The conductance of a potassium chloride solution is measured using the arrangement depicted below. The specific conductivity of the solution n Sm-1, when there is no deflection in the galvanometer, is

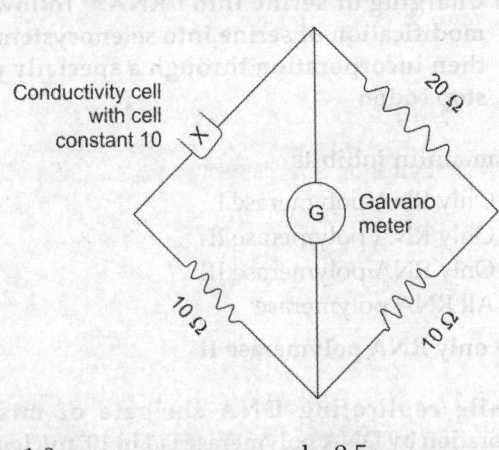

a. 1.0
b. 0.5
c. 2.0
d. 1.5

Ans. (b) 0.5

18. What is the half life of the radio isotope whose activity profile shown below?

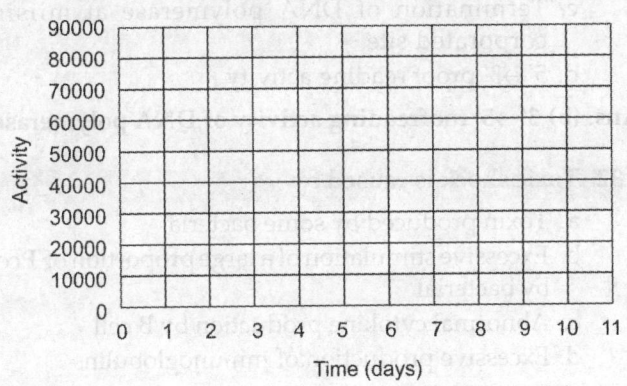

a. 1 day
b. 3 day
c. 2 day
d. 4 day

Ans. (a) 1 day

19. A bell s run before giving food t a dog. After doing this continuously for 10 days, which of the following most likely to happen?

a. The dog learns t ignore the bell
b. The dog salivates on hearing the bell
c. The dog ignores food and runs towards the bell
d. The dog will not eat food without hearing the bell

Ans. (b) The dog salivates on hearing the bell

20. For an elastic material, strain is proportional to stress. A constant stress is applies at time t1. Which of the following plots characterizes the strain n that material?

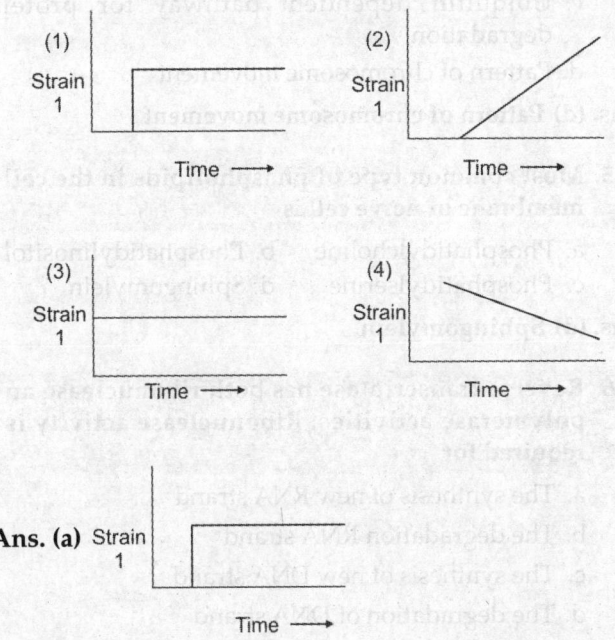

Ans. (a)

21. On the molar scale which of the following interaction in a nonpolar environment provides the highest cntribution to the bio-molecules?

a. Vander walls interaction
b. Hydrogen bonding
c. Salt bridge
d. Hydrophobic interaction

Ans. (c) Salt bridge

22. Michaelis and Menten derived their equation using which of the the following assumption?

a. Rate limiting step in the reaction in the breakdown of ES complex to product an free enzyme
b. Rate limiting step in the reaction in the formation of ES complex
c. Concentration of the substrate can be ignored
d. Non-enzymatic degradation of the substrate is the major step

Ans. (a) Rate limiting step in the reaction in the breakdown of ES complex to product an free enzyme

23. In which form of DNA the number of base pair per helical turn is 10.5?

a. A
b. B
c. X
d. Z

Ans. (b) B

24. In contrast with plant cells, the most distinctive feature of cell division in animal cell is

a. Control of cell cycle transition by protein kinase

b. Enzyme responsible for DNA replication

c. Ubiquitin dependent pathway for protein degradation

d. Pattern of chromosome movement

Ans. (d) Pattern of chromosome movement

25. Most common type of phospholipids in the cell membrane of nerve cell is

a. Phosphatidylcholine   b. Phosphatidylinositol

c. Phosphatidylserine   d. Sphingomylein

Ans. (d) Sphingomylein

26. Reverse transcriptase has both ribonuclease an polymerase activities. Ribonuclease activity is required for

a. The synthesis of new RNA strand

b. The degradation RNA strand

c. The synthesis of new DNA strand

d. The degradation of DNA strand

Ans. (b) The degradation RNA strand

27. The membrane lipids molecules assemble spontaneously into bilayers when placed in water an form a closed spherical structure known as

a. Lysosome   b. Peroxisome

c. Lipososme   d. Endosome

Ans. (c) Lipososme

28. In gene regulation, open reading frame implies

a. Interviening nucleotide sequence in between two genes

b. A series of triplets codons not interrupted by a stop codon

c. A series of triplet codons that begins with a start codon and ends with a stop codon

d. The exonc sequence of a gene that curresponds to 5' UTR of the mRNA and thus does not code for the protein

Ans. (c) A series of triplet codons that begins with a start codon and ends with a stop codon

29. Amino acid selenocysteine is incorporated into polypeptide chain during translation by:

a. Charging of sec in to tRNA^{ser} followed by incorporation through serine codon

b. Charging of Serine in to tRNA^{ser} followed by modification of serine into selenocysteine and then incorporation through serine codon

c. Charging of sec in to tRNA^{sec} and then incorporation through selenocysteine codon

d. Charging of serine into t RNA^{ser} followed by modification of serine into selenocystein e and then incorporation through a specially placed stop codon

Ans. (d) Charging of serine into t RNA^{ser} followed by modification of serine into selenocystein e and then incorporation through a specially placed stop codon

30. α-amanitin inhibits

a. Only RNA polymerase I

b. Only RNA polymerase II

c. Only RNA polymerase III

d. All RNA polymerase

Ans. (b) only RNA polymerase II

31. while replicating DNA the rate of misncorporation by DNA polymerase is 1 in 10^5 nucleotide. However, the actual error rate in the replicated DNA is 1 in 10^9 nucleotide incorporated. This is achieved mainly due to

a. spontaneous excisin of mis incorporation nucleotides

b. 3'→5' roofreading activity of DNA polymerase

c. Termination of DNA polymerase at miisincorporated site

d. 5'→3' proof reading activity

Ans. (b) 3'→5' roofreading activity of DNA polymerase

32. Toxic shock is caused by

a. Toxin produced by some bacteria

b. Excessive stimulation of a large proportion of T cell by bacterial

c. Abnormal cytokine production by B cell

d. Excessive production of mmunoglobulins

Ans. (b) Excessive stimulation of a large proportion of T cell by bacterial

33. Ethylele binding to its receptor does NOT lead to

a. Dimerization of the receptor

b. Phosphorylation of the receptor

c. Actvation of CTR Raf kinase

d. Endocytosis of ethylene receptor complex

Ans. (d) Endocytosis of ethylene receptor complex

34. Graft rejection does not involve

a. Erythrocytes

b. T cell

c. Macrophages

d. Polymorphonuclear leukocytes

Ans. (a) Erythrocytes

35. The blastopore region of amphibian embryo that secretes BMP inhibitor and dorsalizes the surrounding tssue is know as

    a. Bachet's cleft
    b. Nieuwkoop center
    c. Spemann's organizer
    d. Hensen's node

Ans. (c) Spemann's organizer

36. During development of embryo in plants, PIN proteins are involved in

    a. Establishment of auxin gradients
    b. Regulation of gene expression
    c. Induction of programmed cell death
    d. Induction of cell division

Ans. (a) Establishment of auxin gradients

37. Whch of the following maternal effect gene product regulated production of anterior structure in Drosophila embryo?

    a. Bcoiid and Nanos
    b. Bicoid and Hunchback
    c. Biicoid and Caudal
    d. Nanos and Caudal

Ans. (b) Bicoid and Hunchback

38. Which of the floral whorls is affected in agamous mutant

    a. Sepals and petals
    b. Petals and stamens
    c. Stamens and carpels
    d. Sepals and carpels

Ans. (c) Stamens and carpels

39. Which of the following set of cell organelles are involved n the biosynthesis of jasmonic acid through octadecanoid signalling pathway?

    a. Chloroplast and peroxisomes
    b. Chloroplast and mitochondria
    c. Mitochondria and peroxisome
    d. Golgi bodies and mitochondria

Ans. (a) Chloroplast and peroxisomes

40. Which of the following is NOT a prosthetic grou of nitrate reductase

    a. FAD
    b. Heme
    c. Mo
    d. Pterin

Ans. (d) Pterin

41. Chloroplast distribution n a photosynthesizing cell is governed by blue light sensing phototropin 2. When the cells are irradiated with high intensity blue light the chloroplasts

    a. Move to the side walls
    b. Aggregate in the middle of the cell
    c. Are sparsely distributed
    d. Aggregate in small cluster

Ans. (a) Move to the side walls

42. Which of the following acts as a branch point for the biosynthesis of sesquiterpene and triterpenes?

    a. Farnesyl pyrophosphate
    b. Geranyl pyrophosphate
    c. Sopentyl pyrophosphate
    d. Hydroxymethyl glularyl –CoA

Ans. (a) Farnesyl pyrophosphate

43. Which of the following waves is likely to be absent in a normal frog ECG?

    a. P
    b. Q
    c. T
    d. R

Ans. (b) Q

44. The atmosphere in sealed space craft contains

    a. Pure oxygen
    b. A mix of oxygen and nitrogen
    c. Mix of oxygen and CO_2
    d. Pressurise atmospheric air available normally on earth

Ans. (b) A mix of oxygen and nitrogen

45. In a normal human eye, for sharp image formation on the retina, maximum dioptric power is provided by the

    a. Retina
    b. Cornea
    c. Anterior surface of the lens
    d. Posterior surface of the lens

Ans. (b) Cornea

46. In this flow diagram name the chemical A, B, C and D in proper sequence.

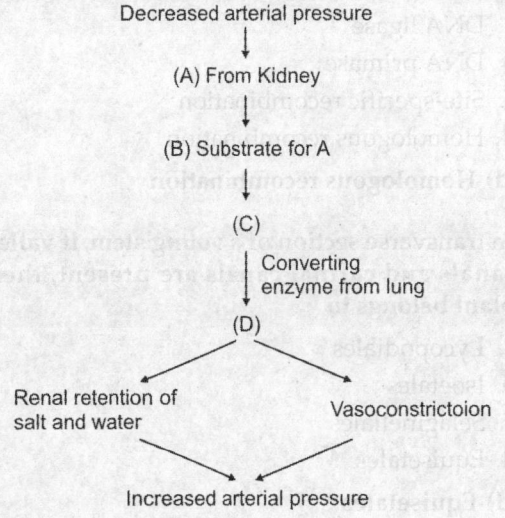

a. Rennin, Angiotensin II, angiotensin I, Angiotensinogen

b. Aqngiotensin I, angiotensinogen, Angiotensin II, rennin

c. Rennin, angiotensin I, Angiotensin II, angiotensinogen

d. Rennin, angiotensinogen, angiotensin I, angotensn II

Ans. (d) Rennin, angiotensinogen, angiotensin I, angotensn II

47. **A plant of the genotype AaBb is selfed. The two genes are linked and are 50 maps unit apart. What proportion of the progeny will haw the genotype aabb?**

    a. 1/2   b. 1/4
    c. 1/8   d. 1/16

Ans. (d) 1/16

48. **The base analog 2-aminopurine pairs with thymine, an can occasionally pair with cytosine. The type of mutation induced by 2-aminopurine is**

    a. Transversion   b. Transition
    c. Deletion   d. Nonsense

Ans. (b) Transition

49. **What kind of aneuploid gametes will be generated if meiotic non-disjunction occurs at first division? ('n' represent the haploid number of chromosome)**

    a. Only n+1 and n   b. Only n-1 and n
    c. Both n+1 and n-2   d. Either n+1 and n-1

Ans. (c) Both n+1 and n-2

50. **A single starnd nick in the parental DNA helix just ahead of a replication fork causes the replication fork to break. Recovery from this calamity requires**

    a. DNA ligase
    b. DNA primase
    c. Site-specific recombination
    d. Homologous recombination

Ans. (d) Homologous recombination

51. **In transverse section of a young stem, if vallecular canals and carinal canals are present, then the plant belongs to**

    a. Lycopodiales
    b. Isoetales
    c. Selaginellales
    d. Equisetales

Ans. (d) Equisetales

52. **Horse shoe crabs belong to the group**

    a. Onychophora   b. Chelicerata
    c. Uniramia   d. Crustacean

Ans. (b) Chelicerata

53. **Which of the following group of species are typical of grassland habitats in India**

    a. Black buck, wolf, great Indian bustard, lesser florican
    b. Spotted deer, dhole, peacock, finch-lark
    c. Sambar, tiger, paradise fly catcher
    d. Otter, cormorant, darter, pelican

Ans. (a) Black buck, wolf, great Indian bustard, lesser florican

54. **Batrachochytrium dendrobatidis, a fungus has been implicated n the decline of population of**

    a. Fish   b. Frogs
    c. Pelicans   d. Bats

Ans. (b) Frogs

55. **The hutchinsonan concept of ecological niche is based on**

    a. Microhabibate occupied
    b. Multidimensional hypervolume
    c. Role played in the ecosystem
    d. A combination of role played and microhabitat occupied

Ans. (b) Multidimensional hypervolume

56. **Which of the following is NOT a physiological characteristic of early successional plants?**

    a. High respiration
    b. Inhibition by far red light
    c. High transpiration rate
    d. Low photosynthesis rate

Ans. (d) Low photosynthesis rate

57. **Aquatic primary production was measured using light and dark bottle technique. If the intitial oxygen concentration was l and final concentration in the light bottle is L and that n the dark bottle D, the gross productivity is given by**

    a. L-D   b. l-D
    c. l-D   d. L-D

Ans. (d) L-D

58. **Wetland are conserved internationally through an effort called as**

    a. Basel convention   b. Rio convention
    c. Montreal convention d. Ramsar convention

Ans. (d) Ramsar convention

59. The first living being on earth were anaerobic because
   a. There was no oxygen in air
   b. Oxygen damages proteins
   c. Oxygen nterferes with the action of ribozyme
   d. They evolved in deep sea

Ans. (a) There was no oxygen in air

60. Which of the following processes interferes in sequence based phylogeny?
   a. Horizontal gene transfer
   b. Adaptive mutation
   c. DNA repair
   d. Reverse transcription

Ans. (a) Horizontal gene transfer

61. The peacock's tail is an example of
   a. Natural selection   b. Dversifying selection
   c. Sexual selection   d. Group selection

Ans. (c) Sexual selection

62. A specialist species has a
   a. Wider niche and high efficiency of niche utilization
   b. Narrower niche and high efficiency of niche utilization
   c. Wider niche and low efficiency of niche utilization
   d. Narrower niche and low efficiency of niche utilization

Ans. (b) Narrower niche and high efficiency of niche utilization

63. To keep them in a totipotent state, embryonic stem cells need to be maintained in a medium supplemented with
   a. Growth hormone
   b. Leukemia inhibiting factor
   c. Nestin
   d. Insulin

Ans. (b) Leukemia inhibiting factor

64. Which of the following feature is NOT shown by glyphosate, a broad spectrum herbicide?
   a. Little residual soil activity
   b. Ready translocation in phloem
   c. Inhibition of a chloroplast enzyme catalyzing the synthesis of aromatic amino acid
   d. Inhibition of early steps in the biosynthesis of branched chain amino acid

Ans. (d) Inhibition of early steps in the biosynthesis of branched chain amino acid

65. The rattans and canes that we use in furniture belong to
   a. Bamboos   b. Palms
   c. Arborescent lilies   d. Legumes

Ans. (b) Palms

66. The presence of salmonella in tap water is indicative of contamination with
   a. Industrial effluents   b. Human excreta
   c. Agriculture waste   d. Kitchen waste

Ans. (b) Human excreta

67. Indirect immunofluoresence involves fllurescently labelled
   a. Immunoglobulin specific antibodies
   b. Antigen specific antibodies
   c. Hapten specific antibodies
   d. Carrier specific antibodies

Ans. (a) Immunoglobulin specific antibodies

68. A sample counted for one minute shows a count rate of 752 cpm. For how many minute should it be counted to have 1% probable error?
   a. 13   b. 5
   c. 2   d. 75

Ans. (a) 13

69. Measurement and mapping with spatial resolution the membrane potential of a cell, which is too small for microelectrode impalement, is done using
   a. Radioisotope
   b. Voltage sensitive dye
   c. pH sensitive chemical
   d. Vital dyes

Ans. (b) Voltage sensitive dye

70. one of the methods for finding common regulatory motif present in a set of co-regulated genes is
   a. prosite   b. MEME
   c. Mat Inspector   d. PSSM

Ans. (b) MEME

71. Equilibrium constant (K) of noncovalent interaction between two non-bonded atoms of two different groups was measured at 27°C. It was observed that K = 100 M-s.the strength of this noncovalent interaction in terms of Gibbs free energy change is:
   a. 2746 kcal/ mole   b. – 2746 kcal/ mole
   c. 247 kcal/ mole   d. – 247 kcal/mole

Ans. (b) – 2746 kcal/ mole

72. If van der waals interaction is described by the following relation

$$\Delta G_{van} = \frac{A}{r^{12}} - \frac{B}{r^6} + \frac{q_1 q_2}{r}$$

Where ΔG_{van} is free energy of the vander waals interaction, A and B are constants, r is the distance between two monbonded atoms 1 and 2 and q1 and q2 are partial charge on the dipoles 1 and 2. In this relation, the parameter A described

a. Electron shell attraction
b. Electron shell repulsion
c. Dipole-dipole attraction
d. Dipole dipole repulsion

Ans. (b) Electron shell repulsion

73. The pH of blood of a healthy person is maintained at 7.40 ± 0.05, Assuming that this pH is maintained entirely by the bicarbonate buffer (pKa1 and pKa2 of carbonic acid are 6.1 and 10.3, respectively), the molar ratio of [bicarbonate]/ [carbonic acid] in the blood is

a. 0.005   b. 1
c. 10   d. 20

Ans. (d) 20

74. The hydrolysis of pyrophosphate to ortho-phosphate is important for several biosynthetic reaction. In *E. coli*, the molecular mass of the enzyme pyrophosphatase is 120 kD and it consists of six identical subunits. The enzyme activity is defined as the amount of enzyme that hydrolyzes 10 μmol of pyrophosphate in 15 minutes at 37°C under standard assay condition. The purified enzyme has a Vmax of 2800 units per milligram of the enzyme. How many moles of the substrate are hydrolysed per second per milligram of the enzyme when the substrate concentration is much greater than Km?

a. 0.05 μmol   b. 62 μmol
c. 31.1 μmol   d. 1 μmol

Ans. (c) 31.1 μmol

75. Denaturation profiles of DNA are shown below

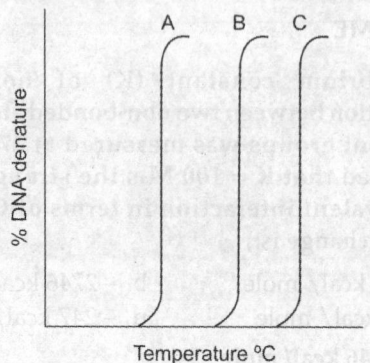

The difference in the profiles arise because

a. The DNA is single stranded but of different sizes
b. A+T content of A>B>A in DNA of comparable sizes isolated from simple genomes
c. G+C content of C>B>A in DNA comparable sizes isolated from simple genomes
d. G+C content is identical but A+T content in A>B>C n DNA of comparable sizes isolated from simple genomes

Ans. (c) G+C content of C>B>A in DNA comparable sizes isolated from simple genomes

76. Biosynthesis of tyrosine is detailed below:

Shikimic acid-A → shikimic acid-5-phosphate –B → C → chorismic acid → prephenic acid → D → transaminase → tyrosine

Identify A,B,C and D

a. ATP, phosphoenolpyruvic acid, 3-enolpyruyl shikimic acid-5-phosphate, p-hydroxyphenyl-pyruvic acid
b. GTP, pyridoxal phosphate, 3-enolpyruvyl shikimic acid-5 phosphate, phenylpyruvic acid
c. NADP, 3-phosphonydroxypyruvic acid, 3-enolpyruvic shikimic acid-5- phosphate, p-hydroxyphenylpyruvic acid
d. ATP, 3- phosphohydroxypyruvic acid, 3 enolpyruvyl shikimic acid-5- phosphate, pyridoxylphosphate

Ans. (a) ATP, phosphoenolpyruvic acid, 3-enolpyruyl shikimic acid-5-phosphate, p-hydroxyphenyl-pyruvic acid

77. A nerve impulse or action potential is generated from transient changes in the permeability of the axon membrane to Na+ and k+ ions. The depolarization of the membrane beyond the threshold level leads to Na+ flowing into the cell and a change in membrane potential to a positive value. The K+ channel then opens allowing K+ to flow outwards ultimately restoring membrane potential to the resting value, the Na+ and K+ channels operate in opposite direction because

a. There is an electrochemical gradient growth generated by proton transport
b. There is a difference in Na+ and K+ concentration on the either side of the membrane
c. Na+ is a voltage gated channel, where as K+ is ligand gated
d. Na+ is dependent on ATP wheras K+ is not

Ans. (b) There is a difference in Na+ and K+ concentration on the either side of the membrane

78. The erythrocyte membrane cytoskeleton consists of a meshwork of proteins underlying the membrane. The principal component spectrin has α,β subunit which assemble to forms tetramers, the cytoskeleton is anchored to the membrane through kinkages with the trnasmembrane proteins band 3 and glycophorin C. the cytosolic domain of band 3 also serves as the binding site of glycolytic enzymes such as glyceraldehydes 3 phosphate dehydrogenase. Analysis of the blood sample of a patient with haemolytic anemia shows spherical red blood cells. The patient carries

a. A mutation in glycophorin C

b. A mutant spectrin with increased tetramerizatioin propensity

c. Mutant β spectin defective in αβ dimerization ability

d. Mutant glyceraldeyde 3 phasphate dehydrogenase

Ans. (c) Mutant â spectin defective in áâ dimerization ability

79. In human, protein coding genes are mainly organized as "exons" and "intron". There are intergenic regions that transcribe into various types of non coding RNA. Some introns may harbour also transcription uints, which are

a. Always other protein coding genes

b. Proteins coding gene and RNA coding genes

c. Always RNA coding genes

d. Pseudo genes

Ans. (b) Proteins coding gene and RNA coding genes

80. Maturation promoting factor (MPF) control the initiation of mitosis in eukaryotic cells. MPF kinase activity requires cyclin B. Cyclin B is required for chromosome condensation degradation is followed by chromosome decondensation, nuclear envelope reformation and exit from mitosis. This requires ubiquitination of a cyclin destruction box motif in cyclin B. RNase-treated Xenopus egg extracts and sperm chromatin were, mixed. MPF activity increased with chromosome condensation and nuclear envelope breakdown. However, this was not followed by chromosome decondensation and nuclear envelop reformation because

a. RNase contamination persisted in the system

b. Cyclin B was missing from the system

c. Ubiquitin ligase had been overexpressed

d. Cyclin B lacking the cyclin destruction box had been overexpressed

Ans. (d) Cyclin B lacking the cyclin destruction box had been overexpressed

81. Many cancers carry mutant p53 genes, while some cancers have normal p53 genes. P53 activates p21 (Waf1) which inhibits G I/S-Cdks, and phosphorylation of the retinoblastoma protein (Rb). Cancers with normal p53 genes could

a. Expressed non-phosphorylatable form of Rb

b. Express high levels of p53-deubiquitinases

c. Express inactive from of G1/S-cdks

d. Express inactive forms of G1/S cyclins

Ans. (a) Expressed non-phosphorylatable form of Rb

82. A fixed smear of a bacteria culture is subjected to the following solutions in the order listed below and appeared red,

1. Carbolfuchsin(heated)

2. Acid-alcohol

3. Methylene blue

Bacteria stained by this method can be identified as

a. Non-acid fast E.coli

b. Acid fast Mycobacterium sp.

c. Gram-positive E.coli

d. Gram-negative Mycobacterium sp.

Ans. (b) Acid fast Mycobacterium sp.

83. In an in vitro experiment using radio labelled nucleotides, a researcher is trying to analyze the possible products using ureapolyacrylamide gel electrophoresis. In one experimental set up RNase H was added(set 1), while in another set no RNase H was added(set 2)

The possible observation of this experiment could be

A. There is no difference in the mobility of labelled DNA fragments between the set 1 and set 2

B. There is distinct difference in the mobility of the newly synthesized labelled DNA fragments between Set 1 and Set 2

C. The mobility of the newly synthesized labelled DNA fragments in case of Set 1 is faster as compared to the Set 2

D. The mobility of the newly synthesized labelled DNA fragments in case of Set1 is slower as compared to the Set 2

Which of the following combination represent correct observation?

a. A and B

b. B and C

c. A and D

d. B and D

Ans. (b) B and C

84. **Synthesis of normal haemoglobin requires coordinated synthesis of a α globin and β globin, Thalassemias are genetic defects perturbed in this coordinated synthesis. Patients suffering from deficiency of β globin chain could also be due to mutation affecting the biosynthesis of β globin m-RNA**

    The following statement describe the genesis of non functional β globin leading to β thalassemia,
    A. Mutation in the promoter region of the β globin gene
    B. Mutation in the splice junction of the β globin gene
    C. Mutation in the intron 1 of the β globin gene
    D. Mutations towards the 3' end of the β globin gene that codes for polyadenylation site
    Which of the following combination is correct?
    a. A, B and D   b. A, B and C
    c. B, C and D   d. C, D and A

    Ans. (a) A, B and D

85. **Pre-m-RNA are rapidly bound by snRNPs which carry out dual steps of splicing that removes the intron and joins the upstream and downstream exons.**

    The following statement described some facts related to this event
    A. almost all introns begin with GU and end with AG sequences and hence all the GU or AG sequences are spliced out of RNA
    B. U2 RNA recognizes important sequences at the 3' acceptor end of the intron.
    C. The spliceosome uses ATP to carry out accurate removal of intron
    D. An unusual linkage with 2' OH group of guanosine with in intron form 'Lariat' structure.
    Which of the following combination is correct?
    a. A and B   b. B and C
    c. C and D   d. D and A

    Ans. (b) B and C

86. **For continuation of protein synthesis in bacteria, ribosomes need to be released from the m-RNA as well as to dissociate into subunits. These processes do not occur spontaneously. They need the following possible condition**

    A. RRF and EF-G aid in this process
    B. An intrinsic activity of ribosome and all uncharged t-RNA are required
    C. IF-1 promotes dissociation of ribosome's
    D. IF-3 and IF-1 Promote dissociation of ribosome
    Which of the following sets is correct?
    a. A and C   b. A and B
    c. A and C   d. B and D

    Ans. (c) A and C

87. **Insulin and other growth factors stimulate a pathway involving a protein kinase mTOR, which in its turn augments protein synthesis, mTOR essentially modifies protein which in their unmodified form act as inhibitors of protein synthesis. The following protein are possible candidate.**

    A. eEF-1   B. eIF-4E-BP1
    C. eIF-4E   D. PHAS-1
    Which of the following sets is correct?
    a. A and B   b. B and D
    c. A and C   d. B and C

    Ans. (b) B and D

88. **Bacteriophage ë has two modes in its life cycle, lytic and lysogenic. In the lysogenic mode, the expression of all the phage genes are repressed while the expression of repressor gene switches between on and off position depending on the concentration of repressor. The following statement are made:**

    A. Repressor may act both as a positive regulator and negative regulator
    B. Expression of repressor gene, cI is independent of the expression of cII and cIII genes
    C. Mutation of cI gene will cause it to it to form clear plaques on both wild type E. Coli and E.coli (λ)
    D. Mutation at operators, O_L and O_R will allow the phage to act as virulent phage.
    The correct statement are
    a. A and B   b. B and C
    c. C and D   d. D and A

    Ans. (d) D and A

89. **Survival of intracellular pathogens depends on the levels of pro-inflammatory and anti inflammatory cytokines in macrophages. In an experimental condition, Mycobacteria infected macrophages were treated with IL-6 or IL-12 for 4 hours at 37°C. untreated cells were used as control. Cells were lysed and nuber of bacteria in each experimental set was counted by measuring colony forming unit (CFU). Which of the following observation is true?**

    a. IL-12 treated cells contain more intracellular bacteria than control
    b. IL-12 treated cells contain less intracellular bacteria than control
    c. IL-6 treated cells contain more intracellular bacteria than control
    d. IL-6 treated cells contain less intracellular bacteria than control

    Ans. (b) IL-12 treated cells contain less intracellular bacteria than control

90. The bacterial flagellar motor is a multi-protein complex. Rotation of the flagellum requires movement of protons across the membrane facilitated by a multi protein complex. The flagella motor proteins combine to creat a proton channel that drives mechanical rotation.

   a. Mutation in tubulin and actin proteins
   b. Mutation in kinesin protein
   c. Mutated H+ ATPase
   d. Mutations in the charged residues lining the ridge of the FliG subunit

Ans. (d) Mutations in the charged residues lining the ridge of the FliG subunit

91. A bacterial response regulator turns on gene A in its phosphorylated form. The amount of "A" shows a sharp and sleep rise at a threshold concentration of the signal sensed by the cognate sensor. This is most likely due to

   a. Increased phosphatise activity of the sensor at the threshold concentration
   b. Decreased phosphorylation of the response regulator by the sensor
   c. Cooperativity in binding of the response regulator to the target gene
   d. A negative feedback in gene A expression

Ans. (c) Cooperativity in binding of the response regulator to the target gene

92. Intracellular transport and cytoskeletal organization of a cell is regulated by nucleotide exchange of different small molecular weight GTPase of Ras super family. Over expression of which of the following GTPase modulates the actin cytoskeleton of HeLa cell?

   a. Ran in GDP bound form
   b. Ran in GTP bound form
   c. Rho in GTP bound form
   d. Rho in GDP bound form

Ans. (c) Rho in GTP bound form

93. You are given a group of four mice. Each mouse is immunized with keyhole limpet heocyanin or azobenzene arsonate or lipopolysaccharide of dextran. Four weeks later, sera were collected from these mice and antigen-specific IgG1 and IgG2a ELISA were performed. Only one of the mice showed positive response. It was

   a. Keyhole limpet hemocyanin-primed mouse
   b. Azobenze arsonate primed mouse
   c. Lipopolysaccharide primed mouse
   d. Dextran primed mouse

Ans. (a) Keyhole limpet hemocyanin-primed mouse

94. Tumour cells were isolated from a breast cancer patient. These cells were injected into nude mice and they were divided into four groups. Group 1 received EGF receptor conjugated with methotrexate. Group 3 received mannose receptor-conjugated with methotrexate; group 4 received same amount of the free drug. In which of the following cases tumorigenic index would be minimum?

   a. Free drug
   b. DGR receptor-conjugated drug
   c. Transferring receptor conjugated drug
   d. Mannose receptor conjugated drug

Ans. (c) Transferring receptor conjugated drug

95. When the prospective neurons from an early gastrula of a frog were transplanted into the prospective epidermis region, the donor cells differentiated into epidermis. However, when a similar experiment was done with the late gastrula of frog, the prospective neurons developed into neurons only. These observation could possibly be explained by the following phenomena.

   A. A early gastrula show conditional development whereas the late gastrula shows autonomous development
   B. The early gastrula show autonomous development whereas the late gastrula shows conditional development
   C. The prospective neurons from the early gastrula are only specified whereas those from the late gastrula are determined.
   D. The prospective neurons from the early gastrula are determined where as those from the early gastrula are determined whereas those from the late gastrula are specified

   Which of the conclusion drawn above are correct?
   a. A and B   b. A and C
   c. A and D   d. B and C

Ans. (b) A and C

96. AP1 (APETLA 1) is one of the floral meristem identifying genes. In wild type Arabidopsis thaliana plants transformed with AP1:GUS, β glucoronidase activity is seen in floral meristem, only after the commitment to flowereing. Ectopic expression of AP1:GUS in the EMBRYONIC FLOWER (emf)mutant background result in GUS activity throughout the shoots in four day old seedlings. These observation suggest that AP1 is:-

   a. Not involved in flowering
   b. Involved in repression of flowering
   c. Involved in promoting flowering
   d. Stimulation of flowering in the emf background

Ans. (b) Involved in repression of flowering

97. In case of morphallactic regeneratioin:

a. There is repatteming of the existing tissues with little new growth

b. There is repatteming of the existing tissues after the stem cell division has taken place

c. There is cell division of the differentiated cells which maintain their differentiated state to finally form a complete organism.

d. There is dedifferentiation of the cells at the cut surface which become undifferentiated. These undifferentiated cells then divide to redifferentiate to form the complete structure

Ans. (a) There is repatteming of the existing tissues with little new growth

98. The decision to become either a trophoblast or inner cell mass blastomere is one of the first decision taken by any mammalian embryo. Below is a diagrammatic representation of the different cells formed during development from the morula with the help of different molecules. Identify the molecules 1-4 sequentially.

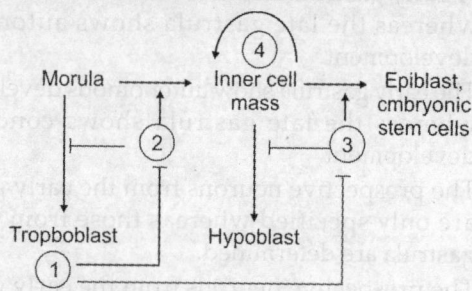

a. Cdx 2, oct 4 ,nanog, Stat 3

b. Cdx 2 , Nanog, Stat 3 , Oct 4

c. Cdx 2, Nanog, Oct 4, Stat 3

d. Cdx 2, Oct 4, Stat 3, Nanog

Ans. (a) Cdx 2, oct 4 ,nanog, Stat 3

99. With respect to the extra embryonic structure formed in the mammals, the possible functional attributes have been designated:

A. Allantoin stores urinary waste and helps mediated gas exchange. It is derived from splanchnopleure at the caudal end of the primitive streak

B. Amnion is a water sac and protect the embryo and its surroucnding amniotic fluid. This epithelium is derived from somatopleure.

C. Chorion is essential for gas exchange is amniote embryos, it is generated from the splanchnopleure.

D. Yolk sac is the last embryonic membrane to form and is derived from somatopleure.

Which of the above statements are correct?

a. A and B
b. A and C
c. B and C
d. A and D

Ans. (a) A and B

100. The figure above represent a late zebrafish gastrula. The following concepts may be proposed during further development of the embryo.

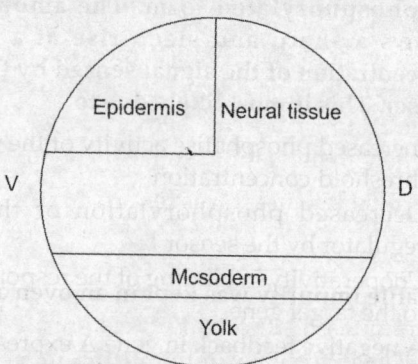

A. The concentration of FGF decrease from the yolk towards the epidermis, along with the increase of BMP activity from the dorsal to the ventral side

B. Increase in FGF activity in the epidermis with concomitant decrease in BMP activity toward the ventral axis.

C. Neural induction in zebrafish is independent of the organizer and depend on activation of BMP signalling

D. In comparison, both Xenopus and chick embryos require activation of FGF for meural induction to occur in addition to BMP inhibition

Which of the above statement are true?

a. A and C
b. B and C
c. A and D
d. C and D

Ans. (c) A and D

Memory Based Paper CSIR NET June 2012

1. Helium and argon gases in two separate containers are at same temperature and so have different root mean square velocities. The two are mixed in a third container keeping the same temperature. The rms velocity of the helium atom in mixture is

   a. More than what it was before mixing
   b. Less than what it was before mixing
   c. Equal to what it was before mixing
   d. Equal to that argon atoms in the mixture

Ans. (c) Equal to what it was before mixing

2. 100 g of inorganic compound $X.5H_2O$ containing a volatile impurity was kept in an oven at 150°C for 60 minutes. The weight of residue after heating is 8 g. The percentage of impurities in X was

   a. 10%   b. 8%
   c. 20%   d. 80%

Ans. (a) 10%

3. Two moles each of oxygen and hydrogen are in two separate continers, each of volume Vo and at temperature 150°C and 1 Atmospheric pressure. The two were allowed to react in third container to form water vapour until hydrogen is exhausted. Then the temperature of the mixture in the tird container was restored 150°C. its pressure become 1 atmospheric. The volume of container must be

   a. Vo   b. 5Vo/4
   c. 3Vo/2   d. 2Vo

Ans. (c) 3Vo/2

4. The mineral talc is used in the manufacture of soap because

   1. Gives bulk to product
   2. Kills bacteria
   3. Gives fragrance
   4. It soft and does not scratch the skin
Which of the following is correct reason?
   a. 4 only   b. 1 and 3 only
   c. 1 and 2 only d. 1 and 4 only

Ans. (d) 1 and 4 only

5. On a certain night the moon in its waning phase was half moon. At midnight the moon will be

   a. On Eastern horizon
   b. At 45°C angular height above the eastern horizon
   c. At the zenith
   d. On western horizon

Ans. (b) At 45°C angular height above the eastern horizon

6. Growth of an organism was monitored at regular intervals of times and shown in the graph below. Around what time is the rate of growth zero?

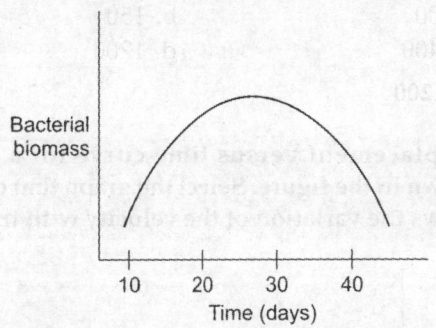

The zero growth rate will be observed during
   a. Close to day 10
   b. On the 20th day
   c. Between 20 and 30 days
   d. Between 30 and 40 days

Ans. (c) Between 20 and 30 days

7. The ends of rope are fixed to two pegs such that rope remains slack. A pencil is placed against rope and moved, such that the rope always remains taut. The shape of the curve traced by pencil would be a part of

   a. A circle
   b. An ellipse
   c. A square
   d. A triangle

Ans. (b) An ellipse

8. Four sedimentary rocks A, B, C and C are intruded by igneous rock R as shown in cross section diagram.

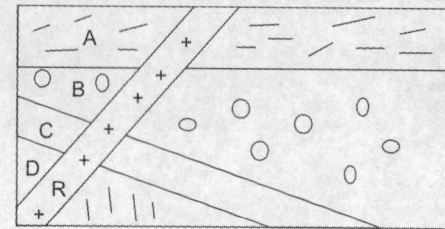

Which of the following is correct about their ages?
a. A is youngest followed by B,C, D and R
b. R is youngest followed by A, B, C and D
c. D is youngest followed by R, A, B and C
d. A is youngest followed by R, B, C and D

Ans. (b) R is youngest followed by A, B, C and D

9. A gemstone is irradiated in a nuclear reactor for 5 days. Ten days after irradiation, the activity of the chromium isotope in gemstone is 600 disintegration per hour. What is the activity of chromium isotope 5 days after irradiation if its half life of is 5 days?

a. 300   b. 150
c. 2400   d. 1200

Ans. (d) 1200

10. Displacement versus time curve for a body is shown in the figure. Select the graph that correctly shows the variation of the velocity with time

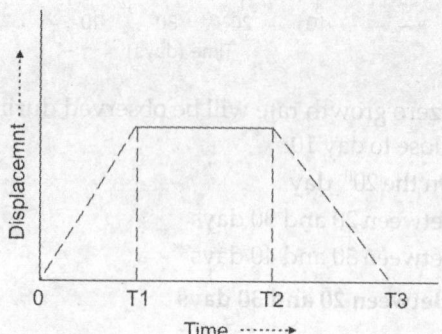

which of the following is correct representation of velocity with respect to time for same body?

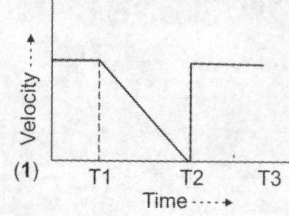

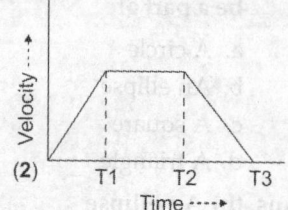

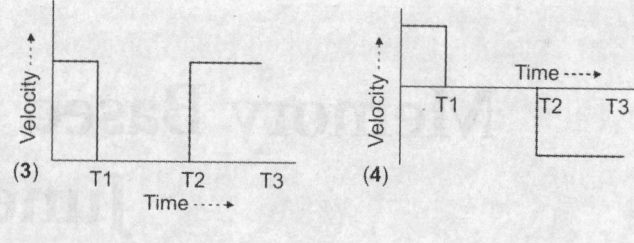

Ans. (d)

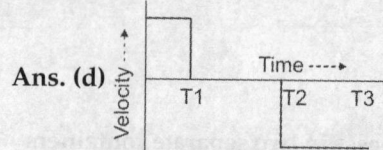

11. The spring balance in figure A reads 0.5 kg and the pan balance in figure B reads 3.0 Kg. If iron block is suspended from spring balance is partially immersed in water in the beaker (figure C). the speing balance now reads 0.4 kg. The reading on the pan balance in figure C is

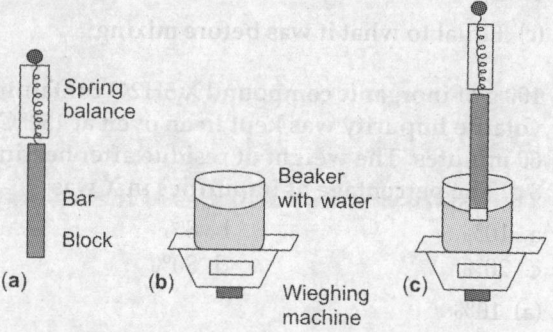

a. 3.0 kg   b. 2.9 kg
c. 3.1 kg   d. 3.5 kg

Ans. (c) 3.1 kg

12. The angles of a right angled triangle shaped garden are in arithmetic progression and the smallest side is 10.00 m. The he total length of the fencing of the garden in m is

a. 60.00 m   b. 47.32 m
c. 12.68 m   d. 22.68 m

Ans. (b) 47.32 m

13. The rabbit population in community A increases by 25% per year while in community B increases at 50% per year respectively. If the present population of A and B are equal, the ratio of the number of rabbits in B to A after two years will be?

a. 1.44
b. 1.72
c. 1.90
d. 1.25

Ans. (a) 1.44

14. AB is diameter of semicircle as shown in diagram. If AQ = 2AP then which of the following is correct

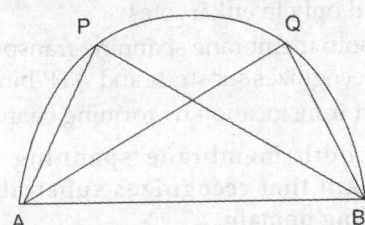

a. Angle APB = 1/2 of angle AQB

b. Angle APB = twice of angle AQB

c. Angle APB = angle AQB

d. Angle APB = 1/4 of angle AQB

Ans. (c) Angle APB = angle AQB

15. A tall plant with red seeds (both dominant traits) was crossed with a dwarf plant with white seeds, if the segregating progeny produced equal number of tall red and dwarf white plants, what would be the genotype of the parents?

a. TrRr X TtRR   b. TtRr X ttrr

c. TTRR X ttrr   d. TTRR X TtRr

Ans. (b) TtRr X ttrr

16. During ice skating the blades of the ice skater's shoe exerts pressure on the ice. Ice skater can efficiently skate on ice because

a. Ice gets converted to water as the pressure exerted on it increase

b. Ice gets converted into water as the pressure exerted on it decreases

c. The density of ice in contact with the blades deceases

d. Blades do not penetrate into ice

Ans. (a) Ice gets converted to water as the pressure exerted on it increase

17. The strain in a solid subjected to continuous stress is plotted

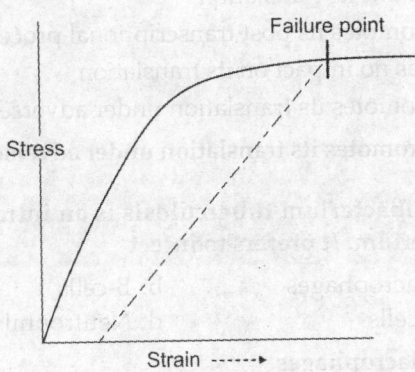

which of the following statement is true?

a. The solid deforms elastically till the point of failure

b. The solid deforms plastically till the point of failure

c. The solid comes back to original shape and size on failure

d. The solid is permanently deformed on failure

Ans. (d) The solid is permanently deformed on failure

18. The area of shaded region in cm^2

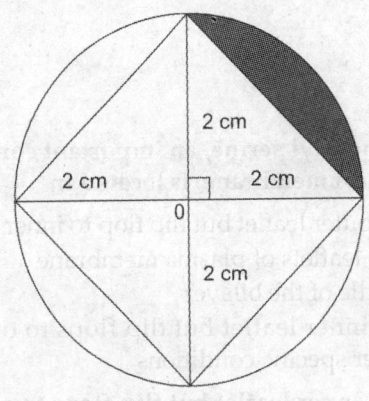

a. $(\pi - \sqrt{2})$ b. $(\pi - 2)$

c. $\dfrac{\pi}{4} - \dfrac{\sqrt{2}}{2}$ d. $(\pi + 2)$

Ans. (b) $(\pi - 2)$

19. Three sunflower plants were placed in condition as indicated below

Plant A: still air

Plant B: moderately turbulent air

Plant C: still air in dark

Which of the following statement is correct?

a. Transpiration rate of plant B > that of plant A

b. Transpiration rate of plant A > that of plant B

c. Transpiration rate of plant C = that of A

d. Transpiration rate of plant C < that of plant A > that of plant B

Ans. (a) Transpiration rate of plant B > that of plant A

20. Which of the following is indicated by the accompanying diagram?

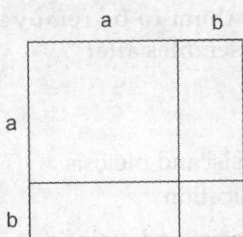

a. $a + ab + ab + \ldots = a[1-b$ for $[b] < 1$
b. $a > b$ implies $a^3 > b^3$
c. $(a + b)^2 + 2ab + b^2$
d. $a > b$ implies $-a < -b$

Ans. (c) $(a + b)^2 + 2ab + b^2$

21. Which nitrogen of adenosine gets protonated if pH of nucleoside is lowered from 7 to 3?

a. N1
b. N3
c. N7
d. N9

Ans. (a) N1

22. Phosphotidyl serine, an important component of biological membrane, is located in

a. The outer leaflet but flip flop to inner
b. Both leaflets of plasma membrane
c. Middle of the bilayer
d. The inner leaflet but flip flops to outer leaflets under specific conditions

Ans. (d) The inner leaflet but flip flops to outer leaflets under specific conditions

23. The oligopeptide, with F-A-R-P-M-T-S-R-P-G-F is treated with trypsin, chymotrypsin and carboxypeptidase B. Apart from original, the number of fragments obtained will be

a. 4   b. 3
c. 2   d. 0

Ans. (c) 2

24. The word "fermentation" is used in biochemistry and Microbial technology to denote different phenomenon. If the former is called C and latter is called T. Which of the following statement is true?

a. All C is T but all T is not C
b. All T is C but C is not T
c. T is always a product of genetic engineering while C is not
d. C is always an aerobic process, while T can be aerobic or anaerobic

Ans. (a) All C is T but all T is not C

25. All cytosolic proteins have nuclear exort signals that allows them to be removed from nucleus when it reassembles after

a. Meiosis
b. Mitosis
c. Both mitosisi and meiosis
d. DNA replication

Ans. (c) Both mitosisi and meiosis

26. ATP binding cassette transporters

a. All are P-glycoprotein
b. Found only in eukaryotes
c. Are both membrane spanning transporter domain that recognizes substrate and ATP-binding domain
d. Affect translocation by forming channels

Ans. (c) Are both membrane spanning transporter domain that recognizes substrate and ATP-binding domain

27. Which one of the following interactions plays a major role in stabilizing B-DNA?

a. Hydrogen bond
b. Hydrophobic interactions
c. Vander wall's interactions
d. Ionic interactions

Ans. (b) Hydrophobic interactions

28. Which of the following statement is NOT true about small interfering RNA(si RNA)?

a. si-RNA has 21-25 nucleotide sequence with 2 nucleotide overhang at 3' end
b. si-RNA is processed by RNA protein complex RISC
c. si-RNA is often induced by viruses
d. si-RNA does not generally act at the level of transcription

Ans. (b) si-RNA is processed by RNA protein complex RISC

29. Regulatory elements for expression of ribosomal RNA gene resides in the

a. Transcribed spacer region
b. Non-transcribe spacer region
c. 5' flanking region of individual ribosomal genes
d. Internal regions with in the genes

Ans. (c) 5' flanking region of individual ribosomal genes

30. Presence of an internal ribosomal entry site in m-RNA

a. Inhibit its translation
b. Promotes its post transcriptional processing
c. Has no impact on its translation
d. Promotes its translation under adverse condition

Ans. (d) Promotes its translation under adverse condition

31. Mycobacterium tuberculosis is an intra-cellular bacterium. It prefers to infect

a. Macrophages   b. B-cells
c. T-cells   d. Neutrophils

Ans. (a) Macrophages

32. Integrin molecule link extracellular matrix to the actin cytoskeleton of cell. Integrin binds to which of the following ECM macromolecules?

a. Laminin
b. Collagen
c. Fibronectin
d. Vitronectin

Ans. (c) Fibronectin

33. Major stimulus for spore formaton in bacteria is

a. Nutrient limitation
b. Heat stress
c. Cold stress
d. pH stress

Ans. (a) Nutrient limitation

34. which of the following matches of oncogene protein product is NOT correct?

a. erbA → thryoid hormoe receptor
b. erb B → Epidermal Growth Factor receptor
c. ras → Guanine nucleotide binding protein with GTPase activity
d. fos → platelet derived growth factor receptor

Ans. (d) fos → platelet derived growth factor receptor

35. Which of the following statement is INCORRECT in relation to treatment of pre-B cell with phorbol ester?

a. Phorbol esters activates NF-kB for translocation into nucleus
b. Phorbol esters activate protein kinase C
c. Phorbol ester leads to phosphorylates of NF-kB
d. Phorbol ester remove the inhibitor from inactive NF-kB complex in the cytoplasm

Ans. (c) Phorbol ester leads to phosphorylates of NF-kB

36. CD 19 is a marker for

a. B-cells
b. T-cells
c. Macrophage
d. Natural Killer cells

Ans. (a) B-cells

37. Given below are fate map of two organism and the pattern by which embryos undergo cleavage. Which of the following is/are the right combination?

a. B only
b. B and A
c. A and C
d. B and D

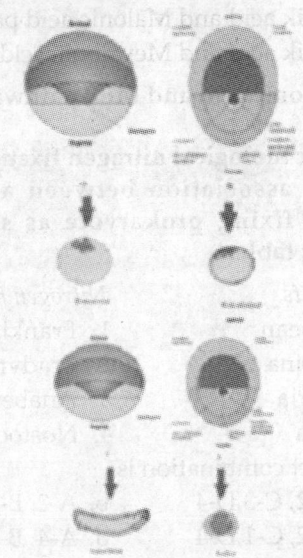

Ans. (a) B only

38. Ced-9 gene appears to be a binary switch that regulates cell survival and apoptosis in nematodes. Considering that CED-9 protein can bind to and inactive CED-4, which of the following would lead to apoptosis?

a. Activation of Ced-9 gene
b. Loss of function of CED-3
c. Loss of function of CED-9 gene
d. Loss of function of CED-4

Ans. (b) Loss of function of CED-3

39. In case of Xenopus levis which cells make up theknewkoop center and Spemann's organizer?

a. Endodermal and mesodermal, respectively
b. Mesodermal and endodermal, respectively
c. Endodermal and ectodermal, respectively
d. Ectodermal and endodermal, respectively

Ans. (a) Endodermal and mesodermal, respectively

40. Photosystem II functions as a light dependent water plastoquinone oxidoreductase. What are the name of two reaction center protein that bind electron prosthetic group, such as P680, pheophytin and plastoquinone?

a. CP43 and CP47
b. D1 and D2
c. 33 kDa and 23 kDa
d. F_A and F_B

Ans. (b) D1 and D2

41. Which one of the following combinations of secondary metabolite biosynthetic pathway result in the biosynthesis of terpenes?

a. Mevalonic acid and MEP pathways
b. Malonic acid and MEP pathways

c. Shikimik acid and Malonic acid pathway

d. Shikimik acid and Mevalonic acid pathways

Ans. (a) Mevalonic acid and MEP pathways

42. Symbiotic biological nitrogen fixation takes place with the association between a plant and a nitrogen fixing prokaryote as shown in the following table:

List of plants	Nitrogen fixing
A. Soyabean	1. Frankia
B. Casurina	2. Bradyrhyzobium
C. Guneria	3. Anabena
D. Azolla	4. Nostoc

The correct combination is

a. A-1, B-2, C-3,D-4   b. A-2, B-1, C-4,D-3

c. A-3, B-2, C-1,D-4   d. A-4, B-3, C-2,D-1

Ans. (b) A-2, B-1, C-4,D-3

43. Plants have evolved with multiple photoreceptors, which can perceive specific wavelength of light. Which of the following statement is correct about photoreceptors?

a. Phytochrome A can receive both far-red and blue light

b. Phytochrome C can receive far-red light

c. Cryptochrome I and phytochrome B are for perceiving blue light

d. Phytochrome B can predominantly perceive far red light

Ans. (a) Phytochrome A can receive both far-red and blue light

44. Which of the following statement describes the process of phloem loading?

a. Triose phosphate is transported from chloroplast to cytosol

b. Sugars are transported into sieve elements and companion cell

c. Sugars are transported from producing cell in msophyll in the vicinity of sieve element

d. Solutes are transported from roots to te shoots

Ans. (c) Sugars are transported from producing cell in msophyll in the vicinity of sieve element

45. Which of the following is responsible for initiation of maternal behaviour in first time pregnant rats after parturition?

a. High prolactin levels in blood

b. Stimulation of sensory receptors during delivery

c. Changes in uterine volume

d. Presence of male rat

Ans. (a) High prolactin levels in blood

46. Which one of the following changes will occur in the cell membrane of nodal tissue of heart, which results in an increasd heart rate due to stimulation of sympathetic nerves?

a. Opening of sodium channels is facilitated

b. Potassium conductance is increased

c. Opening of L-calcium are facilitated

d. 'h' channels are inhibited

Ans. (c) Opening of L-calcium are facilitated

47. A person takes 1.0 ml of insulin injection daily at 8:00 AM. His son gave 1,5 ml of insulin at 8:0 AM considering the father will go to party and eat more during lunch. The father also avoided breakfast, as he planned to eat more during lunch. Which one of the following events will occur?

a. Father will be normo-glycemic

b. Fater will be in hypoglycaemic condition before lunch

c. Fater will be hyperglycaemic condition before lunch

d. Blood glucose of father will be low after taking lunch

Ans. (b) Fater will be in hypoglycaemic condition before lunch

48. A gene encoding t-RNA undergoes a mutational event in its anticodon region that enables it to recognize a mutant nonsense codon and permit completion of translation. Such a mutation is known as

a. Silent mutation   b. Neutral mutation

c. Reversion   d. Non sense suppressor

Ans. (d) Non sense suppressor

49. Mutation at two different loci of the same gene X results in altered function. These two mutated versions of gene X are called

a. Alleles

b. Complementation group

c. Interrupted genes

d. Linkage group

Ans. (a) Alleles

50. Spermatogonial stem cell undergoes extensive metamorphosis to become a spermatozoan. Meiosis leads to the formation of spermatid containing 22 autosomes and one sex chromosome. A male mouse was found in a colony which always produced only female puff upon matting. Which one pf following is a possible reason

a. Spermiogenesis was defective

b. All spermgonial stem cells contained only X and no Y chromosome

c. Activation of Y-chromosome linked post meiotic death related gene may lead to such a situation

d. Activation of X chromosome linked post meiotic death related gene may lead to such a situation

Ans. (c) Activation of Y-chromosome linked post meiotic death related gene may lead to such a situation

51. Two pure line of corn have mean cob length of 9 cm and 3 cm, respectively. The polygenes involved in this trait exhibit additive gene action. Crossing these two lines is expected to produce a progeny population with mean cob length of

    a. 12.0 cm
    b. 7.5 cm
    c. 6.0 cm
    d. 2.75 cm

Ans. (c) 6.0 cm

52. How many genetically different gametes can be made by an individual of genotype AaBbccDDEe?

    a. 3   b. 5
    c. 8   d. 32

Ans. (c) 8

53. A paraphyletic group

    a. Contains unrelated organisms
    b. Includes the most recent common ancestors but not all of its decedents
    c. Includes all the representative of a clade but not the most recent common ancestor
    d. Contains all the representative of a clade and most recent common ancestor

Ans. (b) Includes the most recent common ancestors but not all of its decedents

54. Which of the following organism is widely used as a biocontrol in organic farming?

    a. Rhyzobium tropicii
    b. Trichorderma viridis
    c. Fusarium oxysporum
    d. Nostoc muscorum

Ans. (b) Trichorderma viridis

55. Which of the following is NOT an adaptive modification in a xerophytic plant?

    a. Strongly developed Sclerenchyma
    b. Sunken stomata
    c. Sparse stomata
    d. Presence of Lacunar tissues

Ans. (d) Presence of Lacunar tissues

56. If the misk is left open, lactose is fermented first to produce acid. This is followed by protelytic bacteria which increases the pH. Ultimately milk fats are degraded to produce rancidity. This is an example of

    a. Ecological succession
    b. Antagonism
    c. Interference competition
    d. Microevolution

Ans. (a) Ecological succession

57. Based on per molecule, which of the following gas has the most powerful greenhouse effect?

    a. CO_2 b. CH_4
    c. N_2O d. CFCs

Ans. (d) CFCs

58. The Hardy-wienberg principle comes from considering what happens when medelian gene act on population. The model predicts that there will be no change in alleles frequencies when

    a. Migration into the population occurs at a steady rate
    b. The population suffers a bottle neck
    c. A rare new mutation is associated with a sharp increase in fitness
    d. No evolutionary process is at work

Ans. (d) No evolutionary process is at work

59. Among the following events in history of life

    a. Prokaryotic cell
    b. Eukaryotic cell
    c. Natural selection
    d. Organic molecules
    e. Self replicating molecule

    Which is the correct chronological order?

    a. $d \rightarrow e \rightarrow c \rightarrow a \rightarrow b$ b. $d \rightarrow e \rightarrow a \rightarrow b \rightarrow c$
    c. $e \rightarrow d \rightarrow a \rightarrow c \rightarrow b$ d. $d \rightarrow e \rightarrow a \rightarrow c \rightarrow b$

Ans. (a) $d \rightarrow e \rightarrow c \rightarrow a \rightarrow b$

60. Sexual selection results in variation in the reproductive success of males, often due to female choice with particular phenotypes. This type of sexual selection is because

    a. Males cannot compete with other male
    b. Cost of breeding is higher for females as compared to males
    c. Inappropriate mating results in a similar reduction in fitness of females and males
    d. Males are limiting resource for females

Ans. (b) Cost of breeding is higher for females as compared to males

61. Which is best method for checking mycoplasma contamination in a mammalian cell line?

   a. Southern hybridization b. ELISA

   c. PCR   d. Western Hybridization

Ans. (b) ELISA

62. Major disadvantage of using liposome as targeted drug delivery vehicle is that

   a. It get internalized by phagocytosis inside lysosome

   b. It is very unstable and has low shelf life

   c. It get intercalated in cell membrane

   d. It drug entranment efficiency is very low

Ans. (b) It is very unstable and has low shelf life

63. If 'r' denotes correlation coefficient and 'm' denotes slope of regression line, interchanging X and Y axes would

   a. Change 'm' but not 'r'   b. Change 'r' but not 'm'

   c. Chages both 'r' and 'm' d. Nor change 'r' or 'm'

Ans. (d) Nor change 'r' or 'm'

64. Which of the following statement is NOT true during infection of platn cell by Agrobacterium?

   a. The protein product of virulence genes Vir A and Vir G perceives acetosyringone

   b. The VirB protein forms a connection between Agrobacterium and the plant cell and facilitates T-DNA transfer in to the plant

   c. The T-DNA is excised and bound to Vir D2 protein

   d. The T-DNA after becoming coated with Vir F binds to phosphorylated VIP1, which allows the complex to enter the plant's nucleus

Ans. (d) The T-DNA after becoming coated with Vir F binds to phosphorylated VIP1, which allows the complex to enter the plant's nucleus

65. Which of the following does not represents stategy for phytoremediation?

   a. Phytodegradation

   b. Phytomining

   c. Continous removal through hyper accumulators

   d. Chelate mediated extraction of pollutants

Ans. (b) Phytomining

66. Among existing technologies, which of the following vector system would yor prefer to use for generating a library for 140 kb eukaryotic genomic DNA fragments, while giving due consideration to size as well as stability of insert?

   a. Phage

   b. Cosmid

   c. BAC

   d. YAC

Ans. (c) BAC

67. The use of biotinylated secondary antibody in ELISA?

   a. Increase the sensitivity of assay but compromises the specificity

   b. Increases the sensitivity of assy without compromising the specificity

   c. Does not alter either sensitivity or specificity

   d. Decreases both sensitivity and specificity

Ans. (b) Increases the sensitivity of assy without compromising the specificity

68. Secondary sewage treatment involves

   a. Physical removal of solids from polluted water by filtration and sedimentation

   b. Removal of chemical remains by precipitation

   c. Removal of dissolved organic compounds by activated sludge or trickling filter

   d. Removal of microbial pathogens by chlorination or ozonization

Ans. (c) Removal of dissolved organic compounds by activated sludge or trickling filter

69. Site specific recombination results in precise DNA rearrangement, which is limited to specific sequences. The enzymes that are important to carry out the process are

   a. Restriction endonuclease and ligase

   b. Nuclease and ligase

   c. DNA polymerase and ligase

   d. DNA polymerase and DNA gyrase

Ans. (a) Restriction endonuclease and ligase

70. To replace animal use in testing hepatic toxicity of a drug on trial, which one of the following would be used in vitro to be closest to the in vivo scenario?

   a. Liver cells

   b. Hepatic cell lines

   c. Liver slices

   d. Co-culture of liver parenchymal cell and kupffer cells

Ans. (d) Co-culture of liver parenchymal cell and kupffer cells

71. A plot of V/[S] versus V if generated for an enzyme catalyzed reaction, and a straight line is obtained. Indicate the information that can be obtained from the plot.

   a. Vmax and turnover number Km can be obtained only from a plot of 1/V versus 1/[S]

   b. Km/Vmax from the slope

c. Vmax. Km and turnover number

d. Only Km and turnover number

Ans. (c) Vmax. Km and turnover number

---

72. **Phosphorylation of ADP to ATP occurs through energy metabolixm, comprising oxidative phosphorylation or substrate level phosphorylation or photo-phosphorylatio(in plants). ATP can also be formed from ADP through the action of adenylate kinase, crystal structure determination fo adenylate kinase shows that the C-terminal region has the sequence val-asp-asp-val-phe-ser-gln-val-cys-thr-his-leu-asp-thr-leu-lys.**

What can be a possible conformation of the sequence?

a. A helix that is not amphiphatic

b. Amphipathic helix

c. Leucine zipper helix

d. Beta helix

Ans. (b) Amphipathic helix

---

73. **Consider a 51-residue long protein containing only 100 bonds about which rotation can occur. Assume that 3 orientation per bond are possible. Based on these assumption, how many conformations will be possible for this protein?**

a. 3^{100}

b. 100^3

c. 3^{51}

d. $51 \times 100 \times 3$

Ans. (a) 3^{100}

---

74. **Phosphogluconolactone is added to 0.1 M glucose-1-phosphate (G-6-P). The standard free energy change of the reaction, G-6-P, G-1-{ od 1.8 kcal/mole at 25°C. the equilibrium concentrations of G-6-P and G-1-P, respectively are**

a. 96 mM, 45 mM

b. 100mM, 0mM

c. 45 mM, 96 mM

d. 0 mM, 100 mM

Ans. (a) 96 mM, 45 mM

---

75. **Differential scanning calorimetric study of calf thymus DNA was carried out to measure midpoint of thermal denaturation (Tm). O_ m(enthalpy change at T)m and o_ p (constant pressure heat capacity change). It has been observed that pO = 0, Tm = 75.5°C and o_m = 50,4 kcal/mole. The Gibbs free energy chage at 37°C is**

a. 25.5 kcal/mole

b. 2.6 kcal/mole

c. 0.6 kcal/mole

d. 5.6 kcal/mole

Ans. (a) 25.5 kcal/mole

---

76. **The following reaction are part of the citric acid cycle. The number in parenthesis indicate the number of carbon atoms in each molecule.**

Isocitrate(6) $\overset{A}{\rightarrow}$ L-ketoglutrate(5) $\overset{B}{\rightarrow}$ succinyl CoA(4) $\overset{C}{\rightarrow}$ succinate (4) $\overset{D}{\rightarrow}$ fumarate(4)

Which of the following sequences of the reaction systems A D in correct?

a. $NAD + \rightarrow NADH + H, \rightarrow NAD + , CO_2 \rightarrow NADH + H, GDP, CO_2 \rightarrow GTP, FAD, iP \rightarrow FADH_2$

b. $NAD + \rightarrow NADH + H, \rightarrow NAD + , CO_2 \rightarrow NADH + H, ADP, CO_2 \rightarrow ATP, FAD, iP \rightarrow FADH_2$

c. $NAD + \rightarrow NADH + H, \rightarrow FAD + , CO_2 \rightarrow FADH_2, ADP \rightarrow ATP, NAD, iP \rightarrow NADH + H, CO_2$

d. $NAD + \rightarrow NADH + H, \rightarrow FAD + , CO_2 \rightarrow FADH_2 + H, GDP, CO_2 \rightarrow GTP, NAD, iP \rightarrow NADH + H, CO_2$

Ans. (a) $NAD + \rightarrow NADH + H, \rightarrow NAD + , CO_2 \rightarrow NADH + H, GDP, CO_2 \rightarrow GTP, FAD, iP \rightarrow FADH_2$

---

77. **The respiratory chain is relatively inaccessible to experimental manipulation in intact mitochondria. Upon disrupting mitochondria with ultrasound, however, it is possible to isolate functional sub mitochondrial particles, which consist of broken cristae that have resealed inside out into small closed vesicles, it these vesicles the components that originally faced the matrix are now exposed to the surrounding medium. This arrangement helps in studying electron transport and ATP synthesis because:**

a. It is difficult to manipulate the concentration of small molecules (NADH, ATP, ADP, Pi) in the matrix of intact mitochondria

b. In broken cristae the enzymes and other molecules responsible for electron transport are more active

c. Intact mitochondria are more unstable than broken cristae

d. Purification of intact mitochondria is not possible

Ans. (a) It is difficult to manipulate the concentration of small molecules (NADH, ATP, ADP, Pi) in the matrix of intact mitochondria

---

78. **Cystic fibrosis(CF) trans membrane conductance regulator(CFTR) protein is known to be a cAMP dependent Cl- channel. CF patients (with mutant CFTR proteins) show reduce Cl- permeability and as a result exhibit elevated Cl level in sweat. To prove this, CFTR proteins (both wild type and mutant) are inserted in a model membrane (liposome) and Cl transport is followed with radioactive Cl. It is known that topology of CFTR in membrane is important for its function. Despite no proteolytic degradation of denatureation of**

CFTR proteins, wild type CFTR failed to transport Cl- in liposome.

Which of the following is the correct explanation of this?

a. CFTR protein gest mutated during insertion in liposomes

b. CFTR protein loses affinity with Cl-ions

c. CFTR protein gets wrongly inserted in lipososmes

d. DFTR protein loses channel forming property in lipososmes

Ans. (c) CFTR protein gets wrongly inserted in lipososmes

79. **Which of the following statement regarding aquaporin or water channels is NOT correct?**

a. Aquaporins are found in both plants and animals membranes

b. Aquaporins can not transport uncharged molecules like ammonia

c. Phosphorylation and calcium concentration regulates aquaporin activity

d. Activity of aquaporin is regulated by pH and reactive oxygen species

Ans. (b) Aquaporins can not transport uncharged molecules like ammonia

80. **The intestinal absorption of glucose is impaired by use of ovabain, an inhibitor of Na-K + ATPase. Indicate the correct explanation**

a. The inhibitor has blocked the transport o Na + from intestinal lumen to epithelial cells

b. The inhibitor has blocked the transport of Na + from epithelial cells to intestinal lumen

c. The inhibitor has blocked the transport of Na + form intestinal lumen to intestinal cells

d. The inhibitor has blocked the transport of Na + from intestinal cell to intestinal lumen

Ans. (b) The inhibitor has blocked the transport of Na + from epithelial cells to intestinal lumen

81. **A synthetically prepared m-RNA contains repetitive AU sequences. The m-RNA was incubated with mammalian cell extract which contains ribosomes, t-RNA s and all the factors required for protein synthesis. Assuming no initiation codon is required for protein synthesis , which of the following peptides will most likely be synthesized?**

a. A single peptide composed of the same amino acid sequence

b. A single peptide with alternating sequence of two amino acids

c. A single peptide with alternating sequence of three amino aicds

d. Three different peptides each sequence composed of a single amino acid

Ans. (b) A single peptide with alternating sequence of two amino acids

82. **Hoechst 33342 is a membrane permanent dye that fluoresces when it binds to DNA through intercalating process. It a population of cells is incubated briefly with Hoechst dye and stored in flow cyclometer the cells display various levels of fluorescence in different phases of cell cycles as shown in figure below (marked as X,Y,Z)**

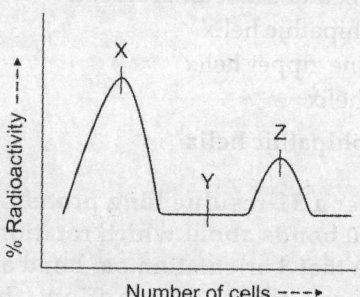

Which of the following is correct?

a. X is G_1 Y is G_2 + M and Z is S

b. X is G_1 Y is S and Z is G_2 + M

c. X is S. Y is G_2 + M and Z is G_1

d. X is S. Y is G_1 and Z is G_2 + M

Ans. (b) X is G_1 Y is S and Z is G_2 + M

83. **During cell cycle regulation in eukaryotes, there are post translational modification of protein factors, which act as switches for different phases of cell cycle, A cell population of yeast was transfected with gene for wee 1 kinase (modifies cdc2 protein). Assuming that the transfection efficiency was 50% only, which of the following graphical representation of the results is most appropriate?**

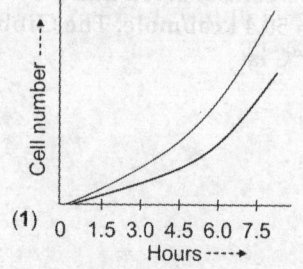

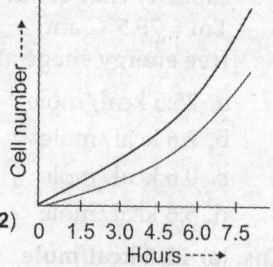

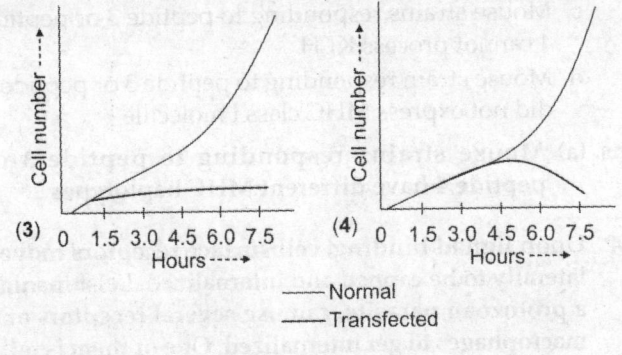

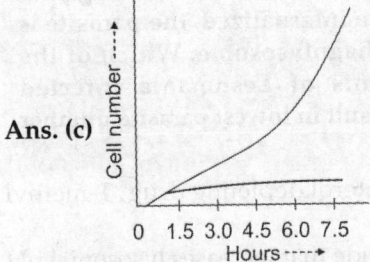

Ans. (c)

84. In semi-conservative mode of DNA replication two parental strands unwind and are used for synthesis of new strands following the rule of complimentary base pairing. Synthesis of complimentary strands require that DNA synthesis proceeds in opposite direction, while the double helix is progressively univngig and replicating in only one direction, one of the DNA strands is continuously synthesised in the same direction s the advancing replication fork and is called leading strand whereas the other strands is synthesised discontinuously in segments and is referred to as lagging strands. These short fragments made discontinuously are labelled as okazaki fragments. These okazaki fragments need to be matured into continuous DNA strand by which one of the following combination of enzymes?

   a. DNA pol III and DNA ligase
   b. DNA pol I and DNA ligase
   c. DNA pol II and DNA ligase
   d. DNA gyrase and DNA ligase

Ans. (b) DNA pol I and DNA ligase

85. The lac operon in E. Coli is controlled by both the lac repressor and the catabolite activation protein CAP. In an in vivo experiment with lac operon, the following observation are made:

   1. c-AMP levels are high
   2. Repressor is bound with allolactose
   3. CAP is interacting with RNA polymerase

Which of the following conclusions is most appropriate based on the above observations?

   a. Glucose and lactose are present
   b. Glucose is present and lactose is absent
   c. Both are absent
   d. Glucose is absent and lactose is present

Ans. (d) Glucose is absent and lactose is present

86. Assunign that the histone octamer forms a cylinder 9 nm in diameter and 5 nm in height and that the human genome forms 32 million nucleosomes, what fraction (approximately) of the volume of nucleus (6 μm diameter) is occupied histone octamers?

   a. 1/22   b. 1/11
   c. 10/21   d. 10/11

Ans. (b) 1/11

87. A reporter cell line with stable integrated retroviral promoter luciferase construct was transfected with an expression vector for a cellular protein. The protein seems to regulate the activation of retroviral promoter as analyzed by luciferase activity assay. Which one of the following techniques will you use to show "in vitro" recruitment of the cellular protein on the integrated retroviral promoter?

   a. Electrophoretic mobility shift assay
   b. RNAse protection assay
   c. DNAse hypersensitivity assay
   d. Chromatin immunoprecipitation assay

Ans. (d) Chromatin immunoprecipitation assay

88. In a tissue, cells are bound together by physical attatchment between cell to cell or between cell to extra cellular matrix. Following are some of the characterstics of cell junction:

   A. Aderens junctions are cell-cell anchoring junctions connecting actin filament in one cell with that in next cell.
   B. Desmosomes are cell-matrix anchoring junctions connecting actin filament to extra cellular matrix
   C. Gap junctions are channel forming junctions allowing passage of small water soluble molecule from cell to cell.
   D. Tight junction are occluding junction, which seal gap between two cells
   E. Hemidesmosomes are cell matrix anchoring junctions connecting intermediate filament in one cell to extra cellular matrix

Which of the following combination of statements is NOT CORRECT?

   a. A and B   b. A and C
   c. C and D   d. D and E

Ans. (a) E and F

89. **A mouse was primed with trinitrophyenyl-lipopolysaccharide(TNP-LPS) whereas another mouse was primed with TNP keyhole limpet hemocyanin (TNP-KLH). after three weeks, these mice were sacrificed and splenic cells were fractionated to B cells and T cells. B cells from TNP-LPS primed mice were co-culture with T cells from TNP-LPS or TNP-KLH primed mice. Similarly. B cells from TNP-KLH primed mice were co cultured with the T cells from TNP-LPS or TNP-KLH primed mice. So, we have four co-culture:**

1. $B^{TNP-LPS} \times T^{TNP-LPS}$ 2. $B^{TNP-LPS} \times T^{TNP-KLH}$
3. $B^{TNP-KLH} \times T^{TNP-LPS}$ 4. $B^{TNP-KLH} \times T^{TNP-KLH}$

Among these co cultures, where do you except the highest IgG production?

a. 1   b. 2
c. 3   d. 4

Ans. (c) 3

90. **A large protein or a pathogenic Bacterium hs been enymatically digested to generate a mixture of peptides ranging in size from 3 to 8 amino acids in length. Peptide mixtures were then admisnstered in experimental animals to generate peptide specific antibodies. In order to develop diagnostic for the bacteria, the antisera were used Western blotting to detect bacterial antigen. Western blotting failed despite the use of a wide range of antisera concentration.**

a. Peptide specific antibody mixture is unstable
b. Peptide specific antibodies were not generated as adjuvant was not administered
c. Peptide specific antibodies were not generated as they were not coupled to a protein carrier
d. Peptide specific antibodies could not recognize the bacterial antigen

Ans. (c) Peptide specific antibodies were not generated as they were not coupled to a protein carrier

91. **Ten different mouse strains were primed with whole keyhole limplet hemocyanin (KLH). KLH was broken into peptides for in vitro stimulation. The splenocytes from ten different primed mouse strains were re stimulated with each of these 10 peptides and responsiveness to these were measured in vitro. It was found that each of these mouse strains had responded to one of the peptide. Where the peptide 3 responder was mated with peptide 4 responder, the splenocyte of F_1 offsprings responded to both the peptide. Which of the following is most appropriate**

a. Mouse strains responding to peptide 3 or peptide 4 have different MHC haplotypes
b. Mouse strains responding to peptide 3 or peptides 4 have either of these T cell receptors

c. Mouse strains responding to peptide 3 or peptide 4 cannot process KLH
d. Mouse strain responding to peptide 3 or peptide 4 did not express MHC class I molecule

Ans. (a) Mouse strains responding to peptide 3 or peptide 4 have different MHC haplotypes

92. **Upon lignad binding, cell surface receptors move laterally to be capped and internalized. Leishmania a protozoan parasite, can use several receptors on macrophages to get internalized. One of them is toll like receptor 2 (TLR2) that binds lipophosphoglycan on Leshmania. Once internalized, the parasite is destroyed in the phagolysosome. Which of the following treatments of Leshmania infected macrophages will result in lowest parasite number in macrophages?**

a. Membrane cholesterol depleting drug, T-methyl cyclodextein
b. Ammonium chloride that increases lysosomal pH
c. Both T-MCD and ammonium chloride
d. Ant TLR2 antibody

Ans. (c) Both T-MCD and ammonium chloride

93. **Oncogenes and tumor suppressor genes are termed as cancer critical genes, increasingly powerful tools are now available for systematically searching the DNA or m-RNAs of cancer cells for either significant mutations or altered expression. To identify independently an oncogene or a tumor suppressor gene, which of the following would be the most convincing tests to be used?**

a. Transgenic mice that overexpress the candidate oncogene and knockout mice that lack candidate tumour suppressor gene
b. Transgenic mice that overexpress the candidate tumor suppressor gene and knockout mice that lack candidate oncogene
c. Transgenic mice that over express the candidate oncogene and tumor suppressor gene
d. Knockout mice that lack the candidate oncogene and tumor suppressor gene

Ans. (a) Transgenic mice that overexpress the candidate oncogene and knockout mice that lack candidate tumour suppressor gene

94. **The functionality of the paxo gene in the formation of optic and nasal structure may be attributed to the following**

1. Paxo makes the optic vesicle competent and allows lens formation
2. The optic vesicle can induce any part of the head ectoderm to form the nasal and optic structures, due to presence of paxo

3. Paxo renders the head ectoderm competent to receive signals from optic vesicle.

4. Apart from the optic vesicle, the head ectoderm may also be induced by BMP and FGF, so paxo is not exclusive for lens formation.

Which of the above attributes are true?

a. 1 and 4

b. 3 and 4

c. 2 and 3

d. 3 only

Ans. (c) 2 and 3

---

95. The pattern of embryonic cleavage specific to a species is determined by two major parameters.

1. The amount and distribution of yolk protein within the cytoplasm.

2. The factors in the cytoplasm that influence the angle mitotic spindles and the timings of its formation.

Which of the following statements are true?

a. Species having teloecithal egg follow a holoblastic cleavage

b. Species having isolecithal egg follow a holoblastic cleavage

c. Species having centrolecithal egg follow a holoblastic cleavage

d. Species having isolecithal egg follow a meroblastic cleavage

Ans. (b) Species having isolecithal egg follow a holoblastic cleavage

---

96. The fate of a cell or a tissue is specified when it is capable of differentiating autonomously on being placed in a neutral environment with respect to the developmental pathway. An embry will show development pattern based on its type of specification:

Based on the above fact it can be said that potency of a cell is:

1. Equal to its normal fate in regulative development

2. Greater than its normal fate in regulative development

3. Equal to its normal fate in mosaic development

4. Greater than its normal fate in mosaic development

Which of the above statements are true?

a. 2 and 3

b. 1 and 4

c. 1 and 3

d. 2 and 4

Ans. (a) 2 and 3

---

97. In the context of the proximal distal growth and differentiation of a tetrapod limb following experiments were visualized

1. If the apical ectodermal ridge(AER) is removed at any time during the limb development, further development of distal limb skeletal elements ceases.

2. If leg mesenchyme is placed directly beneath the wing AER, proximal hind limb structure develop at the end of the limb

3. If an extra AER is grafted on to an existing limb bud, supernumerary structure are formed usually at the distal end of the limb.

4. If leg mesenchyme is placed directly beneath the wing AER, proximal hind limb structures develop at the end of the limb

Which of the bove experiments would show the possible interaction between the AER and the limb mesenchyme directly beneath it during limb development?

a. 1 and 2 only

b. 2 and 3 only

c. 3 and 4 only

d. 1, 2 and 3

Ans. (d) 1, 2 and 3

---

98. The following statements have been proposed for plant vegetative development:

1. Lateral roots develop from epidermal cells.

2. Shoots axillary meristem develops from shoot apical meristem during differentiation of leaf primordial

3. Root cap is made of dead cells.

4. Lateral meristem and cylindrical meristem found in roots and shoots results in secondary growth.

Which of the above statements are true?

a. 1 and 2

b. 2 and 4

c. 1, 2 and 4

d. 3 and 4

Ans. (b) 2 and 4

---

99. Red and far red lights are perceived by plants through various photoreceptors including phytochromes. The activation of phytochromes is caused by?

a. Conversion of Pr to Pfr from through the effect of red light

b. Repression of Pr from through the effect of far red light

c. Equal proportion of red and far red light at same fluence rate

d. Presence of red and far red light at different fluence rate

Ans. (a) Conversion of Pr to Pfr from through the effect of red light

100. Following are some facts regarding localization of photosynthetic supramolecular complexes on plastid lamellae:

1. PSII is preferentially localized on granal lamellae
2. ATP synthae and PS I is preferentially localized in stromal lamellae
3. PS I and PS II are located adjacent to each other in stromal lamellae
4. Cytochrom B_6/f complex is not a membrane bound complex

which of the following combinations of the above statements is true?

a. 1 and 2　　　　b. 3 and 4
c. 2 and 4　　　　d. 2 and 3

Ans. (a) 1 and 2

101. Phenyl ammonia lyase (PAL) and chalcone synthase (CHS) involved in biosynthesis of phenolic compound in plants.

Following are some statements regarding the action of PAL and CHS:

1. Substrate for PAL is phenyl alanine and for CS is chalocone
2. PAL catalyze conversion of phenyl alanine to trans cinnamic acid
3. PAL catalyze conversion of phenyl alanine to p-coumaric acid
4. Coumaryl CoA is converted to chalcone by chalcone synthase

Which of the following combination of above statement is true?

a. 1 and 2　　　　b. 1 and 3
c. 2 and 3　　　　d. 2 and 4

Ans. (d) 2 and 4

102. I[pm absorption of a photon, a chlorophyll molecule get converted to its excited state when the energy of photon is

a. More than that of ground state of pigment molecule
b. Equal to that of pigment molecule's excited state of the pigment molecule
c. Equal to energy gap between ground state and excited state energy

Ans. (d) Equal to energy gap between ground state and excited state energy

103. Following are certain facts about the effect of abcisic acid (ABA) on the development and physiological effect of plant:

1. ABA promotes leaf senescence independent of ethylene.
2. ABA promotes shoot growth and inhibits root growth at low water potential.

3. ABA inhibits gibberellins induced enzyme production
4. Seed dormancy is controlled by ratio of ABA and gibberllin

Which one of the following combination of above statements is true?

a. 1, 2 and 3　　　　b. 2, 3 and 4
c. 1, 2 and 4　　　　d. 1, 3 and 4

Ans. (d) 1, 3 and 4

104. While studying the primary effect of different abiotic stresses on plants, a researcher observed water potential reduction and cellular dehydration, which of the following combination of abiotic stress may cause observed effect?

a. Water deficit, salinity and chilling
b. Salinity, high temperature and flooding
c. Freezing, salinity and water deficit
d. Freezing, chilling and flooding

Ans. (c) Freezing, salinity and water deficit

105. In an experiments, sperm removed from epididymis of a male mouse was added in a dish containing appropriate media and oocyte. No fertilization was seen. However, when sperm from spididymis were directly placed in uterus of an ovulated female, she became pregnant. These observation suggest that

a. The sperm need to travel some distance to attain fertilizing ability
b. The oocyte secrets some biochemicals or factors which help sperm to fertilize
c. The hormones in body help sperm to attain fertilizing ability
d. The contents of female reproductive tract interact with sperm and activate it for fertilization

Ans. (d) The contents of female reproductive tract interact with sperm and activate it for fertilization

106. Level of follicle stimulating hormone(FSH) during infancy and adulthood is the same but spermatogenesis is seen only during adulthood. mRNA levels coding for FSH receptor are also found to be the same in testis of both age groups.

Which of the following investigations will clarify this paradox a little more?

a. Culture testicular cells and add LH to see testosterone production
b. Culture testicular cells and add testosterone to see comparative rise in FSH mRNA from both age groups

c. Culture testicular cells and add FSH to see comparative rise in cAMP production by both age groups

d. Add both LH and FSH to testicular cells and evaluate cAMP production

Ans. (c) Culture testicular cells and add FSH to see comparative rise in cAMP production by both age groups

107. GnRH is secreted during infancy (0.6 month) and puberty onwards (4 years and above) in monkeys, however, i,v. Injection of GnRH during pre pubertal period (about 2 years of age) led to elevated LH and FSH in blood compared to untreated 2 years old monkey. This suggest that

    1. Hypothalamus is active during pre pubertal period
    2. GnRH action on pituitary is age dependent
    3. Pituitary mtures during adulthood
    4. Pituitary is active in all stage of development in monkeys

    which one of the following is true?
    a. 1 and 2
    b. 2 and 3
    c. 3 only
    d. 4 only

Ans. (d) 4 only

108. The stereocilia of auditory hair cells are arranged in rows but the height of stereocilia are not the same in all the rows. Though the height of stereocilia is the same within a particular row, the heights increase in subsequent rows, when the stereocilia of shorter rows are mechanically pushed toward the taller rows, the hair cells are depolarized but a push on opposite direction hyperpolarize them. The significance of this graded height of stereocilia is:

    1. Each row of stereocilia may be displaced independent of other rows in physiological condition
    2. The tip of the taller stereocilia will show greater displacement as compared to shorter ones when all the rwos are moving in same axis
    3. The air cells will be depolarized or hyperpolarized in different grades when the axis of displacement is changed
    4. The taller stereocilia are involved with depolarization and shorter ones are responsible for hyperpolarization

    which of the following is correct?
    a. 1 only
    b. 2 only
    c. 2 and 3
    d. 1 and 4

Ans. (c) 2 and 3

109. A person suffering from thyrotoxocosis has extremely high level of hyroid hormone in blood. There is failure of feedback regulation in hypothalamic pituitary thyroid axis. The detailed blood investifation exhibited high level of the following

    1. Thyroid stimulating hormone
    2. Thyroid stimulating Immunoglobulin
    3. Thyroid releasing hormone
    4. Parathyroid hormone

    In your opinion, which one of the following is the reason for such thyrotoxicosis
    a. 1 only
    b. 2 only
    c. 1 and 3
    d. 3 and 4

Ans. (c) 1 and 3

110. A person has been suffering from night blindness. On consultation, the doctor advised person to eat carrots and/or cod fish oil. After some time having seen no improvement, doctor gave person vitamin A injection. Still no marked improvement was seen. The doctor mooted several suggestions indicating lack of the following enzymes for failure of treatment.

    A. Retinol dehydrogenase   B. Retinal reductase
    C. Retinal isomerise   D. Retinal synthase

    According to your opinion which is correct reason for night blindness in above case?
    a. A only
    b. B only
    c. B and C both
    d. C and D both

Ans. (a) A only

111. The rate of mutation in *E.coli* from lac to lac + are determined using medium containing lactose, as the only sole source of energy. The principle of spontaneity can be said to be violated if:

    a. The rate of mutation increase during starvation
    b. In the presence of lactose the rate of mutation from lac to lac + increases but overall rate of mutation is not
    c. The rate of mutation in lack gene is always greater than in other genes
    d. The rate of mutation in lac gene is always less than in other genes

Ans. (b) In the presence of lactose the rate of mutation from lac to lac + increases but overall rate of mutation is not

112. Three *E. coli* mutant were isolated which require compound 'A' for their growth. The compounds B, C and D are known to be involved in biosynthetic pathway to A. In order to determine pathway, the mutants were grown in a ninimal medium

supplemented with ONE OF THE COMPOUNDS, A TO D. The result obtained are summarized below:

Mutant	Medium supplemented with compound			
	A	B	C	D
1	+	0	0	0
2	+	0	0	+
3	+	0	+	+

'+' = growth on medium

'0' = no growth

Which of the following equation represent the biosynthetic pathway of A?

a. $B \rightarrow C \rightarrow D \rightarrow A$ b. $C \rightarrow D \rightarrow B \rightarrow A$

c. $B \rightarrow D \rightarrow C \rightarrow A$ d. $A \rightarrow C \rightarrow D \rightarrow B$

Ans. (a) B   C   D   A

113. A cell undergoing meiosis produces four daughter cells, two of which are aneuploids, while two are haploid. This can occurs due to:

a. Non-disjunction during first meiotic division only

b. Non-disjunction during second meiotic division only

c. None-disjunction during either first or second meiotic division

d. Non-disjunction during both first and second meiotic

Ans. (b) Non-disjunction during second meiotic division only

114. When two independent pure lines of pea with white flowers are crossed, the F1 progeny has purple flowers. The F2 progeny obtained on selfing shows both pruple and white flower in a ratio on 9 : 7. The following conclusions were made

A. Two different genes are involved, mutation in which lead to formation of white flower.

B. These two genes show independent assortment

C. This is an example of complementary gene action

D. The is an example of duplicate genes

Which of the following conclusion are correct?

a. A and C only   b. A and D only

c. A, B and D   d. A, B and C

Ans. (d) A, B and C

115. **Following are four modes of inheritance**

A. X-linked recessive   B. X-linked dominant

C. Autosomal recessive   D. Autosomal dominant

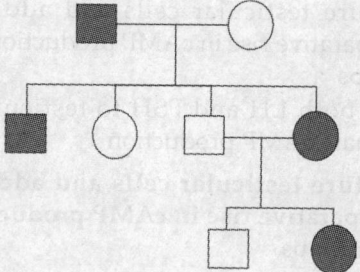

Which of the following modes can be represented by pedigree chart above?

a. A and C

b. B and C

c. C and D

d. D only

Ans. (c) C and D

116. **Four different mutant lines showing similar phenotype were identified from a genetic screen. When genetic crosses amount these mutants were carried out, the first mutant was found to complement the second, third and fourth mutant lines, however, no other complementation groups do the four mutant lines belongs to?**

a. 1   b. 2

c. 3   d. 4

Ans. (b) 2

117. **Why lysogeinc cycle is more beneficial to a virus than lytic cycle under certain circumstances?**

a. The sysogenic cycle prevent local extinction of host while still retaining infectious potential

b. By integrating with the bacterial chromosome, the genetic instructions for the virus become refreshed after one or more replicatioin events during binary fission

c. Lysogenic infection cycles donot harm their host cells, so they can produce virus particles indefinitely

d. Lysogeny causes more mutations to occur in the virus, creating more variants upon which natural selection can operate

Ans. (a) The sysogenic cycle prevent local extinction of host while still retaining infectious potential

118. **Two auxotrophic strains of *E. coli*: A (met bio thr leu thi +) and B (met bio thr leu thi) were incubated together for 18 hours in liquid medium and then ~10^9 cells were plated on minimal medium. Prototrophs were observed at frequency of 1×10^{-7} cells. This may have happened by process of genetic recombination between two strains or by mutation of strains. Which of the following**

control experiment would help rule out the possibility of mutation?

a. Planting strains A and B directly on minimal medium

b. Growing the mixture of strain A and B for 18 hours and then planting on complent medium

c. Growing strins A and B individually in a liquid completer medium for 18 hours and then planting them on minimal medium

Ans. (c) Growing strins A and B individually in a liquid completer medium for 18 hours and then planting them on minimal medium

119. According to fossil record, the earliest fossils of liverworts are found in late Devonian, of mosses in early cretaceous, and vascular plants in the later Silurian/early Devonian. Anthoceros (hornworts) fossils have not been recovered. Reading fossil recores we would say that vascular plants appeared first and then liverworts.

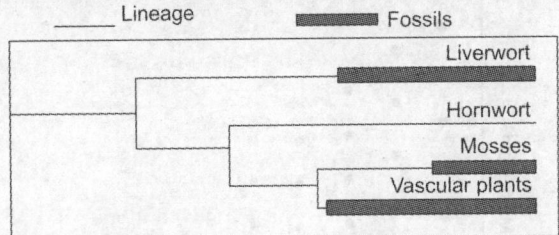

However phylogenetic relationship(shown in figure) suggest otherwise. It may be that

A. Evolutionary history can be read direcly from fossil Devonian

B. Fossil can only set a maximum age fro a lineage

C. Fossil can only sets a minimum age for a lineage

D. The divergence between liverworts and rest of land plants goes back to at least early Ordovician

Which of the following statements in correct?

a. A, B, C and E

b. B, D and E

c. A, B, D and E

d. B, C and E

Ans. (b) B, D and E

120. Which of the following hypothesis best explains the occurrence of Himalayan floral element in Western Ghats of India?

a. Continental drift theory

b. Deccan trap hypothesis

c. Himalayan glaciations theory

d. Coromondal coast hypothesis

Ans. (c) Himalayan glaciations theory

121. In which of the following classes of vertebrates there are group of animals without limbs?

a. Fish, reptiles and mammals

b. Reptiles only

c. Amphibians and Reptiles

d. Amphibian only

Ans. (c) Amphibians and Reptiles

122. Identify 'a', 'b' and 'c' in the figure

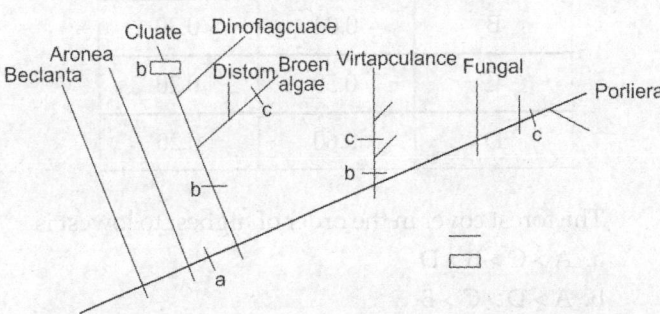

a. a = mitochondria, b = multicellularity, c = chloroplast

b. a = mitochondria, c = multicellularity, b = chloroplast

c. c = mitochondria, b = multicellularity, a = chloroplast

d. c = multicellularity, b = nucleus, a = chloroplast

Ans. (b) a = mitochondria, c = multicellularity, b = chloroplast

123. the schematic section given below of an animal indicates that the animals is

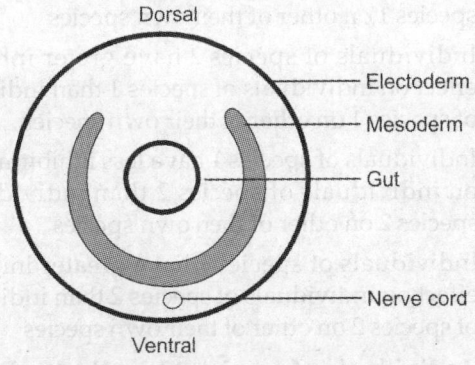

Based on above diagram the organism is

a. Triploblastic, coelomate and invertebrate

b. Triploblastic, acolemate and invertebrate

c. Diploblastic, coelomate and invertebrate

d. Triploblastic, coelamate and vertebrate

Ans. (a) Triploblastic, coelomate and invertebrate

124. A researcher collected information from four forest using sensors to assess their green cover. Observed average spectral values from each of the forest are given in the table below:

Forest	Spectral value	
	NIR	VIS
A	0.50	0.08
B	0.04	0.30
C	0.50	0.20
D	0.60	0.20

The forest cover in the order of highest to lowest is

a. A > C > B > D

b. A > D > C > B

c. B > C > D > A

d. D > A > B > C

Ans. (b) A > D > C > B

125. In Lotka and Volltera's two species competition model:

$$\frac{dN1}{dt} r_1N_1 \frac{K1-N1-N2\alpha12}{K2} \text{ AND } \frac{dN2}{dt} r_2N_2 \frac{K2-N2-N1\alpha21}{K2}$$

Where N represent population size, r growth rate and K maximum carrying capacity for species 1 and 2. The interspecific competition coefficient $L_{12} < 1$ will mean:

a. Individuals of species 2 have less inhibiting effect on individual of species 1 than individuals of species 1 on other of their own species

b. Individuals of species 2 have greter inhibiting effect on individuals of species 1 than individuals of species 1 on other of their own species

c. Individuals of species 1 have less inhibiting effect on individuals of species 2 than individuals of species 2 on other of then own species

d. Individuals of species 1 have greater inhibiting effect on individuals of species 2 than individuals of species 2 on other of their own species

Ans. (a) Individuals of species 2 have less inhibiting effect on individual of species 1 than individuals of species 1 on other of their own species

126. While studying the diversity of 3 communities,5 species and 50 individuals were recorded from each community. The number of individuals under each species was listed as mentioned in the following table. In which of the following community Pielou's Evenness index(e) will be 1?

Community	Species				
		1	2	3	4	5
(1)	A	20	8	7	5	10
(2)	B	10	10	10	10	10
(3)	C	10	12	10	8	10
(4)	D	1	1	1	1	46

Ans. (2)

127. The scatter plot of growth rate and growth yield for 100 reandom environment isolates of bacteria is shown below

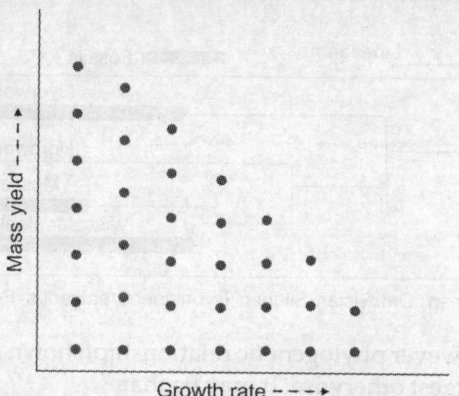

Which of the following can be inferred from data?

a. The two parameter are not related

b. Growth rate is inversely proportional to growth yield

c. Growth yield is negatively correlated with growth rate

d. High growth rate cannot be accompanied by high growth yield

Ans. (d) High growth rate cannot be accompanied by high growth yield

128. A protein contains 2 Trp and 4 Tyr residues. The molecular mass of the protein is 17000 D and that of Trp and Tyr are 204 and 180 D respectively. Values of E 1% 1cm² the absorption coefficient of 1% (g/v) solution of Trp and tyr in 1-cm cell at 280 nm, are 269.60 and 83.33, respectively. The absorption of 1 mg/ml protein solution in 1 cm cell at 280 nm will be

a. 0.1   b. 1.0

c. 0.7   d. 1.7

Ans. (b) 1.0

129. Double stranded DNA replicates in a semi conservative manner. In an invitro DNA synthesis reaction, dideoxy CTP and , dideoxy CMP were individually added in excess(in separate reaction tubes) in addition to dNTPs and other necessary reagents. Rate of DNA synthesis was measured by incorporation of ^{3}H-thymidine. The four graphs drawn below represent the rate of DNA synthesis in two separate reaction tubes.

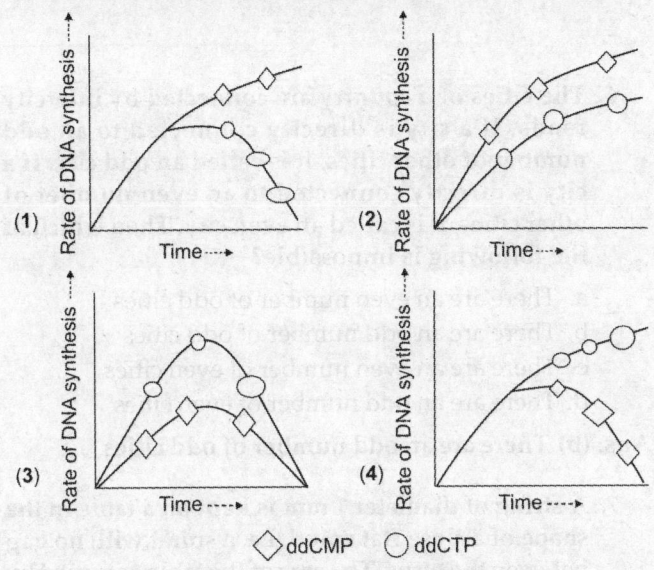

Which of the following graphs represent the expected data?

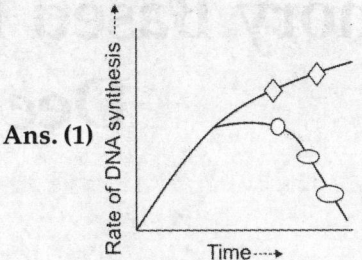

Ans. (1)

130. For the generation f transgenic plant in crop improvement, one important regulatory gene 'X' was overexpressed in a crop plant. Out of 30 transgenic rice plants generated, 22 showed high levels of gene 'X' expression.

However, rest 8 line displaed low level of expression. One explanation of such observation may be:

a. Suppression effect of the transgene

b. Knock down effect of gene X

c. Gene silencing effect

d. Co- suppression effect of transgene

Ans. (d) Co- suppression effect of transgene

Memory Based Paper CSIR NET Dec 2012

1. A granite block of 2m × 5m × 3m size is cut into 5 cm thick slabs of 2m × 5m size these slabs are laid over a 2 m wide pavement. What is the length of the pavement that can be covered with these slabs?

   a. 100 m   b. 200m

   c. 300 m   d. 500 m

Ans. (c) 300 m

2. Which is the least among the following?

   a. $0.33^{0.33}$ b. $0.44^{0.44}$

   c. $\pi^{-1/\pi}$ d. $e^{-1/e}$

Ans. (d) $e^{-1/e}$

3. What is the next number in this "see and tell" sequence?

   1   11   21   1211   111221

   a. 312211   b. 1112221

   c. 1112222   d. 1112131

Ans. (a) 312211

4. A vertical pole of length a stands at the centre of a horizontal regular hexagonal ground of side a. A rope that is fixed that in between a vertex on the ground and the tip of the pole has length

   a. A   b. $\sqrt{2a}$

   c. $\sqrt{3a}$ d. $\sqrt{6a}$

Ans. (b) $\sqrt{2a}$

5. A peacock perched on the top of a 12 m high tree spots a snake moving towards its hole at the base of the tree from a distance equal to thrice the height of the tree. The peacock flies towards the nake in the straight line and they both move at the same speed. At what distance from the base of the tree will the peacock catch the snake?

   a. 16 m   b. 18 m

   c. 14 m   d. 12 m

Ans. (a) 16 m

6. The cities of a country are connected by intercity roads. If a city is directly connected to an odd number of other cities, it is called an odd city. If a city is directly connected to an even number of other cities, it is called an even city. Then which of the following is impossible?

   a. There are an even number of odd cities
   b. There are an odd number of odd cities
   c. There are an even number of even cities
   d. There are an odd number of even cities

Ans. (b) There are an odd number of odd cities

7. A string of diameter 1 mm is kept on a table in the shape of a close flat spiral, i.e. a spiral with no gap between the turns. The area of the table occupied by the spiral is 1 m². Then the length of the string is

   a. 10 m   b. 10^2 m

   c. 10^3 m   d. 10^6 m

Ans. (c) 10^3 m

8. 25% of 25% of a quantity is x% of the quantity where x is

   a. 6.25%   b. 12.5%

   c. 25%   d. 50%

Ans. (a) 6.25%

9. Find the missing letter:

A	EGK	C
?		P
U		R
Q		V
B	OJF	D

   a. H
   b. L
   c. Z
   d. Y

Ans. (c) Z

10. Out of the following hydrogen bonding schemes shown by….., which one corresponds to the weakest hydrogen bond in a given solvent condition?

a. O – H ......O<

b. N – H ....O<

c. O – H ....N<

d. N – H ......N<

Ans. (d) N – H ....N<

11. Which peptide bond (s) marked as a, b, c, d and e will be broken when the following oligopeptide is treated with trypsin at pH 7.0?

$$Lys \xrightarrow{a} Arg \xrightarrow{b} Pro \xrightarrow{d} Lys \xrightarrow{c} Arg \xrightarrow{e} Gly$$

a. a, b, d, e

b. b, d, e

c. d, e

d. d

Ans. (d) d

12. In cellular respiration, which of the following processes occur only inside mitochondria and not in the cytoplasm?

a. Glycolysis and the pentose – phosphate pathway

b. Glycolysis and the citric acid cycle

c. The citric acid cycle and oxidative phosphorylation

d. Glycolysis and oxidative phosphorylation

Ans. (c) The citric acid cycle and oxidative phosphorylation

13. An enzyme catalysed reaction was measured in the presence and absence of an inhibitor, for an uncompetitive inhibition,

a. Only K_m is increased

b. Both K_m and V_{max} are decreased

c. Only V_{max} is decreased

d. Both K_m and V_{max} are not affected

Ans. (b) Both K_m and V_{max} are decreased

14. KCl (100mM) was entrapped inside large unilamellar vesicles. A diffusion potential across the bilayer can be generated by diluting with buffer containing

a. 100 mM KCl and a protonophore

b. 100 mM NaCl and a protonophore

c. 100 mM KCl and a K^+ specific inophore

d. 100 mM NaCl and a K^+ specific ionophore

Ans. (d) 100 mM NaCl and a K^+ specific ionophore

15. Acetylcholine receptor is an archetype for:

a. Ligand gated ion channel

b. ATPase dependent voltage-gated ion channel

c. ATPase dependent Ca^{++} gated ion channel

d. ATPase independent voltage gated ion channel

Ans. (a) Ligand gated ion channel

16. With reference to lac operon, what will be the phenotype of an *E. coli* strain having a genotype $i^-o^+z^+y^-/F'$ $i^+o^cz^-y^+$?

a. Constitutive for both β-galactosidase and lac permease

b. Inducible for both β-galactosidase and lac permease

c. Inducible for β-galactosidase and constitutive for lac permease

d. Constitutive β-galactosidase and inducible for lac permease

Ans. (c) Inducible for β-galactosidase and constitutive for lac permease

17. An organism that has peroxidise and superoxide dismutase but lacks catalase is most likely an

a. Aerotolerant anaerobe

b. Aerotolerant aerobe

c. Obligate anaerobe

d. Facultative anaerobe

Ans. (a) Aerotolerant anaerobe

18. During DNA replication, events at the replication fork require different types of enzymes having specialized functions *except*:

a. DNA polymerase III

b. DNA gyrase

c. DNA ligase

d. DNA glycosylase

Ans. (d) DNA glycosylase

19. Which of the following names is appropriate for the sequences 5' – G/ANNAUG-3' in a mammalian mRNA?

a. Shine dalgarno sequence

b. Kozak sequence

c. Internal ribosome entry sites

d. Translation termination site

Ans. (b) Kozak sequence

20. The specificity of t-RNA recognition by a aminoacyl tRNA synthetase that is intrinsic to the tRNA molecule lies on

a. Acceptor stem

b. Acceptor stem and anticodon loop

c. Anticodon loop

d. D-arm

Ans. (b) Acceptor stem and anticodon loop

21. Viral gene expression after T3 bacteriophage infection is controlled by:

a. Repressor molecule

b. Slow injection of nucleic acid

c. Modification of RNA polymerase

d. DNA polymerase

Ans. (b) Slow injection of nucleic acid

22. **Which of the following factors is NOT true for the low levels of immune response in plasmodium infection?**

    a. Different types of antigens are expressed at various stages of *plasmodium* life cycle

    b. Most of the phases in the life cycle of *plasmodium* are intracellular

    c. Sporozoites are rapidly cleared from blood circulation

    d. *Plasmodium* infection primarily destroys macrophages and dendritic cells

Ans. (d) *Plasmodium* infection primarily destroys macrophages and dendritic cells

23. **Presence of the nuclear localization signal in a steroid receptor indicaes that the receptor resides**

    a. On the nuclear membrane

    b. With in the nucleus

    c. On the cell membrane

    d. In the cytosol

Ans. (d) In the cytosol

24. **Which of the following is an intracellular anchor protein?**

    a. Vitronectin

    b. Vinculin

    c. Integrin

    d. Elastin

Ans. (b) Vinculin

25. **Out of the following matches of oncogenes with the proteins that each spedifies, which one is incorrect?**

    a. Erb A-thyroid hormone receptor

    b. RrbB-epidermal growth factor receptor

    c. Ras-guanine-nucleotide binding protein with GTPase activity

    d. Fos-platelet derived growth factor

Ans. (d) Fos-platelet derived growth factor

26. **capacitation of sperms in humans**

    a. Occurs during copulation

    b. Occurs after the acrosome reaction

    c. Takes place in the ampulla of the oviduct

    d. Takes place in the epididymis of testis

Ans. (c) Takes place in the ampulla of the oviduct

27. **With respect to development of any organism, "autonomous specification" would result in which type of development**

    a. Regulative

    b. Mosaic

    c. Syncytial

    d. Definitive

Ans. (b) Mosaic

28. **The group of cells which generates the vascular tissues including the pericycle in roots of higher plants are called**

    a. Procambium

    b. Protoderm

    c. Ground meristem

    d. Apical meristem

Ans. (a) Procambium

29. **If embryo undergoes 13 cleavage division during embryogenesis, then the size of the embryo compared to zygote**

    a. Increases 13 times

    b. Increases in an exponential fashion

    c. Increases only 6–7 times

    d. Remains almost the same

Ans. (d) Remains almost the same

30. **The chlorosis (yellowing) symptom of iron deficiency is influenced by**

    a. Sodium and potassium

    b. Sodium and phosphorus

    c. Calcium and Nitrogen

    d. Potassium and phosphorus

Ans. (d) Potassium and phosphorus

31. **A plant hormone that promotes the acquisition of desiccation tolerance in developing seed is**

    a. ABA   b. Ethylene

    c. IAA   d. GA3

Ans. (a) ABA

32. **Change in Ca^{+2} concentration can initiate various responses in plants. Which one of the following responses is NOT known to be initiated by change in Ca^{+2} concentration?**

    a. Closure of stomata

    b. Reorientation of growth in pollen tubes

    c. Thickening of cell walls in young tobacco seedlings in res;onse to wind

    d. Lateral root formation

Ans. (d) Lateral root formation

33. Water can move through the soil plant atmosphere continuum, only if water potential (ψ_w) along that path

a. Decreases
b. Increases
c. Remains unchanged
d. Fluctuates rapidly in either direction

Ans. (a) Decreases

34. Which one of the following is responsible for the ejection of milk from mammary glands in mammals?

a. Oxytocin
b. Prolactin
c. Serotonin
d. Melatonin

Ans. (a) Oxytocin

35. A nerve fibre can not be stimulated during the absolute refractory period of a previous stimulus because

a. Sodium permeability remains high
b. Sodium-potassium pump does not operate
c. Voltage-gated calcium channels remains closed
d. Potassium conductance remains low

Ans. (a) Sodium permeability remains high

36. The T-wave of ECG indicates

a. Atrial depolarizatioin
b. Ventricular depolarization
c. Ventricular repolarization
d. Atrial repolarization

Ans. (c) Ventricular repolarization

37. Blood group type A antigen is a complex oligo-saccharide which differs from H antigen present in type O individual b the presence of terminal

a. Glucose
b. Galactose
c. N- acetyl galactosamine
d. Fucose

Ans. (c) N- acetyl galactosamine

38. A cross was made between pure wild type males and brown eyed, curled winged females of *D. Melanogaster*. The F1 females were test crossed, the F2 progeny obtained was as follows:

Wild type	200
Brown eyes, curled wings	150
Brown eyes, normal wings	30
Normal eyes, curled wings	20
Total	**400**

The genetic distance (cM) between brown eye and curled wing loci is:

a. 12, 5
c. 150

b. 50
d. 25

Ans. (a) 12, 5

39. The effect of nonsense mutation could be mollified by reversion as well as suppression. Which of the following processes will help to distinguish between the two kinds of revertants?

a. Complementation
b. Transgenesis
c. Test for allelism
d. Recombination

Ans. (d) Recombination

40. 2-aminopurine induces mutation by

a. Base pair change
b. Frameshift
c. Duplication.
d. Insertion

Ans. (a) Base pair change

41. In a transformation experiment, donor DNA from an *E. coli* strain with the genotype Z^+Y^+ was used to transform a strains of genotype Z Y. the frequencies of transformed classes were:

Z^+Y^+	200
Z^+Y	400
Z^-Y^+	400
Total	**1000**

What is the frequency (%) with which Y locus is cotransformed with the Z locus?

a. 1
c. 33.3

b. 20
d. 40

Ans. (c) 33.3

42. The ' Tribe' refers to a taxonomic group recognized between the ranks

a. Genus and species
c. Order and family

b. Family and genus
d. Class and order

Ans. (b) Family and genus

43. A plant species has been described for the first time by author 'X'. Later, the species has been transferred to some other genus by author 'y'. Then the author citation for the new combination will be

a. X et Y
c. (X) y

b. X ex Y
d. (Y) x

Ans. (c) Family and genus

44. A group which is no longer considered under fungi is

a. Ascomycetes
b. Basidiomycetes
c. Chytridiomycetes
d. Oomycetes

Ans. (d) Oomycetes

45. A character similarity that can be misinterpreted as common descent as called:

a. Symplesiomorphy
b. Symapomorphy
c. Homology
d. Homoplasy

Ans. (d) Homoplasy

46. The following table shows survival and fertility data for a seasonally breeding species.

Season	Proporying surviving	Fertility
0	1.0	0
1	0.5	20
2	0.0	–

Based on above data net reproductive rate (R_0) of the species will be

a. 1
b. 5
c. 10
d. 20

Ans. (c) 10

47. Which of the following is NOT a characteristic of late successional forest plant species?

a. Large seed size, high root to shoot ratio
b. Long seed dispersal distance, long seed viability.
c. Slow growth rate, long maximum life span
d. Low light saturation intensity, high efficiency at low ligh.

Ans. (b) Long seed dispersal distance, long seed viability.

48. Which of the following organisms do not possess the ability to fix nitrogen?

a. Organisms specialized for high altitude
b. Marine plankton
c. Eukaryotic organisms
d. Acidophilic organisms

Ans. (c) Eukaryotic organisms

49. Which of the following greenhouse gases has got highest atmospheric life time?

a. CO_2
b. CH_4
c. N_2O
d. CFCs

Ans. (d) CFCs

50. Which of the following evolutionary processes played an important role in the evolution of complex immune system?

a. Reproductive isolation
b. Adaptive radiation
c. Neutral evolution
d. Co-evolution

Ans. (d) Co-evolution

51. In some species of new world monkeys, only one female reproduces in a group. One or more younger females have suppressed reproduction and assist the reproductive female. This is an example of

a. Sexual selection
b. Group selection
c. Kin selection
d. Reciprocal altruism

Ans. (c) Kin selection

52. In bird species where both parents contribute equally to parental care, generally

a. Males are larger than females.
b. Females are more colourful than males
c. Females are larger than males.
d. Both sexes are morphologically similar

Ans. (d) Both sexes are morphologically similar

53. The idea that an altruistic gene will be favoured if r > C/B, where r is the coefficient of relatedness, B is the benefit to the recipient of the altruism, and C is the cost incurred to the donor, is known as

a. Red queen hypothesis
b. Handicap principle
c. Hamilton's rule
d. Competitive exclusion principle

Ans. (c) Hamilton's rule

54. Use of doubled haploid in plant breeding helps to

a. Reduce generation time while interogressing recessive traits
b. Reduce generation time while interogressing dominant traits
c. Develop somatic hybrids
d. Interogress transgenic traits

Ans. (a) Reduce generation time while interogressing recessive traits

55. For sustained expression of a transgene in the successive generation of a cell line in culture, the ideal gene transfer can be obtained using

a. Lentiviral vector
b. Adenoviral vector

c. Plasmid DNA containing the transgene

d. Only transgenic DNA

Ans. (a) Lentiviral vector

56. *Desulphovibrio desulfuricans* (A) and pseudomonas species (B) are involved in mercury bioremediation, which of the statement below is correct?

a. A converts methyl mercury to mercuric ion, B converts mercury to methyl mercury

b. A converts mercury to methyl mercury, B converts mercury to mercuric ion

c. A convert mercury to methyl mercury, B converts methyl mercury to mercuric ion

d. A converts methyl mercury to mercuric ion, B converts mercury to mercuric ion

Ans. (c) A convert mercury to methyl mercury, B converts methyl mercury to mercuric ion

57. Optical density of a 400 base pair long 1 ml DNA solution was found to be 0.052. how many DNA molecules are present in the solution?

[1 base pair = 650 dalton, optical density of 1.0 D corresponds to 50 μg DNA/ml]

a. 6.023×10^{23}

b. 6.023×10^{18}

c. 6.023×10^{18}

d. 6.023×10^{13}

Ans. (a) 6.023×10^{23}

58. In which of the following techniques does molecular fragmentation offer clues to the covalent chemical structure of biomolecules?

a. MALDI – TOF MS mass spectrometry

b. MALDI – TOF MS/MS mass spectrometry

c. ESI – TOF MS mass spectrometry

d. LC coupled ESI–TOF MS mass spectrometry

Ans. (b) MALDI–TOF MS/MS mass spectrometry

59. The movement of a single cell was required to be continually monitored during development. This cell was marked with a reporter gene. To visualized this movement one would use

a. Phase constrast microscopy

b. Bright field microscopy

c. Fluorescence microscopy

d. Atomic force microscopy

Ans. (c) Fluorescence microscopy

60. The Gibbs free energy of binding of a ligand with a protein is determined using alorimetric measurements at 25°C. the value of DG° thus determined is 1.36 kcal/mole. The binding constant for the ligand-protein association is:

a. 1.30×10^{-12}

b. 0.10

c. 1.00

d. 0.97

Ans. (b) 0.10

61. A is converted to E by enzyme E_A, E_B, E_C, E_D. The K_m(M) values of the enzymes are $10^{-2}, 10^{-4}, 10^{-5}$ and 10^{-4}, respectively, if all the substrates and products are present at a concentration of 10^{-4} M, and the enzymes have approximately the same Vmax the rate limiting step will be

a. $C \underset{E_C}{\rightleftharpoons} D$

b. $D \underset{E_D}{\rightleftharpoons} E$

c. $A \underset{E_A}{\rightleftharpoons} B$

d. $B \underset{E_B}{\rightleftharpoons} C$

Ans. (c) $A \underset{E_A}{\rightleftharpoons} B$

62. The molecular mass of a protein determined by gel filtration is 120 kDa. When its mass is determined by SDS-PAGE with and without β-mercaptoethanol, it is only 60 kDa. What is the most probable explanation for these observations?

a. Protein is a dimer in which two identical chains are cross-linked by disulphide bond (s).

b. Protein is a monomer of molecular mass 60 kDa but it is excluded from the gel matrix due to strong repulsion between the gel matrix and the protein

c. Protein is most likely to be composed of two sub-unit having identical molecular mass.

d. Protein is a monomer but it is nicked into half its size by SDS

Ans. (c) Protein is most likely to be composed of two sub-unit having identical molecular mass.

63. Mouse IgG is left either intact (left lane in A, B, C, D) or digested with papain or pepsin or treated with β-mercaptoethanol and run on non-reducing SDS- PAGE and stained with Coomassie blue. In a separate experiment, papain-digested products are immunoblotted with an anti idiotypic monoclonal antibody. Following four profiles are attributed to each of these treatments

Which one of the following possibilities is correct?

a. A (pepsin), B(papain), C(β-ME). D (papain, followed by anti idiotype immunoblot)

b. A (papain), B(pepsin), C (papain, followed by anti idiotype immunoblot), D(β-ME).

c. A (papain, followed by anti idiotype immunoblot), B (papain), C(pepsin), D (β-ME)

d. A (β-ME), B(papain), C(pepsin), D(papain, followed by anti-idiotype immunoblot)

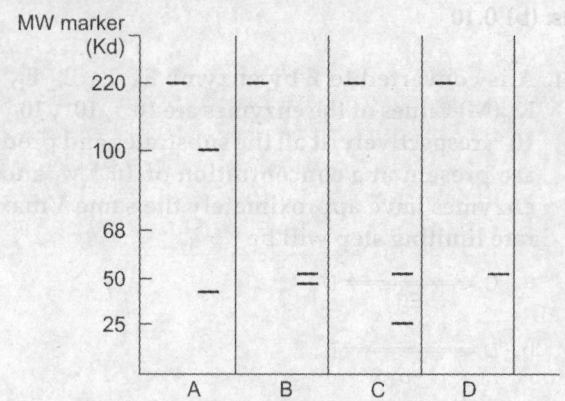

Ans. (a) A (pepsin), B(papain), C(β-ME). D (papain, followed by anti idiotype immunoblot)

64. The citric acid cycle in respiration yields:

a. 1GTP, 3 NADH, 1 FADH$_2$, 2 CO$_2$

b. 2GTP, 2 FADH$_2$, 2 NADH, 2 CO$_2$

c. 4GTP, 6 NADH, 4 FADH$_2$, 2 CO$_2$

d. 32GTP, 2 NADH, 4 FADH$_2$, 4 CO$_2$

Ans. (a) 1GTP, 3 NADH, 1 FADH$_2$, 2 CO$_2$

65. Phosphatidyl serine (PS) is mostly located in the inner bilayer of plasma membrane of red blood cells (RBCs). You have to prove this fact about PS by an experiment. You are provided with PS- Identify the correct sequence of experiments to be carried out to settle this issue

a. RBCs → inside out vesicles → PSE → thin Layer Chromotography

b. RBCs → right side out vesicles → TLC → PSE

c. RBCs → PSE → Inside out vesicles → TLC

d. RBCs → PSE → TLC → Inside out vesicles

Ans. (a) RBCs → inside out vesicles → PSE → thin Layer Chromotography

66. ATP driven pumps hydrolyze ATP to ADP and phosphate and use the energy released to pump ions or solutes across a membrane. There are many classes of these pumps and representatives of each are found in all prokaryotic and eukaryotic cells. Which of the following statements about these pumps is NOT correct?

a. P-type pumps are multipass transmembrane proteins which phosphorylate themselves during pumping and involve in ion transport

b. F-type pumps normally use the H$^+$gradient across the membrane to drive the synthesis of ATP.

c. V- type pumps normally use voltage gradient for transport of small molecules

d. ABC transporters primarily pump small molecules across cell membrane

Ans. (c) V- type pumps normally use voltage gradient for transport of small molecules

67. Following are statements related to the organization of the four major protein complexes of thylakoid membrane

A. Photosystem II is located predominantly in the stacked regions of the thylakoid membrane

B. Photosystem I is found in the unstacked regions protruding into stroma.

C. Cytochrome B$_6$ f complex is confined to stroma only

D. APT synthase is located in the unstacked regions protruding into stroma.

Which one of the following combination of above statements is correct?

a. A, B and C

b. A, B and D

c. B, C and D

d. C, D and A

Ans. (b) A, B and D

68. A bacterial population has a plasmid with copy number 'n'. It was observed that on an average in one out of 2$^{(n-1)}$ cell divisions, there was spontaneous plasmid curing. It was inferred from the observation that:

A. Each cell division does not have equal probability of polasmid curing

B. There is not evidence for any mechanism of plasmid segregation in the two daughter cells

C. Plasmid has an equal chance of being in either of the two daughter cells

Which of the combination of above statements is true?

a. A and B

b. B and D

c. Only A

d. B, C and D

Ans. (d) B, C and D

69. In a given experiment the cells were labelled for 30 minutes with radioactive thymidine. The medium was then replaced with that containing unlabelled thymidine and the cells were grown for additional times. At different time points after replacement of medium the fraction of mitotic cells were analysed. Based on the results obtained, the above figure was drawn which shows the percentage of mitotic cells that are labelled as a function of time after brief incubation with radioactive thymidine.

Considering the above experiment, the following statements were made:

A. Cells in the S-phase of the cell cycle during the 30 minute labelling period contain radioactive DNA.

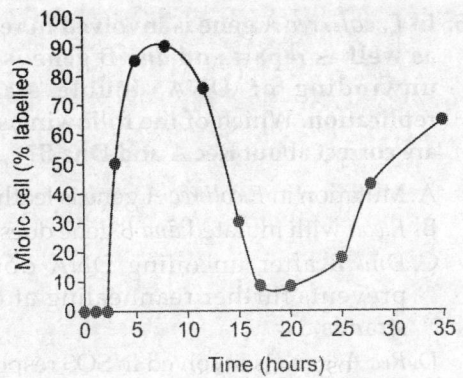

B. It takes about 3 hours before the first labelled mitotic cells appear

C. The cells enter the second round of mitosis at t_{30} hours

D. The total length of the cell cycle is about 27 hours with G_1 being more than 15 hours

Which of the combinations of the above statements is correct?

a. A and B

b. B and C

c. C and D

d. A and D

Ans. (a) A and B

---

70. **Mutants of lac Y (Y⁻) gene of *E.coli* do not synthesize the lactose permease protein. The following statements refer to the behaviour of lac Y⁻ mutants under different experimental conditions.**

A. No synthesis of β-galactosidase when Y⁻ cells are induced with lactose.

B. Synthesis of β-galactosidase when Y⁻ cells are induced with lactose.

C. No synthesis of β-galactosidase when Y⁻ cells are induced with IPTG.

D. Synthesis of β-galactosidase when Y⁻ cells are induced with lactose.

E. The cells induced with IPTG cannot grow in the presence of TONPG (TONPG is a compound, whose uptake is mediated by lactose permease and cleaved by β-galactosidase to release a toxic compound).

F. Cells induced with IPTG can grow in the presence of TONPG.

Which combination of the above statements is correct?

a. A, D and F

b. B, C and E

c. A, C and F

d. A, C and E

Ans. (a) A, D and F

---

71. **The semiconservative nature of DNA replication was established by Meselson and Stahl in their classic experiment with bacteria. They grew bacteria in N^{15} NH_4Cl containing medium, washed and then incubated in fresh medium with N^{14} containing compounds and allowed to grow for three generations. CsCl density gradient centrifugation of isolated DNA established the nature of semiconservative DNA replication. The pictorial representation below shown the position of differentially labelled DNA in CsCl density gradient.**

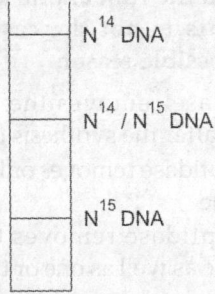

Had the DNA replication been conservative, what would have been the pattern?

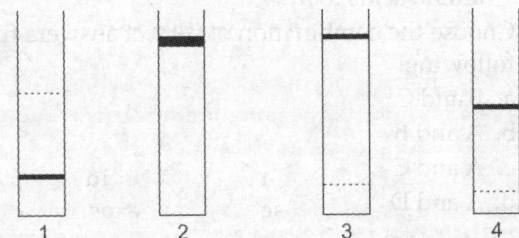

Ans. (3)

---

72. **HeLa cell extract was used to study stranscription of a gene X having six introns, RNA Pol II complex containing all associated proteins was isolated from actively transcribing system and subjected to proteome analysis. Results showed the presence of both splicing and capping enzymes in the complex. When transcription elongation was inhibited by flavopiridol, polymerase complex contained only capping enzymes. When phosphorylation of the CTD domain of Pol II was inhibited by a kinase inhibitor, the complex contained neither splicing nor capping enzymes. From these results, following conclusions were made:**

A. Transcription of gene X is coupled to mRNA capping

B. Transcription elongation is coupled to splicing

C. Phosphorylation of CTD is required for the recruitment of capping and splicing enzymes

D. Both capping and splicing of m-RNA occurs simultaneously

Identify the correct set of conclusions:

a. A, B and C

b. B , C and D

c. C, D and A

d. D, A and B

Ans. (a) A, B and C

73. **In bacteria, N-formyl methionine is the first amino acid to be incorporated into a polypeptide chain Accordingly, one would think that all bacterial proteins have a formyl group at their amino terminus and the first amino acid is methionine, however, this is not the case, because of the following possible reason**

A. Deformylase removes the formyl group only during or after the synthesis of the polypeptides

B. Aminopeptidase removes only the amino terminal methionine

C. Aminopeptidase removes the amino terminal methionine as well as one or two additional amino acids

D. Deformylase removes the formyl group as well as amino terminal methionine and adds one or two amino acids to it

Choose the combination of correct answers from the following:

a. B and C

b. A and B

c. A and C

d. A and D

Ans. (c) A and C

74. **Bacteriophage λ is a temperate phage. Immediately after infection, viral specific mRNAs for N and Cro proteins are expressed followed by early mRNAs. At the commitment phase, either lytic cycle starts with the expression of genes for head tail, and lytic proteins or lysogenisation cycle begins with the expression of repressor and integrase genes. During induction of lysogens both INT and XIS protein are needed along with host factors, out of the four processes below, some govern integration of viral genome and its excitation?**

A. Repression of transcription

B. Retroregulation

C. Rearrangements of viral genome

D. Repression of translation

Identify the correct set of combination

a. A and B

b. B and C

c. C and D

d. D and A

Ans. (b) B and C

75. **In *E. coli*, *rec A* gene is involved in recombination as well as repair and *dna B* gene is involved in unwinding of DNA double stands during replication. Which of the following statement is / are correct about Rec A and Dna B?**

A. Mutation in *E.coli rec A* gene is leathal

B. *E.coli* with mutated *dna B* gene does not survive

C. *Dna B* after uncoiling DNA double strands, prevents further reannealing at the separated strands

D. *Rec A* gene is involved in SOS response and helps DNA repair

The correct option are:

a. B and C

b. A and B

c. B and D

d. A and C

Ans. (c) B and D

76. **The challenges faced by aminoacyl t-RNA synthetase in selecting the correct amino acid is more daunting than its recognition of the appropriate t RNA. In case of amino acids with similar structures like valine and isoleucine, this challenge is met by the enzyme possibly through its**

A. Catalytic pocket

B. Editing pocket

C. Anticodon loop

D. Acceptor arm

Choose the correct set from the following:

a. A and B

b. A and C

c. B and D

d. B and C

Ans. (a) A and B

77. **p24 is an important core protein of HIV. This protein is abundant during active replication of the virus. The serum of an HIV patient was examined for the presence of p24 and antibody against p24 for proper diagnosis of the infection stages. Match the clinical observation in column A with the inferences in column B.**

Column A	Column B
A. p24 is present in the serum	Viarl latence
B. Anti-p24 antibody is high in the serum	Progression of HIVA from latency to lytic stage
C. Anti –p24 antibody begins to decline with corresponding increase in p24	Early stage of infection

Choose the correct matching

a. A-a, B-b, C-c

b. A-b, B-a, C-c

c. A-c, B-a, C-b

d. A-c, B-b, C-a

Ans. (c) A-c, B-a, C-b

78. Epidermal growth factor (EGF) is needed for growth of almost all cells. EGF receptor is a transmembrane protein having an extracellular ligand binding domain, a transmembrane domain and a cytosolic domain of protein tyrosine kinase (PTK). Binding of EGF to the receptor activates PTK resulting in activation of transcription factor through intracellular transducers. In cell type A, much of the extracellular ligand binding domain is deleted by proteases such that cytosolic domain of PTK becomes constitutively active whereas cell type B is having normal EGF receptor, what will be the best fit graph for the growth of the cultures of cell type A and B in complete medium in presence (+) and absence (–) of EGF?

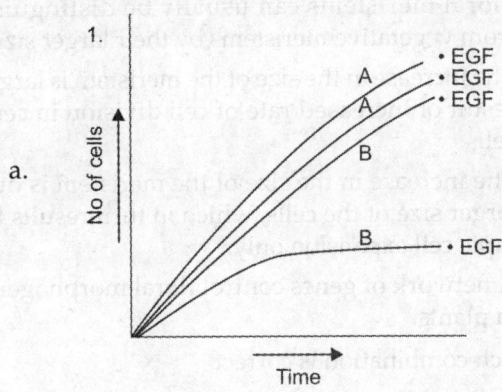

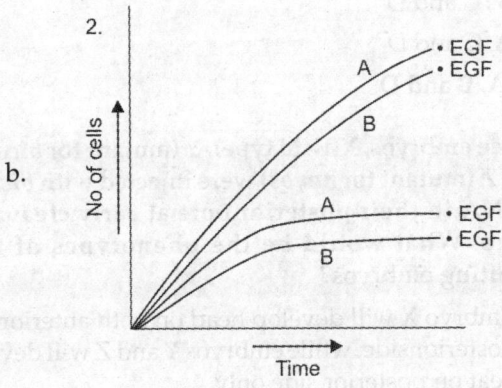

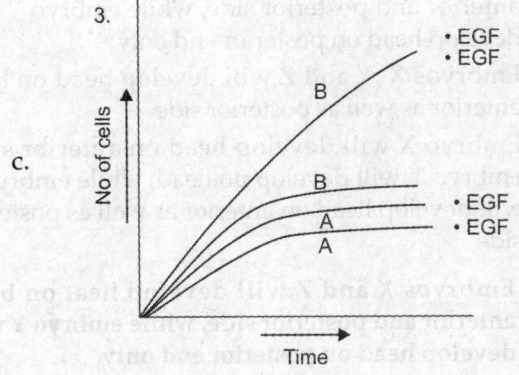

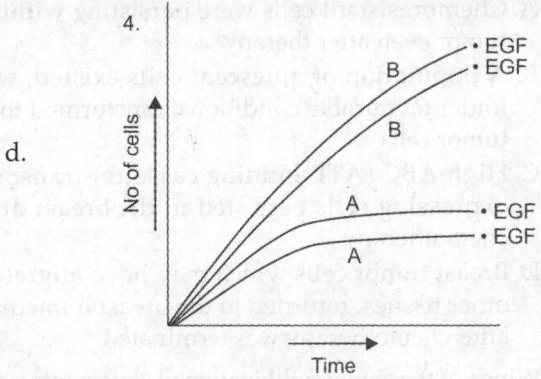

Ans. (a)

79. A particular type of cancer cell undergoes apoptosis by both extrinsic and intrinsic pathways when treated with a chemotherapeutic agent X. Caspase 8 and Caspase 9 are the initiator capases associated with extrinsic and intrinsic pathways respectively. Now, if caspase 9 is silenced in cancer cell by shRNA transfection, what will be the best-fit graph for apoptosis scenario in the cancer cell when trated with agent X?

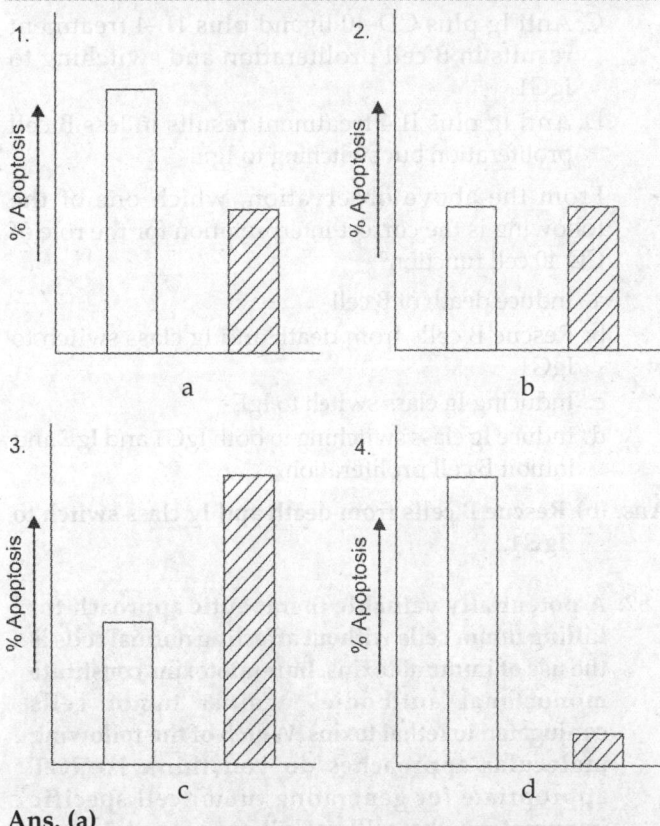

Ans. (a)

80. After successive surgery and chemotherapy, the tumor of a breast cancer patient subsided However, after almost 5 year, the tumor relapsed in a more aggressive manner and did not respond to the conventional chemotherapy delivered earlier, the following postulations were made.

A. Chemoresistant cells were persisting within the tumor even after therapy

B. A population of quiescent cells existed, which under favourable conditions, ransformed to new tumor cells.

C. High ABC (ATP-binding cassette)-transporter expressing cells persisted in the breast during chemotherapy

D. Breast tumor cells which may have migrated to other tissues, returned to the breast immediately after chemotherapy was terminated

Which of the above combination of statements is true?

a. A and D
b. A, B and C
c. Only B
d. B and D

Ans. (b) A, B and C

81. **Following are the experimental observation made on treatment of B cells:**

A. Anti-immunoglobulin antibody treatment results in B cells apoptosis

B. Anti-Ig plus CD 40 ligand treatment results in B cell proliferation

C. Anti Ig plus CD-40 ligand plus 1L-4 treatment results in B cell proliferation and switching to IgG1.

D. Anti Ig plus IL4 treatment results in less B cell proliferation but switching to IgE.

From the above observation, which one of the following is the correct interpretation for the role of CD 40 cell function?

a. Induce death of B cell
b. Rescue B cells from death and Ig class switch to IgG1.
c. Inducing Ig class switch to IgE
d. Induce Ig class switching to both IgG1 and IgE and inhibit B cell proliferation.

Ans. (b) Rescue B cells from death and Ig class switch to IgG1.

82. **A potentially valuable therapeutic approach for killing tumor cells without affecting normal cells is the use of immunotoxins. Immunotoxins constitute monoclonal antibodies against tumor cells conjugated to lethal toxins. Which of the following molecular approaches do you think is NOT appropriate for generating tumor cell specific immunotoxin that will not kill normal cells?**

a. Cell surface receptor binding polypeptide chain of toxin molecule should be replaced by monoclonal antibodies against a particular tumor cell type.

b. Constant region Fc domain of tumor cell specific monoclonal antibody should be replaced by ligation of toxins.

c. Variable region $F(ab)_2$ domain of tumor cell specific monoclonal antibody should be replaced by ligation of toxins.

d. Inhibitor polypeptide chain of toxin should be conjugated to $F(ab)_2$ domain of tumor cell specific monoclonal antibody

Ans. (c) Variable region $F(ab)_2$ domain of tumor cell specific monoclonal antibody should be replaced by ligation of toxins.

83. **Flowers represent a complex array of functionally specialized structure that differ substantially from the vegetative plant body in form and cell types. Following are statements made regarding floral meristems.**

A. Floral meristems can usually be distinguished from vegetative meristems by their larger size

B. The increase in the size of the meristem is largely a result of increased rate of cell division in central cells.

C. The increase in the size of the meristem is due to larger size of the cells, which in turn results from rapic cell expansion only.

D. A network of genes control floral morphogenesis in plants.

Which combination is correct

a. A, B and D
b. A, B and C
c. B, C and D
d. A, C and D

Ans. (a) A, B and D

84. **Three embryos, X(wild type), Y (mutant for *bicoid*) and Z (mutant for *nanos*) were injected with *bicoid* mRNA in their posterior pole at early cleavage stage. What would be the phenotypes of the resulting embryos?**

a. Embryo X will develop head on both anterior and posterior side, while embryos Y and Z will develop heat on posterior side only.

b. Embryos X and Z will develop heat on both anterior and posterior side, while embryo Y will develop head on posterior end only.

c. Embryos X, Y and Z will develop head on both anterior as well as posterior side

d. Embryo X will develop head on anterior side, embryo Y will develop no head, while embryo Z will develop head on anterior as well as posterior side

Ans. (b) Embryos X and Z will develop heat on both anterior and posterior side, while embryo Y will develop head on posterior end only.

85. In *C.elegans* during embryogenesis, an anchor cell and 6 hypodermal vulval precursor cells get involved in forming the vulva. If 3 of the hypodermal VPCs are killed by a laser beam, a normal vulva is still formed. This could be due to the following possible reasons.

A. Six hypodermal VPCs form equivalence group of cells, out of which only 3 participate in vulva formation and 3 cells remain as reserve cells.

B. When 3 hypodermal VPCs are killed, the 3 neighboring hypodermal non VPCs get freshly recruited.

C. Anchor cell functions as an inducer which can induce epithelial cells of the gonad to get recruited to compensate for the loss.

D. Anchor cell acts as an inducer which can spatially induce only 3 hypodermal cells to form the vulva

Which combination of the above statements is correct?

a. A and B
b. B and C
c. C and D
d. A and D

Ans. (d) A and D

86. In tadpoles, if the tail is amputated it can regenerate. However, if the tail is amputated and then exposed to retinoic acid, it develops limbs instead of regenerating the tail. This could be due to the following reasons:

A. Retinoic acid is a morphogen and induces gene responsible for limb formation

B. Retinoic acid raises the positional values in that region for limb development to take place

C. This is a random phenomenon and is not well understood

D. Retinoic acid possible acts as a mutagen and the phenotype observed is a result of several mutations.

Which combination of the above statements is true?

a. A and B
b. C and D
c. B and D
d. B and C

Ans. (a) A and B

87. In sea urchins, a group of cells at the vegetal pole become specified as the large micromere cells, these cells are determined to become skeletogenic mesenchyme cells that will leave the blastula epithelium to ingress in to the blastocoels. This specification is controlled by the expression of pmar 1 which is a repressor of HesC. Hes C represses the genes encoding transcription factor activating skeleton forming genes, the gene regulatory network is given below.

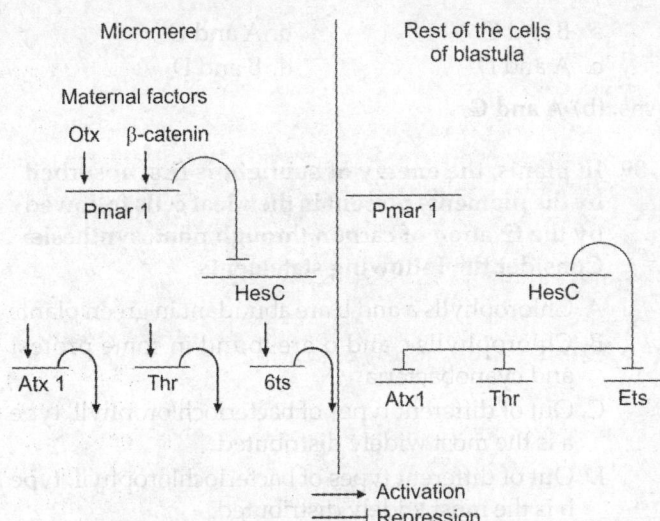

Below, column I list the experiments carried with mRNA/antisenxe RNA of different genes injected into single celled sea urchin embryo while column II lists the developmental outcomes match the following:

Column I (Injection of)	Column II (developmental outcomes)
A. mRNA of Pmar 1	1. All cells will strat ingressing into the blastocoels
B. m RNA of Hes C	2. Skeleton mesenchyme will not be formed
C. Antisense of Pmar 1	
D. Antisense of Hes C	

Which of the following combination is correct?

a. A-2, B-1, C-1, D-2
b. A-1, B-1, C-2, D-2
c. A-1, B-2, C21, D-1
d. A-2, B-2, C-2, D-2

Ans. (c) A-1, B-2, C21, D-1

88. Which of the following cellular communications shown below will override the process of normal development and lead to cancer?

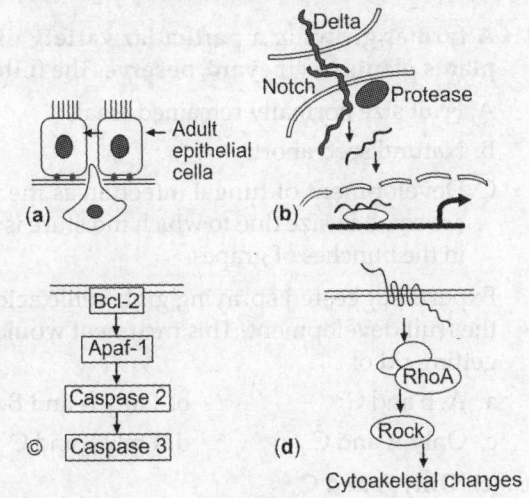

a. B and C

b. A and C

c. A and D

d. B and D

Ans. (b) A and C

89. In plants, the energy of sunlight is first absorbed by the pigments present in their leaf cells followed by the fixation of carbon through photosynthesis. Consider the following statements.

A. Chlorophylls a and b are abundant in green plants

B. Chlorophylls c and d are found in some protest and cyanobacteria

C. Out of different types of bacteriochlorophyll, type a is the most widely distributed.

D. Out of different types of bacteriochlorophyll, type b is the most widely distributed.

Which one of the following combination of above statement is correct?

a. A, B and C

b. A, C and D

c. B, C and D

d. A, B and D

Ans. (a) A, B and C

90. Nitrate reductase is an important enzyme for nitrate assimilation. Given below are some statements on nitrate reductase enzyme:

A. Nitrate reductase of higher plants is composed of two identical subunits

B. One subunit of nitrate reductase contains three prosthetic groups

C. One of the prosthetic groups attached to both subunits is heme.

D. One of the prosthetic groups complexed with pterin is magnesium

Which one of the following combinations of statements on nitrate reductase mentioned above is correct?

a. A, B and C

b. A, C and D

c. B, C and D

d. A, B and D

Ans. (a) A, B and C

91. A farmer growing a particular variety of grape plants plants in vineyard, observes the following :

A. Fruit size normally remained small

B. Natural seed abortion

C. Development of fungal infection as the pedicels are small in size due to which moisture is retained in the bunches of grapes.

Experts suggested spraying gibberellic acid during the fruit development. This treatment would help in getting rid of

a. A, B and C

b. Only A and B

c. Only A and C

d. Only B and C

Ans. (c) Only A and C

92. Light is perceived by various photoreceptors in plants, the photoreceptors predominantly work at specific wavelength of light. Some of the following stagement are related to the function of plant photoreceptors.

A. Phytochrome A predominantly perceives the red and far red light

B. Phytochrome B predominantly perceives red light

C. Cryptochromes regulate plant development.

D. Phototropins are involved in blue light perception and chloroplast movements.

Which one of the following combinations based on above statements is correct?

a. A, B and C

b. B, C and D

c. C, D and A

d. A, B and D

Ans. (b) B, C and D

93. From the following statements:

A. Triose phosphate is utilized for the synthesis of both starch and sucrose

B. Triose phosphate is translocated to cytosol from chloroplast

C. Triose phoasphate is confined to chloroplast and is utilized fot synthesis of starch only

D. Triose phosphate is translocated from cytosol to chloroplast.

Which one of the following combination is correct regarding starch and sucrose synthesis during day time?

a. A and B

b. B and C

c. C and D

d. D and A

Ans. (a) A and B

94. Shown blow, is a graph representing the growth of different plant species subjected to salinity relative to that of unsalinized control. Which of the following statements is NOT true?

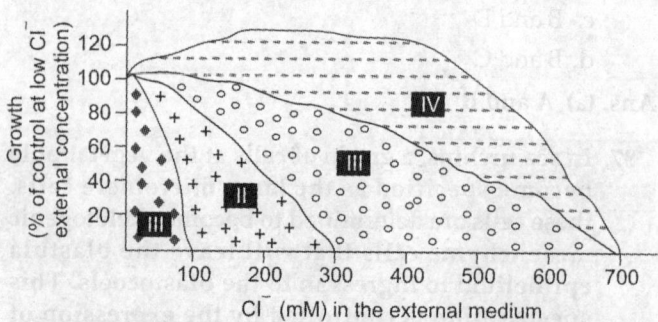

Growth (% of control at low Cl⁻ external concentration) vs Cl⁻ (mM) in the external medium

a. Plants in group IA are extreme halophytes while very salt sensitive species will be part of group III

b. Plants in group IA are very salt sensitive and extreme halophytes will be part of group III.

c. Halophytes, which can tolerate salt but their growth is retarded will be of part of group IB

d. Non-halophytes, which are salt tolerant but lacks salt glands will be a part of group II.

Ans. (b) Plants in group IA are very salt sensitive and extreme halophytes will be part of group III.

95. An experimentalist stimulates a nerves fiber in the middle of an axon and records the following observations. Which one of the observation is correct?

a. Nerve impulse is travelling in a direction towards cell body.

b. Nerve impulse is travelling in a direction towards telodendrons.

c. Nerve impulse are travelling in both the direction opposite to each other.

d. Nerve impulse is not moving in either direction.

Ans. (c) Nerve impulse are travelling in both the direction opposite to each other.

96. Desert animals have longer loop of Henle compared to that of humans, it may be due to the following reasons:

A. Long loop of Henle is associated with with greater amount of vasopressin secreation

B. In long loop of Henle, the counter current exchanger is more effective

C. Long loop of Henle conserves more water

D. Long loop of Henle stimulates production of angiotensin II.

Which of the above reason (s) is/are correct?

a. A and B

b. B and C

c. C and D

d. Only D

Ans. (c) C and D

97. A boy cats a large serving of cheese having high amount of sodium. He hardly drinks any fluid. Inspite of this, the water and electrolyte balance was maintained. Which one of the following explanation is correct?

a. His aldosterone was decreased and alcohol dehydrogenase was increased

b. His aldosterone was increased and ADH was decreased

c. There was no change in either of the hormones

d. His sympathoadrenal system was stimulated.

Ans. (a) His aldosterone was decreased and alcohol dehydrogenase was increased

98. The blood volume decreased when a mammal was bled rapidly. However, the cardiovascular changes resulting from hemorrhage could be minimized by the following compensatory mechanisms:

A. Increased cerebral blood flow.

B. Reduction of baroreceptor activity and stimulation of chemoreceptors

C. Reabsorption of tissue fluid in blood

D. Increased release of enkephalins and beta endorphins.

Which of the above is/are correct?

a. A and B

b. B and C

c. C and D

d. Only D

Ans. (b) B and C

99. The stomach of a person was partially removed during surgery of a gastric tumour, Despite taking a balanced diet, the person developed anemia. Following possible explanations were offered:

A. Lower gastric secreation inhibits folic acid absorption

B. Protein digestion was disturbed in partial gastretomy

C. Lower HCl secretion from stomach reduced iron absorption

D. Lower secretion of intrinsic protein factor from stomach reduced Vit B_{12} absorption

Which of the above explanation were correct?

a. A and B

b. B and C

c. C and D

d. A and d

Ans. (c) C and D

100. The RFLP pattern observed for two pure parental line (P1 and P2) and their F1 progeny is represented below. Further, the P1 plant had red flowers while the P2 had white flowers, the F1 progeny was backcrossed to P2. The result obtained, showing the number of progeny with red and white flowers and their RFLP patterns is also represented below.

	P1	P2	F1	Progeny of the cross between F1 and P2			
Phenotype	Red	White	Red	Red		White	
RFLP pattern	—	—	—	—	—	—	—
No. of progeny				45	5	45	5

Which one of the following conclusions made is correct?

a. The DNA marker and the gene for the flower colour are 10 cM apart

b. The marker and the gene for the flower colour are 5 cM apart

c. The marker and the phenotype are independently assorting

d. The marker and the gene for the colour segregate from one another

Ans. (a) The DNA marker and the gene for the flower colour are 10 cM apart

101. **Wild type T4 bacteriophage can grow on B and K strains of *E. coli* forming small plaques. rII mutants of T4 bacteriophate cannot grow on *E. coli* strains K (non-permissive host), but form large qlaques on *E. coli* strains B (permissive hsot). The following two experiments were carried out:**

Experiment I: *E. coli* K cells were simulataneously infected with two rII mutants (a⁻ and b⁻) several plaque with wild type morphology were formed

Experiment II: *E. coli* B cells were simultaneously infected with the same mutants as above. T4 phages were isolated from the resulting plaques and used to infect *E. coli* K cells, Few plaques with wild type morphology were formed.

Which one is the correct conclusion made regarding the rII mutants, a⁻ and b⁻ from the above experiments?

a. The mutation a⁻ and b⁻ belong to two different cistrons (experiment I) and there is not recombination between them(experiment II)

b. The mutation a⁻ and b⁻ belong to two different cistrons (experiment I)and they recombined (experiment II)

c. The mutation a⁻ and b⁻ belong to two different cistrons (experiment II)and they recombined (experiment I)

d. The mutation a⁻ and b⁻ belong to two same cistrons (experiment I) and they recombined (experiment II)

Ans. (b) The mutation a⁻ and b⁻ belong to two different cistrons (experiment I)and they recombined (experiment II)

102. **The following pedigree represents inheritance of a trait in an extended family:**

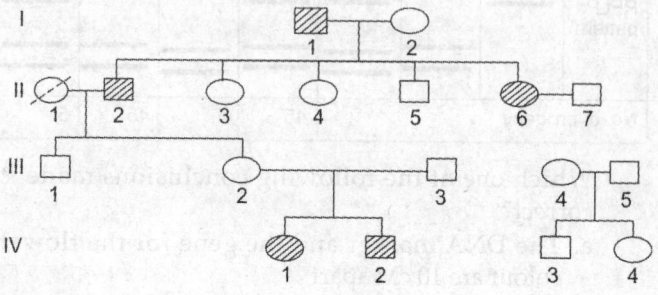

What is the probable mode of inheritance and which individuals conclusively demonstrate this mode of inheritance?

a. Autosomal recessive, III-2, 3 and IV-1,2 conclusively demonstrate the mode of inheritance.

b. Autosomal recessive,I-1,2 and II- 2 conclusively demonstrate the mode of inheritance.

c. Autosomal domiant, III-2, 3 and IV-1,2 conclusively demonstrate the mode of inheritance.

d. X-linked recessive, II- 3,4and 5 conclusively demonstrate the mode of inheritance.

Ans. (a) Autosomal recessive, III-2, 3 and IV-1,2 conclusively demonstrate the mode of inheritance.

103. **Following is the diagram of a paracentric inversion heterozygote ABCDEFG/ABFEDCG involved in recombination during meiosis I:**

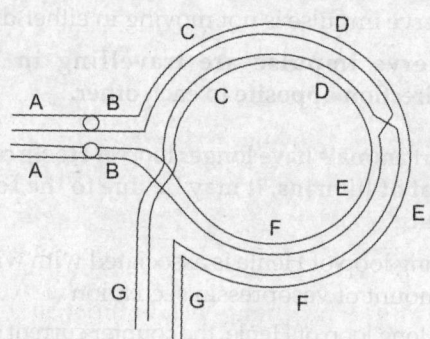

The consequence of this recombination will be the formation of

A. A dicentric and an acentric chromosome in meiosis I as the chiasmata gets terminated.

B. No dicentric or acentric chromosome but appearance of deletion and duplication in both the chromosomes

C. All none viable gametes

D. Non viable gametes from crossover products

Which of the following statements are correct?

a. A and B   b. A and C

c. A and D   d. B and C

Ans. (c) A and D

104. ***Wolbachia* are obligate intracellular bacteria, many different strains of which are abundantly present in insects. They induce mating incompatibility in host, i.e. males infected with one strains can only fertilize females infected with the same strain. No other pathological effects are observed in host. A possible evolutionary consequence of this phenomenon would be:**

a. Exitinction of many insect species

b. Thermination f sexual reproduction in many insect species

c. Co-extinction of host and parasite

d. Reproductive isolation leading to rapid speciation in insects

Ans. (d) Reproductive isolation leading to rapid speciation in insects

105. Twenty small population of a species, each polymorphic for a given locus (T,t) were bred in captivity, in 10 of then the population size was kept constant by random removal of individuals, while other 10 were allowed to increases their population size. After several generations it was observed that in 7 of the size restricted populations only T was present, in the remaining 3 only t was present, it the growing populations 8 retained their polymorphism and in 2 only t was observed. The experiment illustrates

a. Genetic drift which is more likely in large populations

b. Genetic drift which is more likely in small populations

c. Density dependent selection against T

d. Density dependent selection against t

Ans. (b) Genetic drift which is more likely in small populations

106. Some important events in the history of life on earth are given below

A. First vertebrates (jawless fishes); first plants

B. Forest of ferns and conifers; amphibians arise; insects radiate

C. Conifers dominant; dinosaurs arise; insects radiate

D. Flowering plants appear; climax of dinosaurs followed by extinction

E. Radiation of flowering plants, most modern mammalian orders represented

F. Ice Ages, modern humans appear

Match the above with the geological time periods and choose the correct combination,

a. A- Silurian; B-Permian; C-triassic; D-jurassic; ECretaceous; F-tertiary

b. A-ordovician; B-Carboniferous; C-triassic, D-Cretaceous, E-tertiary; F-Quaternary

c. ACambrian; B-Ordovician; C-Silurian; Devonian; E-Permian; F-tertiary

d. A-Devonian; B-Permian; C-triassic;D-Cretaceous; E-tertiary; F-Quaternary

Ans. (b) A-ordovician; B-Carboniferous; C-triassic, D-Cretaceous, E-tertiary; F-Quaternary

107. Microbes produce either primary or secondary metabolites during fermentation. A metabolite production curve is shown below:

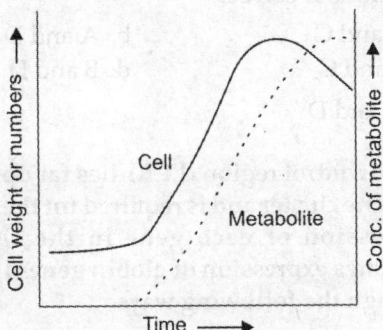

The following statements refer to the above figure:

A. A primary metabolite has a production curve that lags behind the line showing cell growth.

B. A primary metabolite is produced after the Trophophase is completed

C. A secondary metabolite is produced mainly during Idiophase

D. The curve shows the production of Penicillin from mold

Which of the above statement are correct?

a. A and b   b. C and D

c. A and C   d. B and D

Ans. (b) C and D

108. During transgenesis, the location of the genes and their number integrated into the genome of the transgenic animal are random. It is often necessary to determine the copy number of enes and their tissue specific transcription. The following are the possible methods used for the determination.

A. Polymerase Chain Reaction

B. Reverse Transcriptase PCR

C. Southern blot hybridization

D. Western blot

Choose the correct set of combination

a. A and B   b. B and C

c. B and D   d. A and D

Ans. (b) B and C

109. *Agrobacterium tumefaciens*, also known as natural genetic engineers, causes crown gall disease in plants, however, when the same bacteria are used to raise transgenic plants with improved agronomic traits, no such tumor (disease) is observed. This is due to:

A. Vir D_2 gene is mutated in Ti plasmid

B. Disarmed Ti plasmid is generally used

C. Heat shock during transformation destroys virulence

D. Oncogenes have been removed

Which one of the following combination of above statemtns is correct?

a. A and C   b. A and D

c. B and C   d. B and D

Ans. (d) B and D

110. Locus control region (LCR) lies far upstream from the gene cluster and is required for the appropriate expression of each gene in the cluster. LCR regulates expression of globin genes in the cluster through the following ways.

A. LCR interacts with promoters of individual genes by DNA looping through DNA binding proteins.

B. The LCR bond protein attract chromatin remodelling complexes including histone modifying enzyme and components of the transcription machinery

C. LCR acts as an enhancer for global regulation of gene cluster and does not regulate individual genes

D. LCR participates in converting inactive chromatin to active chromatin around the gene cluster.

Choose the correct set of combinations

a. A and B

b. A and C

c. B and C

d. B and D

Ans. (a) A and B

111. A student wrote following statemtns regarding comparison of Restriction fragment Length polymorphism (RFLP), Random Amplified Polymorphic DNA (RAPD), Amplified Fragement Length polymorphism (AFLP) and Simple Sequence Repeats (SSRs) technique used for generating molecular marker in plants:

A. All these techniques can be used for fingerprinting

B. Detection of allelic variation can be achieved only by RFLP and SSRs

C. Use of radioisotopes is required in RFLP and RAPD only

D. PCR is required for all the technique

Which one of the following combination of above statement is correct?

a. A and B

b. B and C

c. C and D

d. D and A

Ans. (a) A and B

112. In order to clone an eukaryotic gene in pBR 322 plasmid vector, the desired DNA fragment was produced by Pst I cleavage and incubated with PstI digested pRR 322 (PstI cleavage site lies within the ampicillin resistant gene) and ligated. Mixure of ligated cells were used to transform *E. coli* and plasmid containing bacteria were selected by their growth in tetracycline containing medium. Which type of plasmid/s will be found?

a. Circular pBR 322 plasmid containing the target gene and resistant to only tetracycline

b. Circular pBR 322 plasmid containing the target gene and resistant to tetracycline only and recircularised pBR 322 plasmid resistant to both ampicillin and tetracycline

c. Circular pBR 322 plasmid containing the target gene and resistant to only tetracycline, recircularised pBR 322 resistant to both ampicillin and tetracycline and concatemerized pBR 322 resistant to both ampicillin and tetracycline

d. Circular pBR 322 plasmid containing the target gene and resistant to both tetracycline and ampicillin

Ans. (c) Circular pBR 322 plasmid containing the target gene and resistant to only tetracycline, recircularised pBR 322 resistant to both ampicillin and tetracycline and concatemerized pBR 322 resistant to both ampicillin and tetracycline

113. During apoptosis, phosphatidyl serine (PS) usually present in the inner leaflet of fhe plasma membrane flips to the outer membrane. Annexin V is a protein that bind to PS, Using this as a tool, we identify the apoptotic cells from necrotic and normal cell populations by FACS using FiTC-Tagged Annexin V, Propidium iodide (PI) is used to stain the nucleus which generally identifies necrotic and late apoptotic cells, in which area of the plot you should get early apoptotic cells by FACS analysis?

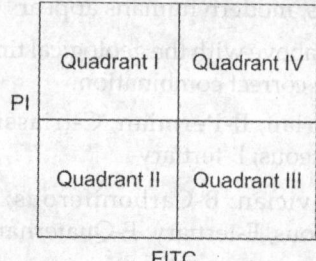

a. Quadrant I

b. Quadrant II

c. Quadrant III

d. Quadrant IV

Ans. (c) Quadrant III

114. The muscle tone was increased after electrolytic lesion of the caudate nucleus in a cat. The muscles tone decreased within seven days. The following explanation were given by the researcher.

  A. The functional recovery was due to plastic changes of nervous system.
  B. The brain tissue surrounding the lesioned area was non functional due to circulatory insufficiency immediately after surgery which led to greater functional loss
  C. The circulatory status in surrounding issue recovered with time resulting in partial functional recovery
  D. The degenerating nerve fibres were regenerated which underlie functional reconvery

  Which one of the folloiwng is correct?

  a. A and B
  b. B and C
  c. C and D
  d. A and D

  Ans. (b) B and C

115. A fluorophore when transferred from solvent A to solvent B results in an increase in the number of vibrational states in the ground state without any change in the mean energies of either the ground or excited state. What would be the chage seen in the fluorophore's emission spectrum?

  a. An increase in emission intensity
  b. An increase in emission bandwidth
  c. An increase in emission wavelength
  d. A decrease in emission wavelength

  Ans. (b) An increase in emission bandwidth

116. You wish to localize a given gene product at sub-cellular levels following immunofluorescence staining. Routine microscopy could not resolve whether the gene product is localized inside the nucleus or on the nuclear membrane. Which of the following will resolve this unambiguously?

  A. Sectioning of cell followed by phase contrast microscopy
  B. A simulation of 3 D picture following confocal microscopy
  C. Optical sectioning and observing each section
  D. Freeze fracturing followed by scanning Electon Microscopy

  a. A and B   b. B and C
  c. C and D   d. A and C

Ans. (b) B and C

117. The Triver-Willard hypothesis states that the physiological state of a female can bias the sex ratio of offspring. In an experiment in the bird species a group of females were fed a diet 30% lower in calories than the control females. After allowing both the groups to mate and breed freely, the ofspring of control 1 group were 22 males and 18 females. The diet restricted females laid a total of 40 eggs. What should be the minimum deviation from the control to conclude that they have significantly female biased offspeing sex ratio (Chi sq [0.05]df = 1 is 3.84)

  a. 18 male   22 female
  b. 20 male   20 female
  c. 15 male   25 female
  d. 10 male   30 female

Ans. (c) 15 male   25 female

Reader's Notes

Reader's Notes